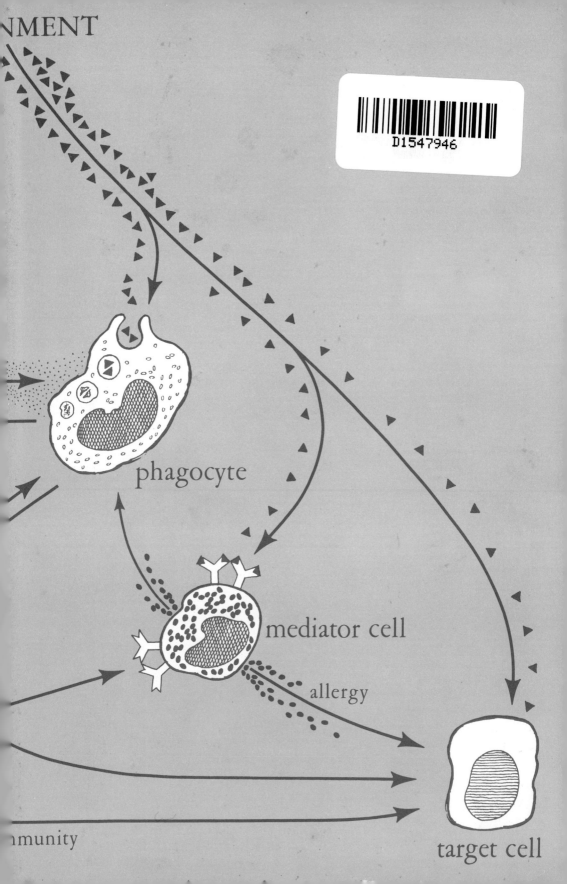

NMENT

phagocyte

mediator cell

allergy

mmunity

target cell

IMMUNOLOGY II

JOSEPH A. BELLANTI, M.D.

PROFESSOR OF PEDIATRICS AND
MICROBIOLOGY AND DIRECTOR,
INTERNATIONAL CENTER FOR INTERDISCIPLINARY
STUDIES OF IMMUNOLOGY

Georgetown University School of Medicine
Washington, D.C.

W. B. SAUNDERS COMPANY
Philadelphia   London   Toronto

W. B. Saunders Company: West Washington Square
                           Philadelphia, PA   19105

                           1 St. Anne's Road
                           Eastbourne, East Sussex BN21 3UN, England

                           1 Goldthorne Avenue
                           Toronto, Ontario M8Z 5T9, Canada

Library of Congress Cataloging in Publication Data

Bellanti, Joseph A   1934–

Immunology II.

Includes index.

1. Immunologic diseases.   2. Immunology.   I. Title.

RC582.B44   616.07′9   77–72808

ISBN 0–7216–1681–X

Listed here is the latest translated edition of this book together
with the language of the translation and the publisher.

Italian (*1st Edition*) – Piccin Editore, Padova, Italy

Spanish (*1st Edition*) – NEISA, Mexico D. F., Mexico

Immunology II   ISBN   0-7216-1681-X

Last digit is the print number: 9   8   7   6   5   4   3   2

This edition is dedicated with affection to my parents, my wife Jacqueline (who gives me hope to carry on), and my children Dawn, Lisa, Jeannine, Loretta, Maria (who helped me with the proofs), Joseph (who was born during the First Edition), and little Tony (who was born during the Second Edition).

A set of 35 mm. teaching slides of drawings and photographs from this book is available through the publisher.

CONTRIBUTORS

JOSEPH A. BELLANTI, M.D.

Professor of Pediatrics and Microbiology, and Director, International Center for Interdisciplinary Studies of Immunology, Georgetown University School of Medicine, Washington, D.C.

Introduction to Immunology; General Immunobiology; Immunogenetics; Antigen-Antibody Interactions; Cell-Mediated Reactions; A Unifying Model for Immunologic Processes; Host-Parasite Relationships; Mechanisms of Immunity to Bacterial Diseases; Mechanisms of Immunity to Viral Diseases; Mechanisms of Immunity to Fungal Diseases; Immune Defense Mechanisms in Tumor Immunity; Immunologically Mediated Diseases; Immunoprophylaxis: The Use of Vaccines; Immunotherapy: The Use of Passive Immunization; Diagnostic Applications of Immunology

GEORGE M. BERNIER, M.D.

Professor of Medicine, Case Western Reserve University School of Medicine, Cleveland, Ohio.

Antibody and Immunoglobulins: Structure and Function; Proliferative Disorders of the Immune System

JOHN J. CALABRO, M.D.

Professor of Medicine and Pediatrics, The University of Massachusetts Medical School, Worcester, Massachusetts.

Immunologically Mediated Disease Involving Autologous Antigens

RAY H. CYPESS, D.V.M., Ph.D.

Professor of Microbiology and Epidemiology, New York State College of Veterinary Medicine at Cornell University, Ithaca, New York.

Mechanisms of Immunity to Parasitic Diseases

ANTHONY S. FAUCI, M.D.

Head, Clinical Physiology Section, Laboratory of Clinical Investigation, National Institute of Allergy and Infectious Diseases, National Institutes of Health, Bethesda, Maryland.

Clinical Aspects of Immunosuppression: Use of Cytotoxic Agents and Corticosteroids

MICHAEL C. GELFAND, M.D.

Clinical Assistant Professor of Medicine, Georgetown University School of Medicine, Washington, D.C.

Organ Transplantation; Immunologically Mediated Disease Involving Autologous Antigens

PETER M. HENSON, Ph.D., B.V.M. & S., M.R.C.V.S.

Department of Pediatrics, National Jewish Hospital and Research Center, Denver, Colorado.

Mechanisms of Tissue Injury Produced by Immunologic Reactions

HERBERT B. HERSCOWITZ, Ph.D.

Associate Professor of Microbiology, Georgetown University Schools of Medicine and Dentistry, Washington, D.C.

Immunophysiology: Cell Function and Cellular Interactions

THOMAS T. HUBSCHER, Ph.D.

Associate Professor of Pediatrics and Microbiology, Georgetown University Schools of Medicine and Dentistry, Washington, D.C.
Antigen-Antibody Interactions

ANNE L. JACKSON, Ph.D.

Director of Research and Development, Kent Laboratories, Ltd., North Vancouver, B.C., Canada
Antigens and Immunogenicity

CHARLES H. KIRKPATRICK, M.D.

Head, Clinical Allergy and Hypersensitivity Section, Laboratory of Clinical Investigation, National Institute of Allergy and Infectious Diseases, National Institutes of Health, Bethesda, Maryland.
Immune Deficiency Diseases

WILLIAM T. KNIKER, M.D.

Professor of Pediatrics and Microbiology, and Chief, Division of Immunology-Allergy, University of Texas Health Science Center at San Antonio, San Antonio, Texas.
Immune Defense Mechanisms in Tumor Immunity

ROBERT H. MCLEAN, M.D.

Assistant Professor of Pediatrics, University of Connecticut Health Center, Farmington, Connecticut.
Complement Activity

JOHN B. ROBBINS, M.D.

Director of Bacterial Products, Bureau of Biologics, Food and Drug Administration, Bethesda, Maryland.
Immunoprophylaxis: The Use of Vaccines; Immunotherapy: The Use of Passive Immunization

ROSS E. ROCKLIN, M.D.

Assistant Professor of Medicine, Harvard Medical School, Robert B. Brigham Hospital, Boston, Massachusetts.
Cell-Mediated Reactions

ROBERT T. SCANLON, M.D.

Clinical Professor of Pediatrics, Georgetown University School of Medicine, Washington, D.C.
Immunologically Mediated Disease Involving Exogenous Antigens (Allergy)

ROBERT J. SCHLEGEL, M.D.

Professor and Chairman, Department of Pediatrics, Charles R. Drew Postgraduate Medical School, and Los Angeles County Martin Luther King, Jr. General Hospital, Los Angeles, California.
Immune Deficiency Diseases

KENNETH J. SELL, M.D., Ph.D.

Scientific Director, National Institute of Allergy and Infectious Diseases, National Institutes of Health, Bethesda, Maryland.
Immunogenetics

SAMUEL D. WAKSAL, Ph.D.

Assistant Professor of Pathology and Medicine, Tufts Cancer Research Center, Tufts University School of Medicine, Boston, Massachusetts.
Immunogenetics; Immunomodulation: Immunopotentiation, Tolerance and Immunosuppression

PETER A. WARD, M.D.

Professor and Chairman, Department of Pathology, University of Connecticut Health Center, Farmington, Connecticut.
Complement Activity; Inflammation

CHESTER M. ZMIJEWSKI, Ph.D.

Associate Professor of Pathology, University of Pennsylvania School of Medicine, and Director, Histocompatibility Laboratory, Philadelphia, Pennsylvania.
Antigen-Antibody Interactions; Immunologically Mediated Disease Involving Homologous Antigens

Drawings for this book were made with skill and insight by JANE A. HURD.

PREFACE

Immunology is the study of those processes used by the host to maintain constancy in his internal environment when confronted with foreign substances. Implicit in this broad definition is the fact that the field embraces both the basic and the clinical sciences. In turn, significant advances in immunology have resulted from the interaction of these disciplines. Thus, in the present text, contributions have come from a wide variety of basic and clinical collaborators. *Immunology II* itself emanates from an interdisciplinary center whose mission of research, education, and patient care is based on the symbiotic relationship among individuals engaged in this multitude of scholarly disciplines.

The book is directed to students at all levels: the undergraduate, the graduate, and the postgraduate. The first edition appears to have been useful in the teaching of a variety of subspecialty areas of medicine, including allergy-immunology, rheumatology, nephrology, infectious diseases, hematology-oncology, otolaryngology, and dermatology. The text has also been applied in the teaching of dentistry, nursing, medical technology, and undergraduate biology. Certainly, it has been the intent of the author and his collaborators in both editions to provide a comprehensive introductory text in immunology, while maintaining a fidelity to a clinical theme.

Although *Immunology II* is organized into the same three basic sections of the first edition—Principles, Mechanisms, and Clinical Applications—the book has been extensively revised and updated. Several new chapters have been added, including 7 (Immunophysiology: Cell Function and Cellular Interaction), 11 (A Unifying Model for Immunologic Processes), and 25 (Clinical Aspects of Immunosuppression: Use of Cytotoxic Agents and Corticosteroids). For a complete and concise overview of the immunologic system, and an understanding of its medical implications, the reader is referred to Chapter 11. I would like to express my sincere appreciation to Ms. Jane Hurd for creating the imaginative figures that illustrate the concepts in this chapter so vividly, as well as for her indefatigable support throughout both editions of the text.

Many persons have contributed to the preparation of the second edition, and I wish to express my indebtedness to them. First, I want to thank Dr. Philip L. Calgagno, who has been most generous in his encouragement. Others who have read sections of the manuscript, or who have made helpful suggestions, include the following: Dr. Lata Nerurkar, Mrs. Barbara Zeligs, Dr. Nancy Balter, Dr. Anne Morris Hooke, Dr. Stephen Peters, Dr. Frederick G. Burke, Dr. Val Abbassi, Dr. Heinz Bauer, Dr. Barbara Bainton, Dr. David Talmadge, Dr. Max Cooper, Dr. Mauricio Sauerbrey, Dr. John E. Salvaggio, Dr. Philip S. Norman, Dr. Franklin N. Adkinson, Jr., Dr. Raymond G. Slavin, Dr. Frank Palumbo, Dr. Lawrence D. Frenkel, Dr. Robert H. Purcell, and Dr. Thomas T. Provost.

My appreciation is also extended to my colleagues at Georgetown and to my clinical and research fellows and house staff, who have contributed to my intellectual life and to the life of the Immunology Center. I owe a special debt of gratitude to students of all ages, for whom the book is written and with whom I share the joy of discovery. It is the questions they ask in the lecture hall, the laboratory, and the clinic and bedside that have provided me with the incentive to write. Although many individuals have contributed information to this text, I alone assume responsibility for any errors found within these pages.

I am deeply indebted to the staff of the Department of Medical and Dental Communications at Georgetown for their assistance in the preparation of the charts and drawings. I wish also to thank Miss Diane Hargrave for her diligent typing of the entire manuscript.

Finally, I wish to express my thanks and appreciation to Ms. Marie Low, Mr. John Hanley, Ms. Patrice Lamb, Mr. Herb Powell, and their colleagues at W. B. Saunders Company for their patience, support, constant nudging, and inspiration during the lengthy preparation of this revision.

JOSEPH A. BELLANTI

CONTENTS

APPROACH TO THE PATIENT WITH IMMUNOLOGIC DISEASE

Section One

THE PRINCIPLES
OF IMMUNOLOGY

INTRODUCTION TO IMMUNOLOGY

Joseph A. Bellanti, M.D.

HISTORICAL BACKGROUND

The concepts of immunology are ancient and pragmatic and are derived primarily from the study of resistance to infection. It was known for centuries before the discovery of the germ theory of infectious disease that recovery from illness was accompanied by the ability to resist reinfection. Thus, the elements of classical immunology preceded bacteriology and contributed to it. Similarly, contributions were made to immunology by anthropologists, anatomists, biologists, chemists, and geneticists. These fields in turn have been enhanced by the application of immunologic phenomena. Shown in Figure 1–1 is a schematic representation of some major milestones important in the development of immunology.

Preceding modern medicine, Chinese physicians in the eleventh century observed that the inhalation of smallpox crusts prevented the subsequent occurrence of the disease. Later, the technique of variolation, the intradermal application of powdered scabs, was used in the Middle East, where its primary intent was "preserving the beauty of their daughters." This primitive immunization reached England in the eighteenth century through Pylarini and Timoni and was later popularized by Lady Mary Wortley Montagu (Fig. 1–2). Wide variations in vaccination procedures, however, occasionally led to death. In addition, the widespread acceptance of herb medicine prevented the full acceptance of this form of therapy.

The future of modern immunobiology was assured when Edward Jenner (Fig. 1–3), as a medical student, made the surprisingly sophisticated discovery that inoculation with cowpox crusts protected man from smallpox. This important finding resulted from Jenner's observation that milkmaids who had contracted cowpox were resistant to infection with smallpox.

The enhancement and further development of preventive immunization was made possible by Louis Pasteur (Fig. 1–4), who coined the term "vaccine" (from *vacca*: L., cow) in honor of Jenner's contribution. Pasteur's researches led to the development of the germ theory of disease from which he developed techniques for the *in vitro* culture of microorganisms. This work produced material that could be used for

3

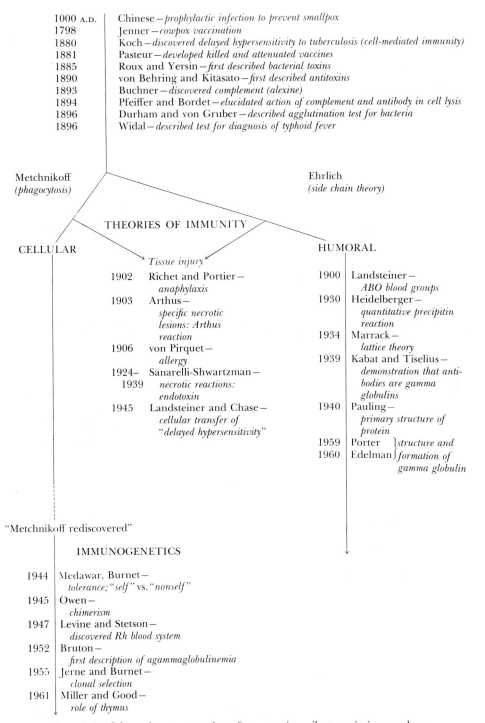

1000 A.D.	Chinese—*prophylactic infection to prevent smallpox*
1798	Jenner—*cowpox vaccination*
1880	Koch—*discovered delayed hypersensitivity to tuberculosis (cell-mediated immunity)*
1881	Pasteur—*developed killed and attenuated vaccines*
1885	Roux and Yersin—*first described bacterial toxins*
1890	von Behring and Kitasato—*first described antitoxins*
1893	Buchner—*discovered complement (alexine)*
1894	Pfeiffer and Bordet—*elucidated action of complement and antibody in cell lysis*
1896	Durham and von Gruber—*described agglutination test for bacteria*
1896	Widal—*described test for diagnosis of typhoid fever*

Metchnikoff
(phagocytosis)

Ehrlich
(side chain theory)

THEORIES OF IMMUNITY

CELLULAR

HUMORAL

Tissue injury

1902	Richet and Portier— *anaphylaxis*
1903	Arthus— *specific necrotic lesions: Arthus reaction*
1906	von Pirquet— *allergy*
1924– 1939	Sanarelli-Shwartzman— *necrotic reactions: endotoxin*
1945	Landsteiner and Chase— *cellular transfer of "delayed hypersensitivity"*

1900	Landsteiner— *ABO blood groups*
1930	Heidelberger— *quantitative precipitin reaction*
1934	Marrack— *lattice theory*
1939	Kabat and Tiselius— *demonstration that anti- bodies are gamma globulins*
1940	Pauling— *primary structure of protein*
1959	Porter ⎱*structure and*
1960	Edelman⎰*formation of gamma globulin*

"Metchnikoff rediscovered"

IMMUNOGENETICS

1944	Medawar, Burnet— *tolerance; "self" vs. "nonself"*
1945	Owen— *chimerism*
1947	Levine and Stetson— *discovered Rh blood system*
1952	Bruton— *first description of agammaglobulinemia*
1955	Jerne and Burnet— *clonal selection*
1961	Miller and Good— *role of thymus*

Figure 1–1.   Schematic representation of some major milestones in immunology.

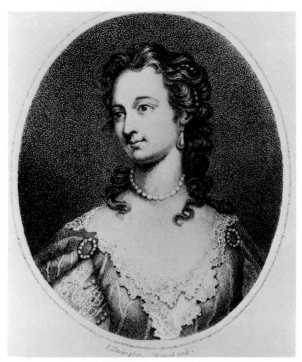

Figure 1–2. Lady Mary Wortley Montagu. (Courtesy of National Library of Medicine.)

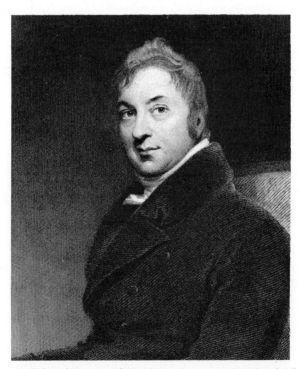

Figure 1–3. Edward Jenner (1749–1823). (Courtesy of National Library of Medicine.)

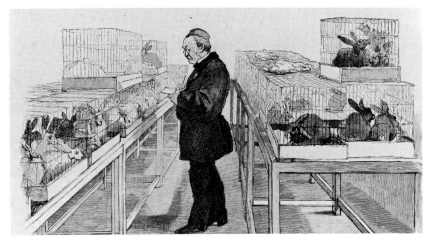

Figure 1–4. Louis Pasteur (1822–1895). (Courtesy of National Library of Medicine.)

vaccines: living, heat-killed, and attenuated (living but with reduced virulence). During these investigations, Pasteur observed that old cultures (attenuated) of fowl cholera organisms when inoculated into fowl produced no disease. Surprisingly, these fowl were resistant to subsequent infection with the organism and were solidly immune. This early use of living attenuated cultures for active immunization is still our therapy of choice in the prophylaxis of many infectious diseases (Fig. 1–5).

Later, Robert Koch (Fig. 1–6), discovered the tubercle bacillus during his studies of the bacterial etiology of infectious diseases. While attempting to develop a vaccine for tuberculosis, he observed the phenomenon known today as delayed hypersensitivity or cell-mediated immunity.

Following the isolation of the diphtheria bacillus, Roux and Yersin demonstrated the existence of a potent soluble exotoxin elaborated by this organism (Fig. 1–7). This toxin was used by von Behring (Fig. 1–8) and Kitasato to inoculate animals who produced in their serum a toxin-neutralizing substance called *antitoxin*. This neutralizing capability could be transferred by the serum to uninoculated animals, a process called passive immunization. Their work forms a model for the modern techniques of preventing disease through passive immunization (immunotherapy). Pfeiffer and Bordet's work differentiated a substance in serum, distinct from antibody, called *complement* that also participates in the destruction of bacteria. The observations of Durham and von Gruber that serum could clump or agglutinate bacteria formed the basis for tests for the diagnosis of infectious specific agglutination reactions, such as the test described by Widal for the diagnosis of typhoid fever (Widal test).

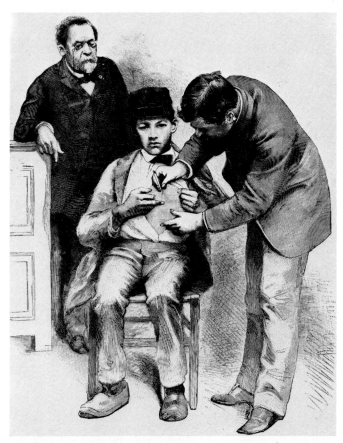

Figure 1–5. Louis Pasteur, to left, watches as an assistant inoculates a boy for "hydrophobia" (rabies). (Wood engraving in "L'Illustration" from Harper's Weekly 29:836, 1885; courtesy of National Library of Medicine.)

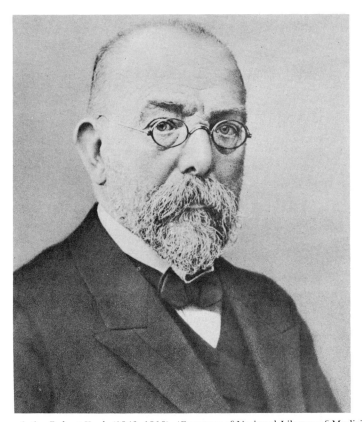

Figure 1-6. Robert Koch (1843–1910). (Courtesy of National Library of Medicine.)

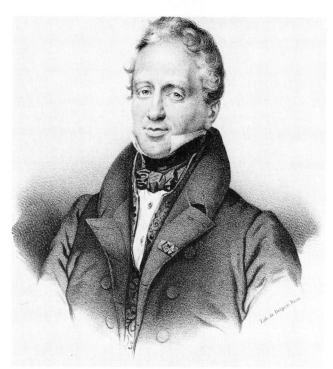

Figure 1-7. Pierre Paul Emile Roux (1853–1933). (Courtesy of National Library of Medicine.)

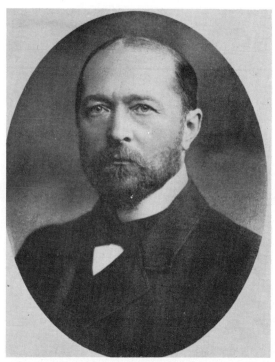

Figure 1-8. Emil Adolf von Behring (1854–1917). (Courtesy of National Library of Medicine.)

Up to the turn of the century, the French and German schools dominated these areas of immunologic research. At that time, there emerged two divergent vantage points from which immunology was observed and later developed: (1) the *humoral*, whose emphasis was the study of chemical products (antibodies) elaborated by cells, and (2) the *cellular*, whose emphasis was the biologic effects of intact cells involved in the host's response to foreignness (see Fig. 1–1). Paul Ehrlich (Fig. 1–9) proposed the humoral theory of antibody formation, and Elie Metchnikoff (Fig. 1–10) almost simultaneously developed the cellular theory of immunity. Both were correct, since in the individual both cellular and humoral factors are intimately interwoven and interdependent.

Ehrlich's side chain theory proposed the pre-existence of receptors on the living cell surface that reacted with toxins; the excess receptors eventually could be released into the circulation as antibody (Fig. 1–11). It is ironic that one of the major areas of immunologic research today is the study of receptors on immunocompetent cells (Chapter 7). Subsequently, the major emphasis in immunology was directed at the identification, characterization, and biologic function of humoral factors (see Fig. 1–1).

Metchnikoff's theories of cellular immunity held that the body's scavenger cells, the phagocytes, were the prime detectors of foreign

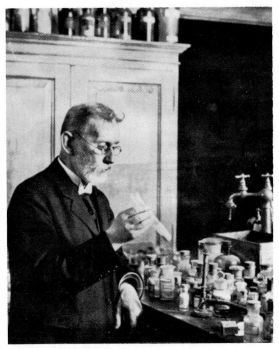

Figure 1–9. Paul Ehrlich (1854–1915). (Courtesy of National Library of Medicine.)

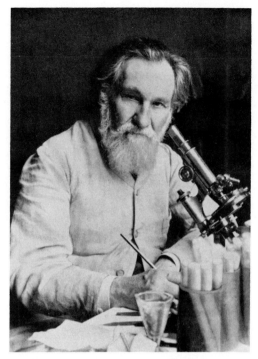

Figure 1–10.   Elie Metchnikoff (1845–1916). (Courtesy of National Library of Medicine.)

material as well as its primary defense system. His concepts went unrecognized for several decades but today represent an area of intensive immunologic research. Both cellular and humoral factors are involved in understanding the principles underlying the immunologic processes that result in tissue injury.

Today, there still remain two schools of immunologic investigation. The humoral school reached its peak with the discovery and characterization of the protein molecules that contain antibody activity, the immunoglobulins. This work has culminated in the elucidation of the total amino acid sequence of some antibody molecules. At the same time, the cellular area is now being actively pursued from the standpoint of protection to infectious agents, graft rejection, and immunity to tumors in man. The cellular-humoral dichotomy is also illustrated by the clinical observations of increased susceptibility to infection seen in individuals with congenital defects of the immunologic system. Some lack the humoral protective function but retain the cellular; others are deficient in cellular but have normal humoral activity; still others are defective in both humoral and cellular functions. Clearly, both areas are of profound importance to man. Although one or the other aspect will be stressed at times throughout this book, cellular and humoral factors of immunity are interrelated and interdependent.

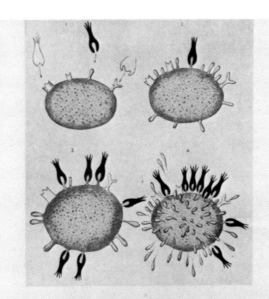

DIAGRAMMATIC REPRESENTATION OF THE SIDE-CHAIN THEORY
(PLATES I AND II)

Fig. 1   "The groups [the haptophore group of the side-chain of the cell and that of the food-stuff or the toxin] must be adapted to one another, *e.g.*, as male and female screw (PASTEUR), or as lock and key (E. FISCHER)."

Fig. 2   ". . . the first stage in the toxic action must be regarded as being the union of the toxin by means of its haptophore group to a special side-chain of the cell protoplasm."

Fig. 3   "The side-chain involved, so long as the union lasts, cannot exercise its normal, physiological, nutritive function . . ."

Fig. 4   "We are therefore now concerned with a defect which, according to the principles so ably worked out by . . . Weigert, is . . . [overcorrected] by regeneration."

Figure 1–11   Diagrammatic representation of the side-chain theory, showing the presence of preexisting receptors on the cell surface (*A*), which when produced in excess (*B*) could be released as antibody. (From Croonian Lecture, "On Immunity with Special Reference to Cell Life," Proc. Roy. Soc. London (Biol.) 66:424, 1906; courtesy of National Library of Medicine.)

Illustration continues on the opposite page

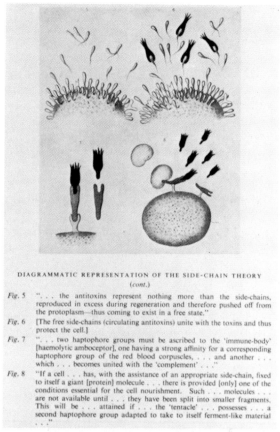

DIAGRAMMATIC REPRESENTATION OF THE SIDE-CHAIN THEORY
(*cont.*)

Fig. 5 "... the antitoxins represent nothing more than the side-chains, reproduced in excess during regeneration and therefore pushed off from the protoplasm—thus coming to exist in a free state."

Fig. 6 [The free side-chains (circulating antitoxins) unite with the toxins and thus protect the cell.]

Fig. 7 "... two haptophore groups must be ascribed to the 'immune-body' [haemolytic amboceptor], one having a strong affinity for a corresponding haptophore group of the red blood corpuscles, ... and another ... which ... becomes united with the 'complement' ..."

Fig. 8 "If a cell ... has, with the assistance of an appropriate side-chain, fixed to itself a giant [protein] molecule ... there is provided [only] one of the conditions essential for the cell nourishment. Such ... molecules ... are not available until ... they have been split into smaller fragments. This will be ... attained if ... the 'tentacle' ... possesses ... a second haptophore group adapted to take to itself ferment-like material ..."

Figure 1–11. *Continued.*

IMMUNITY AND HYPERSENSITIVITY

The term *immune* is derived from the Latin *immunis* (free from taxes or free from burden). In classic usage immunity referred to the relative resistance of the host to reinfection by a given microbe. It is now evident that immune responses are not always beneficial, nor are they solely associated with resistance to infection. On the contrary, they can even confer unpleasant and harmful effects on the host. The noxious effect has been called *hypersensitivity* or *allergy*. Listed in Figure 1–1 are some of the early pioneers who contributed to this field of tissue injury. The immunologic system is equipped not only to perform a *defense* function against infectious agents, but also to concern itself with the more diverse biologic functions of *homeostasis* and *surveillance*.

At the turn of the century, von Pirquet put forward a hypothesis to explain the multifaceted aspects of the immune response. He coined the term "allergy" to mean "altered reactivity" of the host; one change was recognized as immunity, and the other as hypersensitivity. Von Pirquet made no distinction between beneficial and harmful responses and suggested that they were all manifestations of a common biologic process of sensitization which he encompassed by the term allergy. He restricted the use of the term immunity to mean protection from infectious agents and the term allergy for a more generalized reactivity of the host to foreign substances. Over the years the terms allergy and immunity have become reversed in their meanings; immunity has come to mean that which von Pirquet defined originally as allergy, and allergy has come to mean hypersensitivity. Nevertheless, von Pirquet's concepts of the broad scope of the immune response are now accepted in immunology.

IMMUNOLOGY IN THE MODERN SENSE

A contemporary definition of the term immunity would include "all those physiologic mechanisms that endow the animal with the capacity to recognize materials as foreign to itself and to neutralize, eliminate, or metabolize them with or without injury to its own tissues." The responses of immunity may be classified into two categories: (1) *nonspecific* immunologic responses and (2) *specific* immunologic responses. Specific immune responses depend upon exposure to a foreign configuration and the subsequent recognition of and reaction to it. Nonspecific responses, on the other hand, occur following initial and subsequent exposure to a foreign configuration, and while selective in differentiating "self" from "nonself," they are not dependent upon specific recognition. In the modern view, immunologic responses serve three functions—defense, homeostasis, and surveillance (Table 1–1). The first is involved in resistance to infection by microorganisms, the second in removal of worn-out (effete) "self" components, and the third with the perception and destruction of mutant cells.

The first function, defense against invasion by microorganisms, has occupied the thinking of immunologists for more than 100 years. If

TABLE 1–1. Functions of the Immune System

FUNCTION	NATURE OF IMMUNOLOGIC STIMULUS	EXAMPLE	ABERRATIONS *Hyper*	*Hypo*
Defense	Exogenous	Microorganisms	Allergy	Immunologic deficiency syndrome
Homeostasis	Endogenous or exogenous	Removal of effete and damaged cells	Autoimmune disease	—
Surveillance	Endogenous or exogenous	Removal of cell mutants	—	Malignant disease

the cellular elements of defense are deployed successfully, the host will emerge victorious in the struggle with microorganisms. However, when these elements are *hyperactive,* certain undesirable features such as allergy or hypersensitivity, may be seen (Chapter 20). Conversely, when these elements are *hypoactive,* there may be an increased susceptibility to repeated infections in the host, as seen in the immunologic deficiency disorders (Chapter 22).

The second function, homeostasis, fulfills the universal requirement of all multicellular organisms to preserve uniformity of a given cell type. It is this function that concerns itself with normal degradative or catabolic functions of the body charged with the removal of damaged cellular elements, such as circulating erythrocytes or leukocytes. These may be damaged during the course of a normal life span or may arise as a consequence of injury. Aberrations of homeostasis are exemplified by the autoimmune diseases, in which these mechanisms are unduly enhanced (Chapter 20).

The third function of the immune system is the most recently recognized and concerns itself with surveillance. This function monitors the recognition of abnormal cell types, which constantly arise within the body. These mutants may occur spontaneously or may be induced by certain viruses and chemicals (Chapter 19). The immune system is charged with the recognition and disposal of these newly acquired configurations, most of which occur on cell surfaces. Failure of this mechanism has recently been assigned a causal role in the development of malignant disease (Chapter 19).

MODIFYING FACTORS

There are a number of factors that modify immune mechanisms: genetic factors, age factors, metabolic factors, environmental factors, anatomic factors, physiologic factors, and microbial factors (Table 1–2).

Genetic Factors. The whole of the immune response is under

TABLE 1–2. Elements Involved in Immunologic Processes

MODIFYING FACTORS	TYPE OF RESPONSE	TYPE OF ENCOUNTER	EXAMPLES
Genetic Age Metabolic Environmental Anatomic Physiologic Microbial	Nonspecific immunity	All	Phagocytosis, inflammatory response, cellular immunity, fever, acute phase phenomena (CRP, sedimentation rate)
	Specific immunity	Initial and subsequent	Humoral, cell-mediated immunity (delayed hypersensitivity)

genetic control (Chapter 3). It has been shown that genetic differences within species of animals determine whether or not a given animal will respond to a specific stimulus. It has been shown, for example, that certain strains of guinea pigs are capable of responding to a given antigen (responders), whereas others are not (nonresponders). In addition, there are genetic differences in susceptibility to infection that may have similar bases. Strains of rabbits have been bred, one susceptible, the other resistant, to infection with *Mycobacterium tuberculosis.* In man, there are racial differences in susceptibility to tuberculosis; and disease susceptibility is more similar in monozygotic than in dizygotic twins. One of the exciting recent developments in immunology has been the identification of a genetic complex that controls both immune responsiveness and the expression of histocompatibility antigens on cells (Chapter 3).

Age Factors.   Chronologic age influences immunity, and direct evidence is accumulating that a hypofunctional state of the immune system occurs in the very young and the very old. For example, these two age groups are uniquely susceptible to the ravages of infection. Generalized sepsis due to *Escherichia coli* is not an uncommon event in the newborn period. Presumably, this is because of a number of factors, including an incompletely developed specific immune system and deficiencies of nonspecific immunity such as a thin integument and a poor inflammatory response. Similarly, fatal pneumonia due to *Streptococcus (Diplococcus) pneumoniae* is not an uncommon event during old age. This pathogen is more virulent in the elderly who have underlying cardiac, pulmonary, and metabolic derangements (e.g., diabetes mellitus). In addition, direct evidence is accumulating that shows that the functional state of the immune system lessens with age. There is a higher incidence of autoimmune phenomena in the elderly, as well as a decrease in many of the immunologic functions such as immunoglobulin concentrations and cell-mediated immunity.

Metabolic Factors.   Certain hormones have been shown to affect the host immune responses. In both hypoadrenal and hypothyroid states there is a diminished resistance to infection. Patients treated with steroids have been shown to be unduly susceptible to bacterial diseases (e.g., staphylococcal infection) as well as to certain viral diseases (e.g., varicella). Steroids appear to affect many modalities of the immune response, having an inhibitory effect on phagocytosis, inflammation, and antibody formation (Chapters 10 and 25).

Environmental Factors.   The increased rate of infectious diseases owing to poor living conditions is well known. An increased rate of infection may be related to a greater exposure to pathogens, as well as to diminished resistance caused by poor nutrition itself. Recently, in studies conducted in African children, nutritional deprivation at an early age has been shown to be associated with developmental failure of the immune response.

Anatomic Factors.   The first line of defense against invasion by microbes is usually provided by the *skin* and the *mucous membranes*. These tissues act in nonspecific immunity by providing a physical barrier to invasion. The intact skin appears to be a more effective barrier than the mucous membranes. The increased susceptibility to infections following burns or secondary to eczema is a well-known clinical finding. The skin and the mucous membranes may allow penetration by certain pathogens, e.g., the tubercle bacillus, which can pass across the intact gastrointestinal mucosa after ingestion, leading to local infection and regional lymph node enlargement.

Microbial Factors.   Following colonization of the body surfaces, both internal and external, a "normal" flora develops. Not only is this flora essential for the production of metabolites, e.g., vitamin K, but it also contributes to the production of "natural" antibodies to these organisms. The flora also act to suppress the overgrowth and subsequent infection by pathogenic and possibly virulent organisms. The well recognized overgrowth of virulent staphylococci in patients treated with so-called broad-spectrum antibiotics illustrates the effect of a disturbed ecologic microbial balance in man.

Physiologic Factors.   The gastric juice is an unfavorable milieu for many pathogenic strains of bacteria, which are destroyed in the stomach following ingestion. Some bacteria, such as the typhoid bacilli, are not affected, survive digestion, and produce disease. Ciliary action in the respiratory tract is another important physiologic mechanism of resistance. Normal urine flow clears bacteria from the urinary tract, preventing infection. It is well known that the obstructed urinary tract is more susceptible to infection probably owing to the absence of this clearing action.

Certain skin secretions of normal individuals have been shown to be bactericidal; the skin of a cadaver shows no such effect. This is believed to be due in part to the acidity of the skin produced by *lactic acid*. After puberty the skin appears more resistant to infection with certain fungi (dermatophytes). This may result from an increase in saturated fatty acids in the skin. In postpubertal skin, there are also increased amounts of unsaturated fatty acids known to be bactericidal.

Lysozyme is an enzyme that has been shown to have bactericidal activity. The enzyme is found in many types of cells and body fluids and functions by virtue of mucolytic properties that cleave acetylaminosugars, the backbone of both gram-positive and gram-negative bacteria. Certain basic polypeptides (with large amounts of lysine) have been shown to kill anthrax. There are other chemical substances in the body that kill, injure, or inhibit bacteria and viruses.

The blood contains a number of protective substances that act in a nonspecific manner. Bactericidal substances in blood have been demonstrated that do not appear to be specific antibody, since they are present without prior exposure to a foreign configuration. These have been called *natural antibodies.* Their precise origin is not known, and, indeed, the concept of preformed antibodies has been a subject of controversy. For example, in the sera of normal human beings who have never seen a chimpanzee, there exists a naturally occurring "antibody" to chimpanzee red blood cells. This has been explained by the presence of genetically predetermined clones of antibody-producing cells that could be stimulated following exposure to closely related materials. It is known, for example, that isohemagglutinins—the antibody to blood groups—(Chapter 3) may develop as a result of exposure to enteric bacilli containing blood group–like substances in their structure. Recently, this phenomenon has found application to clinical medicine. Bacterial vaccines are being developed that are capable of generating protective antibody against certain pathogenic organisms such as *Haemophilus influenzae* following immunization with antigenically related, cross-reacting organisms such as *Escherichia coli* (Chapter 23).

Another humoral factor described is *properdin.* This substance, a serum protein, exerts bactericidal and viricidal effects in the presence of the third component of complement and magnesium ions. Although originally thought to be a "natural" mechanism of host resistance different from antibody, it is now felt that the presence of minute amounts of "natural" antibody accounts for the properdin effect.

Tissue mucoprotein inhibitors are also viricidal substances that may prevent attachment of certain viruses to susceptible host cells. A protein, *interferon,* acts on host cells to block viral replication (Chapter 16).

Nonspecific Immunity: Inflammatory Response and Phagocytosis

The first encounter of the host with a foreign configuration leads to a stereotyped response that consists of mobilization of phagocytic elements into areas where a foreign configuration has been introduced (Table 1–2). This may occur as an isolated event or as part of the inflammatory response.

Inflammatory Response.   Following any one of a variety of tissue injuries, a spectrum of cellular and systemic events occurs in which the host attempts to restore and maintain homeostasis under the adverse environmental influences. This reaction is referred to as inflammation and is described in greater detail in Chapter 12. Accompanying the inflammatory response are a number of systemic events that involve fever as well as a series of hematologic phenomena. The febrile response is believed to reflect enhanced metabolic activity following injury. One mechanism is believed to be the release of endogenous pyrogen from host leukocytes; an increased leukocyte count occurs during bacterial infections or tissue injury. Tissue necrosis, for example, with myocardial infarction, is associated with a "left shift," i.e., a predominance of polymorphonuclear leukocytes with many young forms, e.g., bands. In general, bacterial products cause more tissue injury than do viruses and induce the greatest febrile response.

Increased blood fibrinogen, activation of the Hageman factor, and increased fibrinolytic activity and erythrocyte rouleaux formation are each associated with one of the most useful indices of the acute phase response—the erythrocyte sedimentation rate (ESR). This parameter is affected by any factor causing erythrocyte rouleaux formation, such as increased gamma globulin. A rapid sedimentation rate is most commonly associated, however, with a raised fibrinogen level.

Other changes in serum globulins occur during illness, such as an increase in the alpha and beta globulins. One of these, the C-reactive protein (CRP), is elevated in the early phases of many illnesses. It was originally discovered by virtue of its interaction with the C substance of *Streptococcus (Diplococcus) pneumoniae,* but it is now recognized that CRP is released from many types of tissues following injury.

Phagocytosis. Once mobilized, the phagocytic cells mount an attack on their target by a process called phagocytosis (cell-eating), a multiphasic act requiring the following steps: recognition of the material to be ingested, movement toward the object (chemotaxis), attachment, ingestion, and subsequent intracellular digestion by a number of antimicrobial mechanisms (Chapter 2). A series of complex biochemical reactions occurs involving utilization of complement, certain humoral antibodies (opsonins), and the enhancement of intracellular metabolic events. Knowledge of these steps has assumed great clinical importance with the recent discovery that there occur in man inborn errors of metabolism involving leukocyte function. This family of neutrophil dysfunction syndromes may involve deficiencies in chemotactic factors, antibody, or intracellular enzymes concerned with antimicrobial activity (Chapter 22).

SPECIFIC IMMUNOLOGIC RESPONSES

Definitions.   The specific immune responses are concerned with the recognition and ultimate disposal of foreignness in a highly discriminatory fashion. The final outcome of the encounter between host and a foreign configuration is dependent upon the properties of the substance (size, structure, chemical nature, amount) and also upon properties of the host (age, genetic constitution) (Figure 1–12). The material may interact with the host in a number of ways. It may become localized or completely removed by phagocytic elements, usually inert particles (i.e., carbon), without any further response. It may lead to a specific immune response in which the material is referred to as an *immunogen* or *antigen* (Chapter 4). On the other hand, after interaction with the host the material may induce a state of unresponsiveness in

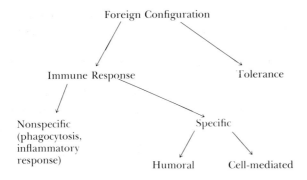

Figure 1–12.   Possible outcome of an encounter of the host with a foreign configuration.

which case it is said to be a *tolerogen*. The resulting condition is referred to as *immunologic tolerance* and will be considered in Chapter 10.

General Characteristics of the Specific Immune Response.   The *specific immune response* is the reaction of the host to a foreign substance and encompasses a series of cellular interactions expressed by the elaboration of specific cell products. There are three general characteristics of the specific immune response that distinguish it from the nonspecific responses: (1) *specificity*, (2) *heterogeneity*, and (3) *memory*.

Specificity is the highly discriminatory selectivity by which the products of the immune response will react solely with the configuration identical or similar to that which initiated the response. Landsteiner first demonstrated specificity and showed that antibody could distinguish closely related substances; it is the property of the immune response which distinguishes one antigen from another. Operationally, the immune response can distinguish and differentiate antigens originating from different species (*species specificity*), from different individuals (*individual specificity*), or from different organs (*organ specificity*).

The second characteristic of the specific immune response is heterogeneity, in which a vast array of cell types and cell products are induced to interact with a diversity of response commensurate with the variety of cell types. The heterogeneity of cell types gives rise to the elaboration of an equally heterogeneous population of cell products (antibody). This heterogeneity of antibody contributes a fine degree of homeostatic control with which the host can respond in a highly variable and specific manner with foreign structures.

The third hallmark of the specific immune response is memory. Memory is the property that results in augmentation of the specific response through proliferation and differentiation of cells upon subsequent exposure to an immunogen. This leads to an enhanced elaboration of cell products.

Nonspecific responses, on the other hand, represent the initial encounter with foreignness, and upon subsequent encounter merely repeat the same general response to the substance. Unlike the specific responses, the nonspecific responses include a limited number of preexistent cell types. The specific responses are characterized by the induction and interaction of a variety of new cell types specific for the inducing antigen. The nonspecific immune responses do not include the property of memory.

EFFECTOR MECHANISMS: COMPONENTS OF THE SPECIFIC IMMUNE RESPONSE

There are two types of effector mechanisms that mediate specific immune responses (Fig. 1–13): (1) those mediated by a cell product of the lymphoid tissues referred to as antibody *(humoral immunity)* and (2) those mediated by specifically sensitized lymphocytes themselves *(cell-mediated immunity)*.

Following an immunogenic stimulus a series of cellular events occurs prior to the expression of the *specific immune response*. For ease of discussion, we may divide these events into two general areas: (1) the *afferent limb*, in which there takes place the processing of the immunogen by macrophages and cellular interactions between lymphocytes and macrophages culminating in the activation of lymphocytes, and (2) the *efferent limb*, in which the specifically activated lymphocytes prolifer-

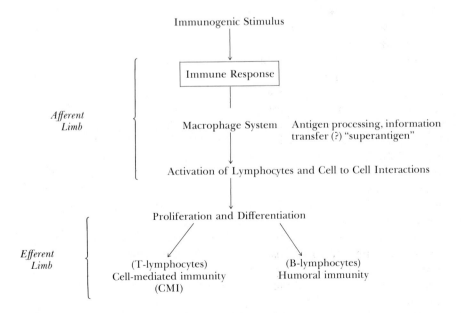

Figure 1–13. Effector mechanisms that mediate specific immunologic responses.

ate and differentiate in the expression of specific humoral and cell-mediated immunity. These events are described in detail in Chapter 7.

Humoral Immunity. Antibody is a product of certain lymphoid elements (B-lymphocytes and plasma cells) and is either cell-bound or secreted as an extracellular product. It has the capability of reacting with the configuration responsible for its production (immunogen or antigen) (Chapter 4). In the human, antibody is associated with five major classes of proteins (immunoglobulins) that can be differentiated from one another on the basis of either size or electrophoretic mobility (Chapter 5). Each immunoglobulin class (antibody) is distinct in its function. The presence of antibody is determined by measuring some functional parameter of the interaction between antigen and antibody (Chapter 8). For example, some antibodies can neutralize the effect of a toxin (antitoxin), others can punch holes in cell membranes (cytolytic antibodies), and still others are measured *in vivo* by eliciting a hypersensitive reaction (anaphylactic antibody) such as the IgE. It is believed that the humoral effector mechanism is derived embryologically in the chicken from the bursa of Fabricius. In the human, the location of this tissue is not known with certainty, but it is nevertheless referred to on occasion as the gut-associated lymphoid tissue (GALT).

Other Humoral Factors: Biologic Amplification Systems. Immunologic reactions may also involve other humoral factors that can augment or amplify the response without the direct participation of cells. The best known example is the complement system in which a variety of factors, both cell-bound and soluble, come into play and set the stage for protective mechanisms and, in some cases, detrimental events. Most complement factors act by triggering the inflammatory response. Under certain conditions this leads to the removal of infective agents; however, under other conditions the result is tissue damage. The complement system will be described in detail in a later section (Chapter 6).

The kallikrein system is yet another component of the amplification system and represents a well-defined system of proteins in plasma, activated by a reaction of antigen with antibody. Presumably through the activation of the Hageman factor and the permeability factor of Miles, the enzyme kallikrein interacts with its substrate, an alpha-2-macroglobulin, to produce at least three different vasoactive peptides—bradykinin, lysylbradykinin, and methionyl-lysyl-bradykinin. Slow reacting substance (SRS-A) is a humoral factor liberated by the interaction of antigen with sensitized cells. All these agents increase capillary permeability.

Certain proteins of the coagulation sequence also may act to amplify the immune response during the interaction of antigen with antibody. Increase in the rapidity of clotting in plasma following such interaction has been attributed to activation of the Hageman factor, although an earlier step in the coagulation sequence may be directly activated by an antigen-antibody complex. Finally, there is some evidence that the fibrinolytic system may be activated in plasma by the antigen-antibody interaction, but the precise mechanism for the conversion of plasminogen to plasmin is unknown.

Cell-Mediated Immunity.   The cell-mediated response is the second major type of effector mechanism underlying specific immunologic immunity (Fig. 1–13). This is mediated by a group of lymphocytes that differentiate under the influence of the thymus and are therefore referred to as T-lymphocytes. This effector arm of specific immunity is carried out directly by specifically sensitized lymphocytes or by specific cell products that are formed upon interaction of immunogen with specifically sensitized lymphocytes. These specific cell products, the lymphokines, include migration inhibitory factor (MIF), cytotoxin, interferon, and several others and are believed to be the effector molecules of cellular immunity (Chapter 9).

CONCEPT OF IMMUNOLOGIC BALANCE

In order to understand immunologically mediated disease, the immunologic system may be viewed as a dynamic multicompartmental collection of elements with ever-changing morphologic components and functions. It should be kept in mind that much of the work in experimental immunology has been performed with nonreplicating antigens. Normally, many immunologic stimuli are self-replicating, such as bacteria, viruses, and organ transplants. Thus, data obtained in the laboratory may not be directly applicable to natural phenomena occurring in humans. A second point is that not all configurations confronting the host are immunogenic, i.e., lead to a specific immune response. Some antigens are taken up by phagocytic cells and may be completely degraded before they can lead to a specific immune response.

As with all physiologic mechanisms, the immunologic response may be viewed as an adaptive system in which the body attempts to maintain homeostasis between the internal body environment and the external environment.

Following confrontation of the host with a foreign configuration (stimulus) there is a period of disequilibrium. Immunologic balance is restored by the appropriate immunologic response. A perturbation occurs if the stimulus and the response are inappropriate for each other. Any derangement in homeostasis results in the production of undesirable sequelae referred to as immunologic imbalance. The clinical appearance of immunologic imbalance is manifested as the immunologically mediated diseases (Chapter 20).

Overwhelming sepsis is an example of a situation in which the amount of replicating antigen exceeds the capacity of lymphoreticular tissue response. Immunologic unresponsiveness or paralysis may also occur when the host is confronted with antigen in a form not easily catabolized, e.g., the pneumococcal polysaccharide. The net result is referred to as "*high-zone paralysis*" (Chapter 10). This may be the mechanism by which the host maintains nonreactivity to its own bodily constituents, i.e., "*self-tolerance.*"

The converse is also seen and occurs when too little antigen leads to an immunologic imbalance. This is known as "*low-dose tolerance.*" The clinical counterpart of low-dose interaction is perhaps best exemplified by the interaction of certain microorganisms with the host. Dermatophytes can establish a type of infection in which insufficient replication occurs to stimulate the immunologic apparatus. Consequently, these organisms live in peaceful coexistence with the host, usually at body surfaces, and persist in this relationship for many years. Disordered homeostasis owing to the magnitude or type of antigen is at present a subject of intense interest in relation to organ transplantation and maternal-fetal interactions.

The second major cause of immunologic imbalance is related to aberrancy of effector cells or products of the immune response. There may be failure to produce sufficient effector cells or cell products, or they may be defective in type. Failure may be congenital, e.g., poor function of polymorphonuclear leukocytes in chronic granulomatous disease (nonspecific immunity) or diminished antibody responses in congenital agammaglobulinemia (specific immunity). The net result is immunologic imbalance, recurrent infections, and a predisposition to malignant tumors and autoimmune disease. These aberrations also occur as a consequence of acquired cases of immunosuppression, e.g., chemical immunosuppressive agents.

Aberrations may involve the production of cell products. There may be overproduction of a product normally present in trace amounts. An example of this is the allergic individual who produces too much IgE immunoglobulin and manifests immediate-type hypersensitivity. Qualitative aberrations may also occur with natural infection; for example, following streptococcal tonsillitis, antigen-antibody complexes may be produced that damage the kidney (acute glomerulonephritis). Lastly, these aberrations may be produced iatrogenically as a complication of vaccines. Certain vaccines may produce hypersensitivity rather than protective immunity. This has been described with rabies and measles vaccines.

SUGGESTIONS FOR FURTHER READING

History of Immunology

Bulloch, W.: The History of Bacteriology. London, Oxford University Press, 1938.
Burnet, F. M.: Cellular Immunology. Cambridge, Melbourne University Press, 1969.
Edsall, G.: What is immunology? J. Immunol., 67:167, 1951.

Ehrlich, P.: On immunity with special reference to cell life. Proc. Soc. London (Biol.), *66*:424, 1906.

Grabar, P.: The historical background of immunology. *In* Fudenberg, H. H., Stites, D. P., Caldwell, J. L., and Wells, J. V. (eds.): Basic and Clinical Immunology. Los Altos, Lange Medical Publications, 1976.

Metchnikoff, E.: Immunity in Infective Diseases. London, Cambridge University Press, 1905.

Immunology in the Modern Sense

Bellanti, J. A., and Dayton, D. H.: The Phagocytic Cell in Host Resistance. New York, Raven Press, 1975.

Davis, B. D., Dulbecco, R., Eisen, H. N., Ginsberg, H. S., and Wood, W. B., Jr.: Immunology. *In* Microbiology. New York, Harper and Row, Publishers, 1973.

Fudenberg, H. H., Stites, D. P., Caldwell, J. L., and Wells, J. V.: Basic and Clinical Immunology. Los Altos, Lange Medical Publications, 1976.

Gell, P. G. H., Coombs, R. R. A., and Lachman, P. T.: Clinical Aspects of Immunology. Oxford, Blackwell Scientific Publications, 1975.

Humphrey, J. H., and White, R. G.: Immunology for Students of Medicine. Philadelphia, F. A. Davis, 1970.

Kabat, E. A.: Structural Concepts in Immunology and Immunochemistry. New York, Holt, Rinehart and Winston, 1975.

Roitt, I. M.: Essential Immunology. Oxford, Blackwell Scientific Publications, 1974.

Rose, N. R., Milgrom, F., and van Oss, C. J.: Fundamentals of Immunology. New York, Macmillan Publishing Co., Inc., 1973.

Sell, S.: Immunology, Immunopathology and Immunity. Hagerstown, Harper and Row, Publishers, 1975.

Chapter 2 _____

GENERAL IMMUNOBIOLOGY
Joseph A. Bellanti, M.D.

ANATOMIC ORGANIZATION OF THE IMMUNE SYSTEM

CELL TYPES AND EFFECTOR MECHANISMS INVOLVED IN NONSPECIFIC IMMUNE MECHANISMS

In order to carry out the functions of immunity, a ubiquitous immunologic cell system has appeared within the vertebrates: the *lymphoreticular system*. This collection of cellular elements is distributed strategically throughout the tissues as well as lining lymphatic and vascular channels. Its cells are housed within the *blood, tissues, thymus, lymph nodes,* and *spleen* (internal secretory system), and in those body tracts exposed to the external environment—the *respiratory, gastrointestinal, genitourinary* systems (external secretory system) (Fig. 2–1).

The tissues contain a variety of cell types, each performing a separate function either directly or through the elaboration of a cell product(s). The system may be activated by a variety of influences that share the common characteristic of being recognized as foreign by the host. The stimuli may be presented to the host either exogenously (e.g., microorganisms) or endogenously (e.g., effete cells or transformed neoplastic cells).

Following activation, a spectrum of cellular and humoral events occurs that comprises the nonspecific and specific immune responses (Chapter 1). The nonspecific immune responses consist of phagocytosis and the inflammatory response; if the stimulus leads to the production of specific cell products (e.g., antibody, lymphokines) by specialized groups of lymphocytes, the foreign configurations are referred to as immunogens or antigens (Chapter 4). A number of effector mechanisms involving several cell types, cell products, and soluble serum factors may be called into play by the host following the encounter and recognition of a foreign configuration (Table 2–1). The cellular constituents include *mononuclear phagocytes, granulocytes, platelets,* and *lymphocytes*. The origins of these cells are pluripotential hematopoietic stem cells located within the bone marrow, fetal liver, and yolk sac of the fetus. The cell types, differentiation, and tissue localization of these cells are shown in Table 2–2. For ease of discussion, these cells will be grouped into a functional classification according to the following categories: *phagocytic cells, mediator cells,* and *lymphocytes*.

26

ORGANIZATION OF THE IMMUNE SYSTEM
(lymphoreticular tissues)

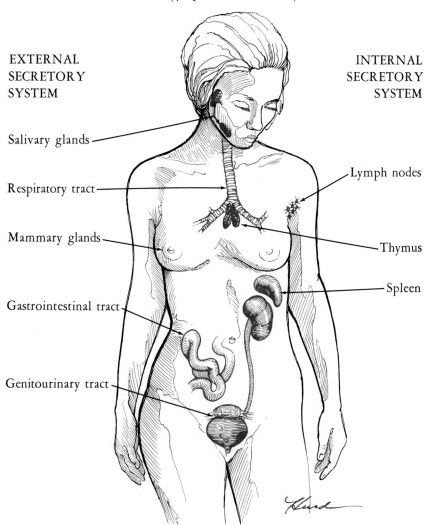

EXTERNAL
SECRETORY
SYSTEM

INTERNAL
SECRETORY
SYSTEM

Salivary glands

Respiratory tract

Mammary glands

Gastrointestinal tract

Genitourinary tract

Lymph nodes

Thymus

Spleen

Figure 2–1.   Schematic representation of the lymphoreticular tissues.

TABLE 2–1.   Cell Types and Effector Mechanisms Triggered
by or Involved in Immune Reactions

| | HUMORAL FACTORS | |
CELL TYPE	Agents Responsible for Mobilization of Cells	Cell Product
Nonspecific		
Mononuclear phagocytes	Chemotactic factors, macrophage activating factor (MAF)	Processed immunogen
Granulocytes		
Neutrophils	Chemotactic factors (complement-associated and bacterial factors) lymphocyte-derived	Kallikreins (producing kinins), SRS-A, basic peptides
Eosinophils	Specific chemotactic factors (e.g., ECF-A), and other chemotactic factors as for neutrophils	Histaminase, aryl sulfatase, phospholipase D, eosinophil-derived inhibitor (EDI)
Basophils	?	Vasoactive amines
Platelets	Factors producing platelet aggregates (thrombin, collagen)	Vasoactive amines
Specific		
B-lymphocytes	Antigen	Antibody
T-lymphocytes	Antigen	Lymphokines, e.g., MIF, interferon, cytotoxin, "transfer factor," and others

TABLE 2–2.   Differentiation and Localization of Cells Involved
in Immune Processes*

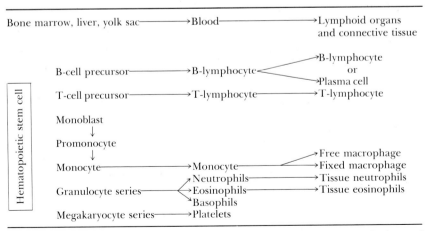

*(Adapted from van Furth, R.: Mononuclear Phagocytes in Immunity, Infection and Pathology. Oxford, Blackwell Scientific Publications, 1975.)

Phagocytic Cells

The process of phagocytosis is part of the nonspecific immune response (Chapter 1) and represents the host's initial encounter with foreignness. Endocytosis is a more general term and includes both *phagocytosis* (ingestion of particles) and *pinocytosis* (uptake of nonparticulates, e.g., fluid droplets). Both represent the process of engulfment and uptake of particles or fluid from the environment, and those groups of specialized cells that carry out these functions are commonly referred to as phagocytic cells. In some cases, subsequent digestion of these materials into smaller fragments facilitates their elimination (Fig. 2–2). In the human, phagocytosis is carried out primarily by *mononuclear phagocytes, neutrophils,* and, to a lesser extent, *eosinophils.*

Mononuclear Phagocytes.   The mononuclear phagocyte system (MPS) consists of a generalized group of cells that are widely distributed throughout the body where they can effectively eliminate foreign materials and debris from the blood, lymph, and tissues. The term MPS has been suggested to replace the less precise term reticuloendothelial system (RES), which was coined by Aschoff to define those morphologic elements of the immune system that are phagocytic as determined by clearance of particles (Fig. 2–3). The mononuclear phagocytes include both monocytes of the circulating blood (Fig. 2–4) and macrophages found in various tissues of the body.

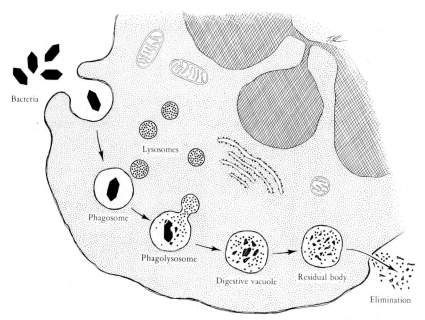

Bacteria

Lysosomes

Phagosome

Phagolysosome

Digestive vacuole

Residual body

Elimination

Figure 2–2.   Schematic representation of phagocytosis showing ingestion process and intracellular digestion.

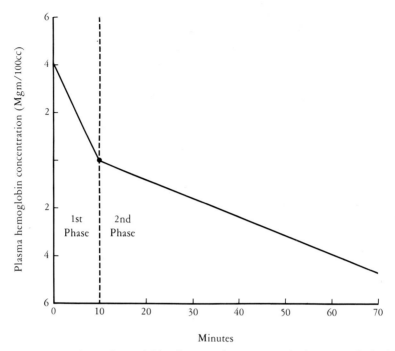

Minutes

Figure 2-3. Plasma hemoglobin clearance in a group of 40 apparently healthy human subjects. (After Gabrieli, E. R., and Snell, F. M.: Reflection of reticuloendothelial function in studies of blood clearance kinetics. J. Reticuloendothel. Soc., 2:141, 1965.)

The mononuclear phagocytes are produced from a stem cell in the bone marrow. Here they undergo proliferation and are delivered to the blood after a period of maturation through a *monoblast* → *promonocyte* → *monocyte* phase. Following a brief time in the blood (approximately one to two days) the monocytes migrate to the main site of their action in the tissues where they differentiate further into macrophages. Here they can divide, thus differing from granulocytes. The blood monocyte serves as an intermediate cell in the monocyte-macrophage transition.

The transition of monocyte to macrophage is also accompanied by morphologic, biochemical, and functional changes. During differentiation, the cell enlarges in size and in the number and complexity of intracellular organelles (e.g., Golgi apparatus, mitochondria, lysosomes, and lipid droplets). In addition, during maturation, the cell increases in

Figure 2-4. Monocyte from peripheral blood. *A,* Light micrograph, Wright-Giemsa stain, × 1400. Note the lobulated nucleus. (Courtesy of Dr. Theodore I. Malinin.) *B,* Electron micrograph, × 16,200, examined for peroxidase. Note the presence of two types of granules (g^1), peroxidase-positive and (g^2) peroxidase-negative; the endoplasmic reticulum (er); Golgi complex (G); the mitochondria (m); the centriole (ce); and the nucleus (n). (From Bainton, D. F.: *In* J. T. Dingle (ed.): Lysosomes in Biology and Pathology. Vol. 5. New York, North-Holland, 1976.)

See illustration on the opposite page

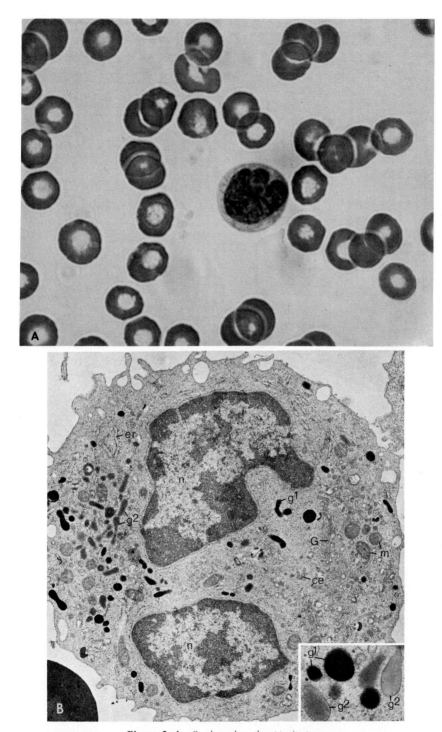

Figure 2-4. *See legend on the opposite page*

the content of lysosomal enzymes such as acid phosphatase, beta-glucuronidase, cathepsin, lysozyme, and aryl sulfatase, as well as related mitochondrial enzymes, e.g., cytochrome oxidase. The energy sources for cells of the MPS are dependent upon the degree of cellular maturity, the level of endocytic activity, and the environment. With the notable exception of the alveolar macrophage, which derives its energy primarily from aerobic metabolism, all other cells of the MPS derive their energy for particle uptake through the glycolytic pathway.

The macrophages are highly specialized to carry out their function in the ingestion and destruction of all particulate matter by the process of endocytosis. These cells remove and destroy certain bacteria, damaged or effete cells, neoplastic cells, colloidal materials, and macromolecules. The phagocytic process is sometimes facilitated by antibody, since particles coated with antibody are ingested more efficiently; complement, a series of sequentially reacting serum proteins, may also be involved as an amplifier of phagocytosis (Chapters 5 and 6). The term opsonin is used to describe this phagocytic-enhancing principle of both antibody and complement. The circulating monocytes are attracted to an area of injury (chemotaxis) by a number of factors, some of which are derived from the complement system or secreted by the T-lymphocytes (Table 2–1). Here they may further differentiate into macrophages and may be activated in a variety of ways — either following endocytosis or through humoral substances, including antibody, complement, or products of lymphocytes (lymphokines) (Chapter 9). Once activated, the cells assume heightened metabolic activity (activated macrophages) and display enhancement of function, e.g., microbicidal activity. Some workers believe that, in addition to a role in defense and surveillance, the macrophage system is important in the initial recognition and processing of antigen, steps which may be necessary for the induction of specific immunologic responses (Chapter 7).

Neutrophils or Polymorphonuclear Leukocytes. In the human the circulating granulocytes comprise three varieties of morphologically identifiable cells that are involved in a number of immunologic reactions in tissue; these include the neutrophil, the eosinophil, and the basophil (Table 2–1). Of these three, only the neutrophil and, to a lesser extent, the eosinophil are primarily phagocytic.

Neutrophils or polymorphonuclear (PMN) leukocytes (Fig. 2–5) normally account for 60 to 70 per cent of the total leukocyte count in the peripheral blood of the adult human. Unlike the macrophage, the neutrophil is an end cell of myeloid differentiation and does not divide. The neutrophils arise in the bone marrow from a common ancestral stem cell and, after a series of divisions, undergo a maturation through a myeloblast → promyelocyte → metamyelocyte → band cell → mature PMN. Unlike the situation with the monocyte-macrophage series, however, there appears to be a large storage compartment in the bone marrow that can be called upon as needed to replenish cells in the circula-

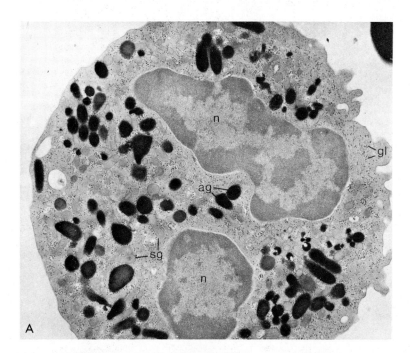

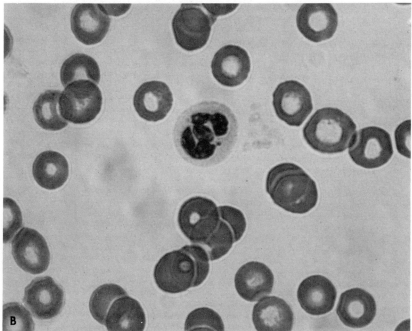

Figure 2–5. Polymorphonuclear leukocyte from peripheral blood. *A*, Electron micrograph, × 13,500, showing a lobulated nucleus (n) and cytoplasmic granules reacted for peroxidase. Note the presence of two types of granules: the peroxidase-positive azurophilic (ag) and the peroxidase-negative specific granules (sg), and the glycogen particles (gl) that are dispersed throughout the cytoplasm. (From Bainton, D. F.: *In* J. T. Dingle (ed.): Lysosomes in Biology and Pathology. Vol. 5. New York, North-Holland, 1976.) *B*, Light micrograph, Wright-Giemsa stain, × 1400, showing fully segmented nucleus. (Courtesy of Dr. Theodore I. Malinin.)

33

tion. After a short period in the blood (about 12 hours), the PMN's enter the tissues where they complete their life span of a few days. Normally, there is no return of these cells from the tissues back to the blood. Some of the cells in the vascular pool do not circulate freely, presumably because they are temporarily sequestered in small blood vessels or adhere to the walls of larger vessels (marginal pool).

With maturation of the cells, there is a sequential appearance of two distinct classes of granules: the primary (azurophilic) and the secondary or specific granules (Fig. 2–5). The primary granules are electron-dense structures approximately 0.4 micron in diameter that appear early in maturation and have many features in common with lysosomes of other tissues. They contain myeloperoxidase, arginine-rich basic (cationic) proteins, sulfated mucopolysaccharides, acid phosphatase, and several other acid hydrolases. The secondary or specific granules are not truly lysosomes; they are smaller (about 0.3 micron in diameter) and are less dense than the primary granules. They are rich in alkaline phosphatase, lysozyme, and aminopeptidase. In the intermediate stage of neutrophil maturation, both populations of granules are seen. As maturation proceeds, however, the secondary granules increase in number and appear to predominate. Both types of granules are important in the breakdown of ingested material and in the killing of microorganisms. Recent evidence suggests that granulocyte production and release may be under the control of cellular and humoral factors.

The Eosinophils.   The eosinophilic granulocytes make up one to three per cent of the circulating blood leukocytes and are distinguished by large cytoplasmic granules that stain intensely red with eosin (Fig. 2–6). They share many features with the neutrophil, arise from a common progenitor cell, and display a similar morphogenesis. In contrast to the neutrophil, however, the eosinophils mature in the bone marrow in three to six days before release into the circulation, following which they circulate with a half-life of approximately 30 minutes. The eosinophils have a half-life of 12 days in tissues where they fulfill their major function. Like the neutrophil, the eosinophils do not return from tissues to the circulation but are eliminated through the mucosal surfaces of the respiratory and gastrointestinal tracts. With maturation of these cells, there occurs a transition from primary (azurophilic) gran-

---

Figure 2–6. *A,* Eosinophilic leukocyte and a small lymphocyte from peripheral blood. Light micrograph, Wright-Giemsa stain, × 1400. (Courtesy of Dr. Theodore I. Malinin.) Note the bilobed nucleus and the prominent granules of the eosinophil. *B,* Electron micrograph of a human eosinophil from normal bone marrow, × 33,000, reacted for peroxidase. Note the presence of large granules that have a predominance of peroxidase staining filling the granule contents except for the area occupied by the crystalline core (arrow). (From Bainton, D. F.: *In* J. T. Dingle (ed.): Lysosomes in Biology and Pathology. Vol. 5. New York, North-Holland, 1976.)

See illustration on the opposite page

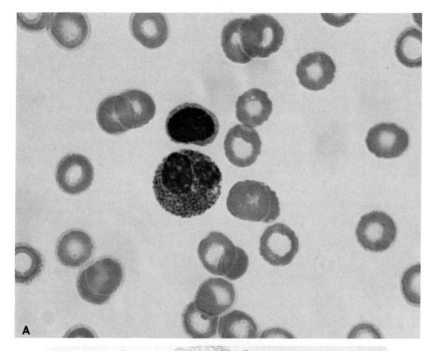

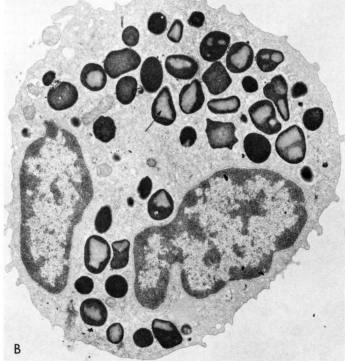

Figure 2-6. *See legend on the opposite page*

ules to large cytoplasmic granules, which have a crystalloid sub-structure (Fig. 2–6). The granules of the eosinophil do not contain lysozyme and phagocytin as found in PMN's. They are rich in acid phosphatase and peroxidase activity. Although the cells have the capacity to phagocytose a variety of particles, including microorganisms and soluble antigen-antibody complexes, the process appears to be less efficient than with neutrophils. In spite of its well known association with allergic and parasitic diseases, the specific role of the eosinophil is not known with certainty. Major roles postulated include the ingestion of immune complexes and their involvement in limiting inflammatory reactions, presumably by antagonizing the effects of certain mediators. For example, aryl sulfatase B from eosinophils has been shown to inactivate SRS-A released by mediator cells (Chapter 13). Recently, the eosinophils have been found to participate in antibody-mediated cytotoxicity reactions of importance in the clearance of certain parasitic organisms, e.g., Schistosoma. As a general rule, eosinophilia is more common in atopic diseases in which increased levels of IgE are found than in other immunologically mediated disorders (Chapter 20).

Mediator Cells

Certain cells of the body also participate in immunologic reactions through the release of chemical substances (mediators) that have a variety of biologic activities including increased vascular permeability, contraction of smooth muscle, and enhancement of the inflammatory response. These cells are referred to as mediator cells and comprise a heterogeneous collection of morphologic types including *mast cells, basophils, platelets, enterochromaffin* cells, and certain of the phagocytic cells, e.g., neutrophils.

Basophilic granulocytes (Fig. 2–7), which make up only 0.5 per cent of the blood leukocytes, and the platelets, the non-nucleated hemostatic elements of the blood, are the two major mediator cells in the circulation. They have been shown to contain a variety of vasoactive amines, such as histamine and serotonin (Chapter 13). The basophils are distinguished by their large purple or blue-black granules that ultrastructurally are electron-dense and homogeneous and when mature show a characteristic banded pattern. These granules contain acid mucopolysaccharides (e.g., heparin), which are responsible for the tinc-

---

Figure 2–7. Basophilic leukocyte from peripheral blood. *A*, Light micrograph, Wright-Giemsa stain, × 1400, showing large granules in the cytoplasm. *B*, Electron micrograph, × 14,800, reacted for peroxidase. Note the unusually large nucleus (n), scattered glycogen particles (gl), and peroxidase-positive granules, some of which may appear speckled (arrow). (From Bainton, D. F.: *In* J. T. Dingle (ed.): Lysosomes in Biology and Pathology. Vol. 5. New York, North-Holland. 1976.)

See illustration on the opposite page

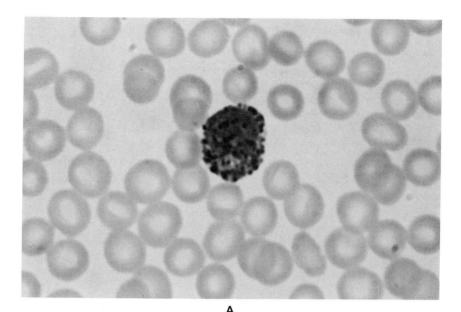

A

B

Figure 2–7.   See legend on the opposite page

torial phenomenon of metachromasia. Little is known of their production, distribution, or life span. Although they resemble the mast cells morphologically, they differ in several respects.

The basophil and mast cell are important sources of mediators, e.g., histamine, which are involved in immediate hypersensitivity (Chapters 13 and 20). The elaboration of these agents is thought to be triggered by contact of these cells with antigen-antibody complexes through complement-dependent or complement-independent mechanisms (Chapter 13). The release of these mediators can occur by direct impact of an environmental agent (e.g., compound 48/80) or indirectly through the interaction of antigen with membrane-bound IgE (Chapter 13). The release appears to be mediated by cyclic $3',5'$-adenosine monophosphate (cyclic AMP) (Chapters 7 and 20). Substances that increase cyclic AMP lead to a decrease in the release of mediators; substances that decrease intracellular levels of cyclic AMP lead to an increased release. These vasoactive amines appear to be involved in tissue injury. Following interaction of antigen with antibody in tissues such as the renal glomerulus, for example, there is a release of these substances that results in permeability changes that lead to accelerated deposition of circulating soluble antigen-antibody complexes. The release of histamine and serotonin therefore appears to be involved in an immunologic cascade, in which there may be amplification of injury mediated by antigen-antibody complexes. The mechanism by which the accumulation of these complexes leads to tissue injury is described in greater detail in Chapter 13. Findings of this nature may have important clinical implications. In animals undergoing experimental forms of immunologic injury (serum sickness), treatment with antihistamines or serotonin antagonists leads to a protection of the animals from immune complex–induced type nephritis (Chapter 13).

Chemotaxis, Phagocytosis, and Metabolic Changes and Antimicrobial Systems of Phagocytic Cells

The primary role of the phagocytic cells in the body economy is the localization and removal of foreign substances, such as microorganisms. Several integrated functions may be required to achieve these goals. First, the cells must reach the site of the foreign configuration (chemotaxis). They must then ingest the foreign substance (phagocytosis). Finally, after a series of metabolic steps, they must destroy the foreign substance or inhibit the replication of the microorganism (microbial killing).

Chemotaxis

There are three phenomena involved in cell movements: *motility*, *locomotion*, and *chemotaxis*. Motility refers to a cell that moves; locomotion refers to movement from one place to another; and chemotaxis refers to unidirectional locomotion toward an increasing gradient of attractant (chemoattractant). A phagocytic cell adherent to glass, for example, can be a highly motile cell but may not be exhibiting locomotion or chemotaxis. A cell that is undergoing random locomotion may not be exhibiting chemotaxis. There are a variety of *in vivo* and *in vitro* techniques for measurement of locomotion and chemotaxis (Chapter 26).

The polymorphonuclear leukocyte responds to at least three different chemotactic stimuli derived from the complement system, as well as bacterial and lymphocyte-derived factors (Table 2–1). The neutrophils also are directly or indirectly involved in the production of a substance known as slow-reactive substance (SRS-A), a humoral factor containing a fatty acid and capable of causing the contraction of smooth muscle (Chapter 13). Other factors produced by the granulocyte include the kinins, small polypeptides that are vasoactive. These substances are important pharmacologic mediators of immediate hypersensitivity reactions (Chapters 13 and 20).

A number of substances chemotactic for monocytes and macrophages have also been described (Table 2–1). These include products of the complement sysem as well as the lymphocyte series, e.g., macrophage activity factor (MAF). Recently, a substance that is inhibitory for chemotaxis of monocytes has been described in extracts of tumor tissues.

There are a number of substances that are chemotactic for eosinophils that are similar to those for neutrophils. These include antigen-antibody complexes; complement-derived chemotactic factors; products of the lymphocyte series, e.g., lymphokines; and an eosinophilic chemotactic factor of anaphylaxis (ECF-A), a substance released from tissue mast cells and peripheral basophils that may be very important in the pathogenesis of immediate-type hypersensitivity reactions (Chapters 13 and 20). Recently, ECF-A has also been shown to be released from PMN leukocytes.

Phagocytosis

The next step in the sequence is phagocytosis, the process by which a particle is ingested by a cell. This process can be divided into two steps: the *attachment phase* and the *ingestion phase*.

During the attachment phase, firm contact is established with the particle. This can occur between the particle and phagocyte directly through unenhanced processes, in which case it is largely dependent upon surface properties of the particle to be phagocytosed, e.g., hydrophobicity and surface tension. In other cases, attachment involves the participation of two types of receptors on the plasma membrane of the phagocyte: (1) a receptor for the Fc fragment of an immunoglobulin molecule; and (2) a receptor for the C3b, a component of complement. These are shown schematically in Figure 2–8.

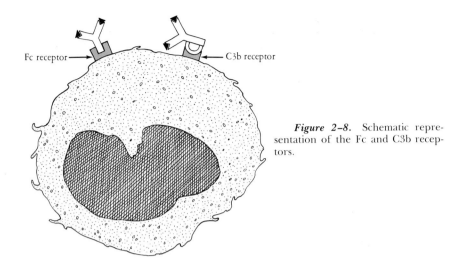

Fc receptor → ← C3b receptor

Figure 2–8. Schematic representation of the Fc and C3b receptors.

Many bacteria that are unencapsulated are rapidly taken up by phagocytes and destroyed. Encapsulated strains such as the pneumococcus, however, are taken up poorly and hence not destroyed. This resistance to engulfment is related to the protective capsule of the bacteria and ensures its survival within the host. When certain serum proteins, e.g., complement or antibodies (opsonins), are present, the attachment of the coated bacterium is facilitated by the surface receptors and the phagocytic uptake is enhanced (Chapter 15).

The ingestion process is the next step of phagocytosis and represents the engulfment of the particle. The phagocyte invaginates its plasma membrane and the particle is then taken up into the cytoplasm and enclosed within a vacuole (phagosome), the wall of which is made up of inverted plasma membrane (see Fig. 2–2). Recently actin- and myosin-like proteins that appear to participate in the ingestion process through the formation of microfilaments have been isolated.

Morphologic Events Associated with Phagocytosis

Following the formation of the phagosome, the membrane enclosing the particle gradually pinches off from the surface membrane and is internalized within the cell, forming the phagocytic vacuole (see Fig. 2–2). The lysosomal granules within the leukocytes come into apposition with this phagosome, and the membranes of the two structures fuse into a phagolysosome. The granules rupture, discharging their enzymatic contents into the vacuole, and come into contact with the ingested particle. This process has been termed degranulation and represents the morphologic counterpart of the transfer of enzymes from the lysosomal granule to the phagosome. The leukocyte granules (primary) are analogous to the lysosomes of other cells and contain several hydrolytic enzymes and other bactericidal substances (Table 2–3). Firstly, these ranges of acidity are achieved by the cell during the "respiratory burst" associated with phagocytosis as described below. Secondly, most of the enzymes found within the primary granules have pH optimum within this acid range. These facts suggest that the fall in pH during phagocytosis might trigger the digestive process by liberating hydrolytic enzymes that function best at a low pH.

Metabolic Events Associated with Phagocytosis

Following the formation of the phagocytic vacuole, a series of biochemical reactions is initiated in phagocytic cells. The metabolic pathways that are primarily involved include the glycolytic pathway and the hexose monophosphate (HMP) shunt (Fig. 2–9). In addition, alveolar macrophages utilize the tricarboxylic acid pathway, which provides their main energy source. Collectively, the stimulation of these pathways is termed the "respiratory burst" and consists of the following: (1) an increase in glycolysis; (2) a marked increase in HMP shunt activity; and (3) an elevation in oxygen consumption and H_2O_2 and lactic acid production. The increase in lactic acid production is in part responsible for the fall in pH within the phagosome, as previously described. Accompanying the respiratory burst is an enhanced RNA and phospholipid turnover, events important in protein synthesis and membrane formation. These changes are most prominent in neutrophils but also are seen to a lesser extent in the mononuclear phagocytes.

The biologic significance of the preferential utilization of these pathways by certain phagocytic cells, e.g., PMN's, may be to facilitate their function in tissues in which oxygen may be limited. In contrast, the

TABLE 2–3. Enzymes and Other Substances Found Within Neutrophils*

Acid phosphatase	Hyaluronidase
Acid ribonuclease	Lysozyme
Acid deoxyribonuclease	Collagenase
Cathepsins B. C, D, E	Aryl sulfatases A and B
Phosphoprotein phosphatase	Phospholipases
Organophosphate-resistant esterase	Acid lipase
β-Glucuronidase	Lactoferrin
β-Galactosidase	Phagocytin and other related bactericidal proteins
β-N-acetylglucosaminase	Endogenous pyrogen
α-L-fucosidase	Plasminogen activator (?urokinase)
α-1,4-glucosidase	Hemolysin(s)
α-mannosidase	Mucopolysaccharides and glycoproteins
α-N-acetylglucosamidase	Basic proteins: (a) Mast cell-active (b) Perme-
α-N-acetylgalactosaminidase	ability-inducing, independent mast cells
Myeloperoxidase	

*(Adapted from Cochrane, C. G.: Immunologic tissue injury mediated by neutrophilic leukocytes. Adv. Immunol., 9:97, 1968.)

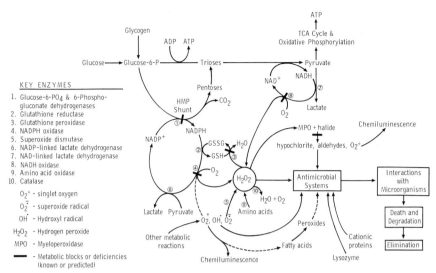

KEY ENZYMES

1. Glucose-6-PO₄ & 6-Phospho-gluconate dehydrogenases
2. Glutathione reductase
3. Glutathione peroxidase
4. NADPH oxidase
5. Superoxide dismutase
6. NADP-linked lactate dehydrogenase
7. NAD-linked lactate dehydrogenase
8. NADH oxidase
9. Amino acid oxidase
10. Catalase

O_2^* – singlet oxygen
$O_2^{\overline{\cdot}}$ – superoxide radical
$OH^{\cdot}$ – Hydroxyl radical
H_2O_2 – Hydrogen peroxide
MPO – Myeloperoxidase
━━ – Metabolic blocks or deficiencies (known or predicted)

Figure 2–9.   Metabolic pathways of leukocytes. (Courtesy of Dr. Lata Nerurkar.)

utilization of the TCA cycle by other phagocytic cells, e.g., alveolar macrophages, may be an adaptation to their aerobic environment.

The precise initiating events that result in the metabolic changes following particle uptake are not known, but appear to involve perturbations of the plasma membrane. Several surface-active agents such as deoxycholate, digitonin, and concanavalin-A can also induce a respiratory burst similar to that seen following particle uptake. The extraordinary feature of this phenomenon is that the initiation of the respiratory burst is detectable within seconds after particle uptake and actually precedes the morphologic events, suggesting that the biochemical changes may be required for subsequent events to occur. In addition, the activation of the macrophages can be produced by several other agents, e.g., adjuvants, closely related microorganisms, lymphokines, and bacterial products (Chapter 14). The features of the enhanced metabolism of this "activated macrophage" are the same as those described with particle uptake.

One of the proposed key enzymes involved in the metabolism of phagocytic cells is NADPH oxidase (Fig. 2–9). This enzyme may serve a twofold function: (1) it provides a source of NADP, which may be the limiting factor regulating HMP shunt activity; or (2) it may be involved in the formation of H_2O_2, which is an essential component in the microbicidal reactions. In addition, NADP also participates in many other metabolic functions, such as glutathione production, RNA and lipid metabolism, and membrane formation, events essential for phagocytic cell function. Other enzyme systems are involved in the conversion of NADPH to NADP, including glutathione peroxidase, which oxidizes reduced glutathione (GSH) to its oxidized form (GSSG) in the presence of H_2O_2. The GSSG is further reduced to GSH and in turn converts NADPH to NADP (Fig. 2–9).

With the respiratory burst there occurs an enhanced production of H_2O_2 or superoxide anion (O_2^-). The superoxide anion undergoes dismutation in the presence of an enzyme, superoxide dismutase, with further production of H_2O_2 (Fig. 2–9). The production of H_2O_2 is more prominent in PMN's than in tissue or alveolar macrophages and appears to be extremely important in microbicidal function of PMN's. Defects in H_2O_2 production associated with failure in the induction of the respiratory burst have been observed in the leukocytes of children with a variety of neutrophil dysfunction disorders, e.g., chronic granulomatous disease (CGD) (Chapter 22). A useful diagnostic test of phagocytic function has been developed based upon these biochemical considerations. The reduction of nitroblue tetrazolium (NBT) to a blue formazan derivative provides a useful functional test of leukocyte HMP activity and is abnormally low in CGD.

Antimicrobial Mechanisms of Phagocytic Cells

In order to successfully destroy and eliminate microorganisms, e.g., bacteria, following their ingestion, the next step in the process is the killing and destruction of the microorganism by the phagocytic cell. The observation that anaerobic conditions only partially impair bactericidal activity led to the discovery that both oxygen-dependent and oxygen-independent antimicrobial mechanisms exist within phagocytic cells. Klebanoff has proposed a classification of these antimicrobial systems on the basis of their oxygen requirements. The oxygen-dependent mechanisms can be further subdivided on the basis of their utilization of myeloperoxidase. This classification of antimicrobial systems of phagocytic cells is shown in Table 2–4.

A system consisting of H_2O_2, halide and MPO has been shown to have powerful microbicidal activity contributing to the microbicidal ac-

TABLE 2–4. Antimicrobial Systems of Phagocytic Cells*

I. *O_2-dependent*	II. *O_2-independent*
a. Myeloperoxidase (MPO)-mediated	a. acid
b. MPO-independent	b. lysozyme
1. H_2O_2	c. lactoferrin
2. superoxide anion (O_2^-)	d. granular cationic proteins
3. hydroxyl radical ($OH^{\cdot}$)	
4. singlet oxygen (O_2^*)	
5. ascorbate-peroxide-metal ion	
6. amino acid oxidation	

*(After Klebanoff, S. J.: *In* J. A. Bellanti and D. H. Dayton (eds.): The Phagocytic Cell in Host Resistance. New York, Raven Press, 1975.)

tion of phagocytic cells, primarily the PMN's (Fig. 2–9). The role of this system in mononuclear phagocytes is less clear. The proposed mechanism of action of the MPO-H_2O_2-halide complex is thought to involve the formation of aldehydes and hypochlorite or halogenation of bacterial proteins, the net effect of which leads to the death of the microorganism. The significance of this reaction is apparent in several clinical disorders of neutrophil function in which a failure of production of H_2O_2 leads to defective bacterial killing and the clinical spectrum of recurrent infection, e.g., CGD, which suggests that there are mechanisms other than the MPO-H_2O_2-halide system operative in antimicrobial activity. These other systems have been referred to as "backup systems." In the case of low concentrations of H_2O_2, the action of MPO can be replaced by catalase. Such alternate pathways may be important in macrophages, in which the role of MPO is less clear. It is of interest that in children with CGD the characteristic spectrum of bacteria causing infection includes those that are catalase-positive and peroxide-negative, e.g., *Staphylococcus aureus.* In contrast, organisms that are catalase-negative and peroxide-positive, e.g., *Haemophilus influenzae*, do not cause serious infection in these children. It has been postulated that these latter organisms can provide an alternate source of H_2O_2 which in effect can partially correct the cellular defects (Chapter 22).

Among the MPO-independent systems, H_2O_2 itself exhibits antimicrobial activity, and since it is produced during the phagocytic event it may in part contribute to the overall killing capacity of the phagocytic cell (Table 2–4). The superoxide radical ($O_2^{\bar{\cdot}}$) that is generated during phagocytosis is formed by the univalent reduction of molecular oxygen and is an extremely toxic and reactive moiety important in bactericidal activity. Subsequent dismutation of $O_2^{\bar{\cdot}}$ by superoxide dismutase (SOD) leads to the formation of H_2O_2.

$$O_2 \xrightarrow{e} O_2^{\bar{\cdot}}$$

$$O_2^{\bar{\cdot}} + O_2^{\bar{\cdot}} + 2H^+ \xrightarrow{SOD} O_2 + H_2O_2$$

The superoxide radical, in addition to its own bactericidal activity, may through dismutation produce H_2O_2, which is microbicidal. This indicates that $O_2^{\bar{\cdot}}$ acts as an intermediate to H_2O_2 production and indirectly contributes to the MPO-mediated system. Singlet oxygen (O_2^*) is an electronically excited state of molecular oxygen that emits light (chemiluminescence) when it reverts to the triplet ground state (O_2). This biochemical finding has also been used in the functional assessment of phagocytic cells. The source of this singlet oxygen (O_2^*) may be an MPO-mediated reaction involving the formation of hypochlorite. Singlet oxygen might also react with certain unsaturated chemical groups, e.g., ethylene groups, forming dioxytanes across double bonds that are unstable, and may be toxic to microorganisms

$$\diagup C = C \diagdown \xrightarrow{O_2{}^*} \diagup C - C \diagdown$$

and thus responsible for the killing by MPO-mediated systems. Other proposed antimicrobial mechanisms include an ascorbate-peroxide system, which may function in synergism with lysozyme and may even be more potent in the presence of metallic ions such as cobalt and copper. The oxidation of amino acids may also add to the generation of H_2O_2.

The mononuclear phagocytes lack significant myeloperoxidase activity and must therefore resort to other microbicidal mechanisms. Although little is known of the microbicidal mechanisms of mononuclear phagocytes at present, they do exhibit the metabolic burst and H_2O_2 and O_2^- generation displayed by PMN's but to a lesser extent.

The oxygen-independent mechanisms also seem to contribute to the killing capacity of the phagocytic cells since anaerobiosis does not totally impair their microbicidal activity (Table 2–4). Although there is evidence that lysozyme may be involved directly in the killing of bacteria, the action of this enzyme may also be to function in a digestive manner after the killing of the bacteria. Lactoferrin, an iron-binding protein, leukin, and phagocytin, found in the specific granules of the PMN but not in mononuclear phagocytes, also have been shown to have bacteriostatic properties. The granular cationic proteins also exhibit antimicrobial activity, presumably after binding to the microorganisms, a function that is also lacking in macrophages. Finally, the formation of lactic acid as a result of the respiratory burst reduces the intracellular pH and thus provides conditions favorable for the action of digestive enzymes rather than functioning directly as a microbicidal agent.

CELL TYPES AND EFFECTOR MECHANISMS INVOLVED IN SPECIFIC RESPONSES

Lymphocytes and Plasma Cells

The lymphoid cells of the immune system differ from the preceding group of cells by their ability to react specifically with antigen and to elaborate specific cell products. The lymphoid cells include plasma cells and lymphocytes (Figs. 2–10 and 2–11). These cells, once sensitized, become "committed" and are referred to as immunocytes. By definition, an immunocyte is a cell of the lymphoid series that can react with antigen with the production of specific cell products called an-

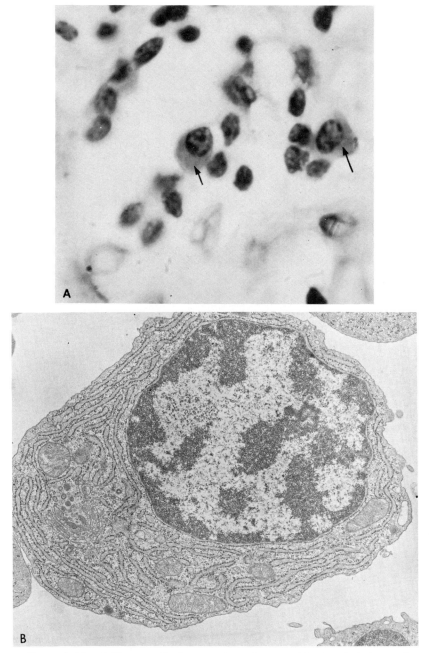

Figure 2–10. *A*, Plasma cells from section of aorta with chronic inflammation. Hematoxylin and eosin stain, × 1000. (Courtesy of Dr. Theodore I. Malinin.) *B*, Electron micrograph of plasma cells showing well developed endoplasmic reticulum, × 11,000. (Courtesy of Dr. Dorothy F. Bainton.)

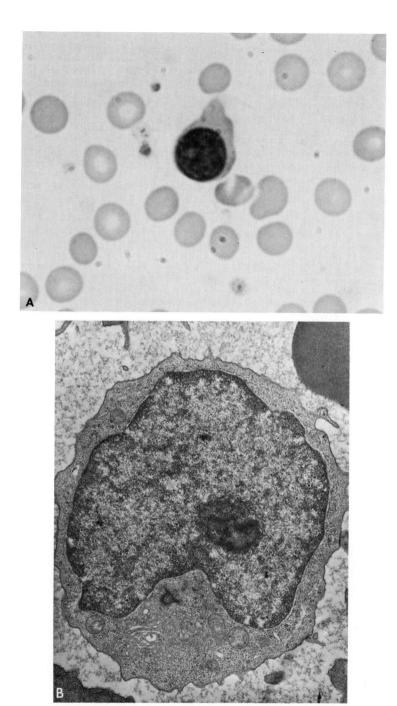

Figure 2–11. *A*, Lymphocytes from peripheral blood. Wright-Giemsa stain, × 1400. *B*, Electron micrograph of a resting lymphocyte × 11,000. (Courtesy of Dr. Dorothy F. Bainton.)

tibody or a cell-mediated event such as delayed hypersensitivity, e.g., tuberculin reaction (Chapter 9).

The traditional classification of lymphocytes as small, medium, and large was based on the concept that morphologically similar cells had the same functions, life cycles, and metabolic behavior. In recent years, however, it has become apparent that even lymphocytes that appear morphologically identical constitute several cell populations that are extremely heterogeneous in function.

The lymphoid cell line traces its origin to a pluripotential stem cell that in the fetus is found within the yolk sac, bone marrow, and liver and in the adult in the bone marrow. These cells produce two classes of committed stem cells: (1) a committed hematopoietic stem cell that can give rise to the erythroid elements, granulocytes, or megakaryocytes; and (2) a committed lymphoid stem cell precursor that can give rise to cells of the lymphoid series (Table 2–2). The commitment to any of these pathways is dependent upon the microenvironments in which these stem cells develop.

Development of the Lymphoid Tissue

Available evidence indicates that the lymphoid system consists of two components: (1) a *central* component involved in the differentiation of the lymphoid stem cells into lymphocytes capable of reacting with antigen (antigen-reactive cell); and (2) a *peripheral* component in which these cells can subsequently react with antigen (Fig. 2–12). The central lymphoid system consists of three components: (1) the *bone marrow*, (2) the *thymus*, and (3) a component whose identity is known with certainty only in birds (the bursa of Fabricius) and that in mammals is designated as the *bursal equivalent tissue*. The peripheral lymphoid system consists

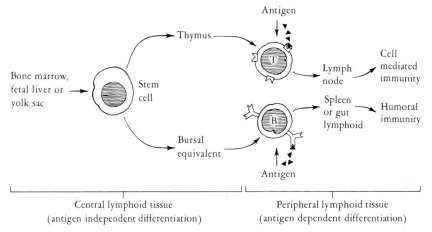

Figure 2–12.   Development of the lymphoid system.

of lymph nodes, spleen, and gut-associated lymphoid tissue. In contrast to the differentiation of lymphocytes in the peripheral component, which is antigen-dependent, the maturation of lymphoid elements in the central component can occur in the absence of antigen (Fig. 2–12).

In higher vertebrates two types of lymphocytes may be found in peripheral lymphoid tissues that are dependent upon their sites of differentiation in the central lymphoid compartment. One type, which develops in the thymus, differentiates into small lymphocytes referred to as T-lymphocytes, which are involved in antigen recognition in cell-mediated immune reactions, including delayed hypersensitivity. The other population of lymphocytes is derived from stem cells, which differentiate in the bursa of Fabricius in birds and in the mammalian equivalent and consist mainly of small lymphocytes referred to as B-lymphocytes, the plasma cells, and their progeny. In higher mammals, although the location of the bursal equivalent is unknown, several sites have been postulated, including the gut-associated lymphoid tissues (GALT), fetal liver, and the bone marrow. Such bursal equivalent– or bone marrow–derived lymphocytes are termed B-lymphocytes. Thus, the bone marrow component of the central lymphoid tissues may serve not only as a site of production of lymphoid stem cells but also as a microenvironment for the differentiation of stem cells into antigen-reactive B-lymphocytes, as well as a site for mature recirculating lymphocyte populations.

Cellular Elements

Lymphocytes thus comprise two lines of immunocompetent cells, one concerned with cell-mediated immunity (T-lymphocytes) and the other with humoral immunity (B-lymphocytes) (Fig. 2–12). Ordinarily, in the absence of stimulation the B-lymphocyte does not replicate. Under an appropriate stimulus, such as antigen, it transforms into a large, metabolically more active, "blast" cell, which has been termed "an active lymphocyte" or "a large pyroninophyllic" cell (Chapter 7). Plasma cells are characterized by their RNA-rich cytoplasm and eccentrically placed nuclei. Ultrastructurally, the cytoplasm contains an extensive system of endoplasmic reticulum studded with ribosomes (Fig. 2–10). This structure is characteristic of cells active in protein synthesis, and the product of these cells is immunoglobulin.

T-lymphocytes are involved in such cell-mediated immune reactions as graft versus host (GVH), delayed hypersensitivity, and tumor rejection, and develop in an alternative pathway of development. These cells are incapable of differentiating into plasma cells but give rise to a cell capable of producing a variety of factors that trigger inflammatory or cell-mediated damaging reactions leading to cell-mediated events. These factors include migration inhibitory factor (MIF), a substance chemotactic for mononuclear and granulocytic

cells, a cytotoxic factor capable of injuring a variety of cell types, interferon, and several other factors whose biologic roles are not yet well
defined (Chapters 9 and 13). Some are released upon interaction of
sensitized lymphocytes with appropriate antigens; others may remain
cell-bound. In either case, they lead to the destruction of foreign target
cells or to the damage and destruction of host cells. Thus, it is apparent
that the lymphocytes possess the most diversified function of all cells of
the immune system.

Following stimulation of either B- or T-lymphocytes, an alternate
pathway of differentiation leads to the production of a subpopulation
termed memory cells. Upon re-encounter with specific immunogens,
these cells have the capacity to proliferate and differentiate into cell
lines responsible for either humoral or cell-mediated immunity
(Chapter 7).

The conversion of small lymphocytes to blast cells provides the
basis for one of the most useful tests employed in clinical immunology,
i.e., the test of immunocompetency of patients suspected of having a
variety of immune deficiency disorders (Chapter 23). In addition, other
tests allow the identification of specific lymphocytes as B- or T-
lymphocytes (Chapters 7, 9 and 26). The transformation of the lymphocyte to the activated lymphocyte can be induced by a variety of stimuli
including specific antigen, in either a soluble or a cell-associated form,
e.g., lymphocytes from a genetically unrelated individual in a mixed
lymphocyte response (MLC), or on a graft in graft rejection, or on a
tumor cell in tumor rejection; or by antilymphocyte sera or by nonspecific mitogens, some of which selectively stimulate B-lymphocytes,
others, T-lymphocytes. These reactions take place by virtue of receptors on the surface of lymphocytes, which are described in greater detail in Chapters 3, 7, and 9.

THE STRUCTURE OF ORGANS THAT HOUSE IMMUNOLOGIC CELLS: THE PERIPHERAL LYMPHOID TISSUE

The immune system contains some cells concerned with the initial
response to foreign configurations and other cells that function in
subsequent encounters. The system is equipped to perform nonspecific
events, such as phagocytosis, as well as responses carried out in a specific manner by cells of the lymphoid tissues.

The lymphoreticular cells are strategically located in areas of the
body best suited to deal with foreign configurations, which may confront the host *exogenously* or may arise *endogenously* (Fig. 2–1). For example, the foreign configuration may be a microorganism entering the
host by such natural portals as the gastrointestinal, respiratory, or genitourinary tract. The lymphoid tissue is arranged in a unique manner in
these areas. When the configuration arises *endogenously* within a host,
e.g., a worn-out erythrocyte or a tumor cell, elements are mobilized

into the lymphatics or the bloodstream where they quickly come into contact with immune effector cells.

The encounter between a configuration and a cellular element involved in immunity appears to be a random event. There are two anatomic features that increase the chance occurrence of these random events. The first feature is that some elements of the system are in constant motion and are recirculating continuously (the phagocytes and lymphoid cells). The second is that certain organs, such as the lymph nodes and spleen, contain a system of conduits through which a continuous recirculation of lymph or blood occurs.

Thus, the system is well organized to carry out its functions in defense, homeostasis, and surveillance. Four types of peripheral lymphatic tissues are important in this regard: (1) the lymph nodules, (2) the lymph nodes, (3) the spleen, and (4) the thymus. Although all four seem to be engaged in lymphopoiesis, only the first three respond actively to antigenic stimulation. The thymus, in contrast, stands autonomous in this regard and appears to be a master central lymphoid organ concerned with embryogenesis and orchestration of the remainder of the peripheral lymphoid tissues.

Lymph Nodule

Lymph nodules consist of collections of lymphoid elements scattered in the submucous tissues of the respiratory passages, the intestine, and the genitourinary tracts. They are particularly well developed in structures such as the tonsils, which stand guard at the entrance of the gastrointestinal and respiratory tracts, and also in the Peyer's patches, collections of lymph nodules in the gastrointestinal tract. Their structure is demonstrated in Figure 2–13. This type of lymphoid tissue is arranged somewhat differently from that in lymph nodes, insofar as it lacks a connective tissue capsule. These nodules are not well developed in the fetus or in germ-free animals, but develop following exposure to antigens. Their development is believed to be related in some way to exposure of the host to antigens in the environment.

Since lymph nodules contain phagocytic elements as well as lymphoid elements, they are capable of reacting in nonspecific as well as in specific immunity. In the lymphoid cells that line these tracts, there occurs synthesis of the secretory IgA immunoglobulins. This class of immunoglobulin has been shown to be important at mucosal surfaces (Chapter 5). These tracts, contiguous with the exterior, elaborate a secretory form of antibody and provide the host with a cell product well suited to function at body surfaces and to deal with pathogens in the external environment. The IgE globulins have also been shown recently to be synthesized by cells in the same locations. Both IgA and IgE globulins are cell products of the external secretory system (Fig. 2–1).

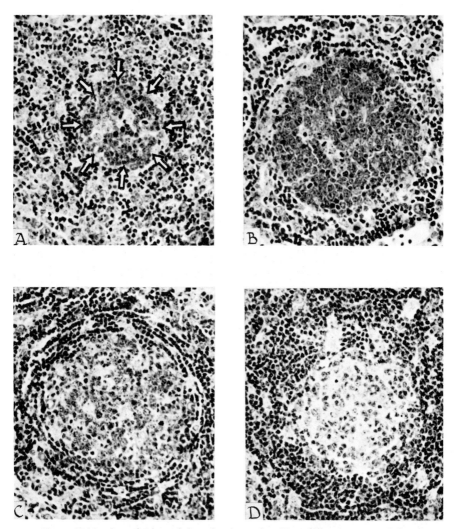

Figure 2-13. Lymphatic nodules of guinea pigs. Note different stages of development following immunization with *Listeria monocytogenes.* Hematoxylin and eosin stain, × 1100. (From Bloom, W., and Fawcett, D. W.: Textbook of Histology. 10th ed. Philadelphia, W. B. Saunders Company, 1975.)

Lymph Nodes

If a foreign configuration can overcome the initial barriers provided by the skin, mucous membranes, and lymph nodules, it may be handled in three additional ways: (1) it may be attached by wandering macrophages in the connective tissue; (2) it may provoke an inflammatory response with cellular accumulations, e.g., neutrophils; or (3) it may be taken up directly into the lymph or blood. The lymph represents a collection of tissue fluids flowing in lymphatic capillaries into a series of even larger collecting vessels called the *lymphatics.* These vessels connect with and pass through a series of structures, the lymph nodes. During this voyage, the lymph becomes progressively enriched with lymphocytes, so that when it finally empties into the bloodstream via the thoracic ducts, the fluid is significantly different from the tissue fluids of its origin. Lymphocytes are also added from postcapillary venules and become part of the *recirculating pool.*

The *recirculating pool* consists of a group of lymphocytes found in the circulating blood, lymph, and lymph nodes which traverse a circumscribed pathway from the blood to the lymph and then back to the blood. The recirculation of lymphocytes from the blood to the lymph occurs through a unique anatomic structure of lymph nodes, the postcapillary venule. These venules, found in the lymph node cortex, are distinguished by their elongated endothelial cell structure. Unlike other interepithelial cell transfers, such as that of the polymorphonuclear neutrophil, the lymphocyte passes from the blood to the lymph by a remarkable process in which the endothelial cell invaginates the lymphocyte and allows it to pass directly through the cell (Fig. 2–14). The recirculating pool of small lymphocytes consists primarily of T-cells that are characterized by their long life spans and are believed to function as memory cells.

Lymph nodes are oval structures distributed throughout the body (Fig. 2–15); through them pass the motile carriers of specific genetic information, the lymphocytes. When enlarged, the lymph nodes be-

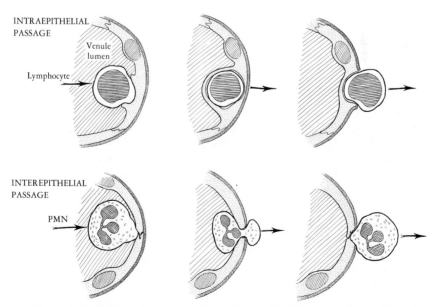

Figure 2–14. Schematic representation of intraepithelial passage of a small lymphocyte and interepithelial passage of a polymorphonuclear leukocyte.

come physically palpable, providing a useful diagnostic sign of infection or malignant disease. The structure of a lymph node is shown in Figure 2–15. It consists of two main portions, an outer portion (cortex) and an inner portion (medulla). The node is surrounded by a connective tissue capsule from which extensions protrude centrally (trabeculae). The capsule provides support and a conduit along which blood vessels run. Weblike structures (reticular fibers) extend from these connective tissue elements into the substance of the node; these contain phagocytic elements of the macrophage system. In the periphery, the node is made up of large numbers of lymphocytes organized into nodules. In the center of the nodules are collections of actively dividing cells termed *germinal centers.* Deeper cortical zones contain the postcapillary venules with their characteristic cuboidal endothelial cells through which passage of lymphocytes from blood lymph occurs (Fig. 2–16). Thus, in the lymph node, lymphocytes enter through both the vascular system and the lymphatics (Fig. 2–16). In mutant strains of mice born without thymuses (nude mice) or following the thymectomy of neonatal animals, there is a depletion of lymphoid elements in these paracortical or subcortical regions; therefore, this region has become known as a *thymic-dependent region* and contains the T-lymphocytes important in cell-mediated immunity. In contrast, upon removal of the bursa of Fabricius (in birds) or the bursal equivalent tissues (in the mammal), there is a failure of formation of the outer cortical regions containing the germinal centers, as well as the deeper medullary region; therefore, these regions have been called the bursal equivalent regions and contain the B-lymphocytes important in antibody synthesis. Following antigen stimulation, antibody synthesis can be noted in both the medullary and the far cortical regions of the node. Although it is tempting to compartmentalize the node according to function, this is undoubtedly an oversimplification of a more complicated process, since elements of each type of tissue may be present in both regions. Nonetheless, the importance of these findings for clinical medicine is illustrated in numerous disease states such as the DiGeorge syndrome, in which T-lymphocytes are absent owing to the congenital absence of the thymus, or X-linked agammaglobulinemia, in which a deficiency of B-lymphocytes occurs as a result of a failure of development of the bursal equivalent tissue (Chapter 22).

There are two basic functions of the lymph nodes. The first function is the filtration of foreign material performed as lymph percolates through the multichanneled structure. This removes particulate matter, and some products of phagocytic degradation become immunogenic.

Figure 2–15. Structure of lymph node, schematic. *A,* circulation; *B,* supporting structures (reticular fibers); and *C,* general areas of thymic-dependent (T-cell) and -independent (B-cell) areas.

See illustration on the opposite page

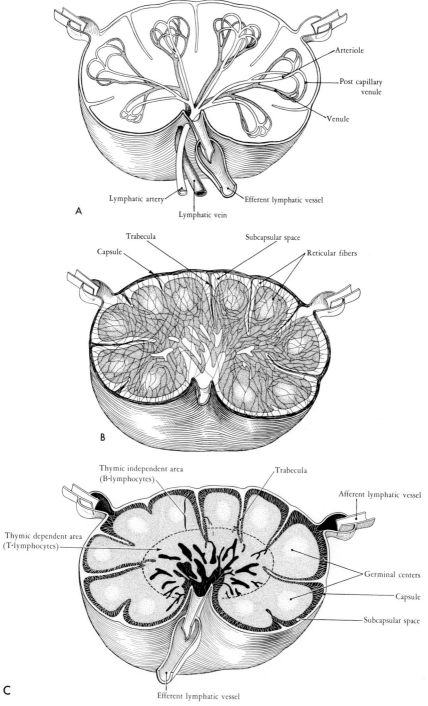

Arteriole

Post capillary
venule

Venule

Lymphatic artery

Efferent lymphatic vessel

Lymphatic vein

A

Trabecula   Subcapsular space

Capsule   Reticular fibers

B

Thymic independent area
(T-lymphocytes)   Trabecula

Afferent lymphatic vessel

Thymic dependent area
(T-lymphocytes)

Germinal centers

Capsule

Subcapsular space

C

Efferent lymphatic vessel

Figure 2–15. *See legend on the opposite page*

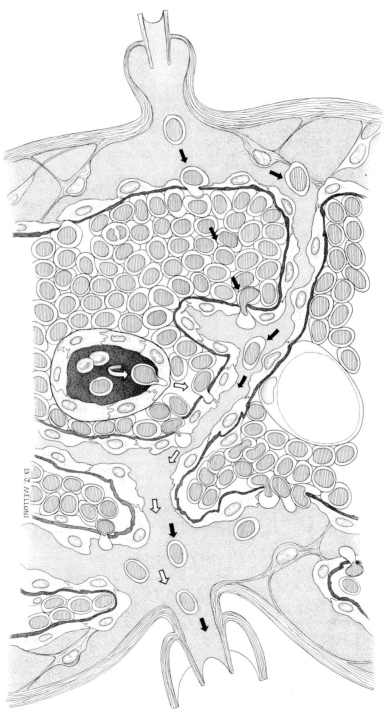

Figure 2–16. Schematic representation of circulation of lymphocytes within a lymph node. Note the dual entry of lymphocytes: from the vascular to lymphatic via postcapillary venule, and from afferent lymphatic vessels.

The second function is the circulation of lymphocytes, which are formed in the central lymphoid pool.

Spleen

If these first two barriers are inadequate, foreign constituents may gain access to the blood, either by direct invasion of small vessels (capillaries, venules) or via lymph stream channels emptying into the blood. The spleen is the sole lymphatic tissue specialized to filter blood. This organ has a number of *nonimmunologic* and *immunologic* functions. It removes effete or worn-out cells from the circulatory system (homeostatic function), converts hemoglobin to bilirubin, and releases iron into the circulation for reutilization. Like the lymph nodes, the spleen is a component of the peripheral lymphoid system, produces lymphocytes and plasma cells, and is important in the mediation of specific immunologic events. Yet the organ is important early in life, when other elements of the lymphoreticular system are incompletely developed. Removal of the spleen has been shown to be associated with overwhelming bacterial infections not only in infants and children but also in young adults.

The spleen is surrounded by a connective tissue capsule from which trabeculae extend into its interior (Fig. 2–17). The interior (pulp) is filled with two kinds of tissue: the *white* pulp and the *red* pulp. The white pulp contains lymph nodules and is the chief site of lymphocyte production in the spleen. The germinal follicles found in this region contain B-lymphocytes and are considered bursal equivalent tissues. Other lymphocytes surrounding the follicles and periarteriolar sheaths of the white pulp contain T-lymphocytes and are referred to as the thymic-dependent regions. Red pulp, on the other hand, surrounds the white pulp and contains large numbers of erythrocytes consonant with its filtration function. The arterial blood supply enters through the hilus and follows along trabeculae until the smaller arteries become surrounded by sheaths or collars of lymphocytes (white pulp). They then give off capillaries to the lymph nodules. The blood passes through the red pulp, containing elements of the reticuloendothelial system active in phagocytosis. These structures are shown in Figure 2–17. In addition to its phagocytic function, the spleen is capable of responding to antigenic stimulation. Following the intravenous injection of rabbits with antigen, one can demonstrate cells actively engaged in antibody synthesis in the sheaths surrounding arteries and also in lymph nodules.

Thymus

The thymus is responsible for the development of lymphocytes involved in cell-mediated immune responses (thymus-derived or T-

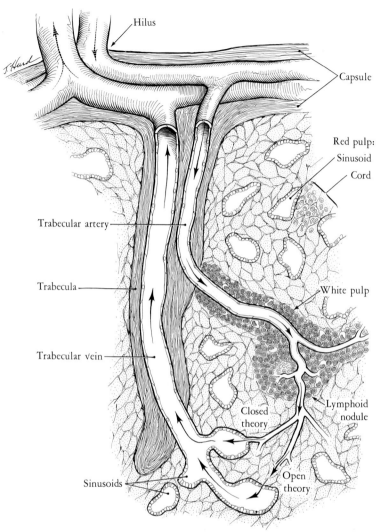

Figure 2–17.   Schematic representation of structure of spleen.

lymphocytes). The gland appears to be a master organ important in immunogenesis in the young and in orchestrating the total lymphoid system throughout life. This central lymphoid organ differs in a number of respects from other lymphoid tissues. All the lymphoid tissues described thus far are advantageously and strategically positioned for contact with foreign configurations that may enter or arise within the host. The thymus, on the other hand, is protected rather than exposed to antigen. In addition, the rate of mitotic activity in the thymus is greater than in any other lymphatic tissue, yet the number of cells leaving it is fewer than the number accounted for by this high rate of mitosis. The assumption made from these findings is that a large number of lympho-cytes produced within the thymus die within its substance. Although originally considered to be a mechanism for removal of "forbidden" autoreactive lymphocyte clones, this function of the thymus probably represents homeostatic activity involved in the production of T-lymphocytes. The role of the thymus in the development of the im-munologic system is described more fully in Chapters 3 and 9.

The thymus consists of two lobes surrounded by a thin capsule of connective tissues (Fig. 2–18). The capsule extends into the substance of the gland, forming septa that partially divide the lobes into lobules. Peripheral portions of the lobule (cortex) are heavily infiltrated with lymphocytes. More central portions (medulla) contain fewer lympho-cytes but more epithelial elements. Within the substance of the thymus are cystic structures containing keratin (Hassall's corpuscles). The thymus is believed to perform two main functions: the production of lymphocytes within the cortex and the production of a humoral sub-stance(s) by epithelial elements of the gland. These humoral substances (or hormones) may induce differentiation of lymphocytes directly within the thymus or may control their differentiation in the periphery. Although the thymus gland has a cortex and a medulla, neither con-tains germinal centers or plasma cells in the normal situation. These may appear when the gland is abnormal, e.g., in thymoma or in certain autoimmune diseases (Chapter 20C).

Unlike other lymphoid organs, the thymus is composed of two tis-sue types: lymphoid and epithelial. The lymphoid cells are of mesen-

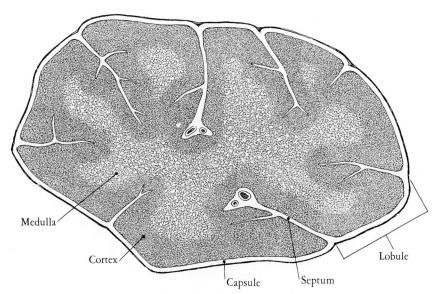

Medulla

Cortex

Capsule

Septum

Lobule

Figure 2–18. Schematic representation of thymus gland, showing division into cortex and medulla.

chymal origin, and the epithelial cells are of endodermal origin. The thymus initially develops as a continuous epithelium of cells from the third and fourth pharyngeal pouches. The process of differentiation in the human begins as a ventral outpocketing from these pouches about the sixth week of fetal life (Fig. 2–19). It is noteworthy that the parathyroids begin their development about the same time from the same pouches. A caudal migration of epithelium occurs with further differentiation. Failure of this migration is seen in one of the immunologic deficiency disorders — thymic dysplasia (Chapter 22). By the tenth week, the thymic epithelium is differentiated into a compact epithelial structure interlaced with a fibrous reticular network. The epithelial cells are secretory cells with a well-developed Golgi apparatus, rough endoplasmic reticulum, and a large nucleus with multiple nucleoli (Fig. 2–20). With further development, the thymus is infiltrated with precursor cells migrating from the liver and yolk sac during fetal life and bone marrow during adult life. Large lymphoblastoid cells first enter the subcapsular cortex and subsequently undergo further differentiation as they migrate through the different areas of the thymus. The clinical importance of the simultaneous embryogenesis of parathyroid glands and the thymus is seen in another of the immunologic deficiency disorders of man, the DiGeorge syndrome (Chapter 22).

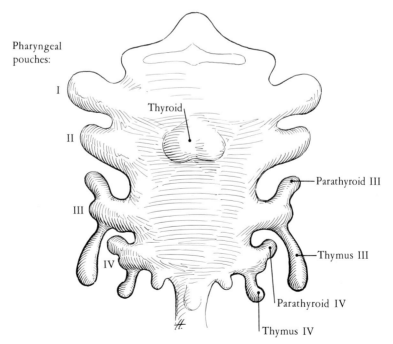

Figure 2–19.   Embryology of the thymus gland from III to IV pharyngeal pouches. Note close proximity of site of differentiation of thyroid gland (II–III) and parathyroid glands (III–IV).

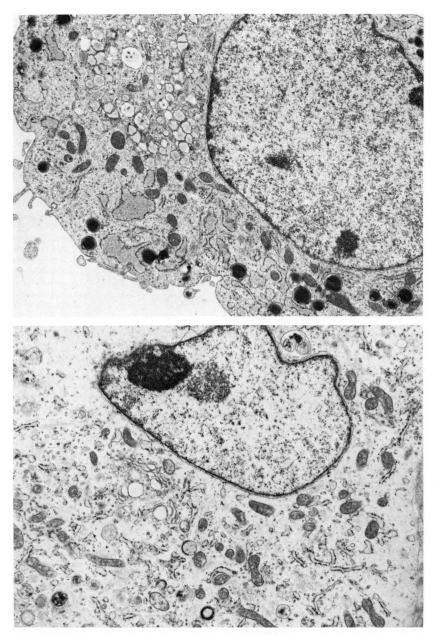

Figure 2-20. Electron micrograph of a thymus epithelial cell in culture. × 11,000. (Courtesy of Sam Waksal.)

Infants with this disorder are born not only lacking in thymic function but also without parathyroid glands. Thus they present with hypocalcemic tetany in the newborn period and with subsequent failure of the development of cell-mediated immunity.

Thymocytes develop within the thymic microenvironment, and autoradiographic studies show that they migrate from cortical areas to medullary areas. This maturation process is characterized by changes in surface (differentiation) antigens as well as functional properties (Table 2–5). In the mouse, one of the more important surface antigens is the Thy-1 (θ) antigen on thymocytes, which also exists on peripheral T-lymphocytes. Less differentiated thymocytes contain large amounts of Thy-1 and TL (thymus leukemia) antigens and small amounts of H-2 antigen on their surfaces. The more differentiated thymocytes contain large amounts of H-2, small amounts of Thy-1, and no TL antigen. The highly differentiated thymocytes in the medullary regions of the thymus acquire GVH reactivity and cortisone resistance. The thymus may exert its control over the differentiation and maturation of prothymocytes by either direct contact with these cells and the thymus epithelium or via the thymic humoral factors. These factors or thymic hormones are putatively secreted by the epithelial cells of the thymus and may be the control mechanism over peripheral T-lymphocytes.

One of the more important recent discoveries in immunology is the recognition that subpopulations of thymic-derived lymphocytes in man and animals exhibit different biologic functions. In the mouse, for example, after emigration from the bone marrow, fetal liver, or yolk sac, prothymocytes differentiate into T-lymphocytes bearing different antigenic markers (Chapter 7). These lymphocytes divide and differentiate into two subpopulations: (1) T-lymphocytes that function as cells that facilitate antibody production ("helper cells") or (2) cells that inhibit antibody production ("suppressor cells") or destroy target cells ("killer cells"). These events will be described more fully in Chapter 7.

After birth, the role of the thymus continues to change. The changes in the size of the gland with age are shown in Figure 2–21. Relative to body size it is largest during fetal life and at birth weighs

TABLE 2–5. Thymocyte Populations (Mouse)

SIZE	Large	Small	Medium
Per cent of Thymus	5–7	85–90	5–7
Location	Subcapsular	Deeper cortex	Medulla
Life span	Rapid turnover	Long-lived	Long-lived
Cortisone sensitivity	Yes	Yes	No
Thy 1 (θ)	+++	++	+
H-2	+	+	++
Per Cent Fc+	<1	10	9

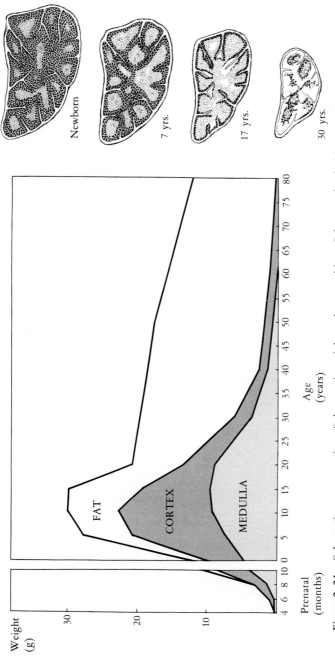

Figure 2–21. Schematic representation of changes in weight and composition of thymus gland with maturation, showing involution of the gland with age. (After Hammar, J. A.: Die Normal morphologische Thymusforschung im letzten Vierteljahrhundert. Leipzig. Barth, 1936.)

from 10 to 15 gm. The gland continues to increase in size, reaching a maximum of 30 to 40 gm at puberty. This follows the same pattern of change that occurs in all lymphoid tissue during childhood. It is of interest that this pattern of growth parallels the sequential appearance of T- and B-cell function during maturation. Following adolescence, the gland begins to involute. The parallel continues in that lymphoid tissues and immunoglobulins also diminish with increasing age. In addition, the development of autoimmune phenomena and malignant disease increases with advancing age with a loss of T-cell (e.g., suppressor) function. Thus the thymus and its associated lymphoid tissues and their

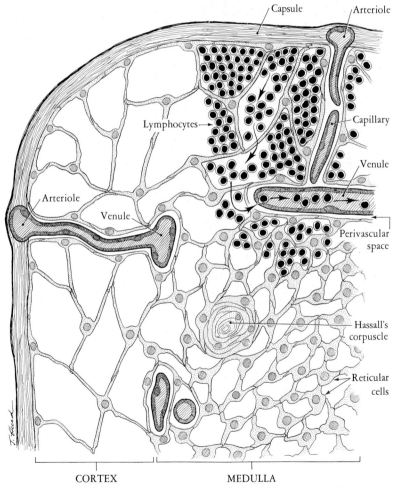

Figure 2–22. Thymus gland. Schematic representation of the perivascular epithelium surrounding blood vessels in the cortex. Note the barrier provided by this sheath and the pathways of lymphocytes formed in the cortex into the blood vessels.

products play a dynamic role from early embryogenesis throughout the life span of the individual.

The thymus thus appears to be equipped to maintain lymphopoiesis while segregated from antigen. This curious finding may be explained in part by the barrier that is made up of a continuous epithelium surrounding blood vessels in the cortex (Fig. 2–22). This epithelial membrane forms a perivascular space between the capillary endothelium and the epithelial sheath. The barrier might prevent macromolecules in the bloodstream from entering the substance of the thymus gland. Although macromolecules may be prevented from entering the epithelial barrier, lymphocytes produced within the cortex are capable of passing freely through this epithelium into the blood system, as in other anatomic sites (e.g., postcapillary venule of the lymph nodes) (Fig. 2–22).

Thus, the thymus may be viewed as a lymphoid organ, anatomically distinct, upon which all other peripheral lymphoid organs are dependent. It is an organ actively engaged in lymphopoiesis but independent of antigenic stimulation. It appears important as a central lymphoid tissue essential for the development and maturation of peripheral lymphoid tissues. Two major functions have been attributed to the thymus: (1) that it acts by the elaboration of a hormone which expands peripheral lymphocyte populations in much the same way as erythropoietin expands erythrocyte populations, and (2) that it acts by direct seeding of peripheral lymphoid tissues with lymphocytes. Recent studies have focused upon the role of the thymus as an endocrine gland, and several thymic hormones from the human and animal sources have been described. Some of these, e.g., thymosin, are receiving clinical trials in the reconstitution of children with a wide variety of immune deficiencies (Chapter 22). Failure of thymic function has also been implicated in the development of neoplasms and autoimmune diseases, e.g., myasthenia gravis.

DEVELOPMENT OF THE IMMUNOLOGIC SYSTEM

The development of the immunologic system may be considered as a series of adaptive cellular responses to a changing and potentially hostile environment (Table 2–6). It may be considered at several levels: *species, individual,* or *cell.*

The effect of the hostile environment ensures by selective pressures the survival of those life forms within the species that are best adapted to that environment. This adaptive process forms the basis for the *phylogeny* of the immune response. The microenvironment in which undifferentiated immunologic progenitor cells exist provides yet another type of inducing stimulus within the developing individual *(ontogeny)*. The immunologically mature individual may be considered as

TABLE 2–6. Effect of Environment on the Development of
the Immune Response

Target	Inductive Environment	Process	Selected Form
Species	Macroenvironment	Phylogeny	Existing life forms
Individual	Microenvironment (thymus, bursal tissues)	Ontogeny	Immunologically mature individual
Cell	Molecular environment (antigen)	Induction of immune response	"Memory" cells

the selected form that resulted from this type of development. Finally, when cells find themselves within the molecular milieu of antigen, a series of proliferative and differentiative events occur that are characteristic of the specific immune response. This leads to the synthesis of cell products such as antibody or mediators of cell-mediated immunity. The "memory" cells that are the result of this process may be considered as the best adapted forms for the environment initiated by antigen. Moreover, the interaction of macrophages, B- and T-lymphocytes involved in immunologic processes, has genetic requirements (Chapter 7). Thus, the development of immune systems at all levels is the result of selective pressures exerted by a type of environment on either a species, an individual, or a cell, the net effect leading to some survival advantage of the evolving form.

DEVELOPMENT OF THE IMMUNOLOGIC SYSTEM IN EVOLVING SPECIES: PHYLOGENY OF THE IMMUNE RESPONSE

Phylogeny of Nonspecific Immunity

The most primitive manifestation of a resistance mechanism is phagocytosis. This event, which is found in the most ancient of the unicellular organisms, served a nutritive function; in higher forms, the process evolved to a *defense* function. This was clearly recorded by Metchnikoff in his writing.

Immunity is a phenomenon which has existed on this globe from time immemorial. Immunity must be of as ancient date as is disease. The most simple and primitive organisms have constantly to struggle for their existence; they give chase to living organisms in order to obtain food, and they defend themselves against other organisms in order that they may not become their prey. When the aggressor in this struggle is much smaller than its adversary, the result is that the former introduces itself into the body of the latter and destroys it by means of infection. In this case it takes up its abode in its adversary in order to absorb the contents of its host and to produce within it one or more generations. The natural history of unicellular organisms, both vegetable and animal, often presents to us these examples of primitive infection.

From the currently identifiable life forms, there arose an increasingly complex immune system, that ranged from the primitive defense of phagocytosis to the humoral and cell-mediated responses characteristic of specific immunity (Fig. 2–23).

As cellular life differentiated into more complex forms, there developed an increasing specialization of the systems concerned with recognition of foreignness. Thus, there evolved ever-increasingly complex immunologic systems. Although phagocytosis was continued as a nutritive function by endodermal cells (sponges, for example), the addition of a newly acquired mesodermal layer added a defense function. *It is the development and specialization of this mesodermal layer in higher life forms, beginning with vertebrates, in which specialization of cells destined for specific immunologic events is seen.*

In higher invertebrates a vascular system developed that allowed phagocytosis to proceed by both *fixed* and *circulating* cells (Fig. 2–23). In man, for example, there are five circulating white cells, three of which are phagocytic (monocytes, polymorphonuclear leukocytes, and eosinophils). Thus, in phylogeny, the two most important nonspecific elements, *phagocytosis* and the *inflammatory response*, were found in primitive life forms. With evolution, these defense mechanisms persisted, and were supplemented and amplified by the addition of new components—*specific immunity* and *biologic amplification systems* (e.g., coagulation system and complement). Thus, these older mechanisms were not replaced with evolution, but rather were continued and reinforced as evolving life forms added new responses.

Phylogeny of Specific Immunity

The first evidence of a specific immunologic system appeared in primitive vertebrates such as the hagfish (Fig. 2–23). It consisted of a dis-

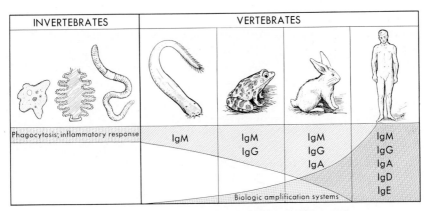

Figure 2-23. Schematic representation of phylogeny of immune response.

seminated lymphoid system, rather than the specialized lymphoid structures that occur in higher forms. In these early species there existed a primitive high molecular weight antibody and cells that could manifest cell-mediated immunity. In the elasmobranchs, for example, a tissue transplant consisting of skin or scales would be promptly rejected. Similarly, the introduction of antigens into these species will elicit a high molecular weight antibody analogous to IgM immunoglobulin of higher forms (Chapter 5). During evolution, there occurred specialization of cells and supporting structures to house these tissues—the lymphoreticular tissues. The thymus is the earliest lymphoid organ to appear in phylogeny and is present in the most primitive of vertebrates. There also appeared in birds a separate anatomic structure arising from the primitive gut, the bursa of Fabricius, which is important in the development of cells that elaborate antibody in avian species. The mammalian equivalent of this organ is not known. In the human, it is useful to consider thymic-controlled tissues that elaborate cell-mediated events as *thymic-dependent* tissues and those that elaborate antibody under a separate influence as *thymic-independent* tissues. Both are important to our understanding of the maturation of immune responses and immunologic deficiency states of man (Chapter 22).

The evolutionary order of appearance of immunoglobulin classes in many respects parallels that seen in the maturing individual (ontogeny). It also recapitulates the sequential appearance of immunoglobulin molecular forms that appear following a single antigenic exposure during the immune response (Chapter 7). These are shown in Figure 2–23. In the most primitive of vertebrates, the predominant antibody is a high molecular weight substance, analogous to the IgM globulins of the human. During phylogeny, a second class of antibody with properties similar to the IgG globulins is elaborated. The IgA immunoglobulins appear as rather late evolutionary events and are restricted to mammals. The development of a novel form of IgA immunoglobulin, the secretory IgA globulins, was also elucidated in mammals. This external antibody system has proved to be of immense importance in defense at body surfaces and appears to be a mechanism by which lower forms, such as the ungulates, receive passive antibody via colostrum. The major transfer of antibody in the human occurs primarily via the placenta; however, breast milk still continues to be a source of IgA antibody. This antibody is not absorbed by the infant's gastrointestinal tract but may be important locally within the intestine (coproantibody). Finally, still later additions seen in man are the IgD and the IgE immunoglobulins. The IgE immunoglobulins, seen also in other mammalian forms, are a unique class of antibody involved in immediate-type hypersensitivity.

With evolution there also occurred the development of an elaborate series of substances that could augment and enhance the efficiency of the ancient resistance mechanisms. These are referred to as biologic amplification systems and consist primarily of the coagulation and the complement systems (Chapter 6).

DEVELOPMENT OF THE IMMUNOLOGIC SYSTEM IN THE DEVELOPING INDIVIDUAL: ONTOGENY OF THE IMMUNE RESPONSE

Available evidence suggests that the maturation of the immune response in the human begins *in utero* sometime during the second to third months of gestation. The differentiation of cells destined to perform both nonspecific and specific immunologic functions seems to have a common ancestral origin. Both cell types appear to arise from a population of progenitor cells referred to as *stem cells* or *hemocytoblasts*; these are located within the hematopoietic tissues of the developing embryo (yolk sac, fetal liver, and bone marrow). Depending upon the type of microchemical environment surrounding the cells, development will occur along at least two avenues: the *hematopoietic* and the *lymphopoietic* (Fig. 2–24).

One type of microchemical environment leads to proliferation and differentiation of myeloid, erythroid, and megakaryocyte precursor

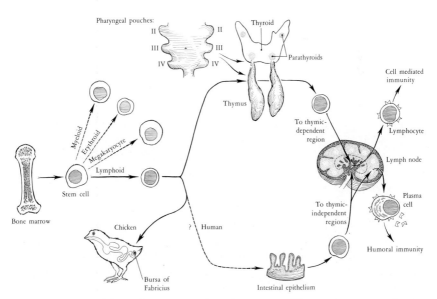

Figure 2–24. Schematic representation of ontogeny of immune response, showing differentiation of progenitor cells into hematopoietic and immunocompetent cells.

cells. The products of these cell lines are the hematopoietic elements of the peripheral blood and tissues and include the *erythrocytes, granulocytes, platelets,* and *monocytes.* A second set of progenitor cells are the lymphoid precursor cells that can differentiate along two additional pathways. The first, under the influence of the thymus, perhaps within the substance of the gland itself, includes a population of small lymphocytes that subserve the function of cell-mediated immunity (thymic-dependent or T-lymphocytes). If the progenitor cells come under a second type of microchemical environment, differentiation will occur to produce a population of lymphocytes and plasma cells concerned with humoral immunity or antibody synthesis. This population of cells comes under the influence of and is expanded within a second anatomic site, whose identity as the bursa of Fabricius is known with certainty only in birds and is referred to as the bursal equivalent or B-lymphocyte (Fig. 2–24).

The functional significance of this *two-compartment system* is important to clinical medicine. It provides a useful basis upon which our understanding of immunologic deficiency disorders rests (Chapter 22). Thus, individuals displaying selective disorders of bursal equivalent tissues, the so-called agammaglobulinemias or dysgammaglobulinemias, present with recurrent bacterial infections. Selective deficiencies of the thymic-dependent tissues, on the other hand, are also seen in man and are manifested with other types of infections, such as fungal and viral diseases. Still a third type of patient presents with combined deficiencies of both thymic-dependent and thymic-independent tissues. These individuals have profound deficiencies in both cell-mediated and antibody-mediated functions and have the most serious sequelae of all the immunologic deficiency syndromes and present with a diversity of infections.

Maternal-Fetal Relationships

One of the most significant developments in phylogeny is the appearance of placentation in the species with the ability to bear live young (viviparity). This occurred in higher forms with the development of the multilayered placenta. One of the challenging problems in biology is the question of how a fetus, who inherits one half of its antigens from paternally controlled genes foreign to the mother, can be tolerated successfully during pregnancy. This has been attributed largely to the barrier function of the placenta. By acting as a mechanical barrier, the placenta usually effectively separates the formed elements of the blood of the mother from that of the fetus. There are elements, however, that do gain access to the fetus and provide protection — antibodies.

There are different pathways of transmission of maternal antibody to the fetus in different species (Table 2–7). In species with large

TABLE 2–7.   Relationship of Type of Placentation with
Character of Maternal-Fetal Transfer of Antibody in Various Species

ANIMAL	NUMBER OF PLACENTAL MEMBRANES	RELATIVE IMPORTANCE OF ROUTE	
		Placental	*Colostral*
Horse	6	0	+++
Sheep, cow	5	0	+++
Cat, dog	5	+	++
Rat, mouse	4	+	++
Rabbit, guinea pig	3	+++	±
Man, monkey	3	+++	0

numbers of membranes intervening between the maternal and fetal circulations, the colostral route seems to be a more important mechanism of transfer. Conversely, as the number of layers of membrane decreases (as in man, for example), the transplacental route seems to assume greater importance. Thus, in man, the predominant transfer of antibody occurs via the passage of the IgG immunoglobulins from the maternal circulation to that of the fetus. This is accomplished by means of an active transport mechanism of this immunoglobulin by virtue of a receptor located on the Fc fragment of the molecule (Chapter 5). In this manner, the fetus receives a library of preformed antibody from its mother, reflecting most of her experiences with infectious agents. Commonly, fetal cells or other proteins may gain access to the maternal circulation and thus actively immunize her to the paternal allotypes (antigen) found on these substances. This process, referred to as isoimmunization, may lead to serious disease in the infant, such as hemolytic disease of the newborn, thrombocytopenia, and leukopenia (Chapter 20B).

The development of serum immunoglobulins during intrauterine life and postnatally is shown in Figure 2–25. If one analyzes the amount and type of gamma globulin found in the blood of the newborn infant at birth, one finds that the levels of immunoglobulin are equivalent to those of the mother and are made up almost exclusively of the IgG immunoglobulins. There is virtually little or no IgA and IgM globulin present in cord sera. This is because the fetus is usually protected *in utero* from antigenic stimuli. If the fetus is challenged *in utero* as a consequence of immunization or infection (e.g., congenital rubella, cytomegalic inclusion disease, toxoplasmosis), it will respond with antibody production largely of the IgM variety. The exclusion of other classes of antibody is beneficial to the fetus in many cases. For example, the exclusion of the IgM isohemagglutinins, leukoagglutinins, or the IgE antibodies of allergy prevents disease that may be produced by these antibodies. However, it also prevents the passage of other maternal antibodies that would be beneficial to the newborn, such as the IgM

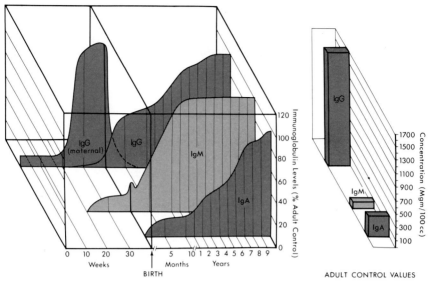

Figure 2–25. Development of serum immunoglobulins in the human during matura-tion. (After Alford, C. A., Jr.: Immunoglobulin determinations in the diagnosis of fetal infection. Pediatr. Clin. North Am., *18*:99, 1971.)

antibodies important in bacterial defense against gram-negative bacteria (opsonins, agglutinins, and bactericidal antibodies). This may explain, in part, the increased susceptibility of the newborn to infection with gram-negative organisms such as *Escherichia coli.*

Since the IgG immunoglobulins are passively transferred, they have a finite half-life of between 20 and 30 days, and therefore their concentration in serum falls rapidly within the first few months of life, reaching the lowest levels between the second and fourth month. This period is referred to as physiologic hypogammaglobulinemia (Chapter 22). During the course of the first few years, the levels of gamma globulin increase because of exposure of the maturing infant to antigens in the environment. There appears to be a sequential development in gamma globulin at different rates. The IgM globulins attain adult levels by one year of age, the IgG globulins by five to six years of age, and the IgA globulins by 10 years of age (Chapter 26). This pattern of appearance of immunoglobulins recapitulates that seen in phylogeny and also appears to parallel that seen following an antigenic exposure during the primary immune response.

It is important to emphasize that the development of immunoglobulin receptors on lymphocytes during fetal life follows the same general pattern as that observed with the appearance of various immunoglobulins in the serum after birth (Table 2–8). It is notable that IgM is present on the surface of cells as early as 10½ weeks. At birth, human immunocompetent cells have become fully responsive to mito-

TABLE 2–8. Maturation of Human T- and B-Cells: Surface Markers and Lymphoproliferative Responses

		Serum Immunoglobulins					Mitogens			Antigens	
	AGE	IgM	IgG	IgA	IgD	IgE	PHA	Con-A	PWM	PPD	SK-SD
Fetal	10 weeks	−	−	−	−	−	+	−	−	−	−
	10.5 weeks	+	−	−	−	?	+	?	−	−	−
	12 weeks	+	+	−	−	?	+	+	−	−	−
	20 weeks	+	+	+	±	±	+	+	+	−	−
	Newborn	+	+	+	+	±	+	+	+	−	−
	Adult	+	+	+	+	+	+	+	+	+	+

gens (Table 2–8). (Mitogens such as phytohemagglutinin [PHA], concanavalin-A [Con-A], and pokeweed [PWM] are substances that will directly stimulate either B- or T-lymphocytes [Chapter 7].) However, the ability of cells to respond to specific antigens, such as tuberculin (PPD) or streptokinase-streptodornase (SK-SD), is limited. Only later do the lymphocytes develop the capability for cell-mediated responses against foreign antigens. Cell-mediated responses can also be measured *in vitro* by the development of lymphotoxin (LT) or macrophage inhibition factor (MIF) (Chapter 9). As can be seen in Table 2–9, at birth, cell-mediated responses are variable; LT can be produced, but MIF cannot.

From the very earliest fetal life, lymphocytes are present that can act both as responders to and stimulators of the mixed lymphocyte reaction (MLR) (Table 2–9). This suggests that the fetus can recognize transplantation antigens even before they can respond to any other foreign antigen, making all the more remarkable the inability of the fetus to react against its mother.

Development of the Immunologic System at the Level of the Whole Organism

It is now well established that the ability to respond to certain antigens is determined by the genetic constitution of the host (Chapter 3). Thus, selected strains of guinea pigs and mice fail to respond with antibody formation following immunization with normally immunogenic polypeptide antigens. The precise mechanism of this *nonresponder state* is not yet known, but is believed to be due to the suppression or deletion of genes important in immune responses.

Recent findings in the mouse indicate an association between certain histocompatibility antigens and the ability to respond to immunogens (Chapter 3). Histocompatibility typing of mice allows the prediction of immune responsiveness to a wide variety of antigens other than histocompatibility antigens. The association between histocompatibility

TABLE 2–9. Maturation of Human T- and B-Cells:
Mixed Lymphocyte Responsiveness and Mediator Production

		MLR		LYMPHOKINE	
AGE		*Responder*	*Stimulator*	*LT*	*MIF*
Fetal	7.5 weeks	+	+	–	–
	10 weeks	+	+	–	–
	12 weeks	+	+	–	–
	20 weeks	+	+	–	–
	Newborn	+	+	+	–
	Adult	+	+	+	+

antigenic composition and immune responsiveness is unknown, but recent data suggest that the expression of certain antigenic phenotypes may also be an expression of an individual immunologic responsiveness.

In the human, the precise analogue of this nonresponder state is not known. However, in certain of the immunologic deficiency states, such as the Wiskott-Aldrich syndrome (Chapter 22), there is an inability to process certain polysaccharide antigens. It would seem reasonable that with the vast heterogeneity of the human species, variations in responsiveness from individual to individual would exist. Indeed, this appears to be the case and is manifested in clinical practice by the frequent encounter of individuals with susceptibility to infectious disease not expressed by other individuals. The susceptibility to certain autoimmune and malignant diseases is also known to occur in children with immunologic deficiency. A genetic basis may be involved in other hypersensitivity diseases of man. Only in certain individuals does acute glomerulonephritis or rheumatic fever occur following infection with group A beta hemolytic streptococci. This may be the human counterpart to the experimental model of serum sickness–type nephritis, which occurs after administration of repeated doses of bovine serum albumin to rabbits (Chapter 13). Such animals could be divided into three groups: good antibody responders, moderate antibody responders, and poor antibody responders. Limited disease was seen in the good and poor antibody responders; the most progressive and chronic forms of glomerulonephritis were seen in animals with moderate antibody production. This was presumably because of the development of antigen-antibody complexes injurious to their kidneys. This model of immunologic injury will be described in greater detail in Chapter 13.

DEVELOPMENT OF THE IMMUNOLOGIC SYSTEM AT THE CELLULAR LEVEL

Antigen itself may be considered as part of the cellular environment that induces the development of an immune responsiveness (Table 2–

6). During the induction of an immune response, antigen comes in contact with an appropriate collection of lymphoid cells, following which a series of proliferative and differentiative steps are initiated (see Fig. 7–2). At the moment of presentation of antigen, at least two, and possibly three, cells are involved. The first is a macrophage, which in some cases is essential for the processing of antigen to a form that can interact with a second series of cells, those of lymphoid type. These latter cells can proliferate and differentiate to become immunocompetent cells, capable of antibody formation or cell-mediated events. Following removal of antigen, there is an involution of this population of immunocompetent cells. However, some cells remain as "memory" cells, capable of carrying out specific immunologic events during any future encounter with the same antigen. These consist of either B- or T-lymphocytes. The whole cellular burst of activity seen in the induction of an immune response may be analogous to genetically controlled differentiation seen in the development of the species or during ontogeny of the individual. The memory cells may be considered as the best adapted forms for this type of environment (Table 2–6).

These processes involve a variety of cell types. As described previously, the lymphoid cell populations that respond to antigens can basically be divided into two populations, the T- and B-lymphocytes, which can act independently as well as in cooperation to produce an immune response (Chapter 7). Specific antigen receptors exist on the surface of both T-cells and B-cells. Certain antigens can directly stimulate the B-cells so that they will subsequently produce plasma cells and antibody; other antigens require the interaction of T-cells, which provide specific and nonspecific helper substances that will allow the B-cell to mature to produce antibody. It is interesting to note that antigen, after processing by macrophages, can lead to the production of activators of helper T-cells. Further, these macrophages must be syngeneic to the T-cells in order for the help to occur. Subsequent to activation, the T-lymphocytes produce a factor (IgT) that can trigger the B-cells. A separate population of T-lymphocytes can also act to suppress the immune response, i.e., suppressor T-lymphocytes. This appears to involve active processes in the suppression of helper T-cells.

The interaction of T-cells, in both their helper and suppressor functions, is under strict genetic control, which is mediated by genes that are located within the major histocompatibility complex. These immune response (IR) genes apparently are related to histocompatibility identity between the various cell types involved in the immune response. Immunoregulation and the multiple interactions between specific cell types are only now beginning to be understood. The future directions of clinical immunology will, we hope, provide for the unraveling of these complex events. In the meantime, the clinician must deal with diseases that result from genetic failure to regulate immune response at each level of interaction.

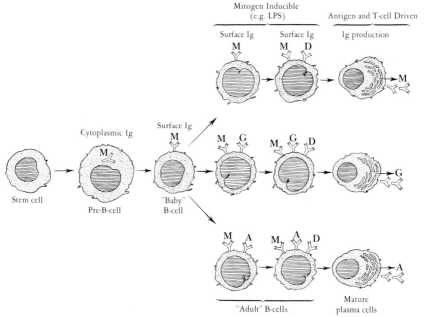

Figure 2-26. Ontogeny of B-lymphocyte system. (Adapted from M. D. Cooper and M. Seligmann: B and T lymphocytes in immunodeficiency and lymphoproliferative diseases. *In* F. Loor and G. E. Roelants (eds.): B and T Cells in Immune Recognition. West Sussex, England, John Wiley and Sons Ltd., 1977.

Based upon evidence obtained from the human and experimental animal, Cooper and his coworkers have proposed a model of B-cell differentiation (Fig. 2-26). In this model, B-cells differentiate from a stem cell to a pre-B-cell that initially expresses only cytoplasmic IgM. The next stage is represented by a cell expressing surface IgM receptors only. This "Baby B-cell" is a pivotal cell for further differentiation of cells that produce immunoglobulins. After this, two stages of differentiation exist: (1) an antigen-independent stage responsive to mitogen and (2) an antigen-dependent T-cell driven stage that requires the presence of an IgD surface marker lost after antigenic stimulation.

To summarize, the whole of the immune response appears to be under developmental (genetic) influences. These range from the controls exerted on the evolving species (phylogeny) to those imposed on the maturing individual (ontogeny), the controls exerted within an individual and on the cell and cell products. Both immune responsiveness and unresponsiveness should be considered as genetic processes. This approach to immunology may better enable the physician to appreciate the pathogenesis of many immunologically mediated diseases, their transmissions within families, and their expected reappearances in future offspring.

SUGGESTIONS FOR FURTHER READING

Anatomical and Functional Organization of the Immune System

Bloom, W., and Fawcett, D. W. (eds.): A Textbook of Histology. 10th ed., Philadelphia, W. B. Saunders Co., 1975.

Cline, M. J. (ed.): The White Cell. Cambridge, Harvard University Press, 1975.

Dingle, J. T., and Dean, R. T. (eds.): Lysosomes in Biology and Pathology. New York, American Elsevier Publishing Co., Inc., 1976.

Gabrieli, E. R., and Snell, F. M.: Reflection of reticuloendothelial function in studies of blood clearance kinetics. J. Reticuloendothel. Soc., *2*:141, 1965.

Van Furth, R. (ed.): Mononuclear Cells in Immunity, Infection, and Pathology. Oxford, Blackwell Scientific Publications, 1975.

Weiss, L. (ed.): Cells and Tissues of the Immune System: Structure, Functions, Interactions. Englewood Cliffs, N.J., Prentice-Hall, Inc., 1972.

Chemotaxis, Phagocytosis, Metabolic Changes and Antimicrobial Systems of Phagocytic Cells

Bellanti, J. A., and Dayton, D. H. (eds.): The Phagocytic Cell in Host Resistance. New York, Raven Press, 1975.

Cline, M. J. (ed.): The White Cell. Cambridge, Harvard University Press, 1975.

DeChalelet, L. R.: Oxidative bactericidal mechanisms of polymorphonuclear leukocytes. J. Infect. Dis., *131*:295, 1975.

Specific Immune Responses

Fudenberg, H. H., Stites, D. P., Caldwell, J. L., and Wells, J. V. (eds.): Basic and Clinical Immunology. Los Altos, Lange Medical Publications, 1976.

Gell, P. G. H., Coombs, R. R. A., and Lachman, P. T.: Clinical Aspects of Immunology. Oxford, Blackwell Scientific Publications, 1975.

Roitt, I. M.: Essential Immunology. Oxford, Blackwell Scientific Publications, 1974.

Suskind, R. M. (ed.): Malnutrition and the Immune Response. Kroc Foundation Series, Vol. 7. New York, Raven Press, 1977.

Phylogeny and Ontogeny

Cooper, E. L. (ed.): Contemporary Topics in Immunobiology. Vol. 4. Invertebrate Immunology. Plenum Publishing Corp., 1974.

Cooper, M. D., and Dayton, D. H. (eds.): Development of Host Defenses. New York, Raven Press, 1977.

Cooper, M. D., and Seligmann, M.: B and T lymphocytes in immunodeficiency and lymphoproliferative diseases. *In* F. Loor and G. E. Roelants (eds.): B and T Cells in Immune Recognition. West Sussex, England, John Wiley and Sons Ltd., 1977.

Friedman, H. (ed.): Thymus factors in immunity. Ann. N.Y. Acad. Sci., *249*:1–547, 1975.

Stites, D. P., Caldwell, J., Carr, M. C., and Fudenberg, H. H.: Ontogeny of immunity in humans. Clin. Immunol. Immunopathol., *4*:519, 1975.

Chapter 3

IMMUNOGENETICS

Kenneth J. Sell, M.D., Ph.D.,
Samuel D. Waksal, Ph.D., and
Joseph A. Bellanti, M.D.

Immunogenetics includes all those processes concerned in the immune response that may have a *genetic* basis. In the past, the term has been largely restricted to mean genetic markers on immunoglobulin polypeptide chains. In the light of recent developments, a more contemporary definition of immunogenetics should include *all the factors that control the immunologic responsiveness of the host to foreignness, as well as the transmission of antigenic specificities from generation to generation.*

Immune mechanisms may be viewed from an evolutionary standpoint as a series of genetic adaptations by the evolving species to changing environmental influences exerted upon it (Chapter 2). This has been referred to as *phylogeny* of the immune response. Similarly, the maturation of the immune mechanisms within the developing individual may be considered, and this has been termed *ontogeny* of the immune response. In a narrower sense, the genetic controls can be considered at a cellular level as the proliferation and differentiation of a variety of cell types in response to antigen (Chapter 7). The action of genes can also be studied at the molecular level in terms of the unlimited variability of immunoglobulin structures that are directly encoded within DNA (Chapter 5). The heritability of antigens themselves, such as the blood group and histocompatibility antigens, is also transmitted within the chromosomes of the germ cells. Finally, of considerable importance are the recent discoveries indicating that the genes that control the expression of certain cellular antigens are closely identical to those that control immune responsiveness.

CLINICAL IMPORTANCE OF IMMUNOGENETICS

A knowledge of the genetic influences exerted on evolving life forms (phylogeny) may seem far removed from the applications of immunology to clinical medicine. An understanding of these phenomena is essential in the practice of medicine, however, since it lends perspective to the coordination and control of the complex immunologic systems that have evolved over 300 million years and that we see in man today. Equally important are the immunogenetic influences that control the development of the immunologic system within the maturing individual (ontogeny). In many respects, the acquisition of various components seen within the developing individual recapitulates what occurred in the evolution of the species. For example, the first antibody seen in the fetus is an IgM antibody, related phylogenetically to more primitive antibodies seen in lower species. Similarly, the genetic variability from individual to individual within a species, although incompletely understood, is assuming great importance in determining genetic susceptibility to infection and predisposition to many of the allergic diseases, the autoimmune diseases, and possibly even malignant diseases.

Knowledge of genetics also provides a powerful tool for the physician in the diagnosis, treatment, and prevention of disease. The power of the pedigree or family history is not to be underestimated in the diagnostic approach to common problems, as well as to rare defects of the immune system. For example, a family history of allergic manifestations such as asthma or allergic rhinitis may help the pediatrician arrive at a correct diagnosis of milk allergy in a small infant who presents with gastrointestinal colic (Fig. 3–1).

Genetics is also helpful in establishing diagnoses in diseases that are less common but nonetheless confront the physician. Inherited defects in immunity may present in children as recurrent bacterial infections of the skin and deeper tissues. Such individuals may have fundamental defects of their phagocytes, as in chronic granulomatous disease, or of their antibody-synthesizing tissues, as in X-linked agammaglobulinemia (Chapter 22). The sex-linked mode of inheritance in many of these diseases can be of assistance to the physician in arriving at a correct diagnosis. Further, if a primary immunoglobulin deficiency exists in a patient, the physician should be alerted to the associated findings in other family members. There is an increased incidence of clinical or serologic evidence of autoimmunity not only in the patient

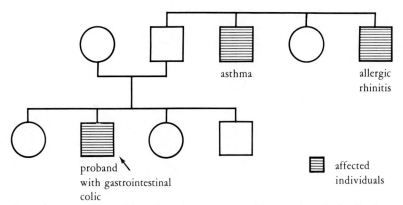

Figure 3–1. Pedigree of an infant who presented with gastrointestinal colic, showing other allergic disorders within the kindred.

with immunoglobulin deficiency but also in his first- and second-degree relatives.

A knowledge of the genetic factors controlling the formation of tissue antigens is also of importance to the physician. The principles governing the antigenic specificities of the major blood groups, for example, provide the basis of our understanding of diseases such as hemolytic disease of the newborn and of forms of therapy such as blood transfusions (Chapter 20). Finally, a knowledge of transplantation immunity involving the genetic control of histocompatibility antigens is of crucial importance in the grafting of tissues. Organ replacement as a form of therapy is now well-established, and the success of the procedure is dependent upon the knowledge of the transmission of these antigenic specificities within families (Chapter 20). Recently, associations of histocompatibility type and disease in man have uncovered new and exciting diagnostic possibilities. Thus, immunogenetics not only interests the theoretical immunobiologist, but also is of practical significance to the physician.

IMMUNOGENETIC PRINCIPLES

The immune system consists of a highly complex network of components, both cellular and soluble, most of which are specifically encoded for by gene products. It is now clear that a large number of specific immune response genes exist that control the specific responses to a variety of antigens (Chapter 4). Also, many genes may control the cellular interactions within the immune system as well as the transmission of antigenic specificities from generation to generation. Studies performed over the last few years have shown associations between histocompatibility type (genetic) and specific disease entities in man.

THE MAJOR HISTOCOMPATIBILITY COMPLEX

The major histocompatibility complex (MHC) in mammals is a single genetic region that determines the strong transplantation antigens and has a major influence on graft rejection. This region controls not only graft rejection but also a number of other immunologic phenomena including immune responsiveness to many types of antigens (Chapter 4) as well as susceptibility to the development of immunologically mediated disease (Chapter 20). The ABO and Rh blood group systems also affect the survival of grafts and will be described below. The two MHC systems most extensively studied are the *histocompatibility (H-2) system in the mouse* and the *human leukocyte antigen (HL-A) system in man.*

Much of what is now known about the MHC systems of both mice and men has been derived from the pioneering work performed in the field of transplantation immunology. The transplantation of tissue involves a complex collection of cells, each of which has myriad antigenic configurations controlled by DNA. Except for identical twins, each individual's chromosomal DNA is unique. This uniqueness of "self" is accompanied by an exquisite sensing mechanism of the host that triggers the genetically controlled immune reactions to foreignness. This recognition of foreignness of any substance, external or internal, evokes the same complex responses we have defined as immunity. Thus, following tissue transplantation, both humoral and cellular mechanisms of immunity are stimulated. We know that humoral mechanisms recognize what are termed the *serologically defined (SD) antigens,* and the cellular mechanisms recognize both a *lymphocyte-defined (LD)* as well as the SD antigens.

The basic goal of transplantation is the long-term survival of the grafted tissue. The success of this procedure depends primarily on the degree of antigenic similarity between recipient and donor. A second factor determining survival time is related to the nature of the transplanted tissue itself, e.g., whether the graft is non-nucleated and incapable of replication, or nucleated and capable of survival. A blood transfusion, for example, may be considered as a type of short-term transplant; however, even with a completely compatible transfusion, these hematopoietic cells will not survive, since non-nucleated cells are incapable of long-term survival.

Thus, the survival of transplanted tissues may be defined in terms of genetic identity (Table 3–1). The closest identity would be a transplant of tissues from one site to another in the same individual. This is referred to as an *autograft.* A similar degree of identity would occur in grafts from one identical twin to another or from one member of a highly inbred strain to another. In these cases, there would be close to 100 per cent acceptability, since there is almost 100 per cent genetic compatibility. Grafts of this nature are referred to as *syngeneic* or *isogeneic grafts* or *isografts.* When the transplantation involves genetically dissimilar members of the same species, they are called *allogeneic grafts* or *allografts.* Finally, a transplant involving two different species, such as the transplantation of chimpanzee kidneys into a human, is referred to as a *heterogeneic (xenogeneic) graft* or *heterograft (xenograft).* Recent advances in mouse genetics have enabled the transplantation immunologist to develop mouse strains that differ only at single genetic regions. These are termed *conisogeneic* or *congeneic strains.* Also, mouse strains that develop genetic crossovers within these regions are termed *recombinant strains.*

MHC of Mice (H-2)

For ease of discussion, the chromosomal fragment controlling immunologic phenomena in the mouse may be visualized as divided into four subregions (Fig. 3–2). The K and D regions encode for surface antigens that are serologically detectable and recognized during graft rejection; the I region may encode for a portion of the specific antigenic receptor on T-lymphocytes and a group of interaction molecules, the Ia or I region-associated molecules, found on the surface of T- and B-lymphocytes and a subpopulation of macrophages; and the Ss-Slp region controls the synthesis of serum complement components.

The H-2 region in the mouse is located on the seventeenth chromosome and covers a length of DNA equivalent to 0.5 recombination unit. The mouse became a useful model for the study of transplan-

TABLE 3-1. Terminology Used in Transplantation Immunology

Name of Graft	Type of Tissue	Genetic Identity	Definition
Autograft	Autologous	Total	Grafts within the same individual
Isograft	Isologous	Syngeneic Isogeneic Congeneic	Grafts from genetically identical or near-identical individual Differs at single genetic regions
Allograft	Homologous	Allogeneic	Grafts from a genetically dissimilar donor of the same species
Heterograft (Xenograft)	Heterologous	Heterogeneic (Xenogeneic)	Graft from donor of a phylogenetically different species

tation genetics only through the development of inbred strains. It is of interest to note that at the turn of the century, as mice were being bred for scientific purposes, there already were stocks of available mice that had been bred for coat color and sold as pets to wealthy patrons in Europe. The first regions of H-2 to be characterized were the K and D regions (Fig. 3–3). These are homologous to the HLA-A and HLA-B in man. These regions code for products that can be detected by antisera using standard serologic methods and that are also known as the

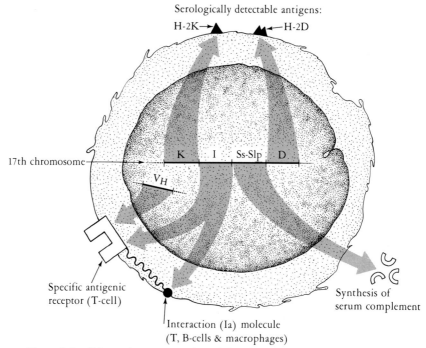

Figure 3-2. Schematic representation of the chromosomal sites and gene products of the major histocompatibility complex of the mouse (H-2).

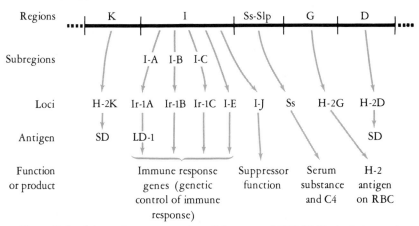

Figure 3–3. Schematic representation of the mouse MHC (H-2), depicting regions, subregions, loci, antigens, and their gene functions and products.

serologically defined SD loci. The H-2 antigens have a molecular weight of 50,000 daltons.

The K and D regions are the regions recognized during allograft rejection by cytotoxic T-lymphocytes (Chapter 9). It has also been shown that when cells are treated with viruses or chemical haptens, they seem to be specifically associated with the SD regions; and cytotoxic T-lymphocytes are lytic only if the target cells that are modified with virus or chemical carry the same modifying antigen and the same K- and D-region molecules as the original stimulating cells (Chapter 9).

For example, experiments by Zinkernagel and Doherty have shown that cytotoxic T-lymphocytes from CBA mice (H-2K) infected with vaccinia virus will kill H-2K fibroblasts if they are infected with vaccinia, but not virus-infected H-2^b cells. A similar phenomenon has been observed by Shearer and his coworkers using the chemical trinitrophenol (TNP) to modify autologous spleen cells. Two hypotheses have been put forward to explain these phenomena (Fig. 3–4). The first is based upon the assumption that the SD regions modified present a new antigenic determinant to the T-lymphocytes. This is called the *altered self hypothesis*. The second hypothesis suggests that cytotoxic T-lymphocytes require dual recognition signals via receptors for (1) the specific antigen and (2) the SD products. This is called the *dual recognition hypothesis*. In both mouse and man, some MHC determinants are found to be noncovalently associated with the β_2 microglobulins (Chapter 7). Molecules encoded for by each locus of MHC also move independently on lymphocyte membranes (Fig. 3–4).

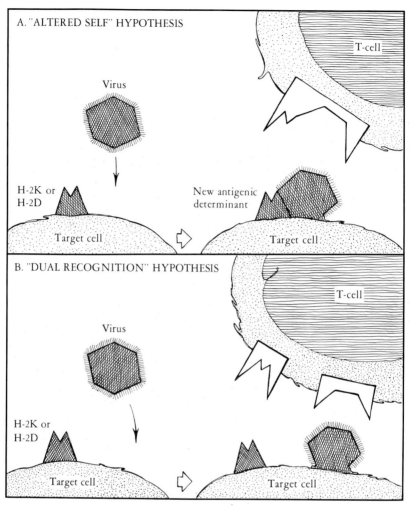

Figure 3-4. Schematic representation of two hypotheses of genetic restrictions concerned with recognition of virus-infected target cells by cytotoxic lymphocytes.

I Region. The I region in the mouse is a region of the major histocompatibility complex (Figs. 3–2 and 3–3) that controls many major immunologic phenomena (Table 3–2). The I region of the mouse and the region around the HLA-D locus in man have many functions in common. Both these regions were initially studied by the use of the mixed-lymphocyte reaction as a means of detecting different alleles. Thus far there are three subregions, I-A, I-B, and I-C, containing loci such as the Ir-1A, Ir-1B, and Ir-1C that control the genetics of immune response to certain defined antigens, e.g., myeloma proteins and synthetic polypeptides. The antigens coded for by this region are termed Ia

TABLE 3–2. Comparison of H-2 and Ia Antigenic Regions

Properties	H-2	Ia
Molecular weight	48,000 D glycoprotein	28,000-32,000 D glycoprotein
Tissue distribution	All tissues except sperm	Sperm T-lymphocytes B-lymphocytes Macrophages Epidermal cells
Human analogues	HLA-A, HLA-B	HLA-D
Function associated with each region	Graft rejection SD antigens Putative receptor for virus and chemical modification	Immune response (Ir) genes Interaction molecules (Ia) Stimulating antigen in the mixed lymphocyte reactions (LD antigens) Graft versus host reactions Immune suppressor activity

(I region-associated) antigens. The Ia antigens have a molecular weight of between 28,000 and 32,000 daltons. While products of the K and D regions (H-2 antigens) of the MHC are located on all tissues except sperm, Ia antigens are located on lymphocytes, macrophages, sperm, and epidermal cells. The fact that Ia antigens are located on sperm cells, which are also involved in complex biologic and cellular interactions, is noteworthy. Other loci encode for the expression of molecules found on the surface of suppressor T-lymphocytes, e.g., I-J, in addition to those that encode for molecules found only on red blood cells, i.e., H_2-G. Using antisera directed against antigens coded for by the I region, it has been shown that it controls such immune functions as genetic control of specific immune responses, graft-versus-host reactions, regulation of immune suppression, and the interaction structures that regulate interactions between T- and B-lymphocytes and macrophages (Chapter 7). The B-lymphocytes, which are Ia-negative, can produce only IgM antibody; those that are Ia-positive can produce IgM or IgG or only IgG antibodies. The T-lymphocytes that are Ia-positive appear to function as suppressor cells. Helper T-lymphocytes produce soluble factors containing Ia molecules but have no Ia antigens on their cell surfaces. Those T-lymphocytes that are Ia-negative function as cytotoxic cells. These antigens have been shown to evoke mainly strong MLR responses in which T-lymphocytes are stimulated by Ia-bearing B-lymphocytes. In order for cooperation to occur between helper T-lymphocytes and B-lymphocytes in the production of antibody, some investigators feel that there must be identity at the I region (Chapter 7). Helper T-lymphocytes have produced a secondary response to a specific antigen when the antigen is presented at the I region by a macrophage that is compatible with the macrophage used for priming.

Two types of factors that contain Ia specificities are produced by helper T-lymphocytes (Fig. 3–5). One is an *antigen-specific T-lymphocyte factor* that consists of the specific T-lymphocyte receptor bound to the specific antigen plus Ia molecules that bind to the acceptor site on B-lymphocytes. This antigen-specific factor can induce a specific antibody response directed against a specific antigen. It has recently been shown that those macrophages that can induce T-cell help also contain Ia molecules involved in macrophage-T-cell collaboration (Fig. 3–5). The second is a nonspecific factor that is produced by T-lymphocytes triggered by a number of agents including allogeneic cells and mitogens. The *nonspecific factor, which has been termed allogeneic effect factor* (AEF), has also been shown to contain Ia-like molecules that can interact with B-lymphocytes resulting in production of antibodies to a variety of antigenic specificities (Fig. 3–5) (Chapter 7).

Genetic Control of Complement. Another region of the MHC in the mouse is the Ss-Slp region, which maps to the left of the H-2D region and controls the synthesis of C4 (Fig. 3–3). The Ss-Slp region involves two genetic traits that control the synthesis of two serum proteins: (1) the Ss or serologically detected serum protein, and (2) the Slp, the sex-limited protein. Both traits control the synthesis of a specific beta globulin, C4. The beta globulin is affected by sex hormones as well as by genes in this region. It is of interest that some of the therapy currently used to enhance complement components in one of the complement deficiencies of man, familial hereditary angioedema, includes the use of the male sex hormones, e.g., testosterone (Chapter 22). Antiserum to the Ss-Slp region was found to inhibit complement activity. In the human, this region appears to be homologous to the genetic region, which is to the left of HLA-B and may control the alternate complement pathway in man.

Immune Response Genes. One of the most important recent observations in immunology has been the discovery of the immune response genes. The immune response genes are divided into two categories. The first includes the histocompatibility-linked immune response genes that are in close association with genes coding for the major histocompatibility antigens. The second is the immunoglobulin allotype-linked immune response genes that appear to determine the structure of the immunoglobulin receptor on B-lymphocytes (Chapters 5 and 7).

The nature of the receptor on the T-lymphocyte is not known with certainty. Evidence is mounting that the T-lymphocyte antigen receptor may consist in part of a dimer of heavy chains, and thus may be structurally similar to the immunoglobulin receptors on B-lymphocytes. The H regions encode for the synthesis of heavy chains of immunoglobulins, which function in part as the antigen-combining sites of the molecule. Recent evidence has shown that antisera generated to the antigen-bind-

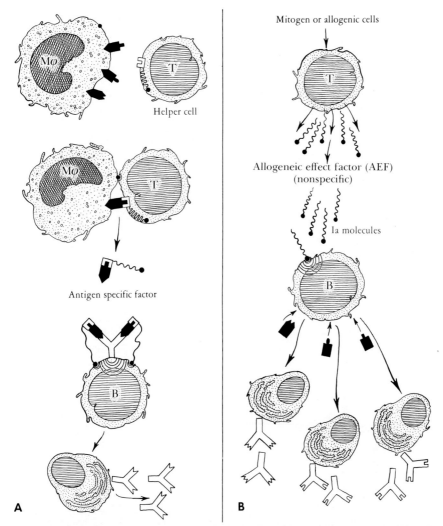

Figure 3–5. Schematic representation of the effects of two types of factors produced by helper T-lymphocytes on antibody production by B-lymphocytes. *A,* An *antigen-specific T-lymphocyte factor* containing the T-lymphocyte receptor, antigen, and Ia molecules, and *B,* an *allogeneic effect factor* (AEF) that contains Ia molecules.

ing site, when reacted with T-lymphocytes, inhibit the ability of helper T-cells to respond to specific antigen. This suggests, therefore, that the antigen-binding receptor on T-lymphocytes and the immunoglobulin receptor on the B-lymphocyte may have structural similarities. Alternatively, the antigen receptor on T-lymphocytes may be encoded for, in part, by the VH region that is associated with the immunoglobulin allotype-linked immune response gene (Fig. 3–2).

Benacerraf and his colleagues took note of earlier experiments that had shown that some animals could be divided into *responders* and *nonresponders* to particular antigens. These workers attached a hapten on poly-L-lysine and injected the complex into guinea pigs. They found that in outbred strains some animals responded while others did not. They then performed simple crosses to find whether there was a genetic basis for the phenomenon. These experiments showed that if two responder animals were bred, the offspring were responders; if two nonresponders were bred, the offspring were nonresponders; if a responder and a nonresponder were bred, the resulting offspring were responders (Fig. 3–6). Thus, immune responses appear to be controlled genetically and inherited as an autosomal dominant trait. It was also shown that the nonresponsiveness was independent of the hapten and dependent only upon the carrier protein. These early experiments thus suggested that the control was at the T-lymphocyte level and that a high responder animal would mount a cell-mediated immune reaction as well as an antibody response to the particular antigen complex. These studies also demonstrated that the genetic control was extremely specific for the antigenic structure.

McDevitt and coworkers found similar genetic control mechanisms in mice in studying responses to synthetic polypeptides. Investigations employing high and low responder strains showed that F_1 progeny of a high and low responder mating were high responders, suggesting once more that the responses to a specific antigen were inherited from a single gene or closely linked group of genes in an autosomal dominant fashion. Utilizing mice that differed only with respect to their MHC region (congeneic strains) or mice that differed at subregions (recombinant strains), McDevitt showed that immune response genes mapped within the (MHC) H-2 region of the mouse and, more specifically, were localized within the I region. The tissue distribution of these genes has been a matter of controversy. Although early studies suggested that the Ir genes are expressed only in T-lymphocytes, more recent evidence has suggested that both T- and B-lymphocytes, as well as macrophages, may express Ir gene products.

Genetic Control of Suppression. Recent studies have also shown that suppressor, but not helper, T-lymphocytes are generated to synthetic antigens in genetic nonresponder mice. These studies confirmed earlier work that demonstrated that tolerance could be more easily induced in genetic nonresponders that in responder mice (Chapter 10). More recently, antisera directed against a single subregion of I, termed the I-J locus (Fig. 3–3), have been shown to inhibit both nonspecific T-lymphocyte suppressors activated by the mitogen concanavalin-A, the specific T-lymphocyte suppression of allotype to carrier hapten conjugates, and T-lymphocyte suppression to other antigens. Thus, it appears that separate genes in the I region are involved in T-lymphocyte help while others are involved in T-lymphocyte suppression of the immune response.

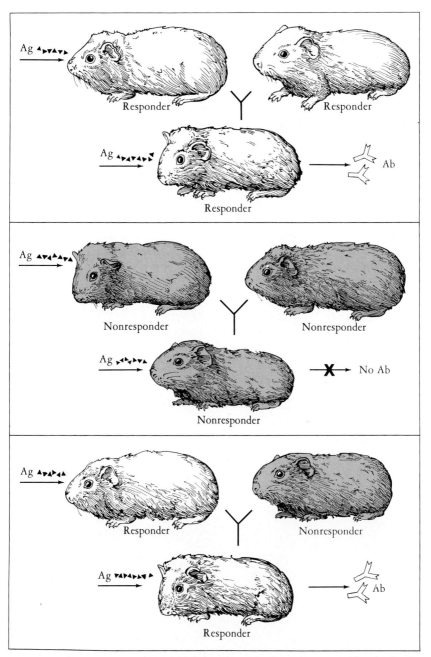

Figure 3–6. Schematic representation of the antibody response to antigenic stimulus by responder animals (upper panel) and the lack of response in nonresponder animals (middle panel), illustrating the autosomal dominant pattern of genetic transmission in F_1 hybrids (lower panel).

MHC of Man (HL-A)

The major histocompatibility system of man, the human leukocyte antigen (HL-A) system, is very complex (Fig. 3–7) and is homologous to the H-2 region in the mouse (Fig. 3–3). Originally, the serologically defined (SD) specificities of the HL-A system were assigned to two linked loci, each with multiple alleles. These two loci have recently been designated as the HLA-A and the HLA-B loci, corresponding to the K and D regions of H-2 in the mouse. A third locus, the HLA-C, has been identified, although only a few of the individual specificities of this locus have yet been identified. A fourth locus, HLA-D, has also been identified by mixed lymphocyte reactions (MLR) and is termed a lymphocyte-defined (LD) antigen. Antisera have been produced that abrogate the stimulating cell (T-lymphocyte) in human MLR and appear to correspond to the anti-Ia sera in the mouse. The specificities (or the antigens) that are controlled by genes at each of these four loci are now identified by numbers. The current practice is to place a lower-case "w" in front of the number when it is first recognized. Later, when general consensus has been reached, and as the specificity is firmly established by the World Health Organization Nomenclature Committee, the "w" is dropped and the number retained. A blank or apparently absent antigen in a genotype might indicate either that an individual is homozygous for single specificity at a locus or, alternatively, an inability to identify an antigen. This is usually clarified by family studies. At present, only the antigens in the HLA-A and HLA-B series are well

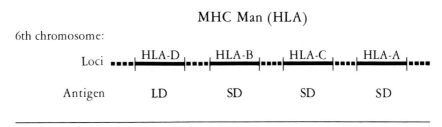

MHC Man (HLA)

6th chromosome:

Loci ▪▪▪▪├─ HLA-D ─┤▪▪▪▪├─ HLA-B ─┤▪▪▪▪├─ HLA-C ─┤▪▪▪▪├─ HLA-A ─┤▪▪▪▪

Antigen   LD   SD   SD   SD

Nomenclature of HLA

NEW	OLD	ORIGINAL
HLA-A	SD1	1st locus
HLA-B	SD2	2nd locus
HLA-C	SD3	3rd locus
HLA-D	LD1	—

Figure 3–7. Schematic representation of the human major histocompatibility complex (MHC), illustrating chromosomal loci (HLA) and their gene products and the lymphocyte detectable (LD) and serologically detectable (SD) antigens.

known (Table 3–3). A comparison of the mouse and human MHC regions is shown in Figure 3–8.

The HL-A system is one of genetic dominance. Thus, two antigens or specificities are possible for each of the four segregating loci. Table 3–3 outlines the 39 specificities that have been recognized at the HLA-A and HLA-B loci. The gene frequencies of each antigen provide good evidence that the distribution of these antigens varies greatly between various racial groups.

The complexity of this system would be emphasized if we were to identify the variations and types available simply by looking at the more than 255 haplotypes that can be recognized within the first two loci of this very complex system. As many as 65,052 genotypes are possible in this system.

Histocompatibility and Disease. Associations between histocompatibility type and disease are of particular importance since these associations can lead to both clinical diagnostic methods and an increased

TABLE 3–3. Recognized HLA Specificities of Man

HLA-A		HLA-B	
New	*Previous*	*New*	*Previous*
HLA-A1	HL-A1	HLA-B5	HL-A5
HLA-A2	HL-A2	HLA-B7	HL-A7
HLA-A3	HL-A3	HLA-B8	HL-A8
HLA-A9	HL-A9	HLA-B12	HL-A12
HLA-A10	HL-A10	HLA-B13	HL-A13
HLA-A11	HL-A11	HLA-B14	W14
HLA-A28	W28	HLA-B18	W18
HLA-A29	W29	HLA-B27	W27
HLA-Aw19	Li		
HLA-Aw23	W23	HLA-Bw15	W15
HLA-Aw24	W24	HLA-Bw16	W16
HLA-Aw25	W25	HLA-Bw17	W17
HLA-A26	W26	HLA-Bw21	W21
HLA-Aw30	W30	HLA-Bw22	W22
HLA-Aw31	W31	HLA-Bw35	W5
HLA-Aw32	W32	HLA-Bw37	TY
HLA-Aw33	W19.6	HLA-Bw38	W16.1
HLA-Aw34	Malay 2	HLA-Bw39	W16.2
HLA-Aw36	Mo	HLA-Bw40	W10
HLA-Aw43	BK	HLA-Bw41	Sabell
		HLA-Bw42	MWA

HLA-C		HLA-D	
New	*Previous*	*New*	*Previous*
HLA-Cw1	T1	HLA-Dw1	LD 101
HLA-Cw2	T2	HLA-Dw2	LD 102
HLA-Cw3	T3	HLA-Dw3	LD 103
HLA-Cw4	T4	HLA-Dw4	LD 104
HLA-Cw5	T5	HLA-Dw5	LD 105
		HLA-Dw6	LD 106

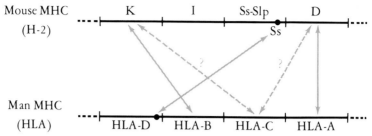

Figure 3-8. Comparison of the MHC of mouse (H-2) and man (HLA).

fundamental understanding of disease processes. These are shown in Table 3–4. Correlations between specific diseases and HL-A type have been made in such diverse disorders as ankylosing spondylitis (HLA-B 27), gluten-sensitive enteropathy (HLA-B8 and Dw3), and multiple sclerosis (HLA-B7 and Dw2). The most powerful of these associations occurs in ankylosing spondylitis, in which more than 90 per cent of affected individuals have HLA-B27. The reasons for these increased (or decreased) gene frequencies have not been established; however, three broad categories of explanation have been made. First, HL-A genes themselves may cause some potentially damaging configurations of the cell. Second, the HL-A gene itself may not be responsible for disease susceptibility but may be closely linked to a gene controlling some other trait, such as immune responsiveness. Third, the HL-A gene may only coincidentally be related to susceptibility and may be found in increased frequency because it would migrate in any population that had a high frequency of an HL-A type and a preponderance of any disease. From an immunologic standpoint, the second of these hypotheses is very attractive since Ir genes closely linked to histocompatibility type have been identified in several mammalian species. Such histocompatibility-linked Ir genes have already been linked to susceptibility to viral oncogenesis in the mouse. These genes, termed RgV-1 by Lilly and coworkers, have been shown to be involved in resistance to Gross, Friend, and related murine leukemia viruses. Although multiple genes (many outside the major histocompatibility complex) are clearly involved in the many human diseases, associations between HL-A and disease are of great power as both illuminators of disease mechanisms and diagnostic tools.

Inheritance of Histocompatibility Antigens. The correctness of Dausset's postulate has been demonstrated in the transmission of histocompatibility within a family. Each histocompatibility complex is located on a single chromosome and contains four loci, each responsible for a group of allelic chains representing HLA-A, HLA-B, HLA-C, and HLA-D. The histocompatibility locus occurs on a pair of chromosomes. Figure 3–9 shows a pedigree in which X and X′ are representative of the major histocompatibility complex present on the pair of chromosomes in the mother and Y and Y′ represent the histocompat-

TABLE 3-4. HLA Antigens and Disease Associations

HLA ANTIGENS	DISEASES	HLA FREQUENCY		RELATIVE RISK FACTORS
		Patients (Positive Reaction, Per Cent)	Controls (Positive Reaction, Per Cent)	
Group 1: Certain Associations				
HLA-B27	Ankylosing spondylitis	81–96	4–8	121
	Reiter syndrome	60–96	4–14	40
	Acute anterior uveitis	55	4	24
	Juvenile rheumatoid arthritis	42	6	11.5
	Psoriatic arthritis	63	8	4.7
	Yersinia arthritis	91	14	*
HLA-B8	Gluten-sensitive enteropathy			11*
	and celiac disease	77–88	20–30	8†
	Grave disease	*	*	11.5
	Myasthenia gravis	38–65	18–31	4.5
	Dermatitis herpetiformis	58–84	17–33	4.3
	Chronic active hepatitis	68	18	3.6
HLA-Bw15	Insulin-dependent	36	10	31
HLA-B8	diabetes mellitus	*	*	16
HLA-A3	Multiple sclerosis	32–40	18–27	24
HLA-B7		35–39	25–26	12
HLA-B18		*	*	12
HLA-B13	Psoriasis vulgaris	11–27	2–5	5
HLA-Bw17		19–36	4–16	4.8
Group 2: Probable Associations				
HLA-B8 and HLA-Bw15	Systemic lupus erythematosus			
HLA-B13	Pemphigus			
HLA-A3	Idiopathic autoimmune hemolytic anemia			
HLA-A3 and HLA-B7	Poliomyelitis			
HLA-B5	Behçet disease			
Group 3: Possible Associations				
HLA-A2 and HLA-B12	Acute lymphoblastic leukemia			
HLA-A2	Chronic glomerulonephritis			
HLA-A2, decreased	Periodontitis			
HLA-Bw35	Infectious mononucleosis			
HLA-B14	Leprosy			
HLA-A10	Hodgkin disease (patients > 45 years of age)			

*In adults.
†In children.
From Ritzmann, S. E.: HLA patterns. J.A.M.A., *236*:2305, 1976.

ibility complex represented on the chromosomes of the father. It can be seen that the genotypes of the grandparents are transmitted to the parents and the grandchildren and these segregate according to mendelian principles of genetics. Each individual carries two alleles that determine the histocompatibility genotype. For example, the X demonstrated in Figure 3–9 might include HLA-A1, HLA-B5, HLA-Cw1, and HLA-Dw1. Any combination of the allelic antigens on each of the four loci is possible in the histocompatibility complex present on a single chromosome. Within a family, the same genotypes recur. Note,

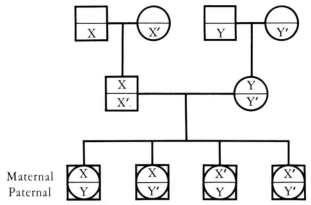

Figure 3-9. Family pedigree, showing inheritance of histocompatibility antigens.

again in Figure 3–9, that there are four possible genotypes inherited from the parents. These are XY, XY′, X′Y, and X′Y′. These are represented as either male or female offspring, since the inheritance of the histocompatibility genetic types occurs irrespective of sex. If a fifth child is born, it must display one of the previous four genotypes. Therefore, the likelihood of identifying a compatible donor for organ transplant or for white cell or platelet transfusion in siblings is much greater than in unrelated donors. Thus, the histocompatibility antigens provide an identification system for the selection of the compatible donors for white cell, platelet, and organ transplantation. It is only through a thorough understanding of these simple immunogenetic principles that the physician and student of medicine will be able to continue to utilize the therapeutic approach for replacement of essential nucleated cells and organs.

GENETICS OF THE BLOOD GROUP SYSTEMS

Another genetic region that has a major influence on immunogenetic responses is that of the major blood group systems, including the ABO and the Rh systems. The erythrocytes contain myriad isoantigenic determinants; however, only a few of them are clinically important, either because of their *immunogenicity* or their *frequency* in the population. The isoantigens of red blood cells that are of clinical importance are those of the ABO system and the Rh system.

THE ABO SYSTEM

For centuries it was known that recipients of blood transfusions often experienced serious or fatal transfusion reactions. The mechanism for these untoward reactions was not understood until the classic work of Landsteiner, who in 1900 defined the major isoantigens of human red blood cells.

Landsteiner performed a very simple experiment in which he collected blood from six members of his laboratory staff. After separating the red cells from the serum of each specimen, he mixed the two reagents in varying combinations in a series of test tubes. By the use of a simple red cell agglutination technique, he observed that the sera of some individuals were capable of clumping the red cells of others, but not their own.

From these experiments, Landsteiner was able to draw several conclusions. First, there were *two* antigenic determinants present on human red blood cells, which he called A and B. Some individuals possessed the A antigenic determinant and were of the A blood group; others contained the B determinant and, hence, belonged to blood group B. There was still another group of individuals who possessed neither of these determinants and belonged to blood group O. However, it was shown subsequently that O type individuals are not deficient in an antigen, but rather, contain a heterogenetic or H antigen. Finally, the work of Landsteiner clearly established that all mature individuals possess antibody in their serum, the so-called "naturally occurring" isoantibodies (isoagglutinins) directed against the antigenic determinant absent from their own erythrocytes. Thus, individuals of blood group A possess anti-B, individuals belonging to blood group B possess anti-A, and those belonging to blood group O have both anti-A and anti-B. Later, the most infrequent blood group was described, blood group AB. Individuals of this group have both A and B antigenic determinants present on their red cells, one of paternal origin and the other of maternal origin. As expected, their serum contains neither anti-A nor anti-B isoagglutinins. These basic studies led to our understanding of the major blood groups of man. They also provided the first clearcut example of self-recognition, which led to later theories of natural tolerance of the host's own antigens (autologous antigens).

Genetic Control of the ABO Isoantigens

The final expression of these antigens is controlled by three allelic genes, A, B and O. The A gene controls the formation of the A substance, and the B gene controls the B substance. The O gene is not expressed (it is an amorph) and is involved in the synthesis of H substance (as described below). The A and B genes are dominant over O. Since man is diploid with two allelic forms at each locus, there is a possibility for four phenotypes and six genotypes. The relationship between genotype, phenotype, red cell antigen, and isohemagglutinins is given in Table 3–5.

Family studies have established the transmission of these blood

TABLE 3–5. The ABO Blood Groups

GENOTYPE	PHENOTYPE	RED CELL ANTIGEN	ISOHEMAGGLUTININS
AO AA	A	A	anti-B
BO BB	B	B	anti-A
OO	O	H	anti-A, anti-B
AB	AB	A,B	none

groups from generation to generation. Thus, all the children of A and O homozygotes (AA × OO) are phenotypically A (genotype AO). However, the mating of the more common heterozygote A parents (AO × AO) would be expected to produce offspring in the ratio of 1AA:2AO:1OO.

H Substance

It is now established that individuals of blood group O do indeed produce a definite isoantigen called H substance or H antigen. The name stems from the fact that this substance is a heterogenetic antigen found in many phylogenetically unrelated species. It is now felt that the H antigen is controlled by a separate genetic locus, independent of the ABO system. This locus controls the synthesis of a mucopeptide backbone structure upon which additional residues may be added to form the A and B substances (Table 3–6).

This backbone structure is similar to the polysaccharide of the type 14 pneumococcus. The H gene results in the formation of an enzyme that adds a fucose to the C-2 position of the terminal galactose residue

TABLE 3–6. Chemistry of the ABO Blood Group Substances

GENE	TERMINAL NONREDUCING END	ANTIGEN SPECIFICITY
O	β-Gal (1→3 or 1→4) GNAc... $\uparrow \alpha$ 1,2 Fuc	H
A	α-GalNAc − (1→3)-β-Gal(1→3 or 1→4) GNAc... $\uparrow \alpha$ 1,2 Fuc	A
B	α-Gal-(1→3)-β-Gal(1→3 or 1→4) GNAc... $\uparrow \alpha$ 1,2 Fuc	B

of the chain, resulting in the formation of the H substance. If an individual is homozygous for the O gene (OO), an "amorph," there is no further gene expression and the synthesis of H substance continues and can be detected on the red blood cells. If an individual has at least one A gene, this results in the formation of an enzyme that attaches a terminal N-acetylgalactosamine to the galactose residue of the H substance, transforming it into A substance. The presence of at least one B gene causes the formation of an enzyme that leads to the addition of another galactose residue to the terminal galactose, transforming it into B substance. The presence of both A and B genes leads to the synthesis of both enzymes with the production of A and B substances. Thus, the blood group substances, of great clinical importance to the physician, are examples of substances whose antigenic expressions are influenced by small structural differences in single sugar residues that are under genetic control.

RH SYSTEM

The second isoantigen of red cells important in clinical medicine is the Rh system. Its discovery occurred with the chance observation of two seemingly unrelated events—one occurring in humans, the other as part of a laboratory effort.

In 1939, Levine and Stetson reported their findings of a newborn infant who was suffering from a severe form of hemolytic disease, consisting of severe jaundice, massive edema, and hepatosplenomegaly, which they termed *erythroblastosis fetalis.* Subsequently, the mother of this affected infant, upon receiving blood from her husband, suffered a massive transfusion reaction.

Fortuitously, at approximately the same time, Landsteiner and Wiener had been immunizing rabbits with red cells of the Rhesus monkey in an effort to define new human isoantigenic specificities. These workers discovered that antibodies generated in this fashion could agglutinate the erythrocytes of 85 per cent of the individuals in New York City, but not of the remaining 15 per cent. These data proved to be crucial to Levine and Stetson's case. It was shown subsequently that although the parents had compatible ABO types, the mother's serum agglutinated the red cells of the husband and of 80 per cent of the population.

The relationship between these isolated clinical and experimental findings was soon borne out and the newly defined determinant was named the Rh_0 factor to indicate the Rhesus species of red cells used in the experimental production of antibody. Thus, a paternal isoantigen on the red cells of the fetus, which was foreign to that of the mother, had entered the maternal circulation with subsequent isoimmunization. The resultant antibodies were passively transferred back to the fetus with the production of a catastrophic hemolytic reaction and erythroblastosis fetalis. The clinical features of this condition are described in Chapter 20B.

Genetic Control of Rh Antigens

The immense complexity of the Rh system has been revealed over the past 30 years with the discovery of many additional Rh antigenic types. Approximately 30 types have been identified; however, the original Rh antigen is by far the most important in terms of immunogenicity and clinical significance.

The lengthy interval between the discovery of the ABO and the Rh blood groups was due, in part, to the serologic properties of the anti-Rh antibodies. Unlike those of the ABO system, Rh antibodies do not occur naturally; rather, they are products of frank immunization either through pregnancy or transfusion. The serologic properties of these antibodies are described in Chapter 8.

There are two theories that have been proposed to explain the inheritance of the Rh antigens. The first of these, suggested by Fisher and Race, proposed that the system consists of five antigenic determinants (D, C, E, c, and e), which are products of genes situated at three distinct, but closely linked, chromosomal loci. The three loci are considered to be so closely linked on the chromosome that crossing over is an infrequent event. It is thought that they are inherited, one set from each parent. It is, in effect, the concept of one cistron controlling the production of one antigenic determinant, the Rh phenotype. This is diagramed schematically in Figure 3–10.

The most important of these loci was called D, and it controls the production of the most clinically significant Rh isoantigen, the D antigen. This isoantigen was responsible for the erythroblastotic infant described by Stetson and Levine and accounts for more than 90 per cent of cases of hemolytic disease of the newborn due to maternal isoimmunization. An alternate allele at this locus was called d (Fig. 3–9). To date, the antigenic product of this hypothetical allele has not been described, and there is considerable doubt that such an antigenic determinant actually exists. The symbol d is used to represent the absence of D, rather than the presence of any known antigenic determinant. A second locus, according to the Fisher-Race scheme, is the position at which one of two alleles, C or c, is located. These genes control the production of either the C or c antigens. Alleles at a third locus, called E, are responsible for the production of the antigenic determinants E or e. These isoantigens occasionally account for isoimmunization.

A second theory of inheritance, proposed by Wiener, differs to the extent that one locus is responsible for the production of several antigenic determinants. This theory utilizes the concept of "multiple complex alleles," in which a single locus on the chromosome controls the production of the Rh antigenic determinants found on the red cell.

Chromosomal loci   Antigenic Determinants

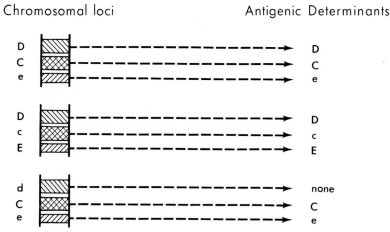

Figure 3–10. Schematic representation of the one cistron–one Rh phenotype concept of Fisher and Race.

At this locus, however, there are a large number of alleles, each being responsible for the production of a single large antigenic structure that encompasses multiple smaller antigenic determinants. The original antigenic determinants were classified as Rh_0, rh' rh", hr' and hr", which corresponds to D, C, E, c, and e of the Fisher-Race scheme (Table 3–7). Each allele is given a symbolic designation, such as Rh, to designate the antigenic specificity it controls. For example, Rh' leads to the production of the antigenic determinants Rh_0, Rh', and hr" on the red cell. Figure 3–11 depicts the same examples used in Figure 3–10, using the Wiener scheme.

Since both nomenclatures are widely used, one should be familiar with them. Table 3–7 presents some of the more commonly encountered Rh isoantigens, together with their controlling allelic forms, employing both system of notation.

According to the Fisher-Race scheme, the isoantigens are con-

TABLE 3–7. Notations of Commonly Encountered Rh Isoantigens and Alleles

ALLELIC FORMS		RH ISOANTIGENS	
Race-Fisher	*Wiener*	*Fisher-Race*	*Wiener*
cDe	Rh_0	D	Rh_0
CDe	Rh_1	C	rh'
cDE Rh^+	Rh_2	E	rh"
CDE	Rh_2	c	hr'
cde	rh	e	hr"
Cde Rh^-	rh'		
CdE	rh_y		

Chromosomal locus   Antigenic Determinants

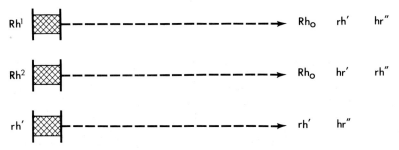

Figure 3–11. Schematic representation of the one-allele multiple determinant of Wiener.

trolled by three linked loci. Since man is diploid, one set of these genetic loci is inherited from each parent. A person is said to be "Rh-positive" if he inherits D from either parent (DD or Dd). In either case, the father can transmit a D to one of his offspring's chromosomes.

For the physician, therefore, the determination of the genotype of an individual is an important consideration when sensitization due to D has occurred in a D-negative (Rh_0-negative) mother. For example, a father who is *homozygous* will transmit D to all the offspring, and each child could suffer from hemolytic disease of the newborn. If, on the other hand, the father is heterozygous, each child has a 50 per cent chance of being negative for D. Thus, by determination of the genotype of the father, the outcome of future pregnancies can be predicted.

SUGGESTIONS FOR FURTHER READING

Bach, F. H., and van Rood, J. J.: The major histocompatibility complex. N. Engl. J. Med., 295:806, 1976.

Benacerraf, B., Kapp, J. A., Debre, P., Pierce, C. N., and Dela Croix, F.: The stimulation of specific suppressor T-cells in genetic non-responder mice by linear random copolymer of L-amino acids. Transplant. Rev., 26:21, 1975.

Dausset, J.: HLA and disease. In Progress in Immunology III. New York, Academic Press, 1978.

Gasser, D. L., and Silvers, W. K.: Genetic determinants of immunological responsiveness. Adv. Immunol., 18:1, 1974.

Katz, D. H., and Benacerraf, B.: The Role of the Products of the Histocompatibility Gene Complex in the Immune Response. New York, Academic Press, 1976.

McDevitt, H. O., and Landy, M.: Genetic Control of Immune Responsiveness. New York, Academic Press, 1972.

Ritzmann, S. E.: HLA patterns and disease associations. J.A.M.A., 236:2305, 1976.

Shreffler, D. C., and David, C. S.: The H-2 major histocompatibility complex and the I immune response region: genetic, variation, formation and organization. Adv. Immunol., 20:125, 1976.

Snell, G. D., Dausset, J., and Nathenson, S.: Histocompatibility. New York, Academic Press, 1967.

Zmijewski, C. M.: Immunobiology. New York, Appleton-Century-Crofts, 1974.

Chapter 4

ANTIGENS AND IMMUNOGENICITY

Anne L. Jackson, Ph.D.

DEFINITIONS

Immunogenicity may be defined as that property of a substance (immunogen) that endows it with the capacity to provoke a specific immune response. This consists of either the elaboration of antibody, the development of cell-mediated immunity, or both. Antigenicity, on the other hand, is the property of a substance (antigen) that allows it to react with the products of the specific immune response, e.g., antibody or specifically sensitized T-lymphocytes. Substances that are immunogenic are always antigenic, but antigens are not necessarily immunogenic. For example, certain low molecular weight substances, referred to as haptens, e.g., penicillin, are not immunogenic unless coupled to a larger *carrier* molecule. Thus, a hapten functions as an antigen but not as an immunogen. Allergens refer to a specialized class of immunogens that induce hypersensitivity (allergic) reactions (Chapter 20A) and include substances that function as immunogens or haptens.

Portions of the three-dimensional structure of every immunogen contain surface groupings, e.g., amino acids in a globular protein or protruding sugar side chains in polysaccharides. These structures are referred to as antigenic determinants and represent exposed active areas of the molecule with which an antibody can combine. Most complex materials, such as red blood cells, tissues, and bacteria, contain numerous antigenic determinants. Because of its small size, an individual antigenic determinant may not be immunogenic and therefore may be considered a hapten. Thus, the immune response to a complex immunogen represents the collective immune responses to a number of antigenic determinants. Of importance to clinical medicine is that new antigenic determinants may appear as a consequence of physical or chemical modification of that material within the body. The significance of this finding is seen in certain immunologically mediated diseases of man, such as drug allergies, the autoimmune diseases, and neoplasia (Chapters 19 and 20).

DEFINITIONS OF ANTIGENIC SPECIFICITIES

Broadly speaking, antigens may be classified into two major types: *exogenous* and *endogenous* (Table 4–1). This is an operational classifica-

TABLE 4–1.   Classification of Antigens

SOURCE	TYPE	EXAMPLE	CLINICAL SIGNIFICANCE
Exogenous	Several	Microorganisms, pollen, drugs, pollutants	Susceptibility to infection, immunologically mediated disease (asthma)
Endogenous Xenogeneic (Heterologous)	Xenoantigen (Heteroantigen)	Forssman antigen, certain tissue antigens that cross-react with exogenous antigens (e.g., renal and cardiac tissues and beta hemolytic streptococcus	Pathogenesis of certain diseases, e.g., glomerulo-nephritis, rheumatic fever
Autologous	Autoantigen	Organ-specific antigens (e.g., thyroid antigen)	Autoimmune diseases, e.g., Hashimoto's thyroiditis
Allogeneic (Homologous)	Alloantigen (Isoantigen)	Blood group, histocompati-bility antigens (HL-A)	Hemolytic disease of the newborn, transfusion re-actions, transplantation immunity

tion of antigens, based upon their applications in immunologically mediated diseases of man (Chapter 20).

EXOGENOUS ANTIGENS

Exogenous antigens are those that are presented to the host from the exterior in the form of microorganisms, pollen, drugs, or pollutants (Table 4–1). These antigens are responsible for a spectrum of human diseases ranging from the infectious diseases to the immunologically mediated diseases of man, such as bronchial asthma (Chapter 20A). There are also genetic mechanisms operating at the level of the exogenous antigens. Influenza virus, for example, which is a major cause of epidemic respiratory disease in man, exists in nature in many antigenic types recognized as A, B, and C. These types represent different mutations of the virus. A susceptible population will be infected by a given serotype. Following recovery and establishment of immunity, the virus can no longer propagate, since there are insufficient susceptibles to establish continued infection. Owing to selective pressure, however, the virus is known to undergo mutation, following which new variants of influenza emerge. These newly acquired variants, when fully virulent, are responsible for new epidemics. Thus, man survives epidemics, and organisms mutate to re-create epidemics.

ENDOGENOUS ANTIGENS

Endogenous antigens are those that are found within an individual and include the following: *xenogeneic* (heterologous), *autologous*, or *allogeneic* (homologous) antigens (Table 4–1).

Xenogeneic antigens are those antigens that are found within a variety of phylogenetically unrelated species. These antigens are also known as *heterogeneic* antigens and are important in clinical medicine, since they give rise to antibody responses associated with or useful in the diagnosis of disease. For example, the cross-reaction of group A beta hemolytic streptococcal antigens and human heart tissue is an example of a relationship between the well-known incidence of rheumatic heart disease and infection. It is believed that tissue damage is due to the cross-reaction of antibody with these heterologous antigens. Other types of heterologous responses are helpful in diagnosis. The best known example of this is the Forssman antigen, which is found in the tissue of many species and is closely related to other ubiquitous antigens such as the A blood group antigen. Because the Forssman antigen itself is not found in the tissues of man, it is possible that the great variety of other tissues or cells that contain this antigen could sensitize man. For example, following infectious mononucleosis, an infection caused by the EB virus (Chapter 16), antibody responses develop, some of which are specifically directed against the EB virus and others against this heterogenetic antigen. This latter reaction, referred to as "*heterophile antibody response*" is a useful test in diagnosing infectious mononucleosis.

Autologous body components are constituents of the host and are recognized as self-components. Under ordinary circumstances, they are nonimmunogenic. It is believed that a change in these body components may cause them to become immunogenic under certain circumstances, and the host mounts an immunologic attack against its own tissues. In some instances, human tissues contain antigens that normally can be recognized by the immune system of the host but are separated from the action of antibodies or immune cells by barriers, such as the basement membrane. In these situations, removal of the barrier, for instance, through the effects of inflammation or acute infection, may release the antigens in such a way as to produce an acute secondary immune response, stimulating the host to mount an immunologic attack against its own tissues. In either case, the final condition is referred to as autoimmunity and is described in greater detail in Chapter 20C.

By far the largest group of antigens significant to the clinician are those known as *allogeneic antigens*. Allogeneic antigens are those genetically controlled by antigenic determinants that distinguish one individual of a given species from another. In man, antigenic determinants of this variety are found on red blood cells, white blood cells, platelets, serum proteins, and the surface of cells making up the fixed tissues of the body, including histocompatibility antigens (Table 4–2). These antigens are known to be *polymorphic*. (Polymorphism is the existence of two or more genetically different forms in one interbreeding population due to an array of alleles at one locus of the chromosome. At any one locus, however, an individual has only two alleles of the entire

TABLE 4–2.   Distribution and Clinical Significance of the Alloantigens of Man

Type	Example of Alloantigens	Clinical Significance
Red blood cell	ABO, Rh_0, blood groups (called isoantigens)	Hemolytic disease of new-born, transfusion reactions
White blood cell	Histocompatibility (HL-A) and neutrophil (NA) antigens	Transplantation immunity
Platelets	Platelet (Pl) antigens	Transplantation, thrombo-cytopenia
Serum proteins	Gamma globulin	Immunologic deficiency
Fixed tissues	Histocompatibility antigens (HL-A)	Transplantation

array that exists in the population.) In Table 4–2 are listed some of the important isoantigens of man with their tissue distribution, and clinical importance. Immunization with any of these antigens can occur and progress to disease. This results when an individual receives an incompatible blood transfusion or a solid graft containing antigenic determinants that are absent in the recipient host. When these specificities are lacking in the recipient, they are perceived as foreign and therefore lead to an immune response. In general, the intensity of the response is proportional to the degree of genetic disparity between immunogen and the host; i.e., the greater the disparity, the more intense the response. These reactions may take the form of a transfusion reaction, as in the case of an incompatible blood transfusion, or the rejection of a solid graft, as in the case of a kidney transplant. Alternatively, immunization can occur during the course of pregnancy when fetal cells (e.g., leukocytes, erythrocytes, platelets) or proteins gain access to the maternal circulation. The maternal production and transplacental transfer of antibody to any of these paternally acquired fetal antigens

TABLE 4–3.   The Reactivity of Sera Prepared Against the Isomers of Tartaric Acid*

	Haptens		
Antisera	l-tartaric acid	d-tartaric acid	m-tartaric acid
Anti-l-tartaric acid	+++	±	±
Anti-d-tartaric acid	0	+++	±
Anti-m-tartaric acid	±	0	+++

*After Landsteiner, K.: The Specificity of Serological Reactions. Cambridge, Harvard University Press, 1956.

can lead to severe anemia, leukopenia, thrombocytopenia, or aberrations in gamma globulin production by the fetus (Fig. 4–1).

STRUCTURE OF AN ANTIGEN

A composite picture of an "antigen" may be seen in the case of the group A streptococcus (Fig. 4–2). The bacterium is composed of several physically and chemically discernible structures, which vary in their immunogenicity. For example, the capsule, which is composed of hyaluronic acid, is relatively nonimmunogenic. This may be accounted for by its close structural similarity to hyaluronates present in animal tissues, and it may not be recognized as foreign by the host. This lack of immunogenicity may also account for the increased virulence of the organism (Chapter 14). The surface antigens, M, T, and R, are found in the cell wall. Of these, the M proteins are the most important biologically since their presence impedes phagocytosis, and they are thought to be the major virulence factor of the group A beta hemolytic streptococcus. Bacteria that are coated with antibody are more readily taken up and destroyed by phagocytic cells. The M proteins are also important diagnostically because they determine the type specificity of the organism. The group-specific "antigens" (A through N) are carbohydrate in nature and are also found within the cell wall of the streptococcal organism. Antibodies to these carbohydrates are not protective but permit the classification of the streptococci into serologic groups, which were first described by Lancefield. In addition, immunogenic extracellular products are elaborated by the streptococcus. These include the erythrogenic toxins, the streptolysins S and O, and a variety of other

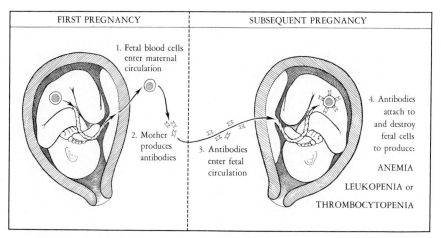

Figure 4–1.   Schematic representation of isoimmunization due to feto-maternal incompatibility.

Living Group A Streptococcus   Dead Vaccine

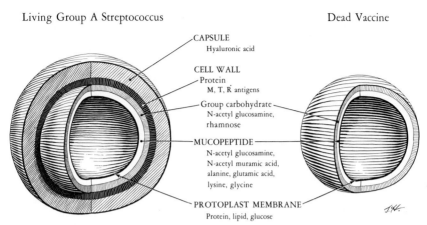

Figure 4–2. Schematic representation of living Group A Streptococcus and the dead vaccine prepared from it. (After Krause, R. M.: Factors controlling the occurrence of antibodies with uniform properties. Fed. Proc., 29:59, 1970.)

toxins. Antibodies to these proteins can serve a protective function (e.g., antierythrogenic toxin in scarlet fever) and may also be of diagnostic aid (e.g., antistreptolysin O). When one considers that each of these immunogens has at least one, and probably more, antigenic determinants, the number of antibodies of different specificity that could be produced following immunization or infection becomes quite large. Not all immune responses are protective to the host, however. In assessing vaccines, it is important to determine the degree of protection produced in a patient by these immunogens (Chapter 23).

GENERAL PROPERTIES OF IMMUNOGENS

FOREIGNNESS

The first and primary requirement for any molecule to qualify as an immunogen is that the substance be genetically foreign to the host. In nature, an immune response will occur to a component that is not normally present in the body or normally exposed to the host's lymphoreticular system. On occasion, however, body constituents may be recognized as foreign, elicit an immune response, and become the adventitious target of injury, as seen in the autoimmune diseases of man (Chapter 20). Under ordinary circumstances, the immune system discriminates between "self" and "nonself." However, not all foreign substances can induce an immune response. For example, exposure to carbon in the form of coal dust will not induce antibodies to these substances; only the phagocytic response is initiated.

In addition to the requirements for foreignness, there is an increasing body of evidence to suggest that the ability to elicit an immune response is under genetic control (Chapter 3). These controls operate both at the level of total immune response, e.g., responders versus nonresponders, and in the control of specific immune products, e.g., IgE antibody. Thus, there exists a genetic requirement with regard to both the immunogen in terms of genetic dissimilarity and the genetic controls of immune responsiveness.

The recognition of a specific immunogen and the commitment to respond to the stimulation by the production of either antibody or cell-mediated immunity or with tolerance also seems to depend on the physical and chemical properties of the immunogen. These responses are mediated by specific receptors on precommitted lymphocytes and will have an influence on the types of cells recruited (Chapter 7). For example, certain immunogens directly stimulate B-lymphocytes with the production of antibody without the requirement for T-cells (T-independent antigens); other types of immunogens require the interaction of T-helper and B-lymphocytes in the full expression of an immune response (T-dependent antigens). Another type of cell cooperation is probably mediated by macrophages (Chapter 7).

PHYSICAL PROPERTIES

SIZE

In order for a substance to be immunogenic, it must be of a certain minimum size; effective immunogens have molecular weights greater than 10,000. Although some smaller molecules, such as insulin (5000 MW) and glucagon (4600 MW), do function as immunogens, the immune response is minimal in most hosts, and these substances function as haptens after combining with tissue proteins. Haptens can induce a strong immune response if coupled to a carrier protein of appropriate size (greater than 10,000). It should be noted that the response to a hapten-protein complex will be directed to (1) the hapten, (2) the carrier, and (3) an area of overlapping specificity involving the hapten and the adjacent carrier constituents. In the case of humoral immunity, specificity is directed primarily to the hapten; in cell-mediated immunity, reactivity is directed to both the hapten and the carrier protein (Chapter 13).

Much of our understanding concerning the specificity of the immune reactions is derived from Landsteiner's studies of haptens. He was able to successfully distinguish antibody in animals immunized with l-tartaric acid from antibody produced in animals immunized with other isomers of tartaric acid (Table 4–3).

It is becoming increasingly clear that although immunogens are usually large substances, only restricted portions of the molecule may be actively involved in the reaction with antibody. Recent studies employing peptide protein complexes have established that peptides the size of a tetra-peptide may be participating in the binding portion of the antigenic determinant with antibody. The subunits of that antigenic determinant appear to contribute unequally to this binding process. The degree to which these components of an antigenic determinant are involved in the reaction with antibody is termed *immunodominance.*

COMPLEXITY

The factors that determine the complexity of an immunogen include both physical and chemical properties of the molecule. The state of aggregation of a molecule, for example, influences immunogenicity. A solution of monomeric proteins may actually induce a refractory state or tolerance when present in monomeric form, but is highly immunogenic in its polymeric or aggregated state (Chapter 10). Several immunogens that do not induce an immune response when isolated in pure form do so when they are a part of a larger particle. Some artificial particles, or adjuvants, such as bentonite or aluminum hydroxide, may also serve to enhance immunogenicity.

CONFORMATION

There is no one molecular configuration that is immunogenic. Linear or branched polypeptides or carbohydrates, as well as globular proteins, are all capable of inducing an immune response. Nonetheless, antibody that is formed to these different conformational structures is highly specific and can readily discriminate these differences. When the conformation of an antigen has been changed, the antibody induced by the original form no longer combines with it. When a determinant group consists of a sequence of amino acids derived from different portions of a folded polypeptide chain, an antibody directed to it cannot, of course, recognize the extended chains when denaturation-unfolding takes place. Figure 4-3 schematically represents the relationships of antibody-combining sites for antigenic determinants. It can be seen that antibody to the first antigen (A) will clearly accommodate its own antigen. Determinant B, which has an additional residue, may not be as easily accommodated with antibody to A.

CHARGE

Immunogenicity is not limited to a particular molecular charge; positive, negative, and neutral substances can be immunogenic. However, the net charge of the immunogen does appear to influence the net charge of the resultant antibody. It has been shown that im-

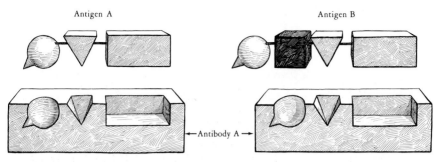

Figure 4-3. Schematic representation of relationships of antibody-combining sites for antigen determinations. (After Sela, M.: Antigenicity: Some molecular aspects. Science, *166*:1365, 1969.)

munization with some positively charged immunogens results in the production of negatively charged antibodies. These data suggest that the production of antibody may be influenced by the overall charge of an immunogen.

ACCESSIBILITY

The accessibility of the determinant groups to the recognition system will determine the outcome of an immune response. Recent developments have allowed investigators to prepare synthetic immunogenic polypeptides that contain a limited number of amino acids and in which chemical structure can be defined. In Figure 4-4, three types of multichain branched synthetic polypeptides are shown. In the first example, alanine side chains are attached to the amino groups of polylysine backbone, and on the outside the immunodominant tyrosine and glutamic acid groups are added. An immune response will occur to

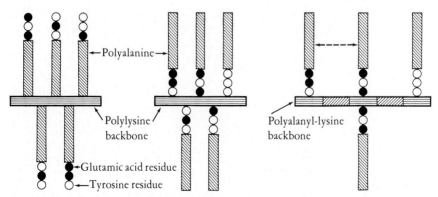

Figure 4-4. Three types of multichain-branched synthetic polypeptides. (After Sela, M.: Studies with synthetic polypeptides. Adv. Immunol., *5*:29, 1966.)

these immunodominant groupings when this polymer is injected into a rabbit. In the center diagram, the immunodominant tyrosine and glutamic acid determinants are placed next to the polylysine backbone, and the alanine side chains or "whiskers" protrude into the outside milieu. No immune response occurs to this configuration. In the third example, however, the spatial configuration of the side chains has been modified by alternating alanine with lysine residues, forming a polylysine-polyalanine backbone structure. Since the side chains can inset only at the location of the lysine groupings, the space between them is greatly lengthened. When injected into an experimental animal, this polymer will induce an immune response. Thus, the accessibility of determinant groupings on an immunogen will influence whether an immune response will occur.

CHEMICAL PROPERTIES

Most organic chemical groupings, with the exception of pure lipids, can be immunogens. The most effective immunogens are those that display diverse chemical and structural characteristics. However, a single amino acid variation in a protein may give rise to a new antibody specificity owing to a profound change in conformation, which might occur as a result of this single substitution.

There are two kinds of chemical structures that appear to influence immunogenicity: (1) the sequential determinants whose specificity is determined by the sequence of subunits within the determinant, e.g., primary amino acid sequence in the case of a protein, and (2) the conformational determinants that are determined by secondary, tertiary, or quaternary structure.

DIGESTIBILITY

In general, a potent immunogen is one that is capable of being phagocytosed and degraded within the host. Recent information has shown, however, that nonmetabolized or noncatabolized substances, such as polystyrene, can also be immunogenic in minute quantities. Moreover, it should be noted that the efficiency with which phagocytosis proceeds appears to determine whether an antigen is eliminated or persists. This outcome is of profound biologic significance, since the elimination of antigens will determine whether an immune response will be beneficial or harmful. With successful elimination of antigen, the outcome is beneficial; if antigen persists, the tertiary manifestations of immunity may result in tissue damage by any of the various mechanisms of immunologic injury (Chapters 13 and 20).

DIFFERENT CHEMICAL TYPES OF IMMUNOGENS

The overwhelming majority of immunogens in nature are protein. These may exist as pure proteins or combine with other substances such as lipids (lipoproteins), nucleic acids (nucleoproteins), or carbohydrates (glycoproteins). Shown in Table 4–4 are some examples of different chemical classes of immunogens.

Some examples of foreign proteins that may be immunogenic include serum and tissue proteins, the structural proteins of viruses, bacteria and other microorganisms, toxins, plant proteins, and enzymes. Antibodies to these substances are sometimes used clinically in immunotherapy (antitoxins) and in the preparation of certain vaccines (Chapters 23 and 24). On the other hand, when they lead to the production of antibodies that are deleterious, they may be responsible for some of the sequelae of the immunologically mediated diseases (Chapter 20). For example, following streptococcal infections, some antibodies that cross-react with cardiac tissue may be associated with some of the disease expressions of rheumatic fever. The lipoproteins are special types of protein immunogens that are found as part of many cell membranes.

Polysaccharides are another class of immunogens. They may occur as pure polysaccharide substances, as in the capsules of bacteria such as the pneumococcus, or they may be lipopolysaccharides occurring within cell walls of gram-negative bacteria (endotoxins). These substances are quite important biologically, since antibodies directed to them may provide protective immunity (antipneumococcal antibody). The lipopolysaccharides account for pathogenicity of certain gram-negative organisms, e.g., cholera endotoxin (Chapter 15).

The best known examples of glycoprotein antigens include the blood group substances A and B and the Rh antigens (Chapter 3). The immunogenicity of these substances has been associated with transfusion reactions and with isoimmunization of pregnancy (Chapter 20). In addition, the histocompatibility antigens (Chapter 3) are also composed of carbohydrate and protein. Polypeptide immunogens have

TABLE 4–4. Chemical Classes of Immunogens

TYPE	SOURCE
Protein	Serum proteins, microbial products (toxins), enzymes
Lipoprotein	Serum lipoproteins; cell membranes
Polysaccharides	Capsules of bacteria (pneumococcus)
Lipopolysaccharides	Cell walls of gram-negative bacteria (endotoxins)
Glycoproteins	Blood group substances A and B
Polypeptides	Hormones (insulin, growth hormones), synthetic compounds
Nucleic acids	Nucleoproteins, single-stranded DNA

been used experimentally in the form of synthetic polypeptides and have contributed to our understanding of many basic principles underlying immunogenicity. They are also used in clinical medicine, e.g., radioimmunoassay of insulin (Chapter 26). Their immunogenicity is at times undesirable, in which case the production of antibodies is associated with refractoriness to therapy, e.g., insulin antibodies.

The nucleic acids were for many years considered nonimmunogenic; however, under certain conditions, they may serve as immunogens, particularly when single-stranded. In patients with the disease systemic lupus erythematosus, circulating antibody to native DNA or other nuclear constituents can be demonstrated. The inflammatory response induced by these antibodies or complexes of DNA–anti-DNA is thought to be responsible for the tissue damage (to blood vessels, glomeruli, and so forth) (Chapter 20) associated with severe forms of the disease.

HOST-RELATED FACTORS

Immunogenicity has profound biologic implications. The response to any given immunogen not only is a function of the physicochemical properties of the substance, but also is connected with several host-related factors, including genetic makeup of the host, age, nutritional status, and any of a number of secondary effects that are derived from disease processes (Chapter 1). It should also be clearly understood that the measurement of any immunologic reactant to an immunogen should not necessarily be equated to a protective function in the host (Chapter 23). For example, it is known that the presence of circulating antibody in many types of localized viral infections does not prevent reinfection with these viruses (Chapter 16). Other factors of immunity also appear to be involved with the total host protection, e.g., secretory IgA antibody, as well as cell-mediated immunity.

It is now well established that live attenuated vaccines have greater clinical efficacy in the prevention of disease than do their killed or inactivated counterparts (Chapter 23). Further, serum antibody levels appear to be of longer duration following the use of live replicating vaccines or natural infection. Possibly owing to the continued persistence of immunogen, replicating agents may provide a more sustained stimulation of the immunologic system through the recruitment of additional immunocompetent cells. The methods used in preparation of an antigen may also have an adverse effect on the immunogenicity of a vaccine. Figure 4–2 shows group A streptococcus from which critical protective immunogens have been removed during processing. As can be seen, the dead vaccine contains neither the capsule nor the M proteins important in inducing protective immunity. Recently, the development of the swine influenza virus vaccine has been shown to lead to a vaccine deficient in neuraminidase, one of the viral antigens important in protective immunity to influenza viruses. Obviously, these are important considerations in the preparation of killed microbial vaccines that may lead to products that are not as effective in inducing protective immunity.

Immunogenicity varies from species to species and, within a given species, from individual to individual (Chapter 3). For example, although nonimmunogenic in the rabbit, the isolated polysaccharide capsule of the pneumococcus can lead to a full immune response in the mouse. However, if polysaccharide is injected as part of a whole bacterial suspension, the rabbit will produce antibody to these polysaccharides. When all physical and chemical requirements for immunogenicity are fulfilled, the capacity of a given individual or inbred strain of animal to respond to various immunogens is genetically determined. The genes controlling the immune response in the mouse (Ir genes) are found within the same complex as the major histocompatibility (H-2) locus. "Responder" and "nonresponder" strains of mice and guinea pigs have demonstrated the exquisite sensitivity of the immune response to minor variations of immunogen (Chapter 3).

The amount of immunogen injected also influences the response. Studies of immunologic tolerance illustrate that a very low or a very high dose of foreign material can inhibit future responses to the subsequent injection of an otherwise immunogenic dose (Chapter 10). Dose and intervals between injections have also been shown to produce antibody populations of differing titer and avidity.

The route of injection can influence the nature of the immune response. For example, certain immunogens, when injected parenterally, e.g., intravenously, lead to the production primarily of circulating antibody; when given intradermally, the same immunogen may also provoke cell-mediated immunity, in addition to circulating antibody. When assessing the immunogenicity of a preparation, the type of test assay must also be evaluated since false negative reactions may occur when test procedures lack sensitivity or specificity.

Finally, an important biologic property of immunogens is the ability of certain antigens to evoke allergic or hypersensitivity responses (Chapter 20). These reactions, which are expressions of the immune response, may either be cell-mediated or humoral. For example, when certain low molecular weight compounds such as the catechols from poison ivy contact the skin, a dermatitis will result that is mediated through sensitized lymphocytes (delayed hypersensitivity). On the other hand, penicillin, when combined with tissue proteins, will evoke an antibody response that may lead to anaphylactic shock or urticarial hives (immediate hypersensitivity). These allergic manifestations are biologic expressions of the immune response that are harmful — the immunologically mediated diseases (Chapter 20).

ADJUVANTS

Certain substances, referred to as adjuvants, enhance the immune response when injected together with an immunogen (Chapter 10). Their function has been considered to increase the surface area of antigen (e.g., alum-precipitated diphtheria toxoid) or to prolong their retention in the body, allowing time for the lymphoid system to have access to the antigen (Freund's adjuvant). Recent evidence suggests that adjuvants may selectively expand T- and B-lymphocyte populations in addition to their classic granuloma-producing effects. The current use of adjuvants in immunotherapy of cancer is described in Chapter 10.

SUMMARY

The term immunogen has been proposed to define any substance capable of evoking an immune response. The properties of an immunogen are determined by the physical, chemical, and biologic properties of the substance, which are in turn related to its primary structure. Certain chemical groupings on the immunogen that determine specificity of the immunologic reaction are referred to as determinant groups, the most potent of which are termed immunodominant points. Implicit in immunogenicity is the requirement for genetic dissimilarity and recognition of foreignness by the host's surveillance system. Thus, immunogenicity represents the net interplay of the physicochemical properties of the immunogen as well as the response of several host-related factors such as age, genetic makeup, and the general state of the host.

SUGGESTIONS FOR FURTHER READING

Borek, F. (ed.): Immunogenicity. North-Holland Research Monographs, Vol. 25, Amsterdam, North-Holland, 1972.

Benjamin, E., Scibienski, R. J., and Thompson, K.: The relationship between antigenic structure and immune specificity. *In* F. P. Inman (ed.): Contemporary Topics in Immunochemistry. Vol. I. New York, Plenum Press, 1972, pp. 1–43.

Goodman, J. W.: Immunogenicity and antigenic specificity. *In* H. H. Fudenberg, D. P. Stites, J. L. Caldwell, and J. V. Wells (eds.): Basic and Clinical Immunology. Los Altos, Lange Medical Publications, 1976.

Kabat, E. A.: Structural Concepts in Immunology and Immunochemistry. 2nd ed. New York, Holt, Rinehart and Winston, Inc., 1975.

Sela, M.: Antigenicity, some molecular aspects. Science, *166*:1365, 1969.

Sela, M.: Studies with synthetic polypeptides. Adv. Immunol., 5:29, 1966.

Williams, R. C., Jr. (ed.): Lymphocytes and Their Interactions. Kroc Foundation Series, Vol. 4. New York, Raven Press, 1977.

ANTIBODY AND IMMUNOGLOBULINS: STRUCTURE AND FUNCTION

George M. Bernier, M.D.

Immunoglobulins are a remarkable collection of protein molecules, which are the effector molecules of the humoral limb of immunity. These proteins share many antigenic, structural, and biologic similarities, but at the same time significant differences in primary amino acid sequence permit their antibody function and biologic activity to be highly specific for their role in bodily defense. Immunoglobulins are not simply molecules that combine with antigens in a "lock and key" fashion; they are very complex proteins with many highly specialized features in addition to their antigen-combining abilities. For example, to be effective, a human antibody to influenza virus might require several different structural capabilities: (1) a portion of the molecule that could combine specifically with the influenza virus and inhibit it; (2) another portion that could facilitate passage into the respiratory tract at the point of viral replication and permit a high concentration of such molecules in that region; and (3) a mechanism to prevent the molecule from being degraded by the proteolytic enzymes that abound in the respiratory tree. The human immune system has developed the kind of sophisticated specialization that permits this remarkable combination of properties to exist in a single molecular species known as secretory immunoglobulin A. Other equally distinctive features are associated with other kinds of immunoglobulins. As knowledge of the structure of immunoglobulins has developed, and in particular as the details of amino acid sequence have been revealed, the chemical basis of these and related phenomena has become more understandable.

HISTORY

The first real chemical information regarding the structure of antibodies was provided by Tiselius and Kabat in the early 1940's. These workers demonstrated that the fraction of serum proteins, the gamma globulins, that migrated most slowly in electrophoresis contained most of the serum antibodies. In the 1950's, Porter treated antibodies with papain, a proteolytic enzyme, which splits the antibody molecules into three fragments; two retained antibody activity and one possessed most of the antigenic features of gamma globulin. In the early 1960's, Edel-

115

man demonstrated that immunoglobulins were multichain structures, and a four-chain model of immunoglobulins was proposed by Porter. Putnam and Titani and Hilschmann and Craig initiated the studies of amino acid sequence of immunoglobulins using Bence Jones proteins, which are excreted in the urine of patients with multiple myeloma (Chapter 21). Determination of the amino acid sequence of the first complete immunoglobulin, an IgG myeloma protein, was completed in 1969 by Edelman and coworkers. In the 1970's, the primary sequence of a great many immunoglobulin molecules, myeloma proteins as well as more normally occurring antibodies, was determined, and it is anticipated that the basic primary structure of all immunoglobulin classes will be known by the end of this decade.

Just as studies into the chemical nature of immunoglobulins were extremely fruitful, investigations into the complex biology of immunoglobulins clarified the function of the various kinds or classes of immunoglobulins.

In all these studies, the proteins elaborated by plasma cell tumors of man and mouse have proved to be of tremendous value in understanding the biologic and particularly the chemical features of immunoglobulins.

THE FAMILY OF IMMUNOGLOBULINS

In man, five different classes of immunoglobulins are known to exist, each with a distinct chemical structure and a specific biologic role. These classes are designated by the letters G, A, M, D, and E following the abbreviation Ig (indicating their immunoglobulin function), or by some writers, following the symbol γ (indicating their electrophoretic mobility as gamma globulins). In Table 5–1, some of the properties of each class of immunoglobulins are listed.

IgG is the most abundant of the immunoglobulins. These molecules achieve significant concentrations in both the vascular and extravascular spaces, have a relatively long half-life (23 days), cross the placenta and are able to activate complement. This class of immunoglobulin is thought to contribute to immunity against many infecting agents that have a blood-borne dissemination, including bacteria, viruses, parasites, and some fungi (Chapters 15, 16, 17, and 18). In addition, it provides antibody activity in tissues. Receptors for IgG exist on human monocytes, on some lymphocytes, and, curiously, on guinea pig skin.

Although IgA is the second most abundant serum immunoglobulin, its most important contribution to the immunity of the individual is in the external secretory system. This important secretory immunoglobulin is produced in high concentrations by the lymphoid tissues lining the gastrointestinal, respiratory, and genitourinary tracts. In these

TABLE 5–1. Some Physical and Biologic Properties of Human Immunoglobulin Classes

Class	Mean Serum Concentration (mg/100 ml)	Molecular Weight	$S_{20,w}$	Mean Survival T/2 (days)	Biologic Function	Heavy Chain Designation	No. of Subclasses
IgG or γG	1240	150,000	7	23	1. Fix complement 2. Cross placenta 3. Heterocytotropic antibody	γ	4
IgA or γA	280	170,000	7, 10, 14	6	1. Secretory antibody 2. Properdin pathway	α	2
IgM or γM	120	890,000	19	5	1. Fix complement 2. Efficient agglutination	μ	1
IgD or γD	3	150,000	7	2.8	1. Lymphocyte surface receptor	δ	2
IgE or γE	.03	196,000	8	1.5	1. Reaginic antibody 2. Homocytotropic antibody	ε	1

secretions (e.g., saliva, tears) IgA is combined with a protein termed *secretory component* that appears to endow the molecule with some protection against the effects of the proteolytic enzymes normally found in these regions. The IgA molecules do not activate complement by the classic pathway but may do so via the properdin system. IgA does not cross the placenta; however, it contributes to the immunity of the newborn by virtue of its high concentration in colostrum.

IgM is the largest of the immunoglobulin molecules and, because of its large size, is restricted almost entirely to the intravascular space. These macromolecules are highly efficient agglutinators of particulate antigens such as bacteria and red blood cells, and they fix complement with a high degree of efficiency (Chapter 6). This class of immunoglobulin seems to be of greatest importance in the first few days of the primary immune response. When a foreign antigen is introduced into a host for the first time, the synthesis of IgM and IgG antibodies begins almost simultaneously; however, the level of IgM antibodies peaks within a few days and then declines more rapidly than the level of IgG antibodies (Chapter 7).

The fourth class of immunoglobulins, IgD, was discovered in the mid-1960's by Rowe and Fahey when they encountered a myeloma protein antigenically and chemically different from the then known immunoglobulins. To date, IgD has not been assigned a clear specific biologic role. Antibody activity has been associated with IgD globulin, for example in cases of penicillin hypersensitivity in the human. This immunoglobulin class is found on the surface of lymphocytes, particularly in neonates, with a frequency that far exceeds its relative serum concentration. Hence, a role for IgD as a specific surface receptor in the initiation of the immune response is possible (Chapter 7).

The reaginic antibody, IgE, is an immunoglobulin present in only trace amounts in serum. It has the ability to attach to human skin (homocytotropic antibody) and to initiate aspects of the "allergic reaction" (Chapters 8 and 13). IgE was initially isolated by Ishizaka, who purified it from vast quantities of serum containing reaginic antibody. Subsequently, a few myeloma proteins of the IgE class have been identified. Like IgA, IgE is produced chiefly in the linings of the respiratory and intestinal tracts and is part of the external secretory system of antibody (Chapter 2). Deficiency of IgE has been inconstantly associated with deficiency of IgA in individuals with impaired immunity who present with undue susceptibility to infection (Chapter 22).

SUBCLASSES

By antigenic analysis, it has been possible to detect relatively minor differences between molecules of a given class of immunoglobulin (Table 5–1). In this way, four different subclasses of IgG have been found and designated IgG1, IgG2, IgG3, and IgG4. In addition, two subclasses each for IgA and IgD globulins have been found and are termed IgA1 and IgA2 and IgD1 and IgD2, respectively. Subsequent chemical analysis has shown that subclass antigenic differences reflect substantial differences in amino acid sequence. As indicated below, important biologic distinctions have been correlated with the various subclasses. For example, IgG4 does not fix complement, whereas the other three IgG subclasses do; and IgG3 globulins have a half-life significantly shorter than that of the other three. A major chemical difference between subclasses is the location and number of interchain disulfide bridges.

CHAIN STRUCTURE OF IMMUNOGLOBULIN

The classification of immunoglobulins, as described above, was made on the basis of antigenic and structural considerations; the real basis for this classification is found in the chemical structure of the molecule. The IgG antibody molecule, for instance, is made up of four polypeptide chains held together by disulfide bonds (Fig. 5–1). Two of the chains are small, with molecular weights of 22,000, and are termed "light chains." The other two, with molecular weights of 55,000, are called "heavy chains." Each immunoglobulin molecule has two identical heavy chains and two identical light chains. A chemically different kind of heavy chain exists for each of the five classes of immunoglobulin and is responsible for the antigenic differences that have been observed between classes. More important, it is the heavy chain that is responsible for the observed biologic differences between the various classes.

Just as there are five kinds of heavy chains, two different *types* of light chains have been found to exist. The light-chain types are called

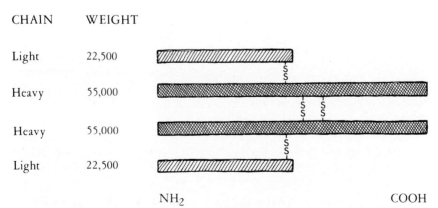

CHAIN	WEIGHT		
Light	22,500		
Heavy	55,000		
Heavy	55,000		
Light	22,500		

NH$_2$ COOH

Figure 5–1. Schematic diagram of human IgG1 showing the location of interchain disulfide bonds. The molecule consists of two light chains and two heavy chains. The amino-terminal end is at the left and the carboxyl-terminal end is at the right. The structure depicted here is also applicable to other immunoglobulins with varying heavy-chain composition and polymerization.

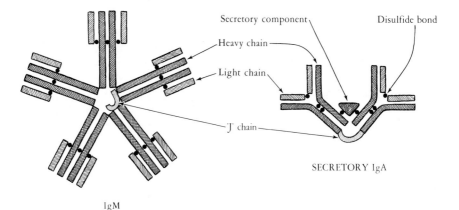

Figure 5-2. Models of IgM and secretory IgA. The former is shown in its usual pentameric form with a J chain involved in the pentamer formation. Secretory IgA is shown as a dimer attached to a secretory component. Note the absence of the light-heavy interchain bonds in the IgA. The IgA predominant in secretions is of the IgA 2 subclass, which lacks such bonds.

kappa (κ) and lambda (λ) (for the pair of investigators who originally observed the two types—Korngold and Lipari). Each type of light chain occurs in association with each kind of heavy chain, i.e., in each of the five classes of immunoglobulins. There are 10 possible combinations of heavy and light chains and all 10 are normally found in any individual. As indicated in Table 5-1, the five kinds of heavy chains are identified by the Greek-letter equivalent of their class name—γ, α, μ, δ, and ϵ. Any immunoglobulin may therefore be designated by its heavy- and light-chain composition, in a manner analogous to the hemoglobin nomenclature. An IgG molecule, for example, would have a formula $\gamma_2\kappa_2$ or $\gamma_2\lambda_2$.

This basic four-chain structural unit is the form in which IgG, IgD, and IgE exist. A four-chain unit is repeated in the higher molecular weight immunoglobulins; IgM generally exists as a pentamer of basic four-chain subunits with each of five subunits held together by disulfide bonds (Fig. 5-2). A relatively small molecule with high sulfhydryl content, the *J chain* participates in the polymerization of IgM. The IgM subunits (180,000 daltons) are each made up of two μ heavy chains (67,000 daltons) and two light chains.

IgA globulin, and occasionally IgG globulin, may also exist in a polymeric form in serum. Serum IgA, like IgM, may be polymerized through a sulfhydryl residue near the carboxyl terminus of the molecule, with the participation of J chain. In secretions, two IgA monomers are linked together by J chain and *secretory component* (another non-immunoglobulin) to produce a complex of high molecular weight (Figs. 5-2 and 5-3).

As described before, it has been possible to classify IgA globulins into two subclasses, IgA1 and IgA2, based upon differences in antigenic structure and variation in the arrangement of interchain disulfide bridges. Whereas the IgA2 is a minor component of serum IgA, this subclass is the dominant form in secretions. Curiously, no covalent bonding exists between light and heavy chains in this subclass (Fig. 5–2). It has been noted that the IgA globulins are synthesized as monomers within plasma cells, which also synthesize J chain and are in contiguity with epithelial cells, containing the secretory component. After passage through the epithelium, IgA is recovered as a dimer, complexed with the secretory component (Fig. 5–3).

Just as the arrangement of interchain disulfide bonds is different in IgA subclasses, so, too, are there differences in the interchain bonds in the various IgG subclasses (Fig. 5–4). The biologic significance of these differences is not readily apparent but they may account for some observed differences in such functions as life span or susceptibility to

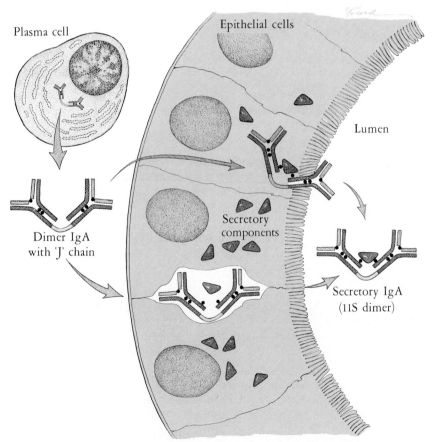

Figure 5–3. Representational drawing depicting the formation of secretory IgA. The IgA globulins are synthesized as monomers but are secreted from the plasma cells as dimers linked by the J chain. As the molecule passes through or in between the epithelial cells, it acquires the secretory component and enters the lumen as the secretory IgA molecule.

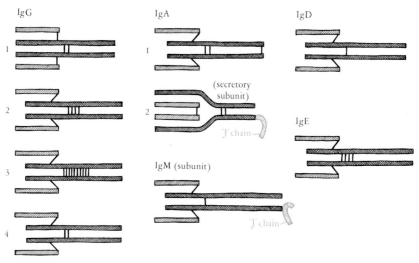

Figure 5-4. Arrangement of peptide chains in various subclasses of immunoglobulins. Disulfide bonds are represented by black bars. In the IgA and IgM subunits, the J chain, in gray, indicates where it would appear in the respective polymeric forms.

proteolytic degradation. For example, the IgG2 subclass has four heavy-heavy interchain bonds and is quite resistant to papain hydrolysis, as will be described below. Pathologically, the differences may be quite important, too. Myeloma globulins of the IgG3 subclass have an asymmetric structure because of the unusually long hinge region, and the abnormal viscosity this imparts to the blood of individuals with myeloma involving this Ig subclass may create serious problems.

ANTIBODY FUNCTION

An antibody produced in response to one antigen obviously must have structural features that are different from an antibody produced in response to any other antigen. Antibody to tetanus, for example, must differ in some chemically definable way from antibody to diphtheria, since both antibodies can be shown to combine specifically with their homologous antigens. This property, known as *specificity*, is determined by the primary amino acid sequence of the antibody molecule. For example, reduction of disulfide bonds and disruption of all noncovalent forces by dispersing agents such as 8 M urea will unfold the polypeptide chains of the molecule, with loss of antibody function. When the molecule is reconstituted by oxidation and removal of the dispersing agent, the antibody will re-form and regain its capacity for combination with its specific antigen.

The "antigen-binding site" or "antibody active site" of the immunoglobulin molecule is the region that combines with a specific an-

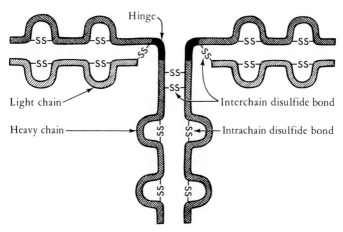

Figure 5–5. Schematic drawing of IgG in T-shaped model. The light chains are shaded by diagonal lines and the heavy chains marked with cross-hatching. The hinge region is depicted in black. Disulfide bridges are represented by –SS–. The intrachain disulfide bonds pinch the chains into loops (domains). Extensive overall similarity is apparent in the placement of these loops between light and heavy chains and between the two portions of the heavy chains.

tigen. In this region, the antibody specificity is determined by the amino acid sequence that permits its combination with the appropriate antigen. Both heavy and light chains share in this site; specifically, the first 110 amino acids from the amino-terminal end of each polypeptide chain are known to house antibody activity. In Figure 5–5, the IgG molecule is represented in a T-shaped configuration. The amino-terminal regions of variability on both the heavy and light chains make up the antibody active sites. It is the amino acid sequence in these regions that dictates the specificity of the antibody. The mechanism by which variability of amino acid sequence occurs, however, is uncertain. In IgG, IgD, and IgE, two antigen-binding sites exist per molecule; in IgM, 10 such sites exist; in dimeric IgA, such as is found in secretions, four combining sites are present.

A feature critical to the understanding of the overall structure of immunoglobulins is the symmetric arrangement of regions or *domains* for each of approximately 110 amino acids. These domains serve their own functions yet share some sequence homology. An immunoglobulin chain is composed of linked domains — two in light chains; 4 in the γ, α, and δ chains; and 5 in the μ and ϵ chains. In heavy chains, a nonhomologous stretch, the hinge region, separates the first two domains of the heavy chain from the other heavy chain domains (Fig. 5–5).

FRAGMENTATION OF IMMUNOGLOBULINS

Knowledge of the structure of the immunoglobulins has been greatly enhanced by the use of proteolytic enzymes, which degrade the

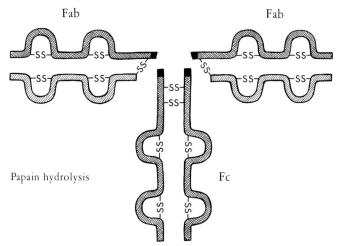

Fab   Fab

Papain hydrolysis   Fc

Figure 5–6. Schematic representation of the fragmentation of the IgG molecule by papain, which results in two Fab fragments and one Fc fragment. The Fab fragments possess one antigen-combining site each and can combine with, but may not give a visible reaction with, antigen. The Fc fragment lacks antigen-binding capabilities but retains many antigenic and biologic properties of IgG.

molecule into definable fragments. *Papain* was shown by Porter to split the heavy chains of IgG in the hinge region, the area of the interchain disulfide bonds, yielding three fragments. One fragment, which can be crystallized, contains most of the IgG specific antigenic determinants of the molecule and is designated the Fc fragment; the other two fragments retain the ability to combine with antigen and are designated the Fab fragments (Fig. 5–6). Although of the same approximate size, the fragments differ strikingly in their function. Table 5–2 lists the composition and biologic activities associated with each. An attempt has been made in this table to describe the structure and function of the fragments in a format that is, if not memorable, at least mnemonic.

Another proteolytic enzyme, *pepsin*, acts upon the IgG molecule by

TABLE 5–2. Fragments of IgG Produced by Papain Cleavage

	FAB	FC
Composition:	1. **A**mino-terminal half of heavy chain and one light chain 2. **Ab**errated sequence	1. **C**arboxyl-terminal half of heavy chain dimer 2. **C**arbohydrate 3. **C**rystallizable (in some species) 4. **C**onstant amino acid sequence
Function:	1. **A**ntigen-binding or **a**ntibody active fragment	1. **C**omplement fixation 2. **C**ross placenta 3. **C**utaneous attachment (guinea pig skin)

$F(ab')_2$

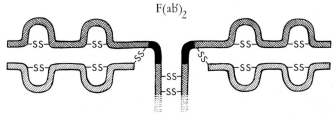

Pepsin digestion

Figure 5–7.   Schematic representation of the degradation of IgG by pepsin. The Fc portion is hydrolyzed below the interchain disulfide bonds, leaving a single fragment with two combining sites intact, the $F(ab')_2$.

degrading the heavy chain, beginning at the carboxyl-terminal end and proceeding to the region of the interchain disulfide bridge (Fig. 5–7). The splitting with *papain* produces univalent antibody fragments that can combine with antigens but not precipitate them; the *pepsin* treatment leaves a fragment that possesses two antigen-binding sites and can therefore still precipitate antigens. This fragment, termed $F(ab')_2$, has lost most of the specific antigenic determinants of IgG, since most of these are located in the carboxyl-terminal half of the γ heavy chain (Fc fragment).

In addition to the Fab, $F(ab')_2$, and Fc fragments, one other portion of the IgG molecule has been named. The term "Fd" is used to designate the amino-terminal half of the heavy chain, i.e., the half of the heavy chain located in the Fab fragment (Fig. 5–8). This region of the heavy chain is of great biologic importance, since it shares in the antigen-binding site, and provides thermodynamically a lion's share of the binding affinity to antigen.

Fd

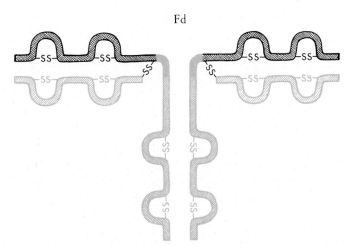

Figure 5–8.   Molecular location of the Fd fragment of IgG is indicated in black. The light chains and the Fc portion of the heavy chain are represented in gray.

Trypsin has been employed in two different ways in the fragmentation of immunoglobulins. Prolonged digestion with trypsin results in cleavage of the peptide chain next to all arginine and lysine residues and the production of "tryptic peptides." These peptides may be examined by a combination of electrophoresis and chromatography, a technique called "fingerprinting" or "peptide mapping." This method has proved valuable in comparing the structure of two or more proteins, since it provides information about the comparative primary amino acid sequence without requiring exhaustive sequence analysis. The technique has been very useful in studies of variant human hemoglobins and in the study of human and animal immunoglobulins. Shorter periods of digestion of IgG or IgM with trypsin produce fragments similar to those derived by papain hydrolysis.

The other immunoglobulins can also be fragmented by proteolytic enzymes, but the fragments produced are not necessarily comparable to those derived from IgG globulin. For instance, papain digestion of IgA globulin often destroys the Fc portion of the molecule. However, in all immunoglobulin molecules, the regions are named according to the system described for the IgG globulin, i.e., Fab, Fc, and Fd.

An enzyme produced by enteric streptococci has been found to have proteolytic activity specific for the IgA1 subclass. This enzyme cleaves IgA1 molecules in the hinge region and produces fragments quite similar in size to the Fab and Fc fragments of IgG. While at first blush this is a tribute to the evolutionary adaptability of enteric streptococci, in fact, the dominant form of IgA in the human intestinal tract is IgA2, a molecule impervious to the protease. Hence, it would appear that the human intestinal tract has emerged as victor in this particular evolutionary battle.

GENETIC FACTORS ASSOCIATED WITH IMMUNOGLOBULINS: GM, INV, AND AM FACTORS

Genetic markers have been found to be carried on immunoglobulin molecules (Chapter 7). The first two identified were designated Gm and Inv factors and were detected by the following indirect method.

The sera of some patients with rheumatoid arthritis agglutinate red blood cells coated with human gamma globulin. The anti-gamma globulin antibody contained in the sera of these individuals is called "rheumatoid factor" (RF) (Chapter 20C). The reaction between the rheumatoid factor from a particular person and gamma globulin–coated red cells was found to be inhibited by preincubation of the rheumatoid serum with serum from some normal persons. Some normal sera inhibited a particular rheumatoid factor reaction; others did not. The ability to inhibit a particular reaction was found to be inherited in a mendelian fashion, and the inhibitory substances in normal serum have been shown to be immunoglobulins. A number of hereditary factors reflecting different loci have been uncovered in this way and are associated with the various IgG heavy chains or with the κ-type light chain. Those factors associated with the heavy chain of IgG are termed Gm (for gamma) and those associated with the κ light chain are called Inv (the abbreviation of a patient's name) or sometimes Km, using analogous reasoning. There are more than 20 recognized Gm factors and three Inv factors. As shown more recently (see Table 5–1), four different subclasses of IgG have been detected, and the various Gm factors are associated with one of these subclasses. The chemical basis for the Gm and Inv factors will be described later. It is important to point out that the Gm and Inv factors are nonallelic—that is, they are inherited independently of each other.

Another independently inherited group of genetic markers associated with IgA has been described. The reagents for identifying such factors have arisen as a result of transfusion. Some patients have been immunized in this way with an IgA genetically different from their own. Anti-IgA allotypic antibodies have thus been inadvertently produced, and their clinical manifestations have been transfusion reactions ranging from mild to severe. Different genetic factors have been found, and the term "Am" (referring to the IgA equivalent of Gm) has been applied to the system.

In all three systems (Gm, Inv. and Am), the detecting antibody is of human origin. In the first two it is frequently a rheumatoid factor but, like the third factor, it is sometimes transfusion-induced. Since chemical differences between allotypes are minimal (one amino acid in

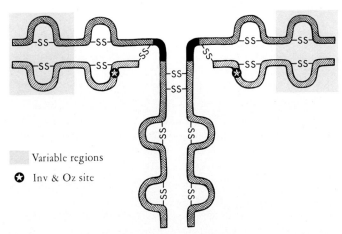

Figure 5–9. In this drawing, the regions of sequence variability are depicted in gray. Note that the variable segment of the light chain is in apposition to the variable segment of the heavy chain—this is the region of antibody specificity. The antigenic markers Inv and Oz are indicated by ✪ . The Gm markers are localized in constant regions of the heavy chains and are probably the result of minor amino acid sequence variation.

the case of the Inv factor), detection has required antibodies generated in the same species. Allotypic differences between proteins of other species have been sought and detected immunologically by immunization within the species, under the assumption that the immunized animal's recognition system will detect minor differences between the immunizing antigen and its own proteins rather than the larger differences existing between proteins of different species.

As might be anticipated, the various Gm factors are associated with specific subclasses of IgG, and the various Am factors are similarly associated with specific subclasses of IgA. To date, in the human system no allotypic markers have been found for the λ light chain or the μ, δ, or ε heavy chain.

PRIMARY STRUCTURE OF IMMUNOGLOBULINS

HETEROGENEITY

An aspect of antibodies that is of paramount interest to the protein biochemist has paradoxically proved to be a major impediment to the understanding of immunoglobulins as protein molecules. This aspect is the unique situation of the extreme chemical heterogeneity of the gamma globulins occurring in the face of a degree of chemical constancy. By way of illustration, albumin, transferrin, and most other serum proteins have a discrete electrophoretic mobility that is a manifestation of chemical homogeneity. Genetic variation in these serum proteins, as in the case of the human hemoglobins, often results in charge differences, which in turn are manifested as different electrophoretic forms. In contrast, the immunoglobulins of all individuals are spread over a very wide electrophoretic range. This electrophoretic variation is most apparent in the case of IgG globulin and is readily illustrated by immunoelectrophoresis, which disperses the IgG molecules from the extreme cathodal end of the electrophoretic field almost all the way to the anode. The extreme electrophoretic heterogeneity of these molecules reflects a degree of variation in primary sequence that is remarkable among protein species. From what has been said before, this heterogeneity is obviously a manifestation of class, subclass, type, and genetic variation. More importantly, however, it reflects the chemical basis of antibody variability, i.e., of those differences, for instance, that distinguish an antitetanus antibody from an antidiphtheria antibody.

Even when antibodies of a single specificity have been isolated, they too have been electrophoretically heterogeneous. It has been, therefore, most difficult to study the basis of chemical variability by analyzing antibodies themselves, because it is virtually impossible to establish the amino acid sequence in regions of variability. Instead, the problem has been approached by analyzing the homogeneous immunoglobulins produced in some malignant conditions that affect lymphocytes and plasma cells, notably in the human disease states of multiple myeloma and macroglobulinemia and in the mouse plasmacytoma system (Chapter 21).

These disorders are characterized by the elaboration of large amounts of homogeneous immunoglobulins by proliferating cells. Such immunoglobulins are found in the serum or urine of affected individuals. The term "monoclonal" has been applied to the homogeneous immunoglobulin, implying that it is a consequence of the proliferation of a single clone of plasma cells. The proteins elaborated may be complete immunoglobulin molecules of IgG, IgA, IgM, IgD, or IgE class, or free light chains (Bence Jones proteins), or both. In very rare human conditions, such as the heavy chain diseases, fragments or portions of immunoglobulin chains or molecules are produced.

Because of their homogeneity and their availability in great abundance, the monoclonal immunoglobulins are chemically suitable for amino acid sequence analysis. Much of the information relating to primary amino acid sequence derived from studies of such proteins has been applied to normal immunoglobulins. The rationale for using these abnormal immunoglobulins as models for normal antibody is based upon the following observations and suppositions:

(1) Each complete monoclonal immunoglobulin appears to be one of the many normal immunoglobulins. The monoclonal proteins differ from pools of immunoglobulin in terms of restricted electrophoretic mobility, restricted expressions of biologic properties, chain type, genetic markers, and physical properties. However, no unique pathologic features, such as novel amino acids, unusual prosthetic groups, or excessive lengths of peptide chains, have been found in any of the complete monoclonal immunoglobulins.

(2) Many monoclonal immunoglobulins have been found to possess antibody activity. Indeed, the frequency of finding monoclonal immunoglobulins with antibody specificity seems proportional to the intensity of the search, and it is likely that all the monoclonal proteins would be *bona fide* antibodies, if only appropriate antigens could be found.

Each monoclonal immunoglobulin possesses distinctive antigenic and chemical features. To date, complete identity has not been established between the monoclonal immunoglobulins produced by any two individuals. Even in the case of free light chains of one type (κ or λ) that have a molecular weight of only 22,500, no two have been identical. The chemical and antigenic differences are termed "idiotypic markers," in contrast to the "allotypic markers" (Gm, Inv, and Am). If one assumes that one monoclonal immunoglobulin differs from another in the same way and to the same extent that one "normal" antibody molecule differs from another, then detailed examination of relatively few monoclonal immunoglobulins would be expected to provide information about the molecular location of variability, the extent of variability, and the genetic mechanisms responsible for the variability. It is of considerable interest that the major antigenic and chemical differences that exist between myeloma proteins occur in that portion of the molecule in which variations between antibodies of different specificities occur.

The sequence of a wide variety of monoclonal immunoglobulins has been determined, and extensive amino acid sequence information is available to aid in the understanding of immunoglobulins.

LIGHT CHAINS

Bence Jones proteins from myeloma patients and from mice with plasmacytomas were the first to be studied in appreciable numbers, and the following generalizations can be made. Two types of light chains exist throughout the vertebrate world: κ and λ. In various species one or the other is a predominant form. In man, approximately twice as many molecules have κ light chains as have λ chains. Light chains have been found to possess a region of constancy and a region of variability. The molecular topography of these regions is illustrated in Figure 5–10, and it is apparent that light chains are composed of two approximately equal halves—one constant and the other variable. The sequence of the carboxyl half of the molecule is virtually constant from one κ-type Bence Jones protein to another, or from one λ-type Bence Jones protein to another. Although a degree of homology is present (approximately 40 per cent), the κ chains are very different from the λ chains in this region, i.e., the constant region or domain.

In the amino-terminal half of the molecule, extensive variability is found between Bence Jones proteins of the same antigenic type. The transition from variable to constant region is an abrupt one. When larger numbers of Bence Jones proteins have been examined, it has become apparent that subgrouping of κ and λ chains is possible, based on overall similarity in the amino-terminal half. The variability in this half within a given subgroup is considerably less and is of the kind that would result from changes in single base pairs. Approximately five different subgroups of each light-chain type have been determined on this basis.

There is one notable exception to the pattern of constancy in the carboxyl-terminal half of light chains. In κ chains, either leucine or valine is found at position 191 and confers one of two genetic factors (Inv1 or Inv3, respectively). The great theoretic importance of this is that by inheritance of these markers the carboxyl-terminal half of the light chain can be shown to be transmitted according to mendelian principles. This will be described later as it applies to the genetic theories of antibody variability.

Another factor, called "Oz", is found in an analogous position in the λ chain (position 190), where an arginine-lysine interchange determines the presence or absence of an antigenic determinant. Unlike the

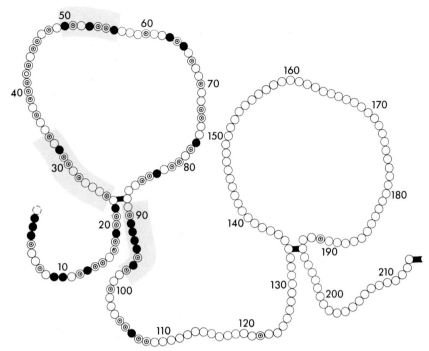

Figure 5–10. Composite drawing of human κ chain sequences illustrating variation in amino acid sequence among several different κ-type Bence Jones proteins. The amino-terminal end of the peptide chain is at the left, the carboxyl terminal at the right. Each circle represents one of the 214 amino acids of the chain. The *white* circles ○ indicate residues where only one amino acid was found. The *shaded* circles ◎ designate positions where two alternate amino acids were detected, and the *black* circles ● indicate positions where three or more different amino acids occurred. Disulfide bonds are indicated by black bars. The variable sequence is confined almost entirely to the amino-terminal half of the molecule. The carboxyl-terminal half is quite constant and the notable variation occurs at position 191, the site of the Inv genetic marker. The gray areas indicate the hypervariable areas that are apparent when sequences of human κ and λ chains and mouse κ chains are compared.

Inv determinant, this is not a genetic factor, since all persons produce some λ chains with the Oz determinant and some λ chains without it.

HEAVY CHAINS

The primary sequence of the heavy chains is different for each of the various immunoglobulin classes, but the amino acid sequence variation of the heavy chains is very similar to that observed in light chains. The amino-terminal end, comprising the first 110 or so amino acids, is the area of variable sequence and is termed the *variable domain* of the heavy chain, or the V_H domain. The remaining residues represent regions of relative constancy and are termed constant regions or *constant domains* (Fig. 5–11). These are named according to the kind of

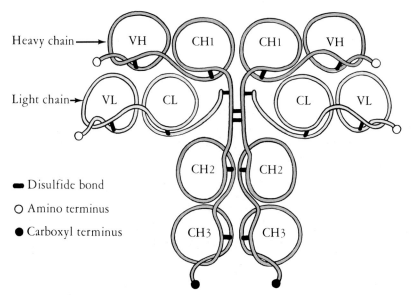

Heavy chain ⟶
Light chain ⟶

VH   CH1   CH1   VH
VL   CL   CL   VL
CH2   CH2
CH3   CH3

● Disulfide bond
○ Amino terminus
● Carboxyl terminus

Figure 5–11. Schematic drawing of IgG in a T-shaped model. Each peptide chain is drawn as a continuous line, and attachments between heavy and light chains and between the two heavy chains are indicated by solid bars. Note the two loops in each light chain and the four loops in each heavy chain. These loops are formed by intrachain disulfide bonds and are termed "domains." In each chain, one domain (V) has a *variable* amino acid sequence depending on the antibody specificity of the molecule. The other domains (C) have a rather *constant* sequence common among molecules of the same class, subclass, and type. They are numbered in sequence from the amino-terminal end.

peptide chain (γ, α, μ, δ, ϵ) and the relative position in the chain sequence (amino to carboxyl terminus). For example, in an IgG molecule, the domains would be identified in order as V_H . . . $C\gamma_1$ . . . $C\gamma_2$ . . . $C\gamma_3$. In the heavy chain of IgM, which is larger by one domain, the order would be V_H . . . $C\mu_1$ . . . $C\mu_2$ . . . $C\mu_3$ . . . $C\mu_4$.

Each constant domain of each kind of heavy chain has a distinctive amino acid sequence. However, there exists a significant degree of homology from constant domain to constant domain within a peptide chain and between heavy chains of various classes. It is interesting, from an evolutionary viewpoint, that greater similarities exist between a given domain in different heavy chains than between two different domains in the same heavy chain. For example, the $C\alpha_2$ is more like the $C\gamma_2$ than the $C\alpha_3$. This would argue that class divergence occurred after basic immunoglobulin structure was established.

Two important points must be made concerning the V_H regions. These domains appear in every kind of heavy chain and are not distinctive for any class. The V_H of a particular IgG molecule may be more like the V_H of an IgM than that of another IgG. Also, just as subtypes of light-chain variable regions are evident from comparative amino acid sequence, so can the variable regions of heavy chains be subgrouped into V_{HI}, V_{HII}, V_{HIII} . . . . Within a given subgroup, the variation in sequence is much less, as is true of the light chains.

Myeloma globulins have provided the prototype models for analysis in establishing these structural considerations. Although the chemical basis was determined by peptide mapping and amino acid sequence analysis, it has been possible to obtain a significant amount of information from immunologic analysis. It is possible, for instance, to recognize the unique variable region of a given myeloma globulin by immunizing rabbits with the monoclonal protein and absorbing the resultant antiserum with normal immunoglobulins. Antisera so prepared often (but not always) continue to react with the variable domains of the immunizing globulin and can distinguish this monoclonal globulin from all others. The antigens recognized in this way are called "idiotypic" antigens and the antisera are termed "anti-idiotype."

By employing antisera made specific for the idiotypic markers of a monoclonal immunoglobulin, it is possible to identify the presence of similar idiotypic markers in cells, on cell surfaces, and in trace amounts in the serum of patients. Anti-idiotypic antibodies have been used to identify antibodies of a common specificity in inbred rabbits.

THREE-DIMENSIONAL STRUCTURE

Immunoglobulins have been visualized by the negative staining technique of electron microscopy. X-ray crystallography has also been applied to the study of immunoglobulins, particularly crystallizable monoclonal immunoglobulins, and electron microscopy has been used in the study of sections of such crystalline IgG molecules. By a variety of physical methods, the IgG molecule appears to be composed of three principal units (one Fc and two Fab's). There appears to be a significant amount of flexibility in the hinge region between the Fc and Fab's, with the molecule able to assume a "Y" or "T" shape, depending on its association with antigen.

Each of the major fragments has dimensions of approximately 50 $\times$ 40 $\times$ 70 Å. Hence the "wing span" of the molecule across the Fab's is approximately 130 to 140 Å (Fig. 5–12).

From hapten-binding studies, as well as physical measurements, the combining site would appear to be a crevice involving the light and heavy chain in the range of 15 Å deep.

Polymeric molecules such as secretory IgA and pentameric IgM have been observed by means of electron microscopy. The striking feature of the IgM molecules is their rosette-like structure, similar to that shown schematically in Figure 5–2.

EVOLUTIONARY ASPECTS

A feature common to both heavy and light chains is the location of the intrachain disulfide bonds. As described earlier, these are so situ-

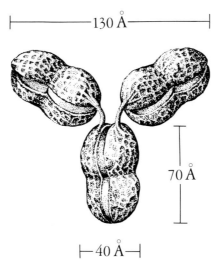

Figure 5-12. Three-dimensional model of IgG showing the close relationship between domains in each of the Fab fragments and in the Fc fragment. The compact areas are linked through the hinge region. This model is based on the studies of X-ray crystallography and electron microscopy.

ated that the peptide chains are "pinched" into a series of loops of approximately 60 amino acids each. Two loops are found in each light chain, four are found in each IgG, IgA, and IgD heavy chain, and five are found in each IgM and IgE heavy chain. The loops are depicted in highly schematic fashion in Figures 5-10 and 5-11. The recurring periodicity of such loops or domains suggests that the complex immunoglobulin molecule has evolved from a primitive peptide chain approximately 110 amino acids long. A significant degree of homology is found among the various domains of light and heavy chains, and this gives credence to the concept of a common primitive progenitor. It is important to point out that as the particular peptide chains exist today, the differences are more pronounced between classes than between species. For instance, the κ chain of man is closer in sequence to the κ chain of the mouse than it is to the λ chain of man. From a phylogenetic point of view, a low molecular weight IgM class of immunoglobulin appears to be the most primitive of the extant immunoglobulins.

Of considerable interest along these lines is β_2 microglobulin, an 11,600 dalton cell surface protein associated with the HLA antigen system. This protein, which is found free in body fluids, has the characteristics of a free domain in that it has a disulfide-bonded loop of 60 amino acids. The β_2 microglobulin has a 20+ per cent homology with virtually every constant domain of every immunoglobulin. It is possible that the earliest forms of immunoglobulins were cell surface–associated protective molecules.

THE GENESIS OF ANTIBODY VARIABILITY

Under appropriate conditions, the introduction of a foreign antigen into a man or an animal results in the production of specific antibody. Two broad mechanisms have been invoked to explain the phenomenon of specificity as it occurs in the immune response. The selection theories hold that cells already committed to production of a particular antibody are stimulated by the introduction of antigen to proliferate and elaborate their product. According to the instructional theories, the antigen interacts in some way with the antibody-forming cells, modifying the antibody that is produced. In their most extreme forms, the selection theory would require a separate germ-line gene for each of the myriad antibodies; and the instructional theory would operate with a single highly plastic antibody. The purely instructional theory is untenable because of (1) the evidence of variable primary sequence derived from the study of monoclonal immunoglobulins and some antibodies, and (2) the dependence of antibody specificity upon primary sequence. This has been shown by experiments already cited, in which activity has been regenerated following initial disruption of the antibody by dispersing agents and disulfide reduction. These experiments indicate that the primary sequence dictates the tertiary one and hence is the most important aspect in determining antibody specificity.

In contrast to the usual "one gene–one polypeptide chain" concept that had been the keystone of molecular biology, a novel theory had to be invoked to explain the origin of antibody variability. A "two genes–one polypeptide chain" concept was proposed to account for the constant and variable portions of the immunoglobulin peptide chain. According to the concept, one gene (a "C" gene) encodes the constant half of the peptide chain and another gene (a "V" gene) encodes the variable half. In some way, the two genes (less likely, the two messengers or the two half-chains) link up, resulting in a complete polypeptide chain product. A person would have relatively few "C" genes, presumably one for each type of light chain (κ and the two kinds of λ) and one for each subclass or class of heavy chain (four for IgG, two each for IgA and IgD, and one each for IgM and IgE). An additional number of "V" genes, however, would have to be present to encode the variable portion of the peptide chain and to confer antibody specificity.

This postulated mechanism is consistent with the observed amino acid sequence variation and was arrived at through consideration of the inheritance of the Inv genetic marker. As was stated previously, the presence of valine or leucine at position 191 of the otherwise constant half of κ chains determines the Inv marker, which is inherited as a simple mendelian trait. For example, a person heterozygous for the Inv marker (Inv 1, 3) mating with another heterozygote has the expected ratio of 1 homozygote (Inv 1):2 heterozygotes (Inv 1, 3):1 homozygote (Inv 3) in the offspring. If the Inv factor were encoded by multiple genes, normal crossing over would prohibit this form of inheritance; all offspring of such a mating would be heterozygous. To account for this kind of inheritance, a single genetic locus must encode for the carboxyl-terminal half of the molecule. By inference, the constant portion of λ light chains and the constant portion of the various heavy chains' subclasses must also be the products of a very limited number of genetic loci.

As mentioned before, it is possible to classify light chains into five or so subgroups, based on common threads of sequence in the variable regions. It appears, therefore, that the "V" genes were relatively few in number at an earlier time, either in the life of the species or in the life of the individual. This can be construed to mean that either (1) a few "V" genes went through evolutionary mutation to achieve their present diversity, and all "V" genes are present in the germ line of each individual; or (2) the germ line of an individual contains relatively few "V" genes (perhaps one for each subgroup), and somatic mutation occurs during the life of the individual. A strict "germ-line" theory would require that information for as many as 10^8 antibodies be present in the germ line. Since light- and heavy-chain V regions contribute to the specificity, 2×10^4 genes could account for the necessary diversity. This would amount to approximately 0.2 per cent of the genetic information in the germ line, certainly not an excessive requirement considering the importance of the immune system to the biology of the individual. Whatever the genetic mechanisms responsible for the variable region, link-up with the constant region would still be necessary.

Another theory that deals with antibody variability is based upon considerations of the precise location of *maximal* sequence variability in the variable region of the peptide chains. When human κ and λ chains, human V_H regions, and mouse κ chains are considered as a group, three stretches of maximal variability occur, at positions 24–34, 50–56, and 89–97. (For the numbering sequence, see Figure 5–10.) The variation among all light chains cannot be fully appreciated from this figure, in which the variation is expressed for only a limited number of human κ chains). In regions 24–34 and 89–97, minor variation occurs in the length of the peptide chain as well. In terms of complementarity of the active site, it is significant that these two stretches are adjacent to each other across a disulfide bond. An insertion mechanism for antibody variability has been proposed in which the information for the amino acid sequence at the active site is contained in some form of extrachromosomal DNA, such as an *episome*. In this proposal, the informational DNA would be inserted into the nucleotide sequence of the structural gene, thus programming the amino acid sequence of short but critical segments of the peptide chain. In the proposed model regions 24–34, 50–56, and 89–97 would be the "active sites" for antigen binding of the light chain, and similar "active sites" would be present on the heavy chain.

Another possible mechanism advanced to explain antibody variability involves cleavage of the DNA at the junction of the C and V genes, partial degradation of DNA by an endonuclease, and subsequent errors in repair leading to alterations in ultimate DNA sequence.

Chromosomal rearrangements such as translocation and recombination have also been suggested as explanations for antibody variability.

It should be clear from the above discussion that at present no single explanation for antibody variability has found wide acceptance. Future studies may be expected to clarify the elusive answer to this most complex of questions in molecular biology.

SUGGESTIONS FOR FURTHER READING

Edelman, G. M.: The covalent structure of a human γ G-immunoglobulin XI. Functional implications. Biochemistry, *9*:3197, 1970.

Hood, L., and Talmage, D. W.: On the mechanism of antibody diversity: germline basis for variability. Science, *168*:325, 1970.

Ishizaka, T., and Ishizaka, K.: Biology of immunoglobulin E: molecular basis of reaginic hypersensitivity. Progr. Allergy, *19*:60, 1975.

Low, T. L. K., Liu, Y-S. V., and Putnam, F. W.: Structure, function, and evolutionary relationships of Fc domains of human immunoglobulins A, G, M, and E. Science, *191*:390, 1976.

Nisonoff, A., Hopper, J. E., and Spring, S. B. (eds.): The Antibody Molecule. New York, Academic Press, 1975.

Putnam, F. W. (ed.): The Plasma Proteins: Structure, Function and Genetic Control. New York, Academic Press, 1976.

Wu, T. T., and Kabat, E. A.: An analysis of the sequences of the variable regions of Bence Jones proteins and myeloma light chains and their implications for antibody complementarity. J. Exp. Med., *132*:211, 1970.

COMPLEMENT ACTIVITY

Peter A. Ward, M.D., and
Robert McLean, M.D.

Although the term complement was originally designated to imply an auxiliary factor in serum that, acting upon an antibody-coated cell (such as a red blood cell or a bacterium), would lead to cytolysis (lysis of the cell), the complement system is now known to be a complex set of interacting proteins. To regard this array of proteins as a single substance would be like considering the maze of proteins involved in the coagulation sequence in plasma as a single factor. It is now known that the complement sequence consists of nine functional entities or 11 discrete proteins (Table 6–1). Until the late 1950's, complement was defined by its cytotoxic (cytolytic) action on sensitized red cells. Precise kinetic data allowed investigators to establish characteristics of the interactions of some of the components: the cationic requirements for two of the steps in the sequence, estimates of numbers of "effective molecules" involved in the various interactions in the sequence, predictions about the numbers of sites of damage on the cell membrane associated with cytolysis, and measurements of levels of hemolytic activity defining some of the individual complement components. With regard to the last category, it has been particularly useful in some clinical situations to be able to obtain titrations of certain complement components as accurate indicators of an adverse, ongoing immunologic reaction (e.g., a certain type of nephritis featuring hypocomplementemia, renal homograft rejection, and systemic lupus erythematosus). In the late 1950's, a new approach to the complement system was introduced that involved the isolation, purification, and characterization of the individual complement components as physicochemical entities. The end result has been the attainment of relatively pure, or nearly pure, proteins, that enable the analysis of individual components by direct immunochemical techniques, e.g., radiolabeling of purified components and studies of interaction in the complement system. It has also been possible to obtain measurements of biologic half-lives of certain of the complement components in patients who have abnormalities in synthesis or catabolism of complement.

138

TABLE 6-1. Properties of Human Complement Proteins*

Properties	C1q	C1r	C1s	C2	C3	C4	C5	C6	C7	C8	C9
Serum concentration (μg/ml)	190	—	22	20–40	1200	430	75	—	—	<10	<10
Sedimentation coefficient (S)	11.1	7.0	4.0	5.5	9.5	10.0	8.7	5–6	5–6	8.0	4.5
Approximate molecular weight	400,000	—	79,000	117,000	185,000	240,000	—	—	—	150,000	79,000
Relative electrophoretic mobility	$\gamma 2$	β	$\alpha 2$	$\beta 2$	$\beta 1$	$\beta 1$	$\beta 1$	$\beta 2$	$\beta 2$	$\gamma 1$	α
Carbohydrate (%)	15	—	—	—	2.7	14	19	—	—	—	—
Reactive SH	—	—	—	2(?)	1–2	—	—	—	—	—	—

*From H. J. Müller-Eberhard: Complement. Ann. Rev. Biochem. 38:389, 1969.

GENERAL TISSUE-DAMAGING REACTIONS REQUIRING COMPLEMENT

At least two complex biologic reactions require complement for their development. In both, tissue damage is associated with the onset of an inflammatory response, which is dependent upon both complement and the neutrophilic granulocytes. In *immunologic vasculitis* (the Arthus reaction), the interaction of antigen and antibody in the wall of a blood vessel leads to complement utilization and its physical fixation, to the immune complex, followed by the rapid extravascular accumulation of circulating neutrophils in and around the deposits of immune complexes. These leukocytes produce tissue-destroying enzymes capable of degrading structural proteins such as elastin, basement membrane, and collagen. In the absence of complement, neutrophils fail to accumulate and little tissue damage develops. It appears rather likely that the complement system somehow functions to cause the accumulation of neutrophils from the circulation (chemotaxis). All these considerations seem to apply equally in the case of *nephrotoxic nephritis*, in which antibody to intrinsic antigens of glomerular basement membrane interacts to trigger the complement sequence, which results in the accumulation of neutrophils and the subsequent destruction of glomerular basement membrane. As in the case of immunologic vasculitis, tissue damage in the nephritis model can be averted if either complement or neutrophils are prevented from taking part in the reaction sequence. Although these experiments do not permit a precise definition of the role of complement, they do indicate its participation in certain tissue-damaging reactions. The clinical applications of these phenomena will be discussed more fully in Chapters 13 and 20. The complement-derived mediators considered to be involved in these reactions are described later.

PROTEINS OF THE COMPLEMENT SEQUENCE

Listed in Table 6–1 are the various physicochemical characteristics of the nine complement components. The numerical designation of these components, as in the case of the coagulation factors, is related not to the order of interaction in the sequence, but to the order of discovery. Most of the components are present in serum in very small quantities (less than 10 μg per ml). It is possible, however, to quantify several components, namely Clq, C2, C3, C4, and C5, by immunochemical analysis. It should be noted that the level of C3 is tenfold greater than that of any other component, except for C4, which is present in a concentration one third that of C3. Advantage is taken of this information in the clinical laboratory, C3 being the most commonly measured component when it is cell-attached (Coombs' testing of red cells, immunofluorescence in tissues). Measurement of C3 in serum is also used clinically, and its reduction reflects clinical states in which complement is decreased, e.g., acute glomerulonephritis and lupus nephritis. The first component consists of three protein subunits termed C1q, C1r, and C1s, which are held together by a calcium ion that acts as a ligand. C1q has an affinity for receptors on the heavy chain of IgG and IgM globulins and seems to function as a binding factor for C1, which becomes fixed to antibody-coated membranes. C1r attached to C1q interacts with C1s to cause activation of the latter subunit (i.e., chemical conversion of the *proesterase* enzyme of C1s to an active *esterase*). When this occurs, the C1 complex is termed "activated" (referred to as C$\overline{1}$). Because of its esterase activity, C$\overline{1}$ is able to act upon C4 and C2, which are its substrates. The interaction of C4 with C2 requires magnesium ions. Interaction of C$\overline{1}$ with C4 and C2 results in proteolysis, with one large and one small cleavage product each from both C4 and C2. Natural association of the large C4 fragment with large C2 fragment results in the entity C$\overline{42}$, which exerts enzymatic (proteolytic) activity on the next component, C3, and its electrophoretic migration changes with its conversion to a more acidic or anodal protein. It is for this reason that C$\overline{42}$ is referred to as "C3 convertase." "Activated C3" (the larger fragment of C3, known as C3b) may be bound to the cell surface or may appear in free solution. There is some evidence obtained by means of synthetic substrates that the activated C3 molecule has enzymatic activity referred to as "C3 peptidase." The sequential interaction with the next component (C5) leads to cleavage of C5. The remainder of the sequence has not been identified in terms of cleavage products or other chemical changes in the complement components. In all likelihood, however, several of the remaining four components undergo fragmentation or "unfolding" as the sequential interaction of the complement sequence progresses to termination. It might be added that C5, C6, and C7 naturally form a single complex in serum. Even though individual sequential interactions involving these proteins occur, under certain circumstances, this trimolecular complex may interact as a single molecular entity with the remaining terminal components.

THE ALTERNATIVE (PROPERDIN) COMPLEMENT SYSTEM

Renewed interest in the alternative or properdin complement system has resulted in a better understanding of the mechanisms and the clinical importance of this system. The alternative C pathway is so named because C3 activation occurs without the early C components, C1, C4, or C2, and without immunoglobulins. This alternative C3 activation step can result in terminal C-component activation (C5, C6, C7, C8, C9), as is seen following activation of the classical system. Components of the alternative C system include magnesium, Factor A (C3 or C3b), Factor B (C3 proactivator), properdin, initiating factor, Factor D, and possibly other components. The role of properdin appears to be unique since it prolongs the biologic half-life of the C3 activating factor that results from activation of the alternative complement pathway (C3b Bb). Several lipopolysaccharides and aggregated immunoglobulins can activate the alternative C systems *in vitro;* the release of C3b by various mechanisms may trigger the alternative pathway *in vivo* and *in vitro.* Several diseases are characterized by decreased serum levels of C3 and alternative C-pathway components (such as mesangioproliferative glomerulonephritis). In addition, the patients with complete absence of early C components may be dependent on the integrity of the alternative C pathway for activation of C3–C9. Unanswered questions about the alternative complement pathway concern what starts it off *in vivo* and of what importance it is in human diseases.

BIOACTIVE PRODUCTS OF THE COMPLEMENT SEQUENCE

C1,4

The only biologic activity ascribed to the interaction of the first two complement components deals with herpes simplex virus, which has been sensitized by addition of IgM antibody. The subsequent addition of C1 and C4 results in neutralization of the virus, i.e., the inability of the virus to grow in tissue culture. Addition of the next two reacting components (C2, C3) does not augment the neutralization. Presumably, the effect is due to molecules of complement bound to the surface of the virus, although no direct evidence for this conclusion has been presented. There is yet no information that explains the action of C1 and C4 in neutralization of the virus.

C1,4,2

Using indirect approaches, it has been suggested that a kinin-like material is generated at some step along the sequence of interactions involving the first two or three components. This kinin-like substance will contract smooth muscle and cause increased vascular permeability that is resistant to the effects of antihistamines. There is a suggestion that the kinin-like factor may be a C4 cleavage product, but this is not yet proven.

C3

The product of C3 produced by interaction with $\overline{C142}$ represents one of the most economic steps in the complement system since the smaller and the residual (larger) fragments have biologic activity. The larger fragment, termed C3b, represents about 96 per cent of the original molecule and either remains membrane-bound, at which point it renders the particle or the cell immediately susceptible to phagocytosis by leukocytes (Fig. 6–1), or appears in free solution after being generated at a site on the cell surface. The result of C3b binding to the cell surface is advantageous, especially if the coated cell is a bacterium. If it is a red cell, rapid red cell destruction, recognized clinically as an autoimmune hemolytic disorder, may result. In addition, the presence of C3b on the surface of a cell such as a platelet, a red cell, or a leukocyte will bring out the phenomenon of *immune adherence*, in which each cell will cause the attachment (adherence) to normal mammalian red cells, leading to agglutination *in vitro*. It is possible for viruses coated with antibody and complement to adhere to platelets or red cells, resulting in a large aggregate that will be removed by the reticuloendothelial system. However, there is recent evidence that C3 is not an absolute requirement for immune adherence, since almost normal immune adherence occurs in patients completely deficient in C3. The small cleavage product of C3 (C3a) has at least two different biologic activities, although it is not proven that every small cleavage product of C3 is, in fact, structurally identical. The biologic activities of C3a include anaphylatoxic activities (Fig. 6–2) and the induction of leukocyte chemotaxis (Fig. 6–3). In the former case, the peptide has three distinct actions: contraction of smooth muscle, increased vascular permeability, and release of histamine from mast cells. The second biologic activity, leukocyte chemotaxis, involves the attraction of neutrophilic granulocytes in a unidirec-

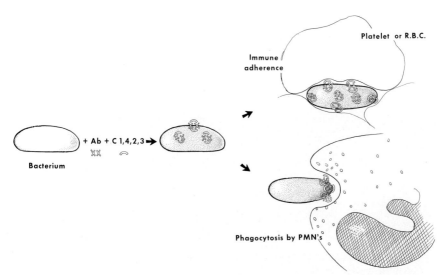

Figure 6–1. Schematic representation of the phagocytic-promoting activity and immune adherence function of complement, associated with the fixation of C3b to the cell surface.

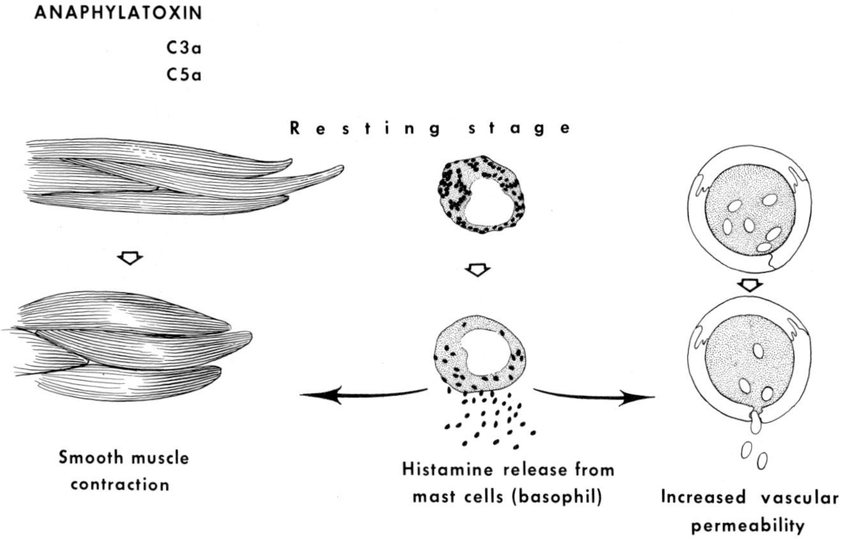

ANAPHYLATOXIN

> C3a
> C5a

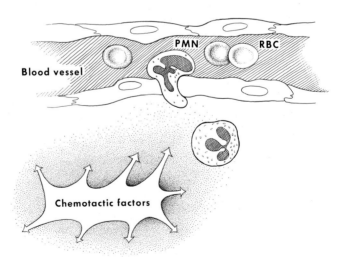

R e s t i n g   s t a g e

Smooth muscle
contraction

Histamine release from
mast cells (basophil)

Increased vascular
permeability

Figure 6–2. Biologic (anaphylatoxic) activities of complement cleavage products C3a and C5a on smooth muscle, mast cells, and blood vessels.

CHEMOTACTIC FACTORS

> C3a
> C5a
> $\overline{C567}$

Blood vessel

PMN   RBC

Chemotactic factors

Figure 6–3. Chemotactic product of the complement system. Schematic representation of their effect in the body.

tional manner. In the intact human or animal, the sum of these two biologic activities is the compromise of vascular integrity and neutrophil accumulation, in other words, acute inflammation. C3a may be cleaved from the parent molecule by sequential interaction of the complement sequence; by artificial cleavage, e.g., trypsin, plasmin or a factor in cobra venom (together with a serum beta globulin co-factor); or by a natural protease existing in a variety of tissues. A realization of the array of enzymes that are capable of cleaving biologically active fragments from C3 has resulted in the concept of the *complement bypass* (Fig. 6–4), in which a large number of enzymes can produce C3a in a manner that requires only one complement component. From these findings, reinforced by similar information on C5, it has been postulated that the complement system may play a major role in the production of mediators of acute inflammation in a way that does not involve conventional interaction of the complement sequence, i.e., by antigen-antibody interaction.

C5

In a manner analogous to the events seen with C3, a cleavage product of C5, termed C5a, has anaphylatoxic as well as chemotactic properties for granulocytes. The peptide can be cleaved from C5 by either the interaction of the first five complement components, the direct action of trypsin, or the presence of an enzyme in lysosomal granules of neutrophilic leukocytes. The latter context implies that neutrophils, once in an extravascular site, carry an enzyme that, in contact with its

BIOACTIVE PRODUCTS OF THE COMPLEMENT SYSTEM GENERATED IN SEQUENCE AND IN BYPASS

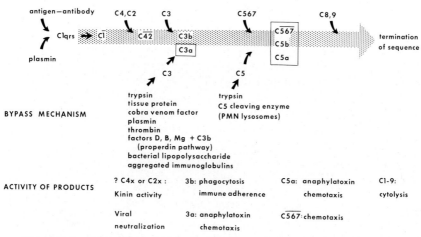

Figure 6–4. Composite of biologic functions of the complement system and methods by which biologically active products can be generated.

substrate (C5), can produce a mediator capable of intensifying and exacerbating the inflammatory reaction.

Until very recently, the information on the phagocytosis-promoting activity of the complement system seemed rather firm—C3b was the only product of complement involved. Now, however, there is indirect information that complicates the picture. Several families have been described whose members have a chemotactic and a phagocytic defect, the latter being measured as the ingestion of yeast particles by blood leukocytes. The phagocytic defect, as well as the chemotactic defect, has been corrected *in vitro* by the addition of purified human C5 to the serum of the patient. From these studies has come the conclusion that C5 plays a role in some phagocytic systems. In line with these observations are the reports that C5-deficient mice are extraordinarily susceptible to challenge by pneumococci and meningococci. In contrast, cogeneic mice that have sufficient C5, but are otherwise genetically identical to the C5-deficient mice, are resistant to challenge by these microorganisms. These findings indicate that C5, probably in the form of C5b, is important in some phagocytic systems.

$\overline{C567}$

As indicated above, these three components form a natural complex that, if "activated" through its interaction with the first four complement components, acquires chemotactic activity for neutrophils. In such a state, the product $\overline{C567}$ is termed the "activated trimolecular complex." This material, unlike C3a and C5a, has a relatively large molecular weight and probably is not free to diffuse quickly from its site of generation. On the other hand, if $\overline{C567}$ is produced in an extravascular location, a more stable gradient of concentration may be established, resulting in extended biologic activity (leukocyte accumulation). Considerable information about the interaction of $\overline{C567}$ with the neutrophil is available. For instance, three enzymes in the leukocyte must be available if the cell is to respond chemotactically. Of particular interest is the fact that one enzyme exists in the leukocyte in precursor form, i.e., as a proesterase. By an unknown mechanism, interaction of the cell with $\overline{C567}$ leads to conversion of the proesterase to an active form (esterase). This probably stands as the first known biochemical signal that can be correlated with the chemotactic response of the neutrophil. A recognition of these enzymes and an understanding of their biochemical interrelationship may eventually permit the development of more specific anti-inflammatory therapy.

C8, C9

No defined products of the interaction of either of these components with the earlier portion of the complement sequence are known.

CYTOLYTIC (CYTOTOXIC) EFFECT OF COMPLEMENT

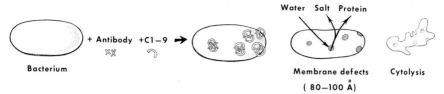

Figure 6-5.   Schematic representation of the cytotoxic effects of complement on cell membranes.

If the terminal interactions do in fact occur in proximity to a cell surface, a cytotoxic effect is produced that may be related to electron-microscopic alterations in the membrane (Fig. 6–5). As a result, the functional integrity of the cell is lost and intracellular constituents pour out of the cell. The cell is thus rendered irreversibly damaged.

NATURAL INHIBITORS OF THE COMPLEMENT SEQUENCE

Just as the coagulation system has a complex array of inhibitors, the complement system is also endowed with similar homeostatic controls. At least three different specific inhibitors are recognized, including those that act on C1, C3, and C6. Several more inhibitors of complement components probably exist in serum. The only well-defined inhibitor is the "C1 esterase inhibitor" that interferes, in a stoichiometric manner, with the esterase activity associated with C1s. At present, the function is complicated by indications that this inhibitor not only blocks C1s, but also blocks the activation of the precursor form of kallikrein, the action of plasmin, and the activation of the Hageman factor. Patients who lack this inhibitor, or contain it in a form that is nonfunctional, have frequent life-threatening episodes of angioedema, especially involving the larynx (Chapter 22). In view of the diverse actions of the C1 esterase inhibitor, it is difficult to determine which mediators are most important in the clinical episodes of angioedema. Too little is known about the other complement inhibitors to dwell on them. It should be pointed out that, in addition to the inhibitors that stop interaction of the complement sequence and prevent generation of inflammatory mediators, the mediators themselves (C3a, C5a, and $\overline{C567}$) have a short half-life and are quickly removed from the circulation. The fact that the body does not tolerate the presence of these mediators for extended periods of time can be considered another part of the balance (homeostasis) of the complement system. At least two different enzymes contained in normal plasma can account for this destruction. The first is plasmin, or fibrinolysin, which destroys $\overline{C567}$ through hydrolysis, although it is not known whether the nonactivated form (C567) is also susceptible. C3a and C5a are susceptible to destruction through hydrolysis of a C-terminal lysine or arginine by a naturally oc- curring enzyme in plasma called the "anaphylatoxin inactivator," which probably represents an agent in plasma functioning to maintain ho- meostatic control.

DEFICIENCIES OF THE COMPLEMENT SYSTEM

Abnormalities of the complement system can be broadly divided into congenital deficiencies of complement components or complement inhibitors and acquired deficiencies of complement components. The latter category, those abnormalities that are acquired, has been recog- nized since early in the 20th century. An association between post- scarlatina nephritis, serum sickness, and low serum complement was noted by early investigators. With the availability of specific immuno- chemical and hemolytic assays, serum levels of the individual comple- ment components in several diseases have now been described. Diseases that are felt to represent antibody-antigen immune complex disease, such as systemic lupus erythematosus, are characterized by low early C component C1, C4, C2, and C3. Depression of the classic C compo- nents is seen during activity of the disease process and a return toward normal is seen as disease activity diminishes. Components of the alter- native C pathway are also decreased during active disease. Although the cause is still uncertain, this decrease may represent secondary ac- tivation of the alternative systems owing to the release of the C3 break- down product, C3b. Other human diseases that are felt to represent immune complex injury, but for which the evidence is less definite than

TABLE 6-2. Congenital Abnormalities of Complement

DEFECT	ASSOCIATED DISEASE
C1q	Combined immunodeficiency disease
C1s	Systemic lupus erythematosus (SLE)
C1r	SLE-like
C2	Some normal
	Some with glomerulonephritis
	Some with SLE-like diseases
C4	SLE-like
C3	Recurrent pyogenic infections
C5	SLE-like disease
C5 dysfunction	Syndrome in infants with diarrhea,
	Dermatitis, infections
C6	Gonococcemia
C7	Raynaud's phenomenon
C8	Gonococcemia
C1s inhibitor deficiency	Hereditary angioneurotic edema
C3b inactivator deficiency	Recurrent infections (also known as Type 1 C3 hypercatabolism)
C3 hypercatabolism, Type 2	Partial lipodystrophy, glomerulonephritis

in lupus, are also associated with characteristic patterns of depression of certain C components. The assessment of individual C components is now a valuable adjunct in the diagnosis of certain diseases.

To date, complete deficiencies have been reported for each C component except C9 (see Table 6–2). These diseases are rare. Absence of the C̄1s inhibitor is the most common and C2-deficiency is the second most common. Most patients with C abnormalities are recognized because of clinical illness, but it seems clear that the frequency of clinical abnormalities among complement-deficient patients is higher than can be explained by chance alone. Particularly common among C-deficient patients is a disease that resembles systemic lupus erythematosus. The association between the genetic loss of some C components and certain histocompatibility loci is now recognized. This association suggests that genetic predisposition to certain diseases may be another important factor—in addition to the complement-deficient state—that determines whether certain diseases occur. Increased susceptibility to bacterial infections is common in patients with "terminal" complement deficiencies, i.e., of C3, C5, C6, and C8.

AN OVERVIEW

The tendency to consider the complement system as a serologic technique to demonstrate the consumption of complement following the interaction of antigen and antibody has undergone considerable change in the past 15 years. Just as with any other complex biologic system of interacting proteins (e.g., the coagulation sequence), the complement system has seemed to evolve essentially for protective functions. The coating of foreign particles and infective agents with the first four components of complement renders the particles immediately susceptible to phagocytosis. The complement interaction at this point, however, or at least up to the C5 step, can also generate C3a or C5a, which in turn will mediate an acute inflammatory response and attract circulating leukocytes to the area of the invading microorganism. It is also possible that the complement system is involved in the surveillance of cancer cells; it may provide factors leading to direct (cytolytic) or indirect destruction of these dangerous cells. Just as the coagulation system may suddenly proceed through its activation sequence in an unchecked manner, resulting in the serious consequences of intravascular coagulation, the complement system may also be triggered by a variety of agents with an outcome that is of little benefit to the individual. In the case of systemic lupus erythematosus, the interaction of DNA and anti-DNA results in complement consumption and the apparent production of phlogistic factors at sites where complexes have lodged. If this occurs in renal glomerular loops or in the walls of blood vessels, the result is immunologic injury (Chapter 13). If, by accident, the body makes antibody to its own red cells, the complement system has no way to distinguish the coated red cells from any other foreign cell. The interaction of complement with antigen-antibody complexes on the cell surface leads to destruction of red cells through phagocytosis or direct cytolysis. The complement system is indifferent to these complexes, insofar as either antigen or antibody may be of host origin, but the outcome is destruction of what are regarded as foreign cells.

It is possible then to regard complement as an array of substrates from which mediators of the acute inflammatory response can be generated. It is these mediators, whether for the benefit or the harm of the individual, that are now beginning to define the system termed complement.

SUGGESTIONS FOR FURTHER READING

Hunsicker, L. G.: Abnormalities of the complement system in acquired renal disease. Transplant. Proc., 6:77, 1974.
Kabat, E., and Mayer, M.: Experimental Immunochemistry, 2nd ed. Springfield, Illinois, Charles C Thomas, Publisher, 1961.
Lachmann, P.: Genetics of the complement system. J. Med. Genet., 12:372, 1975.
Müller-Eberhard, H. J.: Chemistry and reaction mechanisms of complement. Adv. Immunol. 81:1, 1968.
Pillemer, L., Blum, L., Lepow, I. H., et al.: The properdin system and immunity. I. Demonstration and isolation of a new serum protein. Science, 120:279, 1954.
Ward, P. A.: Leukotaxis and leukotactic disorders. Am. J. Pathol., 77:519, 1974.

Chapter 7

IMMUNOPHYSIOLOGY: CELL FUNCTION AND CELLULAR INTERACTIONS

Herbert B. Herscowitz, Ph.D.

INITIATION OF THE SPECIFIC IMMUNE RESPONSE

The specific immune response may be produced in two ways: either (1) through natural exposure or immunization of the host to a foreign configuration _(active immunity);_ or (2) by the passive acquisition of preformed antibody, specifically sensitized lymphocytes, or their products, e.g., transfer factor or informational RNA _(passive immunity)._ The basic differences between active and passive immunity are shown in Table 7–1.

ACTIVE IMMUNITY

Active immunity depends upon the participation of the host after an encounter with the immunogen. It involves proliferation and differentiation of immunocompetent cells in lymphoreticular tissues, which leads to synthesis of antibody or the development of cell-

TABLE 7–1. Comparison of Active and Passive Immunity

	ACTIVE	PASSIVE
Genesis:	Active host participation after exposure to immunogen either naturally (subclinical or clinical disease) or by immunization (vaccine)	No host participation; transfer of preformed substances (antibody, transfer factor, thymic graft) from an actively immunized host to a nonimmune host
Components:	Humoral and cell-mediated immunity	Humoral and cell-mediated immunity
Onset of action:	Only after a latent period	Immediate
Duration:	Long-lived	Transitory
Application:	Vaccination	Immune deficiency

151

mediated reactivity, or both. The onset of this type of immunity is seen only after a specified time lapse subsequent to administration of the immunogen. The duration of active immunity is relatively long and is measured in terms of months or even years. This type of immunity may be the result of exposure to immunogens in nature or the use of vaccines (Chapter 23).

PASSIVE IMMUNITY

Passive immunity occurs without the active participation of the host and is the result of the transfer of substances from an actively immunized host to a nonimmunized host. The passive transfer of immunity from mother to fetus, the use of preformed gamma globulin in immunoprophylaxis, and the use of transfer factor in immunotherapy are examples of passive immunity. Since this type of immunity involves the transfer of preformed materials, the onset of action is immediate; but because there may be no stimulus for continued production, its effect is usually transitory.

RESPONSE OF THE HOST: THE FATE OF IMMUNOGEN

Foreign substances may enter the body either naturally or artificially. Most frequently, they gain entrance through the respiratory or gastrointestinal tract, although they may enter naturally through any body surface, including the mucous membranes and skin, or by transplacental passage. Artificial introduction of foreignness is usually accomplished by either injection (e.g., vaccine) or surgical intervention (e.g., transplantation).

METABOLIC FATE

The fate of an immunogen within an animal can be followed by the use of radioactively labeled materials. Following intravenous injection of a foreign material (e.g., human serum albumin), three phases of disappearance are readily distinguishable (Fig. 7–1). The first phase involves the *equilibration* of the foreign material between the intravascular and extravascular compartments of the plasma protein pool by a process of diffusion. The process is rapid and of similar duration whether the injected material is autologous or foreign. The second stage of clearance, referred to as *catabolism*, occurs over a period of three to seven days and involves the gradual degradation and digestion of the material. The duration of this phase is determined by both the biologic half-life of the material and the enzymatic capabilities of the host for the particular type of substance. Certain substances will survive in the circulation for fairly long periods of time if the host is deficient

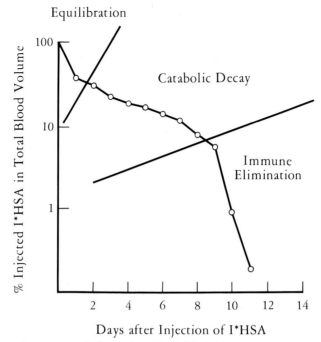

Figure 7–1.   Rate of elimination of radiolabeled immunogen from blood.

in the metabolic machinery required for their degradation (e.g., poly D-amino acids, polysaccharide). In the third phase there is further rapid removal of the immunogen, referred to as *immune elimination.* This stage is the result of the newly synthesized antibody combining with circulating antigen and producing antigen-antibody complexes that are phagocytosed and degraded. Antigen-antibody complexes, particularly when formed in antigen excess, have clinical significance since they may result in tissue injury (Chapter 13). At the end of the third phase, free antibody appears in the serum. Although the curve shown in Figure 7–1 reflects almost complete elimination of the immunogen, absolute removal may take weeks, months, or years, if it ever occurs. Thus, persistence of a portion of the immunogen may provide continued stimulus to the cells involved in the immune response.

ORGAN DISTRIBUTION OF IMMUNOGEN

When injected intravenously, the immunogen is initially found at sites where fixed phagocytic cells are numerous, e.g., the liver, spleen, bone marrow, kidney, and lung. When injected by other routes (e.g., intradermally), the major portion of the material either remains at the site of administration or is localized in the draining lymph node.

Whereas in the case of intravenous injection, clearance of the immunogen from the bloodstream appears to be similar for both soluble and particulate materials, localization of the injected immunogen is more prominent with particulate materials than soluble materials.

Cellular Distribution of Immunogen

Most immunogens are readily taken up by the endocytic processes (phagocytosis or pinocytosis) of the cells of the *mononuclear phagocytic system* within the lymphoid organs. Macrophages in the medullary cords of lymph nodes and in the red pulp of the spleen remove much of the injected material in animals that have not previously been exposed to the foreign substance. In previously immunized animals, the immunogen can be found associated with dendritic macrophages of the lymph node cortex. There is conflicting information regarding the precise intracellular localization of the endocytosed material, because of the breakdown of internally labeled proteins used in such studies and the reutilization of the radiolabeled amino acids in new cellular components. The majority of the evidence points to an intracytoplasmic location of the immunogen, usually in small or large granules, where it may persist. It should be pointed out that there is some controversy about the phagocytic function of macrophages in the immune response. While some investigators feel that the major function of the phagocytic cell is to degrade and eliminate the foreign substance, thereby preventing an immune response, others suggest that this cell is necessary for the "processing" of foreign substances for presentation in a form that will initiate the immune response.

ANTIBODY FORMATION IN THE WHOLE ANIMAL

Primary Response

The injection of a single dose of a foreign substance into an immunocompetent animal will cause specific antibody to appear in the serum after a definite time lapse. First exposure to an immunogen evokes the *primary response* (Fig. 7–2). Immediately after introduction of the immunogen, little or no antibody is detected in the serum. This period is referred to as the *inductive* or *latent* period. It is during this period of time that the immunogen is recognized as foreign and processed, and an unknown signal is transferred to the appropriate cells destined to make antibody. This period is characterized by cellular proliferation and differentiation. The duration of this period is variable and depends upon (1) the immunogenicity, quantity, form, and solubility of the stimulant; (2) the animal species into which it is injected; (3) the route of immunization; and (4) the sensitivity of the assay used to

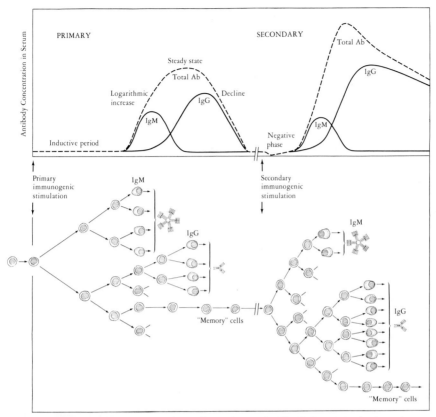

Figure 7–2. Schematic representation of humoral and cellular events in the primary and secondary (anamnestic) antibody responses.

detect the newly formed antibody. For example, antibodies can be detected three to four days after the injection of foreign erythrocytes (e.g., transfusion reaction), five to seven days after soluble proteins, and 10 to 14 days after bacterial cells.

Following the appearance of the first antibody at the end of the induction period, there is a time of active biosynthesis of antibody that can be further subdivided into three phases. In the first, the *logarithmic* phase, the antibody concentration increases logarithmically for 4 to 10 days, again depending upon the nature of the immunogen, until it reaches a peak. During this phase, the doubling time (that required to achieve a twofold increase in serum antibody concentration) has been reported to be as short as five to eight hours. Peak antibody titers against heterologous erythrocytes are usually attained in four to five days, against soluble proteins in 8 to 12 days, and against toxoids prepared from toxins of gram-positive bacilli (e.g., *Corynebacterium diphtheriae*) in as long as two to three months. On a cellular basis, the number of differentiated plasma cells increases soon after immuniza-

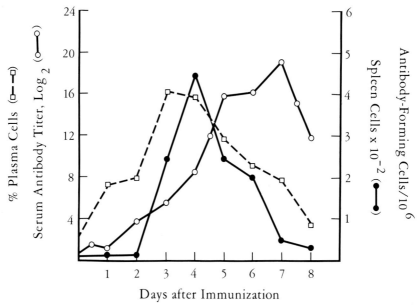

Figure 7–3.   Relationship between appearance of antibody-producing cells and serum antibody following a single injection of immunogen. (After Abramoff, P., and Brien, N. B.: Studies of the chicken immune response. I. Correlation of the cellular and humoral immune response. *J. Immun., 100*:1204, 1968.)

tion, while peak cellular synthesis of antibody precedes the peak serum antibody response by several days (Fig. 7–3).

The level of circulating antibody attained after primary immunization is a reflection of the difference between the antibody's rates of synthesis and catabolism. When these rates are the same, the serum antibody concentration is constant, as shown in Figure 7–2 as a *plateau* or *steady state*. This second phase of the response is highly transitory and in some cases almost nonexistent. The rate of antibody synthesis is dependent upon the number of antibody-forming cells, which can be influenced by the conditions of immunization. The rate of antibody catabolism, however, is a reflection of the half-life of the class of immunoglobulin (Chapter 5).

Finally, a *decline* phase is observed in which the rate of antibody catabolism is greater than that of its synthesis. The duration of this phase is also variable, since there may be varying degrees of difference between rates of synthesis and catabolism.

The early primary response to most immunogens is characterized by the predominance of IgM antibody; the IgG class of antibody appears somewhat later. IgM antibody production is usually transient, and within two weeks after the initiation of the immune response IgG antibody predominates. Whether or not IgM antibodies are always produced in greater quantity before their corresponding IgG counterparts is subject to question. The basis for this controversy is the fact that the IgM antibody is more readily detectable because of the greater sensitivity of the IgM assay methods. Administration of the immunogen in adjuvant (Chapter 10) usually results in the continued synthesis of both IgM and IgG antibodies for several months.

The antibodies formed early in the immune response usually have a low *affinity* (the attractive force between complementary conformational sites on the antibody and antigen that causes them to combine); the affinity of late antibodies is usually greatly increased. Differences in affinity are readily observed with IgG antibodies since such changes can be a thousandfold. In addition to increases in affinity with the passage of time, there is also an increase in *avidity* (the strength of the binding of antibody to antigen); in other words, antigen-antibody complexes formed with late antisera are less dissociable. These changes are related to the diverse antigenic determinants on the immunogen that give rise to a variety of antibody specificities, which appear after different latent periods. As a consequence of these changes, the *cross-reactivity* of a given antiserum also increases with time, probably owing to the fact that high-affinity antibodies can react with closely related antigenic determinants more readily than their low-affinity counterparts can. The compilation of all of these changes exemplifies the fact that the humoral immune response is *heterogeneous*, the manifestation of a population of antibodies with differences in Ig class, affinity, avidity, and specificity.

SECONDARY RESPONSE

Upon a second exposure to the same immunogen, weeks, months, or even years later, there is a markedly enhanced response that is characterized by the accelerated appearance of immunocompetent cells and antibody (Fig. 7–2). If antibody is still present in the serum at the time of the second injection of immunogen it disappears at a faster rate than in the decline phase of the primary response. This *negative phase* is due to the immediate reaction of pre-existing antibody with newly injected immunogen, resulting in the formation of complexes. If the second dose of immunogen is very small, an enhanced immune response may not occur, possibly because all of the newly injected immunogen is consumed in antigen-antibody complexes, phagocytized, and effectively removed, so that the antibody-forming cells are deprived of a stimulus. However, if the dose of immunogen is sufficient to allow the material that remains after complex formation to stimulate the immune system, then a typical *secondary (anamnestic* or *recall)* response is initiated. This enhanced response serves as the principle for giving booster doses of vaccines (Chapter 23).

The differences between the primary and secondary responses are

TABLE 7–2. Relative Differences Between Primary and Secondary Response

	PRIMARY	SECONDARY
Latent period	Long	Short
Rate of antibody synthesis	Low	High
Peak antibody titer	Low	High
Persistence of antibody titer	Short	Long
Affinity of antibody	Low	High
Cross-reactivity of antibody	Low	High
Presence of memory cells	Few (?)	Many
Predominating Ig class	IgM	IgG
Dose of immunogen to elicit	High	Low

summarized in Table 7–2. In contrast to the primary response, the secondary response is characterized by a shorter latent period, a more rapid rate of antibody synthesis, and a higher peak titer of antibody that persists for a longer period of time. The shorter latent period and more rapid rate of antibody synthesis, in spite of the fact that doubling times are similar in primary and secondary responses, are related to the number of antigen-sensitive cells, called *memory* cells, present at the time of secondary stimulation. The scheme presented in Figure 7–2 shows that upon primary stimulation the precursor cell divides and differentiates into a number of antibody-forming cells producing either IgM or IgG immunoglobulins. During this process, a small number of memory cells are also produced. Following secondary challenge the proliferative events appear qualitatively similar, but the number of antigen-sensitive cells is greatly increased over that present in the primary response; the result is a greater pool of antibody-forming cells and thus an increased amount of antibody is synthesized. Serum antibody formed in the secondary response may reach levels as high as 10 to 12 mg/ml and is predominantly of the IgG class, although some IgM memory is also expressed.

The dose of immunogen required to elicit a secondary response is far less than that required for the initiation of the primary response. Again, this is related to the number of antigen-sensitive cells bearing high-avidity receptors available for secondary stimulation and to the presence of circulating antibody remaining from the primary response. This circulating antibody will form complexes with the newly introduced material; antigen-antibody complexes formed in antigen excess are extremely immunogenic. The magnitude of the secondary response depends on other factors, including the interval between stimuli. Both short and long intervals result in decreased responses, the former owing to complete removal of immunogen and the latter possibly as a result of cell senescence. Immunologic memory may persist for many years and thereby provide long-lasting immunity against infection.

Indeed, in the case of some bacterial and viral infections, immunity to reinfection may be lifelong. It is postulated that this immunity is related to the restimulation of long-lived memory cells by persisting antigen or newly introduced antigen. As in the primary response, antibody produced late in the secondary response has higher avidity and affinity for antigen than that synthesized earlier. Late antibodies also appear to exhibit broad specificity. This may be attributed to the appearance of antibodies against certain antigenic determinants that do not stimulate antibodies early in the response (e.g., minor antigenic determinants). Therefore, the apparently broader specificity occurs because late antibodies exhibit a greater degree of *cross-reactivity* with structurally related substances than do early antibodies.

A secondary response can be initiated by an immunogen that is closely related to the primary stimulating agent. In this case, the major portion of the antibodies produced will react more effectively with the first than with the second immunogen. This phenomenon, referred to as *"the doctrine of original antigenic sin,"* was first noted in studies of the response to influenza virus. It was observed that booster immunization with influenza vaccines induced antibodies that were directed mainly against strains of the virus that the individual had previously experienced, and the immune response to the booster vaccine was weaker. A possible explanation for this phenomenon is that the high-affinity antibody-forming cells are selectively stimulated in a population consisting of both low- and high-affinity antibody-producing cells.

IMMUNOLOGIC MEMORY

It appears that both B- and T-cells display immunologic memory. This finding was obtained from studies of cell cooperation in the immune response to hapten-carrier complexes. Although the hapten-carrier conjugates used in these studies may be considered unnatural immunogens, they are, in fact, true analogues of antigens that occur in nature, since the latter are also composed of multiple antigenic determinants, each of which can be considered a hapten. Under ordinary circumstances, when an animal is given a primary immunization with a hapten-protein conjugate, e.g., dinitrophenyl coupled to bovine serum albumin (DNP-BSA), and is given a second injection of the same immunogen at a later time, antibodies against the hapten (DNP) are formed at a rate typical of the secondary response (Fig. 7-4A). If the second injection is given with DNP coupled to a noncross-reacting protein carrier, e.g., ovalbumin (OA), a secondary anti-DNP response is not usually manifested (Fig. 7-4B). However, if the animal that receives the second injection of DNP-OA has been previously primed with OA itself, then a substantial anti-DNP response will be elicited (Fig. 7-4C). This phenomenon, referred to as the *carrier effect,* suggests that recognition of both hapten and carrier is required for the secondary response.

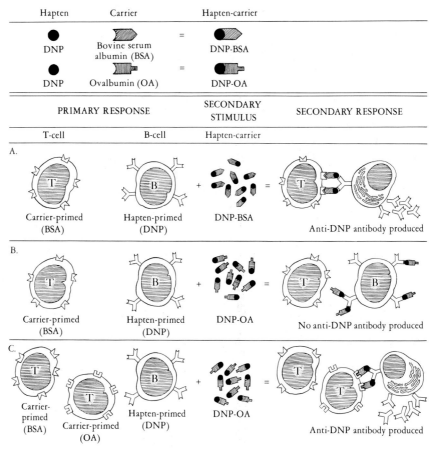

Figure 7-4. Schematic representation of carrier effect in the secondary antihapten antibody response.

Further experiments have shown that T-cells recognize the carrier determinant and B-cells are responsible for recognition of the hapten.

The carrier effect is not always operative in secondary anti-hapten responses. In some cases, up to two years after animals have been given a primary injection with DNP-BSA, a potent secondary anti-DNP response can be induced with DNP coupled to a noncross-reacting carrier such as hemocyanin. This suggests that memory resides in B-cells. Evidence for T-cell memory comes from the inability of the so-called T-independent antigens (e.g., lipopolysaccharide, pneumococcal polysaccharide) to induce a secondary IgG response. Further, data obtained from studies with the congenitally athymic mouse strain (nude, nu/nu) suggest that T-cells regulate secondary responses of the IgG class.

Secondary stimulation of the immune response is not entirely without untoward effects, especially when soluble immunogens or haptens capable of binding to autologous substances are used. A portion of the antibody produced, as well as certain classes of antibody (e.g., IgE) made following primary stimulation, has the ability to fix to tissue cells. These cell-associated antibodies can bind the secondarily injected antigen; and, in some instances, this event can initiate a series of reactions that may be injurious or lethal to the individual. This antibody-mediated tissue injury is based on a secondary response and is further described in Chapters 13 and 20.

CELLULAR EVENTS INVOLVED IN THE SPECIFIC IMMUNE RESPONSE

FUNCTIONAL CELLS

Much of our current information regarding the nature of cells and cellular interactions involved in the immune response has been obtained from studies of the "experiments of nature" that take the form of human immune deficiency diseases (Chapter 22). The results of these studies have shown that there is a functional division of the immune system involving two lines of immunocompetent cells, one concerned with humoral immunity and the other with cell-mediated immunity. Although the early events occurring in the *afferent* arm of both divisions are essentially similar, as depicted in Figure 7–5, the products of the *efferent* arm are different; specific antibody is the product of humoral immunity and specifically sensitized lymphocytes and their lymphokines are the products of cell-mediated immunity (Chapter 9).

According to our current knowledge, at least three types of cells are involved in the immune response. Two of these cells belong to the lymphocytic series, are morphologically indistinguishable, and have been classified, on the basis of their site of differentiation, *thymus-derived* (T-cell) and *bursa-derived* (B-cell) (Chapter 3). The third cell type, which is phagocytic, is often referred to as an *accessory cell* (A-cell) and is thought to be a macrophage. Tables 7–3 and 7–4 summarize some of the major characteristics of these cell types.

LYMPHOCYTES

Cell Surface Antigens

Lymphocytes originate in the bone marrow, pass through the bloodstream, and enter other tissues (Chapter 2). Those cells that enter the thymus (thymocytes) may be modified therein or pass through the organ and be eliminated. It has been suggested that maturation of lymphocytes in the thymus may be influenced by one of several soluble hormones elaborated by the epithelial cells of the thymus, e.g., *thymosin*.

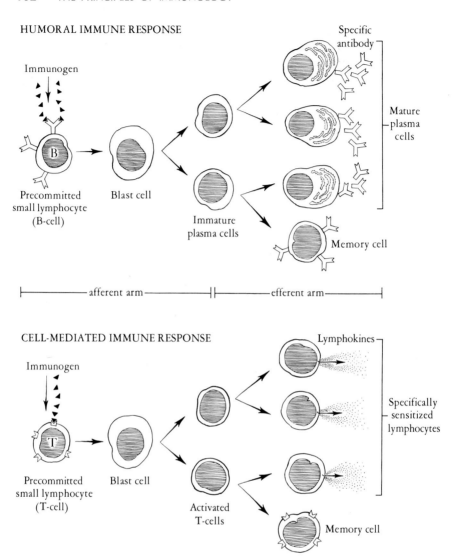

Figure 7-5. Schematic representation of the activation of immunocompetent cells by immunogen for humoral and cell-mediated immune responses.

Evidence for a thymic humoral factor is derived from experiments in which animals made immunologically deficient by thymus ablation were rendered immunologically competent after transplantation of fetal thymus tissue contained within a chamber that is impermeable to cells. Attempts have been made to use a similar thymic factor to reconstitute humans with congenital T-cell defects with some reported success (Chapter 22).

In recent years, with sensitive immunologic techniques (e.g., immunofluorescence, rosette formation), it has become possible to describe characteristic markers useful for the detection of B- and T-cells. In murine systems, some of the lymphocytes that enter the thymus acquire a surface alloantigen formerly called *theta* (θ) that occurs in two allelic forms now referred to as Thy 1.1 and Thy 1.2. This antigen is found on lymphocytes that leave the thymus (thymus-derived or T-cells), on brain cells, and on skin and fibroblast cells in very small amounts, but is absent from B-cells. The presence of the theta antigen is detected by an antiserum prepared by immunizing mice not carrying the specific antigen with thymus cells from mice that do. This antiserum, in the presence of complement, can be used to deplete lymphocyte populations of theta-bearing cells. T-cells express different concentrations of the theta alloantigen on their surface at different stages of their maturation. In the cortex of the thymus, thymocytes express the greatest amount of theta. The more mature thymus medul-

TABLE 7-3. Characteristics of Human Lymphocytes and Macrophages

	T-Cells	B-Cells	Macrophages
Site of differentiation	Thymus	Bone marrow (bursa of Fabricius)	Bone marrow
Surface markers:			
Specific surface antigen	HTLA (theta-like)	B	Mϕ
Specific antigen-binding receptor	Controversial	Immunoglobulin	–
Receptor for SRBC (E-rosette)	+	–	–
Receptor for Fc (EA-rosette)	–	+	+
Receptor for C3b (EAC-rosette)	–	+	Some
HL-A alloantigen	+	+	+
Location: per cent lymphocyte			
Peripheral blood	70–80	20–30	+
Thoracic duct	90	10	+
Lymph node	80	20	+
Spleen	65	35	+
Bone marrow	Few	Abundant	+
Thymus	Abundant	Few	Few
Tissue location:	Cortex of lymph node	Germinal centers	Sinuses
Blast transformation induced by:			
Phytohemagglutinin (PHA)	+	+	–
Concanavalin-A (Con-A)			
soluble	+	–	–
insoluble	+	+	–
Lipopolysaccharide (LPS)	–	±	–
Pokeweed mitogen (PWM)	+	+	–
Anti-immunoglobulin	–	+	–
Antigen	+	+	–
Susceptible to inactivation by:			
Corticosteroids	+	++	–
X-irradiation	+	++++	–
Antilymphocyte serum (ALS)	++++	+	±
Immunosuppressive drugs	+++	+++	–

TABLE 7–4. Immunologic Functions of T-Cells, B-Cells, and Macrophages

	T-CELL	B-CELL	MACROPHAGE
Humoral response:	Helper cell	Differentiate into antibody-forming cell	Accessory cell in afferent limb
Cell-mediated response:	Effector cell	?	Accessory cell in both afferent and efferent limbs
Specificity:	Clonally restricted	Clonally restricted	Nonspecific
Products elaborated:	Lymphokines, regulatory factors	Antibody	Informational RNA, regulatory factors
Memory:	Present	Present	Absent
Can be made tolerant?	Yes	Yes	No

lary lymphocyte expresses a lesser amount of the theta antigen and even less is expressed on circulating (peripheral) T-cells. An analogous thymus alloantigen in humans, called *human thymus lymphocyte antigen* (HTLA), has been used for the preparation of a cytotoxic antiserum that has immunosuppressive capabilities.

Other alloantigens have been detected primarily on the surface of T-cells. Among these is the *Ly series*, Ly 1, 2, 3, 5, which is restricted to the T-lymphocyte population, although Ly 4 is also found on B-cells. The *TL alloantigen* is present on lymphocytes within the thymus of genetically TL^+ mouse strains and is lost as these cells mature into T-cells. The TL antigen also appears on T-cells of leukemic mice in TL^- strains, suggesting that derepression of a previously existing gene occurs. In humans, alloantibodies against T-cells are found in the sera of patients with infectious mononucleosis and systemic lupus erythematosus, which suggests antigenic modulation of the cell surface or derepression of genetic information for expression of that antigen.

B-cells arising in the bone marrow differentiate in the bursa of Fabricius of avian species or in the gut-associated lymphoid tissues (GALT), bone marrow, and fetal liver of mammals (Chapter 2). Alloantigens on B-cells with a similar relationship as that which theta has for T-cells have not yet been described. In murine species, a *mouse B-lymphocyte antigen* (MBLA) has been used for the preparation of anti-B-cell antisera. This antiserum was used in studies of B-cell function only after it had been absorbed extensively with mouse tissue to remove cytotoxic activity against thymus cells. Another murine alloantigen, referred to as *PC.1*, is found on the surface of plasma cells, the terminal differentiation product of the antigen-stimulated B-cell, and on certain murine myeloma cells. This antigen is thought to be a differentiation antigen. Although several attempts have been made to generate antisera against human B-cells, they have been unsuccessful for the most part because of the lack of identification of a unique B-cell alloantigen. The most useful marker to aid in the identification of B-cells is the presence of immunoglobulin on the cell surface.

Macrophages also arise from bone marrow precursor cells that find their way into the bloodstream as monocytes (Chapter 2). These cells wander through tissues and, together with their fixed-form counterparts, serve a phagocytic function. Antisera have also been raised against macrophages that show specificity only after extensive absorption with other tissues, suggesting that there is a cell surface antigen unique to macrophages.

The histocompatibility antigens of the species are expressed on the surface of B- and T-cells and macrophages. A detailed description of these alloantigens is found in Chapter 3.

Surface Receptors

Receptors for several substances can be found on the surface of cells that participate in the immune response. Methods have been developed for detection of these receptors and indirectly serve as a means of evaluating the quantity or quality of the participating cells. One such method involves the formation of *rosettes* consisting of either a lymphocyte or a macrophage surrounded by an appropriate indicator cell. Three types of rosettes can be distinguished that correspond to different cell surface receptors (Figure 7–6). T-lymphocytes from normal individuals that are mixed with sheep erythrocytes (E) form spontaneous rosettes (Fig. 7–6A). The basis for the formation of these nonimmune *T-rosettes* (also called E-rosettes) is uncertain, as is the nature of the receptor; however, these rosettes have proved to be useful for the quantitation of T-cells in peripheral blood. A second class of receptor that participates in rosette formation binds antigen-antibody complexes or aggregated immunoglobulin through the Fc portion of the IgG molecule (Fig. 7–6B). These *Fc receptors* are present on B-cells and macrophages and form *EA-rosettes* (immune rosettes) with sheep erythrocytes that have been coated with specific anti-SRBC antibody (A). The third type of receptor, found on some B-cells, some macrophages, and a limited number of other cell types, recognizes the C3b component of complement (C) when it is bound to either IgG or IgM antibody (Figure 7–6C). These *EAC-rosettes* are formed with SRBC coated with specific antibody and complement. Lymphocytes bearing this receptor for the third component of complement are referred to as *complement receptor lymphocytes* (CRL). Since the activity of none of these receptors is

| | SHEEP RED BLOOD | |
| PARTICIPATING CELL | CELL INDICATOR | ROSETTE |

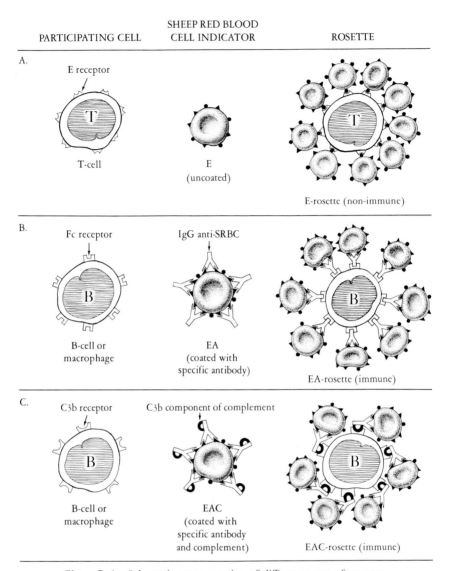

Figure 7–6. Schematic representation of different types of rosettes.

inhibited by treatment of the cells with anti-immunoglobulin antisera, they probably are not immunoglobulin in nature.

Antigen-Binding Receptor on B-Cells. The initiation of the immune response is dependent upon recognition of the foreign configuration of the immunogen by specific receptors on B- and T-cells. The antigen-binding receptor on the B-cell is immunoglobulin. B-cells contain approximately 100,000 immunoglobulin molecules per cell. These are restricted to a single class, subclass, allotype, and probably idiotype.

Antisera prepared against most of the antigenic determinants on immunoglobulins are capable of inhibiting antigen binding by B-cells. The immunoglobulin receptor on the B-cell is a reflection of the antibody ultimately produced by the plasma cell as a consequence of antigen stimulation of the B-cell bearing that receptor.

Specific immunoglobulin classes may be associated with B-cells. In humans and mice, IgM-bearing cells are more common than those bearing IgG. The relative proportion of κ and λ light chains on the surface of B-cells corresponds to that expressed on serum immunoglobulins. However, whereas the major serum immunoglobulin expresses the γ heavy chain, the major immunoglobulin expressed on B-cells bears the μ heavy chain. The cell surface IgM appears to exist predominantly in the monomeric form as IgM$_s$ (8S) and lacks some of the carbohydrate moieties found in pentameric serum IgM. A significant number

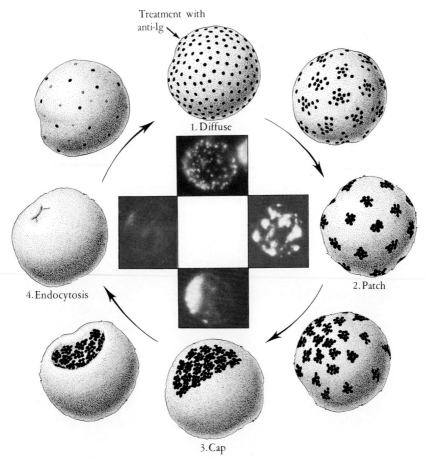

Treatment with anti-Ig

1. Diffuse

2. Patch

3. Cap

4. Endocytosis

Figure 7–7. Redistribution of surface immunoglobulin as a consequence of treatment with anti-Ig. Inserts show cells treated with fluorescein-labeled anti-immunoglobulin. (Photomicrographs courtesy of Dr. Joseph Davie.)

of cord blood and tonsillar lymphocytes express IgM and IgD simultaneously on their surface. IgD is also present on the surface of leukemic cells and on other poorly differentiated cells. Although the function of surface IgD is unclear, its presence has generated a great deal of interest in its potential role as the antigen receptor in humans and has led to the provocative speculation that IgD, rather than IgM, might represent the earliest class in the phylogenetic evolution of the immunoglobulins.

The surface immunoglobulins are neither rigidly held in fixed position nor loosely bound; in fact, there is fluidity and movement of these molecules. For example, when a radiolabeled or fluorescein-labeled anti-immunoglobulin serum is reacted with living B-cells, changes can be observed at the cell surface (Fig. 7–7). If the reaction is carried out at low temperature (4° C), the labeled material can be seen in a *diffuse* arrangement over the entire cell surface, indicating that the surface immunoglobulin is uniformly distributed. As the temperature is raised, the labeled material assumes a distribution of spots or patches over the surface. *Patch formation* is independent of cell metabolism but is dependent upon the divalence of antibody (e.g., F(ab')$_2$). This reaction is thought to depend upon cross-linking of the receptors. After a short time the label coalesces into a cap over one pole of the cell. *Cap formation* is an energy-dependent process. Following this the cap is either released or internalized within the cell, where the material is seen in vesicles. The cell surface remains devoid of immunoglobulin for a period of time before newly synthesized receptors can be detected. The same phenomenon can be demonstrated when B-cells expressing specific receptors bind a multivalent antigen. It has been suggested by some that these events are crucial to the triggering of cell differentiation and proliferation required for the initiation of the immune response; others suggest that the above events function solely to remove excess antigen from the cell surface.

Antigen-Binding Receptor on T-Cell. Based upon our understanding of the specificity of the antigen-antibody reaction, it would be logical to conclude that the T-cell receptor must also be represented by immunoglobulin. However, the nature of the T-cell receptor is controversial and, at present, uncertain. Immunoglobulin can be detected on the surface of T-cells, but only in trace amounts (100 to 1000 molecules per cell) and it is uncertain whether this is passively acquired from B-cells or made by the T-cell. The fact that anti-immunoglobulin antisera do not readily block the immunologic functions of these cells argues against the receptor being an immunoglobulin. Those who favor the immunoglobulin nature of the T-cell receptor suggest that it is located deeper in the cell membrane than that of B-cells, that it is sterically hindered by other surface components, or that it belongs to a class of hitherto unidentified immunoglobulins, referred to as "IgT." Moreover, several soluble factors have been derived from cultured T-cells that have been reported to be the T-cell receptor. One of these resembles monomeric IgM and has antigen-specific activity that can be blocked by anti-μ serum. Another factor also has antigen-specific activity, which, however, can be blocked only by antisera prepared against the product of the major histocompatibility region. Recent studies of the genetic control of antibody formation have shown that many specific immune responses are controlled by genes closely linked to the major histocompatibility locus, called Ir genes (Chapter 3). Although it is still unclear what the specific Ir genes code for, the linkage of Ir to the histocompatibility locus has suggested that the Ir gene product may be the elusive T-cell receptor.

In the human, an additional substance is associated with the cell surface. The material is a low molecular weight protein fragment found in association with the histocompatibility antigens (HL-A). This β_2 *microglobulin* in many ways resembles the homology regions of immunoglobulins; its amino acid sequence is very similar to the homology regions in the constant portion of the light chain (C_L) and the heavy chain (C_H3) of IgG. It has been suggested that the β_2 microglobulin functions as the T-cell receptor by serving as the recognition site for B- and T-cell interactions or some regulatory substance. Its similarity in structure to immunoglobulin and its close association with HL-A suggest an important evolutionary interaction between the products of the immune system and the histocompatibility system.

Blast Transformation. The recognition of an immunogen by specific receptors on B- and T-cells leads to the initiation of a series of events in which the cells increase in size, the nucleolus enlarges, rough endoplasmic reticulum and microtubules become prominent, the rate of DNA synthesis increases, and mitosis ensues. Figure 7–8 shows a typical blast cell. This process of *blast transformation* can also be induced by the addition of divalent F(ab')$_2$, but not of monovalent Fab fragments of anti-immunoglobulin or antiallotype antisera to cultures of immunoglobulin-bearing lymphocytes. The addition of other agents, including certain plant proteins and endotoxin, called *mitogens,* to cultures of nonsensitized lymphocytes may also initiate blast transforma-

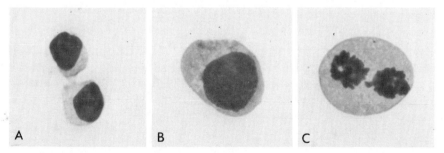

A   **B**   **C**

Figure 7–8. Photomicrographs of lymphocytes in the process of blast transformation, Giemsa stain, ×900. *A,* Unstimulated small lymphocytes; *B,* PHA-stimulated blast cell; *C,* PHA-stimulated lymphocyte in mitosis. (Courtesy of B. Zeligs.)

tion. These observations suggest that some membrane perturbation induced by the cross-linking of certain surface macromolecules stimulates the lymphocyte to divide.

Plant mitogens have the potential to bind to and activate large subpopulations of lymphocytes. These polyclonal mitogens have specificity for sugar moieties of surface glycoproteins (e.g., concanavalin-A [Con-A] binds to glycoproteins containing α-mannosyl moieties). Some of the mitogens have specificity for T-cells, others for B-cells, and some induce changes in both. It is important to note that a given mitogen will have diverse effects on lymphocytes obtained from a different species. For example, whereas the lipopolysaccharide (LPS) of gram-negative bacteria is a potent mitogen for murine B-cells (but not for T-cells), it does not induce blast transformation in rabbit B-cells. Currently, there is question as to the mitogenic effect of LPS on human B-cells. Some believe that LPS induces a clonally restricted response in human B-cells (i.e., similar to that induced by any specific immunogen), but a recent report suggests that after an initial culture period in the absence of LPS, human B-cells will respond to the addition of LPS in a polyclonal manner. It is thought that the initial culture period is necessary to remove the influence of suppressor T-cells. Pokeweed mitogen (PWM) stimulates both B- and T-cell subpopulations of mouse and human lymphocytes. It has been suggested that stimulation of human B-cells by PWM depends on the presence of T-cells. Both phytohemagglutinin (PHA) and Con-A, in their soluble forms, selectively stimulate murine T-cells to synthesize DNA, divide, and produce a nonspecific factor that can replace the T-cell helper function in some immune responses. When rendered insoluble by attachment to large particles, Con-A and PHA induce blast transformation in both B- and T-cell subpopulations. It appears that both human T- and B-cells are stimulated by PHA. In this case, B-cell stimulation could be indirect since nonspecific products elaborated by PHA-stimulated T-cells initiate the activation of B-cells.

In addition to stimulating DNA synthesis in both T- and B-cells, certain mitogens, such as insoluble Con-A, will initiate synthesis and secretion of IgM in cultures of B-cells, and others, such as PHA, will induce lymphokine production (Chapter 9) in cultures of T-cells. The reaction of lymphocyte populations to the various mitogens (Table 7–3) may, with caution, be used by the clinician to identify the type of cell (T or B) and to reveal developmental or functional deficiencies (Chapter 22).

Various clues regarding the possible triggering events of antibody formation have been obtained from studies with lymphocytes activated nonspecifically by mitogens. The initial event observed following the stimulation of lymphocytes by mitogens is the formation of polar caps of mitogen receptors. It has subsequently been shown that capping can occur on cells that do not undergo blast transformation and that cells can divide after stimulation without the formation of polar caps. The

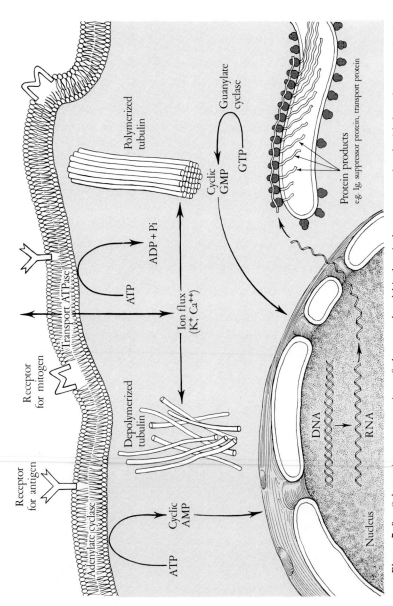

Figure 7–9. Schematic representation of the postulated biochemical events associated with lymphocyte activation that result from the interaction of mitogen or antigen with surface receptors.

critical initial event leading to lymphocyte activation, which appears to occur after stimulation with PHA or anti-immunoglobulin serum, is endocytosis of the receptors. Figure 7–9 shows some of the biochemical changes thought to be involved in lymphocyte activation. The very early events of lymphocyte activation include an increase in membrane transport associated with increased turnover of membrane phospholipids. The permeability for nucleosides, amino acids, or sugars is increased and, at the same time, the flux rates for Ca^{++} or K^+ are enhanced. It has also been shown that the fluidity of the membrane increases within minutes after the addition of mitogen to lymphocytes. Several mechanisms have been proposed to explain the transmission of these membrane changes to an intracellular process that initiates cell activation. One of these has focused on the role of cyclic nucleotides as "second messengers" through their activation of specific cyclic nucleotide-dependent protein kinases. While the expression of some genes is dependent upon elevated levels of cyclic AMP, the expression of other genes can be antagonized by similar levels of this cyclic nucleotide. It has been demonstrated, for example, that cyclic GMP can reverse the effects of cyclic AMP. Moreover, following mitogen stimulation of lymphocytes, a decrease in intracellular levels of cyclic AMP occurs, but intracellular levels of cyclic GMP may rise fiftyfold. It is known that agents that increase levels of intracellular cyclic AMP also suppress mitogen-induced lymphocyte proliferation. Hence, it appears that a delicate balance between the intracellular levels of cyclic AMP and cyclic GMP may control gene expression involved in lymphocyte activation. In addition to the relationship between cyclic nuleotides and protein kinase activation, these agents are involved in the reversible polymerization of tubulin into microtubules, which are necessary for the secretion of stored materials. For example, it has been suggested that cyclic GMP increases the assembly of microtubules from tubulin, whereas increases in cyclic AMP levels result in depolymerization of microtubules. There is also evidence to suggest that a close relationship exists between calcium ions and cyclic nucleotides, since these divalent cations have an effect on intracellular processes responsible for cyclic GMP accumulation. It is interesting to note that mediator release is also under the control of the cyclic nucleotide system (Chapter 20). Additional studies on this complex picture of biochemical interactions will, we hope, provide future insights into our understanding of lymphocyte activation and release of biologically active mediators.

MACROPHAGES

Although the involvement of macrophages in both *in vivo* and *in vitro* immune responses has been known for many years, their precise function still remains unclear. The basic functional property of a macrophage is its ability to engulf and remove foreign and effete materials. The endocytic processes of macrophages appear to be initiated by the interaction of the foreign material with the cell membrane. Phagocytosis can be facilitated by the presence of antigen coated with its specific antibody, a process called *opsonization*. In addition, antibodies of a variety of specificities can be attached to the macrophage surface through its Fc receptor. This *cytophilic* antibody endows the macrophage with enhanced abilities to recognize, engulf, and destroy antigenic substances.

Evidence for the role of the macrophage in humoral responses has been provided by numerous *in vivo* studies using irradiated animals, reticuloendothelial blockade, and antimacrophage serum. The essentiality of macrophage participation in the *in vitro* immune response has been shown by experiments in which mouse spleen populations were separated into adherent (macrophage-rich) and nonadherent (lymphocyte-rich) populations. Neither of these populations by themselves can respond to antigen; however, when they are combined, an antibody response equivalent to that of the unseparated spleen cell population is obtained.

Numerous functional roles have been ascribed to macrophages participating in the immune response. In early experiments, it was thought that macrophages "*processed*" antigens into an immunogenic form that was recognized by a particular lymphocyte subclass. Processing appears to be an important event associated with the initial steps of the immune response to particulate materials; it is thought that this event may expose determinants otherwise available to react with lymphocytes or change pre-existing determinants into a recognizable form. In support of this concept, it has been shown that aggregation of soluble antigens leads to more efficient phagocytosis, which also results in enhanced immunogenicity.

A second function attributed to the macrophage is antigen "*presentation*." It has been amply demonstrated that after incubation of antigen with macrophages, a portion of the antigen remains associated with the macrophage surface. This macrophage-bound antigen is more immunogenic than an equivalent amount of free antigen. It is not clear whether the surface-bound antigen is derived from material taken up by the macrophage and subsequently exocytosed or whether it is a result of direct interaction of the material with components (e.g., antibody affixed to Fc receptors) on the macrophage membrane. This surface-associated antigen appears to be tightly bound and can be recovered in macromolecular form after limited treatment of the cell surface with proteolytic enzymes.

It has also been suggested by some that processing of antigen by macrophages results in the production of a new class of macrophage-derived RNA that carries genetic information. Two fractions of macrophage-derived RNA have been described; however, one of these contains a portion of the original antigen. This antigen-RNA complex is more efficient in stimulating an immune response than the original antigen and has been referred to as a *super antigen*. In this case, the enhanced immunogenicity has been attributed to the adjuvant properties of the component nucleic acid.

The second class of RNA has been shown to be free of antigen fragments and is thought to have messenger RNA activity. It is referred to as *informational RNA* (i-RNA). This RNA has a molecular weight between 400,000 and 750,000 and selectively induces the formation of IgM antibody. Support for an informational role of macrophage-derived RNA was obtained from the following type of experiment (Fig. 7–10). If, after incubation with antigen, macrophage RNA is prepared from cells of a strain of animal that produces antibody with a unique allotype marker (b^4b^4) and is added to lymphoid cells obtained from another animal that produces antibody of a different allotype (b^5b^5), the antibody molecules formed will be of the allotype of the macrophage donor animal (b^4b^4). Recent evidence has also shown that this i-RNA can direct the synthesis of 19S protein of a particular allotype in cell-free extracts, suggesting that the i-RNA functions as messenger RNA.

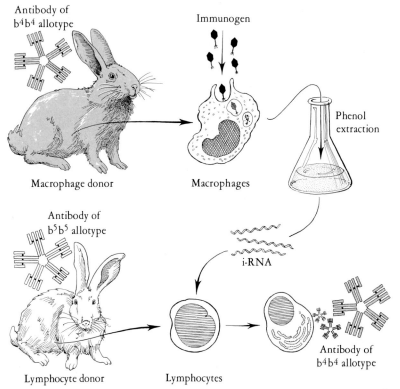

Figure 7–10. Schematic representation of the synthesis of specific allotypic antibody following the transfer of informational RNA (i-RNA).

An additional function attributed to macrophages is the production of factors that influence the activity of lymphocytes. Macrophage extracts or supernatant fluids from macrophage cultures can substitute for the function of intact macrophages. However, it has also been shown that macrophages can be replaced by 2-mercaptoethanol (2-ME) during the induction of the *in vitro* immune response to SRBC by

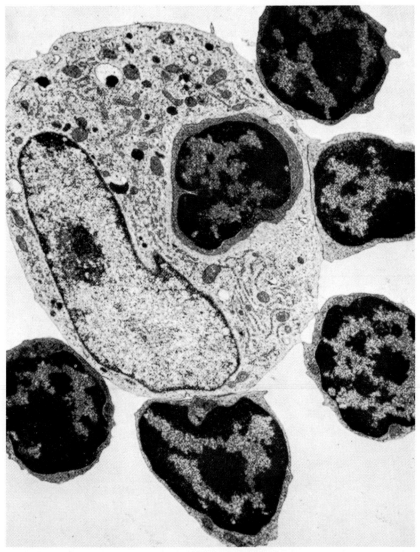

Figure 7-11. Photomicrograph of macrophage-lymphocyte interaction. (Reproduced from Lipsky, P. E., and Rosenthal, A. S.: Macrophage-lymphocyte interaction. I. Characteristics of the antigen-independent-binding of guinea pig thymocytes and lymphocytes to syngeneic macrophages. J. Exp. Med., *138*:900, 1973.)

mouse spleen cells. It has been suggested that in these systems 2-ME can substitute for macrophage function by acting in combination with a serum component in tissue culture media, leading to the activation of T-cells. Therefore, 2-ME appears to fulfill the same function as the macrophage—to stimulate T-cells. Recently, a factor obtained from macrophage cultures was shown to stimulate the proliferation of thymocytes and mature lymphocytes. Substances have also been found that stimulate the differentiation of memory B-cells into antibody-forming cells and enhance helper function T-cells. Whether all these activities are associated with the same factor or are different, and what the mechanism(s) of their action may be, are still subject to investigation.

Although all of the above postulated functions of macrophages are worthy of further consideration, attention has been directed toward the surface membrane of the macrophage. Macrophage-bound antigen is highly immunogenic for T-cells. The fact that maximal stimulation is achieved when the macrophage and lymphocyte share common histocompatibility antigens suggests that something more than antigen is required. Indeed, in several systems direct contact between macrophages and lymphocytes has been observed and suggests the necessity of cell surface interaction or the transfer of information from one cell to the other (Fig. 7–11).

CELL INTERACTIONS IN THE INITIATION OF ANTIBODY FORMATION

The clonal selection theory of antibody formation proposed by Burnet states that an immunologically responsive cell (small lymphocyte) contains within its genome the genetic information to respond to a single immunogen (or a few related ones) even before the cell encounters the foreign configuration. Thus, the lymphocyte population of an individual is preprogrammed to contain a diverse library of cells, some of which respond to one antigen, others to a second, and so forth. The encounter between the immunogen and the precommitted cell results in its proliferation and the generation of a clone of differentiated antibody-forming cells (Fig. 7–12). This hypothesis implies that an antiserum prepared against a complex immunogen (e.g., bacterium) consists of a population of different antibodies, each produced by separate clones preprogrammed to respond to a particular antigenic determinant on the complex microorganism. In order to provide experimental evidence to support this hypothesis, attempts were made to determine the number of antibodies produced by single cells. It was found that a single plasma cell made only one class and allotype of heavy chain and one type (λ or κ) and allotype of light chain, which display unique variable regions (idiotypes). In other words, *one cell, one antibody*. The uniformity in primary structure of the antibody produced

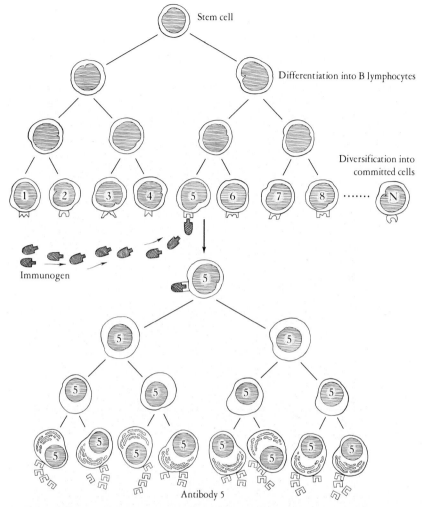

Stem cell

Differentiation into B lymphocytes

Diversification into committed cells

Immunogen

Antibody 5

Figure 7–12. Schematic representation of clonal expansion of committed lympho-cytes as a consequence of subsequent encounter with immunogen.

by a single cell is similar to that of the myeloma protein produced in multiple myeloma and suggests that the immunoglobulin molecule is subject to *allelic exclusion;* that is, the cell expresses only one of its sev-eral alleles for the different polypeptide chains of the immunoglobulin molecule. One possible exception to the one cell–one antibody rule is the finding of a small number of single cells in a population that produce both IgM and IgG or that have IgM on their surface and IgG internally. Since the early immune response is characterized by the predominance of IgM followed later by IgG, it has been suggested that cells undergo an *IgM → IgG switch* during the course of the immune response. This concept is still controversial, but there is immunologic evidence for its support, based mainly on the finding of a patient with a biclonal myeloma. This patient produced both homogeneous IgM and IgG paraproteins. Analysis of these proteins revealed identities in primary amino acid sequence in all regions of the immunoglobulins except for the C_H region, which was μ in one protein and γ in the other. This switch can be explained on a genetic basis whereby in making IgM, the cell expresses genes for V_L, C_L, V_H, and $C\mu$ regions (Fig. 7–13). To initiate the transition to IgG synthesis, only the $C\mu$ gene would be turned off (repressed) and the gene for $C\gamma$ would be turned on (derepressed). Aside from immunologic evidence to support this concept, an interesting analogy can be drawn from the development of high organisms. In humans, there is a complex chain of events that occurs at the time of puberty. Although the information is present at birth, it is not until puberty that certain cells are turned on to produce various substances (e.g., hormones) that have profound influences on morphology (e.g., hair, breast changes) and biochemical functions (e.g.,

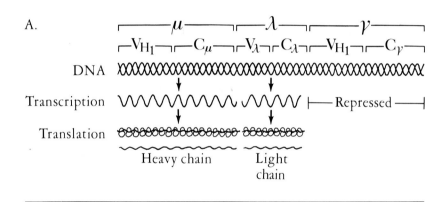

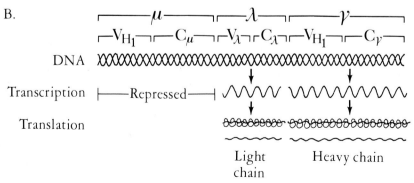

Figure 7–13.   Possible genetic mechanism(s) involved in the IgM → IgG switch in a single cell.

menstruation, ovulation). The mechanism by which hormonal maturation occurs may be analogous to that of antigen stimulation of the precommitted lymphocyte to undergo maturation from IgM to IgG production.

COMPARTMENTALIZATION OF THE IMMUNE RESPONSE

Studies concerning the number of cells required for antibody formation have generated a vast amount of literature in the past decade. It was found that removal of the bursa of Fabricius from neonatal chickens, by either surgical or hormonal methods, resulted in an impairment of the ability of these animals to synthesize antibodies. Similarly, injection of neonatal mice with anti-μ chain antiserum resulted in animals with severe deficiencies of the humoral immune response. The clinical diseases observed in such animals are virtually identical to those seen in children suffering from a congenital sex-linked disease called Bruton's agammaglobulinemia (Chapter 22). In none of the above situations is there impairment of cell-mediated immunity. On the other hand, removal of the thymus gland from neonatal animals resulted in a severely impaired cell-mediated response concomitant with variable deficiencies in the humoral response. Congenitally athymic (nude) mice display similar immunologic deficiencies of the cell-mediated response, although they respond normally to some immunogens and poorly, if at all, to others. In humans, a congenital development anomaly called the DiGeorge syndrome (Chapter 22) results in the birth of children lacking a thymus and displaying severe defects in cell-mediated immunity, along with variable defects in humoral immunity. Integration of these laboratory and clinical findings, which showed on the one hand a division of the immune response into humoral and cell-mediated immunity and, on the other, combined immunodeficiencies related to the absence of the thymus, suggested, even before the nature of B- and T-cells was known, that cooperation between the cells of the two *central lymphoid organs* (bursa and thymus) was required for full expression of humoral immunity.

The current information regarding the mechanisms of cell cooperation involving macrophages, B-cells, and T-cells has been obtained from both *in vivo* and *in vitro* experiments. In 1966, it was first shown that thymus and bone marrow cells act synergistically in the restoration of the immune response of immunodeficient animals, and that if either population was omitted, a response did not take place. Subsequently, it was shown that depletion of spleen cell populations of adherent cells (macrophages) resulted in marked suppression of the immune response to SRBC and that this response could be restored by the addition of macrophages. Elegantly designed experiments showed that B-cells are the specific precursors of the antibody-forming cells and that T-cells, even though they do not differentiate into antibody-producing cells, can be stimulated to divide in response to antigen, can be specifically *educated* (have the ability to be primed by antigen and recognize it at a later time), and provide a specific *helper* function for the enhancement of the humoral response. Further understanding of the functions of B- and T-cells was obtained from studies of the carrier effect, in which it was shown that two receptors were involved in the elicitation of a secondary antihapten response — one hapten-specific, the other carrier-specific — and that B-cells carried the former while T-cells carried the latter.

CELL COOPERATION

In discussing potential mechanisms of antibody formation, two points should be addressed: the first is the mechanism by which the antigen-sensitive cell recognizes the immunogen, and the second is the nature of the signal required to trigger the B-cell to produce antibody. Regarding the first point, evidence has been presented that B-cells express clonally restricted immunoglobulin on their surface capable of reacting with a specific immunogen, and that this reaction leads to changes in the surface membrane, possibly initiating proliferation and differentiation into an antibody-forming cell. While the nature of the T-cell receptor remains elusive, evidence has also been presented that shows that T-cells are capable of recognizing specific immunogens and responding to them.

INFLUENCES OF THE THYMUS ON IMMUNOGENICITY

There is growing evidence that the triggering of B-cells requires either one complex signal or two separate signals. Bacterial lipopolysaccharide, which has been shown to be mitogenic for murine B-cells, has the ability to activate B-cells nonspecifically. Such activation results in a *polyclonal* response, in which many clones of B-cells are activated in the absence of their specific antigen to make small amounts of their appropriate antibodies. Thus, a B-cell mitogen can provide a *nonspecific* signal to trigger B-cell activation. It is thought that the antigenic determinant carries a *specific second signal* that activates specific clones to produce large amounts of antibody. Thus, the triggering of B-cells appears to require two signals, a specific signal represented by the antigenic determinant that is recognized by the Ig receptor on the precommitted cell and a nonspecific signal that may be recognized by the same or another receptor and influences the differentiation and proliferation of the clone. The specific signal is referred to as *immunogenicity* and the nonspecific signal as *mitogenicity* or *adjuvanticity*.

In recent years, by means of *in vitro* systems, some interesting observations have been made concerning the idea that the nature of the immunogen may influence the types of cells that interact in the im-

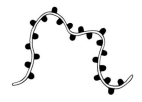 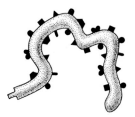

A. T-independent antigen - contains many copies of identical antigenic determinants (e.g., levan, pneumococcal polysaccharide, lipopolysaccharide)

B. T-dependent antigen - few copies of many different antigenic determinants (e.g., RBC, bacterium, protein)

Figure 7–14.   Schematic representation of T-independent and T-dependent antigens.

mune response. A small number of immunogens appear to elicit B-cell responses in the absence of T-cell help. These so-called *T-independent antigens* have been characterized as polymeric substances having a large number of repeating identical determinants that are relatively resistant to degradation and include such substances as dextran, levan, polyvinylpyrrolidone, lipopolysaccharide, polymerized flagellin, and pneumococccal polysaccharide (Fig. 7–14*A*). The immune response to these materials is characterized by the almost exclusive production of IgM with little or no immunologic memory being produced. In addition to the lack of a requirement for T-cell help, it was also thought that the immune response to these materials was independent of macrophage function. Recently, however, experiments using highly selective methods for the depletion of macrophages have suggested that these cells are required, albeit in small numbers, for responses to certain T-independent antigens. Interestingly, it has also been found that T-cells may even play a suppressive role in the response to certain T-independent antigens (e.g., pneumococcal polysaccharide S-III), since removal of these cells by thymectomy or by treatment with antilymphocyte serum results in enhanced antibody production. Therefore, although these antigens appear to be independent of T-cell helper function, they may not be totally T-cell independent in that T-cells may still play a regulatory role. To explain the triggering of B-cells it has been postulated, although not without controversy, that T-independent antigens carry both the specific and nonspecific signals. The presence of the nonspecific signal may be attributed to the fact that those T-independent antigens that are mitogenic for B-cells carry intrinsic adjuvanticity (Fig. 7–15).

   Almost all of the immunogens encountered in nature are not polymers of repeated antigenic determinants. Indeed, they are usually made up of a single or a few copies of diverse antigenic determinants (Fig. 7–14*B*). These substances induce immune response, potentially in-

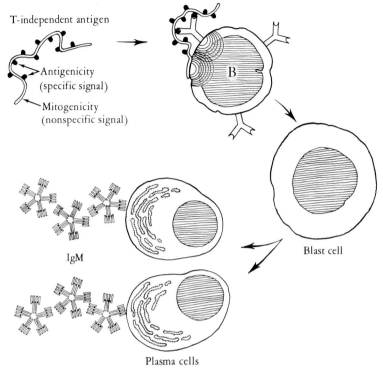

Figure 7–15. Schematic representation of a postulated mechanism for direct stimulation of B-cells by a T-independent antigen. Note that the molecule has the capacity to generate two signals.

volving all of the immunoglobulin classes and immunologic memory, and require T-cell help. Cells, proteins, glycoproteins, and hapten-carrier combinations are but a few examples of substances that make up the class of *T-dependent antigens.* It has been shown that the immune response to these antigens in T-cell-deficient animals is greatly suppressed and limited, for the most part, to the IgM class of antibody, suggesting that T-cells are involved in the transition from IgM to IgG antibody synthesis.

It is now becoming clear that there are subsets of T-cells that influence the activity of other T-cells, as well as B-cells. These T-cell subpopulations have been defined through the use of antisera prepared against alloantigens described earlier in this chapter. The antisera have also provided insight into the ontogeny of lymphoid cells undergoing thymus-dependent differentiation. Three T-cell subsets have been defined by cytotoxic antisera prepared against the murine Ly alloantigens, which are coded for by two unlinked genetic loci (Ly-1 and Ly-2/Ly-3). These subsets have been designated as Ly-1,2,3$^+$, Ly-1$^+$, and Ly-2,3$^+$. Of the T-cells found in peripheral lymphoid tissue, about 50 per

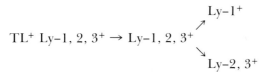

$$TL^+ \, Ly\text{--}1,\, 2,\, 3^+ \rightarrow Ly\text{--}1,\, 2,\, 3^+ \nearrow \begin{array}{c} Ly\text{--}1^+ \\ \\ \searrow \\ Ly\text{--}2,\, 3^+ \end{array}$$

Figure 7–16. A proposed model of T-cell subset differentiation in the mouse.

cent are Ly-1,2,3$^+$, 33 per cent are Ly-1$^+$, and less than 10 per cent are Ly-2,3$^+$.

The Ly-1,2,3$^+$ cells are the earliest to appear in ontogeny and are found in greatly reduced numbers in peripheral tissue shortly after adult thymectomy. The Ly-1$^+$ and Ly-2,3$^+$ subsets appear in peripheral lymphoid tissues later, and their numbers are relatively unaffected by adult thymectomy. The precursor of these subsets, designated as a TL$^+$Ly-1,2,3$^+$ cell, directly differentiates into the Ly-1,2,3$^+$ cell. At present, it is believed that the Ly-1$^+$ and Ly-2,3$^+$ cells arise from the Ly-1,2,3$^+$ cell as two separate lines of differentiation rather than from sequential stages with one maturing into the other (Fig. 7–16).

Cytotoxic antisera have been used to selectively deplete lymphoid cell populations of specific Ly-bearing cells in an attempt to define unique immunologic functions associated with these subpopulations. These studies revealed that the T-cell subsets were precommitted to serve a particular immunologic function during a process of thymus-dependent differentiation, which occurs before the cells encounter specific antigens. In other words, maturation of these cells is independent of antigen stimulation.

The Ly-1$^+$ cell responds to immunogenic stimulation by proliferating and elaborating various factors (specific and nonspecific) that co-

TABLE 7–5. Properties of Ly$^+$ Subsets of Murine T-Lymphocytes

	Ly Subset		
Property	Ly-1$^+$	Ly-2,3$^+$	Ly-1,2,3$^+$
Per cent of T-cells in peripheral blood	33	5–10	50
Ontogeny	Late	Late	Early
Affected by adult thymectomy	−	−	+
Killer potential	−	+	± (precursor)
Killer activity	−	+	±
Helper function	+	−	−
Influence killer precursors (Ly-2,3$^+$)	+	−	+
Suppressor function	−	+	−
Respond to Ia molecules in MLC	+	−	−
Stimulate monocytes and macrophages for delayed-type hypersensitivity	+	−	−
Respond to H2–K/H2–D antigens in MLC	−	+	−

operate with B-cells for the initiation of the humoral response to T-dependent antigens. Thus, the Ly-1$^+$ cell is the carrier-specific T-cell in the hapten-carrier response and is the cell responsible for T-cell helper function. In addition, this cell also elaborates a factor that stimulates the clonal expansion of Ly-2,3$^+$ cells. These Ly-2,3$^+$ cells function as killer cells in cell-mediated immune responses and are involved in the destruction of tumor cells and transplanted allogeneic cells. Thus, there is synergy between Ly-1$^+$ and Ly-2,3$^+$ T-cells in cell-mediated immune responses. It has also been suggested that the Ly-2,3$^+$ cells function as suppressor cells in the regulation of B-cell responses. Although the precise function of the Ly-1,2,3$^+$ cell remains unclear, it has been suggested that it is the precursor of killer cells that destroy virus-infected cells having altered self antigens (Chapter 16). In addition, these cells appear to interact with the Ly-2,3$^+$ cells for other killer functions. Table 7–5 summarizes the properties of these T-cell subsets.

Models of Antibody Formation

In addition to its requirement for T-cells, the complete immune response to many, if not most, of the T-dependent antigens also requires the presence of macrophages. Several models of cell cooperation involving either direct cellular contact or the elaboration of soluble factors have been proposed to explain the mechanism of T- and B-cell interaction. Many of these models also include macrophages.

An *antigen-focusing hypothesis*, based on the carrier effect, suggests that there is simultaneous binding of complex antigens by T- and B-cells. In this model, the T-cell presents a polyvalent pattern of hap-

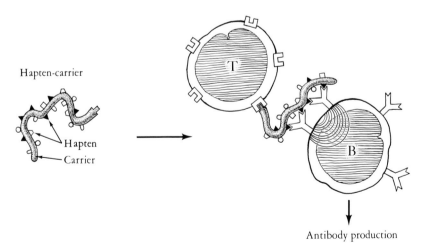

Hapten-carrier

Hapten
Carrier

Antibody production

Figure 7–17. Schematic representation of the antigen-focusing hypothesis. Note the presentation of antigen by T-cells to B-cells, resulting in the cross-linking of two adjacent Ig receptors.

ten determinants whose critical function is the cross-linking of hapten-specific Ig receptors on the surface of B-cells (Fig. 7–17). Present evidence suggests that T-cells play an active role in cell collaboration, rather than the passive role described above. T-cells have been shown to exert regulatory influences on the response of B-cells (e.g., IgM$\longrightarrow$ IgG switch, suppression of response to T-independent antigens). In addition, it is now clear that the production of IgE, and probably IgA, also requires the T-cell helper function. Recent evidence suggests that T-cells exert their effects both through contact with B-cells and by the elaboration of active factors that act at short range with B-cells. In addition, there appear to be certain genetic restrictions on the occurrence of optimal cell interactions, based on similarities of the major histocompatibility antigens of the cooperating cells (e.g., T-cells, B-cells, and macrophages).

Two classes of soluble factors produced by T-cells have been shown to influence the activity of B-cells. The first of these factors is nonspecific (produced by T-cells in response to nonspecific stimuli) and can be generated in several ways. These factors have been used to replace the requirement for a carrier in antihapten secondary responses. One such factor has been produced by injection of allogeneic lymphoid cells into an animal primed with a hapten-carrier complex (Fig. 7–18). For example, if animals primed with DNP-BSA are injected with allogeneic lymphoid cells from a donor whose cells will attack the host's cells in a graft versus host reaction, and if at a later time they receive a second injection of DNP coupled to a noncross-reacting carrier

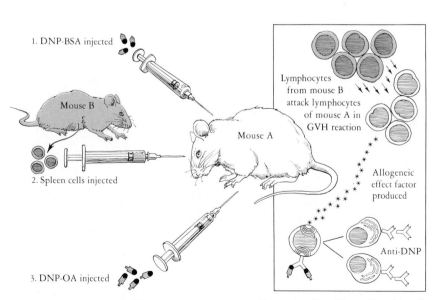

1. DNP-BSA injected

Mouse B

2. Spleen cells injected

Mouse A

Lymphocytes from mouse B attack lymphocytes of mouse A in GVH reaction

Allogeneic effect factor produced

Anti-DNP

3. DNP-OA injected

Figure 7–18. Schematic representation of the allogeneic effect, illustrating the activation of B-cells by *nonspecific factors* derived from T-cells.

such as OA, then a secondary anti-DNP response can be elicited in the absence of OA-primed T-cells. The factor responsible for this so-called *allogeneic effect* is referred to as the *allogeneic effect factor*. (AEF). The active factor appears to be a bimolecular complex consisting of 35,000- and 12,000-dalton subunits. The AEF contains determinants coded for by genes of the major histocompatibility complex of the mouse, since its activity can be removed by absorption with antisera prepared against the product of these genes, specifically anti-Ia. Similar nonspecific factors can be prepared from supernatant fluids of short-term cultures of histoincompatible mouse spleen cells that have participated in an *in vitro* mixed leukocyte reaction or from supernatant fluids of cells stimulated *in vitro* with T-cell mitogens such as Con-A or PHA. Together with the hapten-specific signal, these nonspecific factors are thought to function as a second signal in triggering the activation of B-cells.

T-cells have also been shown to elaborate antigen-specific factors, which cooperate with B-cells in immune responses. One such factor, referred to previously, is monomeric IgM, released from T-cells. This factor has the capacity to bind the specific antigen used to activate the T-cells and also has the ability to bind to the membrane of macro-

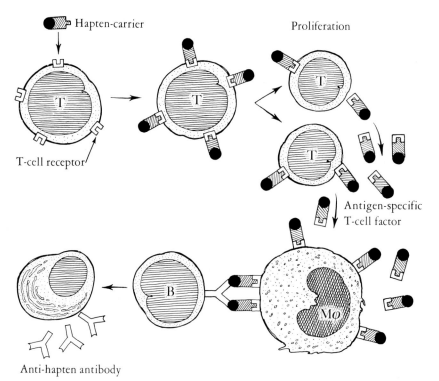

Figure 7–19. Schematic representation of the activation of B-cells by *antigen-specific factor* elaborated by T-cells (After Feldmann).

phages, probably through an Fc receptor. Using *in vitro* systems in which B- and T-cells were separated by a membrane permeable only by molecules, it was shown that upon stimulation with antigen, the T-cells release their IgM receptors complexed with antigen that can diffuse across the membrane and become associated with macrophages. The macrophage-bound antigen-antibody complex induces B-cells to respond specifically to the hapten determinants present on the molecule (Fig. 7–19).

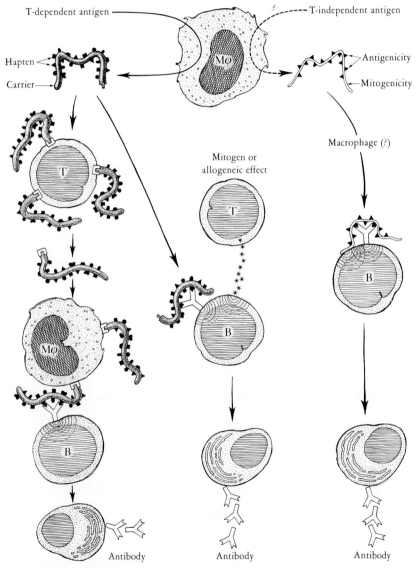

Figure 7–20. Various postulated models of cell cooperation in the generation of humoral immune responses. (After Basten and Howard).

Other factors elaborated by T-cells that both enhance and suppress humoral responses have been reported. However, at present there is a great deal of controversy regrding the role of these factors in immune responses and therefore their description will await the results of further investigation.

Utilizing the information described above, it is now possible to present a model of antibody formation that illustrates the interactions of T-cells, B-cells, and macrophages (Fig. 7–20). This model is based on *in vitro* events and may be subject to massive revision as ideas change and new concepts continuously arise in this rapidly proliferating area of immunobiology. In many cases, the initial events of antibody formation may involve the interaction of the immunogen with a macrophage in a nonspecific manner, leading to the processing of this material into an immunogenic form. In the case of T-dependent anitgens, the first specific recognition event involving carrier determinants occurs at the level of the T-cell and is mediated by the ill-defined T-cell receptor (e.g., IgT, IgM_s, or a product of the Ir gene). The T-cell receptor containing antigen is then released and becomes associated with the membrane of the macrophage through Fc receptors for cytophilic antibody. As a consequence of this binding, a lattice of repeating antigenic determinants is created resembling that found on T-independent antigens. Thus, both types of antigens are presented to B-cells in an analogous manner. The precommitted B-cell recognizes the haptenic portion of the molecule through its surface immunoglobulin. The B-cell becomes activated by a specific signal represented by the hapten and by a nonspecific signal represented by a product of the T-cell or macrophage, or by the specific interaction between cell surfaces. The activated B-cell then goes through a series of events involving its differentiation into a plasma cell, accompanied by proliferation of a clone of antibody-forming cells.

CONTROL OF ANTIBODY FORMATION

It soon becomes apparent that there must be some regulatory mechanism(s) operating to control antibody formation. If this did not occur, antigen stimulation might lead to proliferation of antibody-forming cells comparable to that seen in neoplasia. Several potential mechanisms are described below.

GENETIC CONTROL OF CELL COOPERATION

As indicated in Chapter 3, the immune response is under genetic influence at various levels, including that which encompasses cellular interactions. Such control can exist at the level of antigen processing (macrophage), antigen recognition (T- and B-cells), and cell cooperation.

Advances in our understanding of the genetic control of cell cooperation were made possible by studies of the immune response of inbred animals, mainly mice and guinea pigs (Chapter 3). Specific responses to some antigens have been shown to be under the influence of autosomal dominant genes that are linked to the *major histocompatibility complex* (MHC), a multigenic system determining the structure and expression of a number of cell-surface proteins. In the mouse, the H-2 is the major histocompatibility complex. Within the H-2 complex are two regions, *K and D*, which are approximately 0.5 centimorgan apart, a distance sufficient to include the genetic information for up to 2000 structural genes. The products of the K and D regions are ubiquitously distributed cell-surface glycoproteins that appear to be in close association with β_2 microglobulin. These gene products are serologically defined antigens that elicit graft rejection, specific antibody, strong cytotoxic responses, and weak mixed lymphocyte reactions. Genetic markers have been identified between the K and D regions. The *Ss-Slp marker* appears to control either the structure or levels of the first four components of complement (C1, C4, C2, C3). Located between the K and Ss-Slp regions is the *I region*, which controls immune responsiveness. The I region has been further subdivided into at least three parts: I-A, I-B, and I-C. Recent evidence has suggested that additional subregions exist; these have been tentatively designated as I-J and I-E. There is some question about the existence of the I-E region, based on studies suggesting that cooperation between I-A and I-C reflect I-E function. The gene products of the I region are referred to as I region–associated or *Ia antigens*. These polymorphic Ia antigens are expressed in greatest proportion on B-lymphocytes and only in very small amounts on the various subsets of T-lymphocytes. They are also detected on macrophages, sperm cells, and epidermal cells but not on red blood cells. The Ia antigens are surface glycoproteins that are thought to have an influence on the interactions of T- and B-cells and have been mapped in most, if not all, of the I subregions. It has been suggested that there are specific cell-interaction (CI) genes located within the MHC that code for molecules responsible for mediating cellular interactions. The I region also contains the immune response genes, called *Ir genes*, that control the ability of an animal to respond to a specific antigen as well as the magnitude of that response.

Specific Ir genes have been delineated by measuring immune responses to structurally defined immunogens (Chapter 3). For example, the immune response to the synthetic branched copolymer of tryosine, glutamic acid, alanine, and lysine, called (T,G)-A—L, has been shown to be under genetic control. Mice of the C57B1 strain (responder) produce high titers of both IgM and IgG antibody to this T-dependent antigen. Mice of the CBA strain (nonresponder) produce a normal IgM primary response but do not produce IgG antibodies in the primary or secondary response. Thymectomized mice of responder strains react like nonresponders, thereby suggesting that the product of the Ir gene is associated with the T-cell, since these cells appear to be needed for IgG production.

Additional information has been obtained from studies of the immune response of guinea pigs to poly-L-lysine (PLL). Inbred strain 2 guinea pigs (responder) respond well to DNP-PLL, giving high antibody titers to the haptenic (DNP) portion with cell-mediated hypersensitivity and helper activity to the PLL portion. Strain 13 animals (nonresponder) do not give the above responses. As with F_1 generations of responder × nonresponder mice, F_1 hybrids of strain 2 × strain 13 guinea pigs are all responders, as are about 50 per cent of the progeny of the backcross of hybrids to low-responder strains. Both nonresponder mouse and guinea pig strains will make antihapten responses like that of responder strains if the hapten is administered as a complex with an immunogenic carrier such as BSA (e.g., DNP-PLL-BSA or (T,G)-A—L-BSA). These findings suggest that the Ir gene product is concerned with the recognition of the carrier portion of the immunogen, a function normally ascribed to T-cells.

Although the above evidence suggests that the Ir gene product is expressed only on T-cells, recent studies have established that Ir gene functions are also expressed on B-cells. The evidence can be summarized as follows: (1) with a limiting-dilution assay in an adoptive transfer system, it was shown that the frequency of antigen-sensitive cells in responders and nonresponders was different with some antigens in the thymus but not in the bone marrow populations, and with other antigens the strains differed in bone marrow but not thymus populations, indicating that a genetic defect is not entirely at the T-cell level and may be at the B-cell level; (2) in some systems, effective cooperation between B- and T-cells occurs only when these cells share identity in the major histocompatibility region; and (3) semiallogeneic (F_1) T-cells can cooperate with responder B-cells but not with nonresponder B-cells. The finding that T-cells from nonresponder animals are capable of binding antigen to which the animal does not respond, coupled with the evidence given above, suggests that the product of the Ir gene may not be directly involved in antigen recognition (i.e., it may not be the T-cell receptor) but is involved in cell cooperation.

Recently, it has been shown that (T,G)-A—L-activated spleen cells release an antigen-specific factor after *in vitro* challenge with the same material. This factor replaces the specific T-cell helper function and reacts with antisera prepared against molecules specified by genes located on the left side of the H-2 complex, specifically the I-A region. It has been demonstrated that both responder and nonresponder T-cells produce this "antigen recognition" factor. On the other hand, this factor, whether it was derived from responder or nonresponder animals, will cooperate effectively only with B-cells from responder animals. It has also been suggested that B-cells carry an "acceptor" site for T-cell factors. Thus a genetic defect that gives rise to a nonresponder animal may also be found at the level of the "acceptor" site on the B-cell. In examining several strains for their ability to produce the "antigen-recognition" factor (T-cell) or the "acceptor" site (B-cell), strains have been found that are defective in T-cell factor, B-cell "acceptor," and both. These results suggest that two I region genes are involved in the control of the response to $(T,G)-A-L$; one, expressed in T-cells, codes for an "antigen recognition" factor and is coupled to an "interaction" factor, and the other, expressed in B-cells, codes for the "acceptor" site. It is the "interaction" factor that reacts with the B-cell "acceptor" site and thus facilitates cell cooperation.

There are data to suggest that there is genetic control at the level of the interaction of antigen with macrophages. Macrophages from low-responder strains have been shown to be more active and to degrade antigen more efficiently than those from a high-responder strain. The macrophages from low responders take up more antigen and have greater lysosomal enzyme activity and less surface-bound antigen than those from high responders. It is suggested that since antigen is more readily removed by these macrophages this could account for lower responsiveness in these animals.

Figure 7–21 presents an additional model of cellular interactions involved in antibody formation, based on the factors described above. These interactions appear to be under the control of genes of the major histocompatibility complex. In this model, the initial event involves the activation of T-cells by antigen. This can be accomplished by direct interaction of antigen with the T-cell recognition factor, which is thought by some to be specificed by the Ir gene and by others to be intimately associated with the Ir gene product. T-cell activation can also be initiated by macrophage-bound antigen; some systems require that the cooperating cells share common antigens of major histocompatibility complex. In other systems, however, efficient T-cell activation can be achieved with antigen bound to the surface of allogeneic macrophages. Once activated, T-cell factors can cooperate with B-cells by one of three possible mechanisms. In the first, the activated T-cell can release its specific "recognition" factor, which is coupled to an "interaction" factor (coded for by an I region gene). This soluble complex reacts with a B-cell carrying an Ig receptor and an "acceptor" site (also coded for by an I region gene) for the T-cell "interaction" factor. Since there is no direct contact betwee B- and T-cells, there may not be a requirement for sharing common histocompatibility antigens. Indeed, efficient cooperation between soluble T-cell factors and B-cells has been achieved with various combinations of allogeneic cells. A second mechanism involves presentation of B-cells with the same T-cell factors bound to macrophages. In this case, as in the case of activation of T-cells by macrophage-bound antigen, shared histocompatibility an-

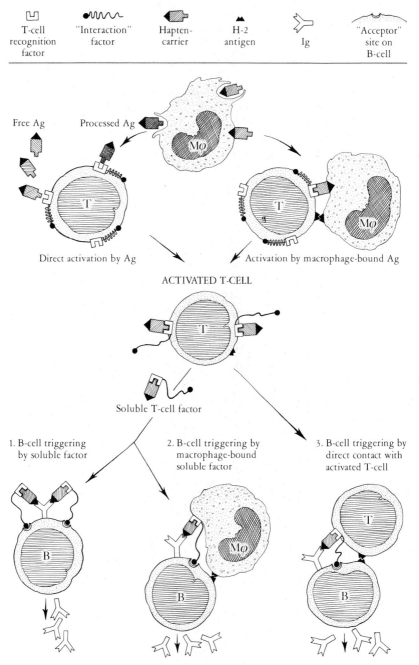

Figure 7–21. Schematic representation of the genetic control of cell corporation. Note that T-cells can be activated in three ways: (1) by free antigen (Ag), (2) by macrophage-processed antigen, or (3) by macrophage-associated Ag. In turn, B-cells may be triggered to produce antibody in three ways: (1) by a soluble Ag-specific T-cell factor, (2) by a macrophage-associated cell factor, or (3) by direct contact with the Ag-bearing activated T-cell.

tigens may or may not be required. A third mechanism of B-cell triggering may involve the direct interaction of activated T-cells with B-cells carrying the Ig receptor and "acceptor" site. In this case, sharing of the major histocompatibility antigen appears to be necessary for optimal antibody formation.

Our understanding of Ir genes, their control of complex cellular interactions in the immune response, and their relationship to the antigenic makeup of the individual is in a very early stage. This area of immunology is destined to have a strong impact on our understanding of disease processes.

ANTIGENIC COMPETITION

The injection of an animal with two unrelated immunogens in some cases results in the synthesis of antibody against one of the antigens but not against the other. This phenomenon, called *antigenic competition,* is defined as the inhibition of the immune response to one antigen or determinant as a consequence of the administration of another antigen or determinant. Although the mechanism is not completely understood, it has been suggested that T-cells are involved, since essential cooperating sites on the macrophage surface are occupied by T-cell helper factors induced by and specific for the immunogen to which antibody is produced, thereby precluding antibody formation to the other immunogen.

Antigenic competition is of both theoretic and practical importance. For the immunologist, it is important to understand the mechanism by which two unrelated immunogens interfere with each other. This is difficult to understand if we accept the premise of the clonal selection theory, which states that antigen-sensitive cells are precommitted to produce antibody of one specificity. This phenomenon has been used as a major argument for multipotentiality of antigen-sensitive cells. For the clinician, antigenic competition has practical significance when vaccination programs are considered (Chapter 23). For example, if appropriate dose adjustments of diphtheria and tetanus toxoids are not made in the DPT vaccine given to children, antigenic competition would occur. The clinician must also consider the immunosuppressive effects of this phenomenon in relation to disease processes. For example, in murine systems it has been shown that infection with leukemia viruses results in an immunosuppressed animal. Similarly, in humans certain virus infections (e.g., measles) result in an immunosuppressed host.

PASSIVE ANTIBODY

It has been shown that the passive administration of specific antibody can suppress the initiation of the immune response to the antigen that combines with the antibody administered without affecting the responses to other materials. Inhibition by passive antibody is pronounced when the antibody is in relative excess. In this case, immunosuppression is attributed to the efficient degradation and rapid removal of antigen-antibody complexes. The clinician has made use of this phenomenon in the prevention of severe hemolytic disease of the newborn due to Rh incompatibility. Preformed antibody prepared against Rh^+ red blood cells is injected into Rh^- mothers at the time of delivery of Rh^+ babies. This antibody binds to and enhances the elimination of Rh^+ red blood cells that enter the maternal circulation as the placenta separates. This procedure prevents the immunization of the mother, who, if untreated, would produce a secondary IgG response to Rh^+ red blood cells in a subsequent pregnancy. These IgG antibodies are capable of crossing the placenta and could result in the destruction of fetal red blood cells (Chapter 24). In addition to the desirable immunosuppressive effect of passive antibody described above, the clinician must be aware of undesirable effects that may occur naturally. For example, the placental transfer of maternal antibody against certain viruses (e.g., polio and measles) could interfere with the initiation of an active immune response against these agents in the young child. Therefore, the clinician must adjust the immunization timetable to allow for the disappearance of maternal antibody if successful active immunization is to be achieved. Although the mechanism of action of this *feedback* effect is not clear, it has been suggested that passive antibody acts by blocking antigenic determinants so that the appropriate antigen-sensitive cells cannot be stimulated.

SUPPRESSOR T-CELLS

Recently, it has been demonstrated that in adddition to the helper function provided by T-cells, the presence of these cells can also result in a reduction in the magnitude of a normal immune response or the level of immunoglobulin synthesis. The concept of a suppressor T-cell population was initially derived from studies involving the transfer of normal or immune cells to tolerant (Chapter 10) hosts and of tolerant cells to normal irradiated hosts. It was found that, as a result of the encounter of antigen with T-cells during the induction of tolerance, B-cells were "turned off" and could no longer cooperate with normal syngeneic T-cells to induce an immune response. This phenomenon is termed *infectious tolerance* and suggests a role for suppressor T-cells in the induction of tolerance.

Additional support for the presence of a population of suppressor T-cells can be summarized as follows: (1) in the immune response to T-independent antigens, removal of the thymus or treatment with anti-lymphocyte serum results in enhanced antibody formation; (2) the immune response of congenitally athymic mice (nu/nu) to T-independent antigens is significantly greater than that of their nu/$^+$ or $+/+$ litter-mates; (3) T-cells from animals displaying chronic allotype suppression will cause allotype suppression by normal cells either *in vitro* or when passively transferred *in vivo;* (4) T-cells stimulated nonspecifically by mitogens (e.g., Con-A) suppress *in vitro* immune responses; (5) on the basis of studies of the hapten-specific IgE response, it appears that T-cells determine the class of immunoglobulin produced following antigenic stimulation; and (6) genetically defined nonresponder strains of animals appear to possess this characteristic owing to the presence of cells capable of suppressing immune responses to specific antigens.

Although there is evidence to support the presence of a suppressor T-cell population, the mechanism by which it exerts its effect remains unclear. Here are but a few of the potential functions of these cells: (1) interfere with cell interactions; (2) prevent recognition of antigen; (3) inhibit antigen-induced biochemical changes in B-cells; (4) interfere with differentiation of B-cells into antibody-forming cells; and (5) inhibit B-cell proliferation.

The importance of suppressor cells is finding its way into clinical medicine. It has been shown that certain patients with common variable immunodeficiency (CVI) appear to have an increase in suppressor cell activity. This has been shown by the inhibition of immunoglobulin synthesis by normal cultured cells after the addition of lymphocytes from CVI patients. It has also been suggested that there is an enhancement of suppressor cell function in patients with multiple myeloma. The normal polyclonal response of the myeloma patient may be suppressed by these cells, with an increased susceptibility to infection resulting. Further, there is evidence to indicate that suppressor cells are closely involved in the control of autoimmune disease. It is thought that with advancing age there is a decrease in number or function of suppressor T-cells that allows for the expression of autoimmune disease. A similar argument has been advanced to explain the higher incidence of cancer in aging patients.

Suppressor T-cells not only regulate the activities of B-cells but also appear to regulate the activities of other T-cells (e.g., GVH reactions). Suffice it to say that the role of T-cells in regulating immune responses is becoming more evident with each passing day.

ANTIBODY FORMATION AT THE MOLECULAR LEVEL

The IgG molecule is a multichain protein that, upon partial reduction, yields two heavy chains and two light chains (Chapter 5). In addition, each chain is composed of a variable sequence of amino acids associated with its antigen-binding activities and a constant sequence of amino acids reflective of that particular class of polypeptide chain. The observation that immunoglobulin polypeptide chains of the same type have identical sequences in the constant region but different sequences in the variable region seems difficult to reconcile with the dogma of molecular biology that states: "one gene, one polypeptide." Based on work done with the inheritance of allotypic markers, it was concluded that each constant-region sequence is coded for by a single structural gene. In order to account for the great diversity of antibody specificities, it was postulated that there were multiple V region genes and each V subgroup must be specified by at least one gene. It is now believed that one of many V region genes becomes associated with a single C region gene for the synthesis of a single immunoglobulin chain (Chapter 5). Therefore, a departure from dogma exists and we now speak of, "two genes, one polypeptide."

The early molecular events preparatory to the formation of antibody follow established patterns of protein synthesis. Following stimulation of the antigen-sensitive cell, there is a period of cellular proliferation accompanied by differentiation. The cells begin to synthesize DNA in as little as three hours after stimulation, and peak synthesis occurs three to four hours thereafter. Increases in RNA synthesis parallel those of DNA, with both mRNA and ribosomal RNA synthesis occurring. The use of inhibitors of nucleic acid synthesis during this time results in marked suppression of the immune response. Morphologic changes become apparent, with the cell displaying a well-developed endoplasmic reticulum and Golgi apparatus.

In the same manner that myeloma proteins have aided in our understanding of the structure of immunoglobulins, studies of their synthesis have also aided in our understanding of the molecular events of antibody formation. After transcription and processing in the nucleus, the mRNA is transported into the cytoplasm where it becomes associated with membrane-bound ribosomes to form the rough endoplasmic reticulum (Fig. 7–22). The individual polypeptide chains of the immunoglobulin molecule are made on separate polyribosome units. The immunoglobulin heavy chain is synthesized as a complete unit on heavy polysomes (16 to 18 ribosomes) having a sedimentation coefficient of 270S. Similarly, the light chains are synthesized as complete units on light polysomes (seven or eight ribosomes) having a sedimentation coefficient of 190S. The newly formed L chains are released from the polysomes and enter an intracellular pool of free L chains. Although there is some assembly of L to H chain at the level of the heavy polysomes, most of it occurs postribosomally as the individual chains pass through the cisternae of the endoplasmic reticulum. Assembly into the fully assembled molecule containing two identical heavy chains and two identical light chains (H_2L_2) occurs by means of a variety of covalently linked intermediates. The H chains, and in some cases the L chains, are glycosylated in both the rough and smooth endoplasmic reticulum. The assembled molecules traverse the Golgi apparatus and then move toward the cell surface. As they are transported to the cell

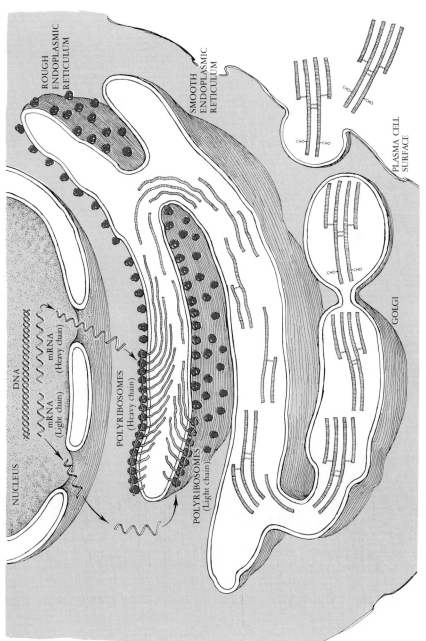

Figure 7–22.   Schematic representation of immunoglobulin biosynthesis at the cellular level. (Adapted from Scharf.)

surface in secretory vesicles, interchain disulfide bonds are formed and sugars are added successively to form oligosaccharide groups of the complete molecule. Most of the immunoglobulin molecules are secreted into the membrane and remain there for several hours before being released.

In the case of IgM and IgA, polymerization occurs with the addition of the J chain either shortly before or simultaneously with secretion of these molecules from the plasma cell.

THEORIES OF ANTIBODY FORMATION

The observation that an animal can produce antibody molecules not only against pathogenic microorganisms but also against foreign proteins and synthetic configurations has led to many speculations regarding the mechanism of antibody formation. The theories proposed fall into two categories that are based on the action of the immunogen, which can be either *selective* or *instructive* in the process of antibody formation.

In 1900, in what we would consider the dark ages of immunology, before the nature of the antibody molecule was known, before the nature of the reactions of antigen and antibody were known, before the nature of the cells that made antibody were known, Ehrlich proposed a theory of antibody formation that was remarkably similar to currently accepted ideas (see Figure 1–11). He proposed that all cells of the body possess side-chains on their surface, termed "haptophores" (antibody) that function as receptors for metabolites, termed "toxophores" (antigens). As a result of the reaction between the metabolite and the receptor, the receptor is consumed and the cell compensates by synthesizing new side-chains in excess, some of which are released into the circulation. Ehrlich's concept of selection of cells with pre-existing receptors for antigen was challenged in the 1930's by the work of Landsteiner, who showed that an animal could respond, by producing antibody, to a large number of synthetic haptens that it would never be expected to meet in nature.

At about the same time, instructive, or template, theories became popular. One of these theories proposed that antigen directs the formation of antibodies from its precursor molecules. Breinl and Haurowitz suggested that under the influence of antigen, the subunits of the antibody molecule (subunit structure was unknown at that time) combine with each other in an anomalous manner so that a specific antibody is formed. This modification was due to the presence of antigen within the antibody-forming cell and thus the antigen served as a direct template. This view was expanded by Linus Pauling, who suggested that all antibody molecules have identical primary structure and differ from each other only in the conformation of their peptide chains. He proposed that antigen within the cell at the time of antibody synthesis serves as a template to stabilize a specific complementary conformation on the antibody molecule. These theories implied that antibody-forming cells are multipotent; that is, they can make all types of antibody specificities. They also predicted that antibody activity would be recovered from denatured antibody by renaturation only in the presence of specific antigen. When it was shown that antibody specificity resides in the primary sequence of amino acids in the antibody molecule, that antibody-forming cells have restricted potentiality, and that renaturation, in the absence of antigen, restores antibody activity, the direct template theory was modified.

An indirect template theory was put forth in which it was suggested that antibody specificity is influenced indirectly through the action of antigen on DNA. This implies an alteration in the sequence of events in protein synthesis from the usual DNA → RNA → protein. It also implies that the antigen can function as a mutagen. These theories are untenable in view of our current knowledge of molecular biology.

In 1955, Jerne proposed a modern view of the selective theory in which he suggested that the population of antibody-forming cells is endowed with a finite number of randomly distributed specific receptor molecules that arise spontaneously in the absence of antigens. These specific receptor molecules (natural antibodies) are released from individual cells, and antigen selects these specific receptors, thereby initiating antibody formation (natural selection). This hypothesis suggested that there are separate genes coding for each antibody molecule and that the entire library of genes required for all antibodies is present in each potential antibody-forming cell. This idea served as the basis for *germ-line* theories.

Burnet evolved the basic principles of the above theory into the modern *clonal selection theory*. This theory suggested that there are a large number of previously programmed clones in the adult, each one carrying specific receptors on its surface capable of reacting with a specific immunogen. The outcome of the reaction between receptor and immunogen is either antibody formation or repression (death of the clone if stimulated during fetal development or tolerance, Chapter 12). Burnet suggested that the progenitor cells of the immune response are highly mutable omnipotent cells. He postulated that the diversity of specificities formed is the result of *somatic* mutation. Somatic development results in the differentiation of a population of individual antigen-sensitive cells, each of which has the capacity to respond to one or a limited number of configurations. The antigen selects a specific precursor cell that then proliferates into a clone of cells producing specific antibody. Although this theory, in its present form, leaves the explanation of certain immunologic phenomena unanswered, it is the most widely accepted among immunologists.

SUGGESTIONS FOR FURTHER READING

The Fate of Immunogen

Ada, G. L., Nossal, G. J. V., and Pye, J.: Antigens in immunity. II. Distribution of iodinated antigens following injection into rats via the hind foot pads. Aust. J. Exp. Biol. Med. Sci., 42:295, 1964.

Campbell, D. H., and Garvey, J. S.: Nature of retained antigen and its role in immune mechanisms. Adv. Immunol., 3:261, 1963.

Dixon, F. J.: The metabolism of antigen and antibody. J. Allergy, 25:487, 1954.

Ehrenreich, B. A., and Cohn, Z. A.: Pinocytosis by macrophages. J. Reticuloendothel. Soc., 5:230, 1968.

Antibody Formation in the Whole Animal

Abramoff, P., and Brien, N. B.: Studies of the chicken immune response. I. Correlation of cellular and humoral immune response. J. Immunol., 100:1204, 1968.

Dixon, F. J., and Maurer, P. H.: Specificity of the secondary response to protein antigens. J. Immunol., 74:418, 1955.

Eisen, H. N., and Siskind, G. W.: Variations in affinities of antibodies during the immune response. Biochemistry (Wash.), 3:996, 1964.

Fazekas de St. Groth, S., and Webster, R. G.: Disquisitions on original antigenic sin. I. Evidence in man. J. Exp. Med., 124:331, 1966.

Mitchison, N. A.: The carrier effect in the secondary response to hapten-protein conjugates. II. Cellular cooperation. Eur. J. Immunol., 1:18, 1971.

Uhr, J. W., and Finkelstein, M. S.: The kinetics of antibody formation. Prog. Allergy, 10:37, 1967.

Cellular Events in the Specific Immune Response

Ada, G. L., and Ey, P. L.: Lymphocytic receptors for antigens. The Antigens, 3:190, 1975.

Bach, J. F.: Evaluation of T cells and thymic serum factors in man using the rosette technique. Transplant. Rev., 16:196, 1973.

Cunningham, B. A.: β_2 Microglobulin: An immunoglobulin domain associated with cell surfaces. Prog. Immunol. II, 1:5, 1974.

Friedman, H., ed.: RNA in the immune response. Ann. N.Y. Acad. Sci., 207, 1973.

Greaves, M.: Surface markers for human T and B lymphocytes. Curr. Titles Immunol. Transpl. Allergy, 1:193, 1973.

Greaves, M., and Janossy, G.: Elicitation of selective T and B lymphocyte responses by cell surface binding ligands. Transplant. Rev., 11:87, 1973.

Möller, G., ed.: T and B lymphocytes in humans. Transplant. Rev., 16, 1973.

Nelson, D. S., ed.: Immunobiology of the Macrophage. New York, Academic Press, 1976.

Nussenzweig, V.: Receptors for immune complexes on lymphocytes. Adv. Immunol., 19:217, 1974.

Oppenheim, J. J., and Rosenstreich, D. L., eds.: Mitogens in Immunobiology. New York, Academic Press, 1976.

Pernis, B., Formi, L., and Amante, L.: Immunoglobulin spots on the surface of rabbit lymphocytes. J. Exp. Med., 132:1001, 1970.

Raff, M. C.: Surface antigenic markers for distinguishing T and B lymphocytes in mice. Transplant. Rev., 6:52, 1971.

Reif, A. E., and Allen, J. M. V.: The AKR thymic antigen and its distribution in leukemias and nervous tissue. J. Exp. Med., 120:413, 1964.

Rosenthal, A. S., ed.: Immune Recognition. New York, Academic Press, 1975.

Singer, S. J.: Molecular biology of cell membranes with application to immunology. Adv. Immunol., 19:1, 1974.

Taylor, R. B., Duffus, W. P. H., Raff, M. C., and DePetris, S.: Redistribution and pinocytosis of lymphocyte surface Ig molecules by anti-Ig antibody. Nature [New Biol.], 233:225, 1971.

Unanue, E. R.: The regulatory role of macrophages in antigenic stimulation. Adv. Immunol., 15:96, 1972.

Vitetta, E. S., and Uhr, J. W.: Immunoglobulin—receptors revisited. Science, 189:964, 1975.

Warner, N. L.: Membrane immunoglobulins and antigen receptors on B and T lymphocytes. Adv. Immunol., *19*:67, 1974.

Cell Interactions in the Initiation of Antibody Formation

Brent, L., and Holborow, J., eds.: Progress in Immunology II, Vol 3, 1975.

Cantor, H., and Asofsky, R.: Synergy among lymphoid cells mediating the graft-versus-
host response. II. Synergy in graft-versus-host reactions produced by Balb/c lymphoid cells of differing anatomic origin. J. Exp. Med., *131*:135, 1970.

Claman, H. N., Chaperon, E. A., and Triplett, R. F.: Thymus-marrow combinations:
Synergism in antibody production. Proc. Soc. Exp. Biol. Med., *122*:1167, 1966.

Feldmann, M.: Cell interactions in the immune response *in vitro*. V. Specific collaboration
via complexes of antigen and thymus-derived cell immunoglobulin. J. Exp. Med.,
136:737, 1972.

Katz, D. H., Paul, W. E., Goidl, E. A., and Benacerraf, B.: Carrier function in antihapten
responses. III. Stimulation of antibody synthesis and facilitation of hapten-specific
secondary antibody responses by graft-versus-host reactions. J. Exp. Med., *133*:169,
1971.

Lawton, A. R., III, and Cooper, M. D.: Modification of B lymphocyte differentiation by
anti-immunoglobulins. Contemp. Top. Immunobiol., *3*:193, 1974.

Miller, J. F. A. P., Basten, A., Sprent, J., and Cheers, C.: Interactions between lymphocytes in immune responses. Cell. Immunol., *2*:469, 1971.

Mishell, R. I., and Dutton, R. W.: Immunization of dissociated spleen cell cultures from
normal mice. J. Exp. Med., *126*:423, 1967.

Mosier, D. E.: A requirement for two cell types for antibody formation *in vitro*. Science,
158:1573, 1967.

Nossal, G. J. V., and Ada, G. L.: Antigens, Lymphoid Cells and the Immune Response.
New York, Academic Press, 1971.

Rajewsky, K. V., Schirrmacher, V., Nase, S., and Jerne, N. K.: The requirement for more
than one antigenic determinant for immunogenicity. J. Exp. Med., *129*:1131, 1969.

Schimpl, A., and Wecker, E.: Replacement of T cell function by a T cell product. Nature
[New Biol.], *237*:15, 1972.

Sercarz, E. E., Williamson, A. R., and Fox, C. F., eds.: The Immune System: Genes,
Receptors, Signals. New York, Academic Press, 1974.

Smith, E. E., and Ribbons, D. W., eds.: Molecular Approaches to Immunology. New
York, Academic Press, 1975.

Waldmann, H., and Munro, A. J.: The interrelationships of antigenic structure, thymus
independence and adjuvanticity. Immunology, *28*:509, 1975.

Waldmann, H., Munro, A. J., and Hunter, P.: Properties of educated T cells. The ability
of educated T cells to facilitate the immune response to noncross reacting antigens *in
vitro*. Eur. J. Immunol., *3*:167, 1973.

Williams, R. C., ed.: Lymphocytes and Their Interactions. New York, Raven Press, 1975.

Control of Antibody Formation

Baker, P. J., Stashak, P. W., Amsbaugh, D. F., Prescott, B., and Barth, R. F.: Evidence for
the existence of two functionally distinct types of cells which regulate the antibody
response to type III pneumococcal polysaccharide. J. Immunol., *105*:1581, 1970.

Benacerraf, B., and Katz, D. H., eds.: The Role of Products of the Histocompatibility
Gene Complex in Immune Responses. New York, Academic Press, 1976.

Gershon, R. K.: T cell control of antibody production. Contemp. Top. Immunobiol., *3*:1,
1974.

Gershon, R. K.: Immunoregulation by T cells. *In* Smith, E. E., and Ribbons, D. W. (eds.):
Molecular Approaches to Immunology. New York, Academic Press, 1975.

Katz, D. H., and Benacerraf, B.: The regulatory influence of activated T cells on B cell
responses to antigen. Adv. Immunol., *15*:1, 1972.

Liacopoulous, P., and Ben Efriam, S.: Antigenic competition. Prog. Allergy, *18*:97, 1974.

McDevitt, H. O.: The evolution of genes in the major histocompatibility complex. Fed.
Proc., *35*:2168, 1976.

McDevitt, H. O., and Landy, M., eds.: Genetic Control of Immune Responsiveness. New
York, Academic Press, 1972.

Möller, G., ed.: Suppressor T lymphocytes. Transplant. Rev., Vol. 26, 1975.

Pross, H. F., and Eidinger, D.: Antigenic competition. A review of nonspecific antigen-induced suppression. Adv. Immunol., *18*:133, 1974.

Shreffler, D. C., and David, C. S.: The H-2 major histocompatibility complex and the I immune response region: Genetic variation, function and organization. Adv. Immunol., *20*:125, 1975.

Taussig, M. J., Munro, A. J., Campbell, R., David, C. S., and Staines, N. A.: Antigen specific T-cell factor in cell cooperation. Mapping within the I region of the H-2 complex and ability to cooperate across allogeneic barriers. J. Exp. Med., *142*:694, 1975.

Unanue, E. R.: The regulation of the immune response by macrophages. *In* van Furth, R. (ed).: Mononuclear Phagocytes. Oxford, Blackwell Scientific Publications, 1975.

Uhr, J. W., and Möller, G.: Regulatory effects of antibody on the immune response. Adv. Immunol., *8*:81, 1968.

Weigle, W. O.: Cyclical production of antibody as a regulatory mechanism in the immune response. Adv. Immunol., *21*:87, 1975.

Antibody Formation at the Molecular Level

Buxbaum, J. N.: The biosynthesis, assembly and secretion of immunoglobulins. Semin. Hematol., *10*:33, 1973.

Parkhouse, R. M. E.: Biosynthesis of polymeric immunoglobulins. Prog. Immunol. II, *1*:119, 1974.

Scharff, M. D., and Laskov, P.: Synthesis and assembly of immunoglobulin polypeptide chains. Prog. Allergy, *14*:37, 1970.

Scharff, M. D., Birshtein, B., Dharmgrongartama, B., Frank, L., Kelly, T., Kuehl, W. M., Margulies, D., Morrison, S. L., Preud'Homme, J. L., and Weitzman, S.: The use of mutant myeloma cells to explore the production of immunoglobulins. *In* Smith, E. E., and Ribbons, D. W. (eds.): Molecular Approaches to Immunology. New York, Academic Press, 1975.

Sherr, C. J., Schenkein, I., and Uhr, J. W.: Synthesis and intracellular transport of immunoglobulin in secretory and nonsecretory cells. Ann. N.Y. Acad. Sci., *190*:250, 1971.

Stevens, R. H.: Distribution of immunoglobulin mRNA in mouse lymphocytes. Prog. Immunol. II, *1*:119, 1974.

Williamson, A. R.: Biosynthesis of immunoglobulins. *In* Porter, R. R. (ed.): Defense and Recognition. London, Butterworth, *10*, 1973.

Theories of Antibody Formation

Burnet, F. M.: The Clonal Selection Theory of Acquired Immunity. Nashville, Vanderbilt University Press, 1959.

Ehrlich, P.: On immunity with special reference to cell life. Proc. R. Soc. Lond. (Biol.), *66*:424, 1900.

Haurowitz, F.: The problem of antibody diversity. Immunodifferentiation versus somatic mutation. Immunochemistry, *10*:775, 1973.

Jerne, N. K.: The somatic generation of immune recognition. Eur. J. Immunol., *1*:1, 1971.

Pauling, L.: A theory of the structure and process of formation of antibodies. J. Am. Chem. Soc., *62*:2643, 1940.

Chapter 8

ANTIGEN-ANTIBODY INTERACTIONS

Chester M. Zmijewski, Ph.D.,
Thomas T. Hubscher, Ph.D.,
and Joseph A. Bellanti, M.D.

The reactants of the specific immune response are either antibody, a product of the B-lymphocytes, or specifically sensitized T-lymphocytes. This chapter will deal with the reactions of antigen with antibody—the antigen-antibody interactions. The expressions of antigen with specifically sensitized T-lymphocytes and other cellular reactions, i.e., cell-mediated reactions, will be described in Chapter 9.

DEFINITIONS

Antigen-antibody interactions can be divided into three categories: (1) the *primary*, (2) the *secondary*, and (3) the *tertiary* (Fig. 8–1). The primary or initial interaction of antigen with antibody is the basic event and consists of the binding of antigen with an antibody molecule.

The measurement of *primary* antigen-antibody interactions can be ascertained by several techniques, including the ammonium sulfate precipitation method (Farr technique), equilibrium dialysis or visualization by immunofluorescence, ferritin labeling, and radioimmunoassay or enzyme immunoassay (Fig. 8–1). These methods are assuming clinical value in the measurement of antibodies important in disease processes, e.g., anti-DNA antibody in lupus erythematosus determined by fluorescent techniques, and hepatitis virus B antigen (HB_sAg) or HB Ag antibody by radioimmunoassay.

The *secondary* manifestations of the antigen-antibody reaction include *precipitation, agglutination, complement-dependent reactions, neutralization,* and *cytotropic effects.* These reactions are of practical importance to the physician, since they form the basis of a number of laboratory tests used in the detection and identification of antigens, antibodies, or antigen-antibody complexes involved in disease processes.

The antigen-antibody interactions are sometimes expressed as *tertiary* manifestations (Fig. 8–1). Such reactions are by definition biologic expressions of the antigen-antibody interaction and at times may be helpful to the patient, but at other times lead to disease through im-

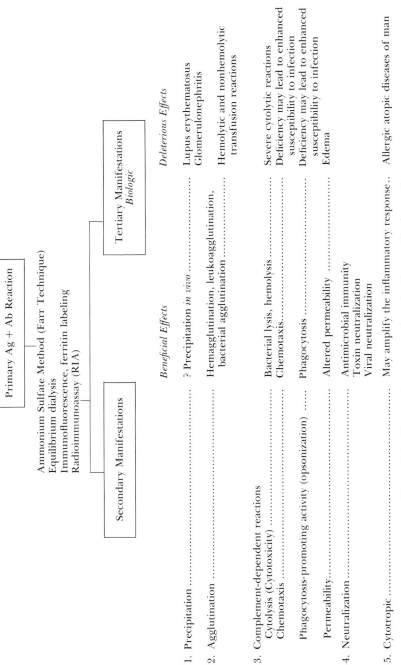

Figure 8–1.   Schematic representation of antigen-antibody reactions.

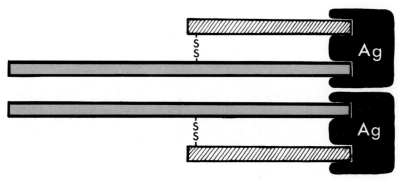

Figure 8–2. Schematic representation of the binding of antigen to antibody sites.

munologic injury. Since the *in vivo* tertiary manifestations of the immune response that are harmful will be described in Chapters 13 and 20, this chapter will be concerned only with the *in vitro* manifestations of the interaction of antigen with antibody.

PRIMARY MANIFESTATIONS OF THE ANTIGEN-ANTIBODY INTERACTIONS

The primary interaction of antigen with antibody consists of the initial binding of antigen with the two or more available antigen-binding sites on any given antibody molecule. This is shown schematically in Figure 8–2. The primary interaction of antigen with antibody is rarely directly visible, and visualization is usually accomplished by labeling antibody or antigen with fluorescent, radioactive, electron-dense, or enzymatic markers. These methods include both *quantitative* assays performed on sera and *immunohistochemical* techniques performed on tissues (Table 8–1).

TABLE 8–1.   Clinical Applications of Primary Antigen-Antibody Interactions

| | TYPE OF ASSAY | |
LABEL	*Quantitative Methods*	*Immunohistochemical Methods*
Fluorescent	Immunofluor method for quantitation of immunoglobulins	Fluorescent antibody method
Radioactive	Radioimmunoassay (RIA)	Autoradiography
Electron-dense	–	Ferritin labeling
Enzyme	Enzyme immunoassays, e.g., enzyme-linked immunosorbent (ELISA)	Immunoperoxidase labeling

QUANTITATIVE METHODS FOR THE MEASUREMENT OF ANTIGEN OR ANTIBODY BASED ON PRIMARY MANIFESTATIONS OF THE ANTIGEN-ANTIBODY INTERACTION

At present, the most widely used quantitative assay for the measurement of antigen-antibody reactions is the *radioimmunoassay* (RIA), in which a radioactively labeled substance (radioligand) is employed either directly or indirectly for the quantitative measurement of the unlabeled substance by a binding reaction to a specific antibody or other receptor systems. Even substances that are not immunogenic by themselves (e.g., haptens) can be measured in these assays if they are coupled to larger carrier substances capable of inducing antibody to the low molecular weight material. Originally introduced as a method for the measurement of plasma insulin concentrations by Berson and Yalow, the technique has had an explosive impact upon all areas of medicine and has made possible the accurate measurement of small concentrations of a wide range of biologic substances, some of which could not be accurately measured previously, e.g., digoxin (Table 8–2). Although the vast majority of these assays employ an antigen-antibody reaction, some substances, e.g., hormones, may be assayed by virtue of their binding to hormone receptors on cells or receptor proteins in the serum, e.g., thyroxin-binding protein (radioreceptor assay). These latter assays differ only in that receptors rather than antibody are used to bind the radioactive ligand. Radioimmunoassays are carried out either in solution, e.g., *liquid- or soluble-phase radioimmunoassays*, or on a supporting matrix to which the antigen (ligand) or antibody is adsorbed or covalently linked, e.g., *solid-phase radioimmunoassay* (Table 8–3).

TABLE 8–2.   Examples of Substances Measurable by Radioimmunoassay

Serum proteins	Angiotensin
IgE (RIST, PRIST)	Bradykinin
IgE antibody (RAST)	Calcitonin
Anti-DNA	Glucagon
Carcinoembryonic antigen (CEA)	Kinins
Microbial agents	*Drugs*
Hb_sAg or Hb_sAb	Digoxin
	Morphine
Hormones	
Insulin	*Metabolites*
ACTH	Cyclic AMP
Growth hormone	Cyclic GMP
Steroid	Folic acid
Estrogen	Vitamin B_{12}
Testosterone	Intrinsic factors
Thyroid hormones	

TABLE 8–3. Quantitative Radioimmunoassay Procedures

Type	Principle	Example
Liquid or soluble phase	Radioimmunoprecipitation	Ammonium sulfate method (Farr technique)
	Double-antibody method	
Solid phase	Competitive binding	Radioimmunosorbent test (RIST)
	Noncompetitive binding (sandwich)	Radioallergosorbent test (RAST) Paper radioimmunosorbent test (PRIST) Hb_sAg, C1q, DNA
	Competitive inhibition of binding	RAST inhibition assay

Liquid-Phase RIA

The basic principle of the liquid-phase RIA is that the ligand to be measured (Ag) is assayed indirectly through its competition with a labeled derivative (Ag*) for binding a limited amount of antibody (Ab). This is shown schematically in Figure 8–3.

The assay is performed by reacting a standard quantity of Ag* with Ab in the presence of varying concentrations of unlabeled Ag in order to establish a standard curve (Fig. 8–4). In a similar fashion, the Ag containing the unknown is reacted with a standard quantity of Ag* plus Ab in a separate reaction mixture. When the reaction comes to equilibrium it is necessary to remove the Ag*Ab from the free Ag* in order to estimate the amount of unlabeled Ag present in the unknown. In the soluble phase, radioimmunoassay can be accomplished by the selective precipitation of the Ag*Ab complex from the solution by physicochemical techniques, e.g., ammonium sulfate method (Farr technique) or by the specific-antibody (double-antibody) method in which a second antibody is directed at the first. The amount of Ag in the unknown is then determined indirectly by the degree of binding of Ag* in the Ag*Ab complex from the standard curve.

Labeled antigen (ligand)	Specific Antibody or Binding Receptor		Labeled antigen-(ligand-) antibody complex
Ag* +	Ab	$\rightleftharpoons$	Ag*Ab
	+		
	Ag	unlabeled antigen	(in standard or unknown)
	$\updownarrow$		
	Ag-Ab unlabeled antigen- antibody complex		

Figure 8–3. Schematic representation of the competitive-binding radioimmunoassay.

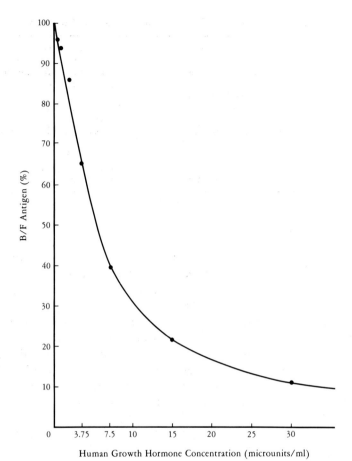

Figure 8-4. Standard curve for use in the radioimmunoassay of human growth hormone. (Courtesy of Dr. Malcolm M. Martin.)

Solid-Phase RIA

In addition to being performed in solution, the RIA assays have been modified so that the Ag or Ab can be immobilized or attached to a supporting medium (solid-phase RIA) (Table 8-3). The main advantage of this technique over the liquid phase is the simplicity of performance and the ease with which the Ag*Ab can be separated from the unreacted Ag*, either by washing or by centrifugation. One example of the competitive binding technique is the radioimmunosorbent test (RIST) for the quantitative measurement of IgE, which is represented schematically in Figure 8-5.

Other types of solid-phase RIA are the noncompetitive binding techniques for the measurement of Ag or Ab (Table 8-3). In this technique, represented schematically in Figure 8-6, either antigen or antibody is attached to a supporting matrix, and then the unknown speci-

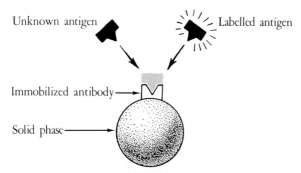

Figure 8-5. Schematic representation of the competitive binding RIA technique, e.g., RIST.

men is added. When antibody is being analyzed, the antibody-containing specimen is added to the antigen-coated matrix, following which a second radiolabeled anti-gamma globulin reagent is added. When antigen is to be determined, antibody is immobilized on the matrix, the antigen-containing specimen is added, and a radiolabeled antibody to the antigen is added (Fig. 8-6). By means of this sandwich technique, which is a noncompetitive direct binding technique, specific antibody or antigen can be detected in a patient's serum. Examples of this technique include the radioallergosorbent test (RAST) for the measurement of specific IgE antibody to a variety of allergens, the PRIST test for the direct measurement of IgE globulin, and the measurement of hepatitis B antigen (HB_sAg) or specific HB_sAg antibody in the sera of patients with hepatitis (Chapter 20). In some cases, the sandwich may be expanded to include an additional layer(s) (noncompetitive indirect binding technique) to increase the sensitivity

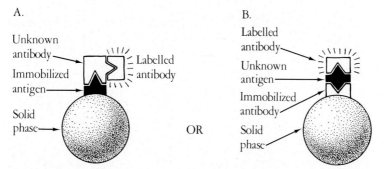

Figure 8-6. Schematic representation of the noncompetitive (direct) RIA binding technique illustrating the use of the test (*A*) in detecting unknown antibody, e.g., RAST and Hb_sAb, in which case antigen is immobilized, or (*B*) in detecting unknown antigen, e.g., PRIST and Hb_sAg, in which case antibody is immobilized onto the solid phase.

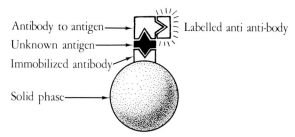

Figure 8–7. Schematic representation of the noncompetitive (indirect) RIA binding ("sandwich") technique.

of the assay or to allow the detection of antibody to antigens that cannot be readily attached to solid surfaces, e.g., penicillin RAST (Fig. 8–7).

Another modification of the solid RIA has been developed for the standardization of biologically active substances. This technique is illustrated in Figure 8–8 and consists of a two-step reaction: a solid-phase antigen is reacted with a known amount of Ab and radiolabeled antihuman gamma globulin, as in the direct sandwich technique described above; and (2) the unlabeled antigen to be assayed is added in a separate reaction mixture. The degree of inhibition of the reaction is used to quantitate the substance. The RAST inhibition assay is an example of this technique, which is currently being utilized for the standardization of allergenic extracts for use in immunotherapy of allergic disease in the human (Chaper 20).

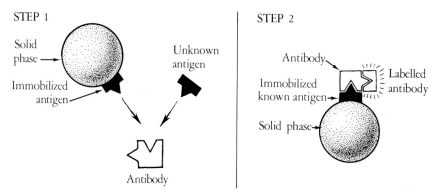

Figure 8–8. Schematic representation of competitive inhibition of binding, e.g., RAST inhibition assay. The assay is performed in two steps: (1) a known quantity of antibody is allowed to react in a competitive reaction between antigen immobilized on a solid phase and the unknown antigen to be measured and (2) the bound antibody is measured in a standard noncompetitive (direct) RIA assay allowing the quantitation of the unknown antigen.

Another radioimmunoassay technique, the immunoradiometric assay, has been developed in which purified antibody is radiolabeled and employed either in a liquid- or solid-phase radioimmunoassay. The primary advantage of this technique is its improved sensitivity and specificity; its main disadvantage is the complexity of the sophisticated techniques required for antibody purification.

Other markers have been developed for the quantitative measurement of primary antigen-antibody interactions (Table 8–1). One of these methods, enzyme-linked immunosorbent assay (ELISA), utilizes an enzyme-linked antibody, e.g., alkaline phosphatase, and the endpoint of measurement is the enzymatic generation of a product that can be measured colorimetrically. Another method is the immunofluor, in which fluorescein-labeled antibody is used as a marker that can be measured fluorimetrically.

IMMUNOHISTOCHEMICAL TECHNIQUES

In addition to quantitative methods for the detection of antigen-antibody reactions, the manifestations of primary antigen-antibody interactions also form the basis of a wide variety of immunohistochemical techniques (Table 8–1). These include the use of fluorescent-labeled antibody (e.g., immunofluorescence), the use of enzymes (e.g., immunoperoxidase), electron-dense markers (e.g., immunoferritin labels), and radioactive markers (e.g., autoradiography).

DETECTION OF IMMUNE COMPLEXES

Recent evidence indicates that antigen-antibody complexes play a major role in the pathogenesis of certain autoimmune diseases, in the modulation of graft and tumor rejection, and in several chronic infectious diseases, including the slow virus infections of man (Chapters 16, 19, and 20). Several techniques are now available for the detection of these immune complexes and are listed in Table 8–4. The clinical usefulness of these techniques has been rather limited since several of them are research tools and are not readily performed. However, newer techniques, e.g., the measurement of C1q, or monoclonal 19S anti-IgG, or the binding of immune complexes to surface receptors on

TABLE 8–4. Techniques for the Detection of Immune Complexes

Physicochemical methods (ultracentrifugation; gel filtration)
Precipitin reaction with C1q or monoclonal anti-IgG
Platelet aggregation
Binding to surface receptors of cultured RAJI cells
C1q binding test
Radioimmunoassays with monoclonal RF (MRF) or polyclonal RF (PRF)

cultured lymphoblasts (RAJI cells), have been developed that may allow new approaches to the elucidation of these obscure diseases, which heretofore have been diagnostic and therapeutic orphans.

SECONDARY OR *IN VITRO* MANIFESTATIONS OF THE ANTIGEN-ANTIBODY INTERACTIONS

The humoral immune response to an immunogenic stimulus results in the production of circulating antibody belonging to one or more of the five major immunoglobulin classes: IgM, IgG, IgA, IgD, and IgE. Evidence for the presence of this type of response may be obtained from any of several serologic assay systems, listed in Figure 8–1, that are based upon secondary manifestations of the antigen-antibody interaction.

PRECIPITATION, AGGLUTINATION, PHAGOCYTOSIS, CYTOTOXICITY, AND TOXIN NEUTRALIZATION

The type of assay system used to detect antibody depends not so much on the antibody produced as on the physical and chemical form of the antigen in question. Soluble antigens, when combined with their specific antibody, will lead to precipitation, in which the antigen-antibody complexes form large insoluble aggregates. The same antigens, if naturally or artificially attached to particulate matter, e.g., bacterial cells, red cells, latex particles, or bentonite particles, will form agglutinates or clumps. This process is referred to as agglutination. If living phagocytic cells, such as polymorphonuclear leukocytes, are added to the assay system, engulfment or phagocytosis of the antigen-sensitized particles may occur. Complement may or may not participate in this reaction; however, should antibody interact with cell-bound antigen to initiate the entire complement cascade, then cytotoxicity (cell death with lysis) may take place.

Toxin neutralization, the ability of specific antibody to neutralize toxin, forms one of the oldest of serologic reactions. It may be demonstrated *in vitro* or *in vivo*. The serum to be tested is first added to a potent toxin *in vitro* and then injected into a living animal or tissue culture system. The survival of the animal or the tissue culture is used as an index of toxin neutralization (LD_{50}) and will occur when antibody (antitoxin) is present in the test serum. On certain occasions, when a toxin is mixed *in vitro* with its specific antiserum, visible precipitation or flocculation will occur because of toxin-antitoxin formation. The Schick test for the detection of antibody to diphtheria toxin and the Dick test for the detection of antibody to tetanus toxin are examples of *in vivo* toxin neutralization.

To some degree, precipitation and agglutination may be consid-

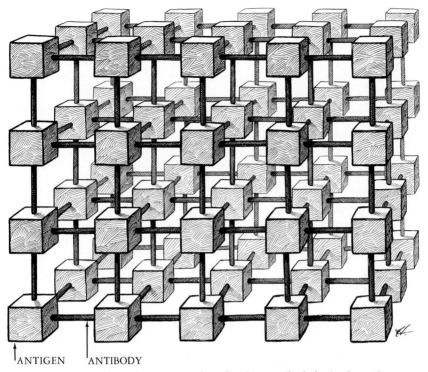

ANTIGEN   ANTIBODY

Figure 8–9. Schematic representation of antigen-antibody lattice formation.

ered as manifestations of the same antigen-antibody interaction, the only difference being the physical form of the test antigen. In both, a two-stage reversible chemical union takes place. In the first stage, antibodies present in the immune serum react with specific antigenic determinants present on the ligand. The ease of combination depends on several factors, notably pH, ionic strength, and temperature. For this reason, *in vitro* antigen-antibody reactions are carried out at specific temperatures in buffered media containing electrolytes. The union between antigen and antibody is accomplished by means of noncovalent binding, e.g., van der Waals forces. When the primary coupling reaction has reached equilibrium, the second stage, or *lattice formation,* takes place. During this phase, the unbound receptor sites on the antibody molecules attach to suitable receptors on additional antigen molecules, forming a lattice. This is represented schematically in Figure 8–9.

As in the first stage of the reaction, the second stage is also specific. Since two antigenic receptor sites of divalent antibody molecules are identical, an antibody with one specificity can link only identical antigens or antigenic determinants on the same molecule, never dissimilar ones. An illustration of this specificity can be noted in the following example:

TABLE 8–5. Sensitivity of Quantitative Tests Measuring Antibody Nitrogen of High-Avidity Antibody

Test	mg Ab N/ml or Test
Precipitin reactions	3–20
Immunoelectrophoresis	3–20
Double diffusion in agar gel	0.2–1.0
Complement fixation	0.01–0.1
Radial immunodiffusion	0.008–0.025
Bacterial agglutination	0.01
Hemolysis	0.001–0.03
Passive hemagglutination	0.005
Passive cutaneous anaphylaxis	0.003
Antitoxin neutralization	0.003
Antigen-combining globulin technique (Farr)	0.0001–0.001
Radioimmunoassay	0.0001–0.001
Enzyme-linked assays	0.0001–0.001
Virus neutralization	0.00001–0.0001
Bactericidal test	0.00001–0.0001

When red blood cells from individuals belonging to blood groups A and B are mixed and then exposed to an immune serum containing only anti-A, the aggregates will be composed only of A cells. The B cells remain free in suspension.

In precipitation, the antigen is a soluble molecule. Therefore, a fairly large lattice must be formed before a visible aggregate is seen. In order to build a lattice of sufficient magnitude, a larger number of antibody molecules are required and the reactants must be present in optimal proportion. In agglutination, on the other hand, the antigen is part of a large insoluble particle, such as a red cell or a bacterial cell, and relatively fewer molecules are required for visible aggregation. Consequently, agglutination is a more sensitive serologic assay for antibody detection than precipitation. This is an important consideration when choosing and interpreting serologic assay systems such as hemagglutination and bacterial agglutination. Sometimes it may become necessary to convert an ordinary precipitating system to an agglutinating system in order to increase the sensitivity of the assay. Shown in Table 8–5 are relative sensitivities of various antigen-antibody tests. In addition to the physical properties of the antigen, the nature of the antibody is also important. On a molar basis, the IgM antibodies are more efficient agglutinators than the IgG antibodies because of the greater number of antibody-combining sites on the IgM molecule; the IgG, on the other hand, are better precipitins than the IgM.

QUANTITATIVE PRECIPITIN REACTION

If increasing amounts of soluble antigen are mixed with a constant amount of antibody and the resultant precipitate is measured quantitatively, a dose-response relationship will be seen similar to that shown in Figure 8–10.

Initially, no precipitate will be formed. As the amount of antigen increases, small amounts of precipitate will result and gradually increase until the amount of precipitate is maximal. With continued addition of antigen, the amount of precipitate slowly diminishes until none is observed. This curve can be divided into the three zones shown in Figure 8–10.

In the first stage of the reaction, there is relative *antibody excess* (Fig. 8–10). Each of the two antigen-combining sites of an antibody molecule can react with a molecule of antigen, resulting in the formation of complexes composed of one antibody holding two antigens. No antigen is available for further union with the excess antibody, and therefore continued lattice formation with subsequent precipitation ceases. If the supernatant fluids are examined, it becomes evident that no free antigen exists. The composition of the supernatant fluids is shown in the accompanying inset of Figure 8–10.

In the middle zone, the concentrations of antigen reach optimal proportions or the equivalent zone (Fig. 8–10). Here the relative concentrations of antigen and antibody are such that maximal precipitation can occur. If, after removing the precipitates, the supernatant fluids are examined, it becomes evident that neither free antibody nor

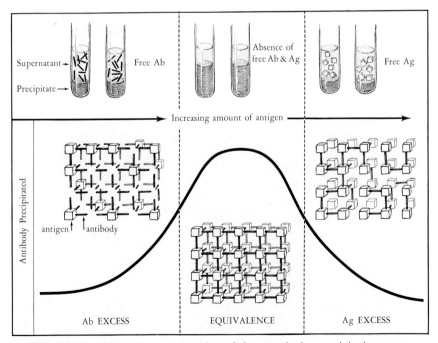

Figure 8–10. Schematic representation of the quantitative precipitation curve.

free antigen remains (Fig. 8–10). The multivalent antigen molecules are tightly held in a three-dimensional lattice by divalent antibody molecules.

The area to the right is known as the *region of antigen excess* (Fig. 8–10). Here, little precipitate is formed, although free antigen can be found in the supernatant. At this point, there is too little antibody to combine with all the antigenic receptor sites. Examination of the supernatant fluid will reveal that free antigen is present in excess.

These relationships of antigen and antibody in precipitin reactions are most relevant to clinical medicine. Phagocytosis is efficient in the removal of aggregates that are formed in the region of optimal proportions. Antigen-antibody complexes formed in relative antigen excess, however, have the capability of initiating a sequence of destructive inflammatory damage, characteristic of the serum sickness type of disease (Chapter 13). These complexes are small enough to remain soluble in the circulation but large enough to produce immunologic injury of tissues through complement activation.

Precipitation assays, apart from being performed in liquid media, are also carried out in semisolid media, e.g., agar, in which one or both constituents are allowed to diffuse into or toward the other. A solution of agar is placed in a Petri dish; wells are cut into the gel; and antigen and antibody are placed in them. During incubation, both antigen and antibody diffuse toward each other from the wells and interact to form precipitins in the agar. A schematic representation of this reaction is shown in Figure 8–11. It can be seen that as diffusion progresses, concentration gradients of both antigen and antibody are established. When optimal concentrations are attained, a precipitate will form that is visible through the agar as a distinct band or line (Fig. 8–11). If the reaction is allowed to continue, the precipitin line may decrease in intensity or actually disappear owing to an excess of antigen or antibody.

The precipitin reaction is a useful analytic tool for the identification of unknown antibodies or antigens. If two different antigens, A and B, are each allowed to diffuse in agar from adjacent wells toward their specific antibody (anti-A or anti-B) in different plates, lines of precipitation will be obtained for each antigen-antibody system. The

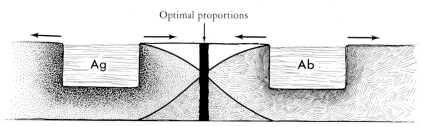

Figure 8–11.   Schematic representation of Ouchterlony double diffusion method.

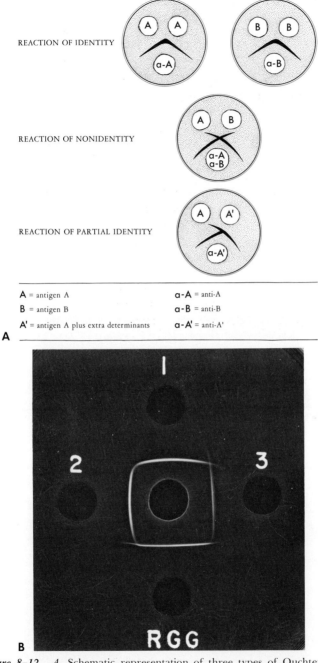

Figure 8–12. *A,* Schematic representation of three types of Ouchterlony double diffusion reactions. *B,* Ouchterlony double diffusion plate showing the reaction of identity between fractions 1 and 2, the reaction of partial identity between whole rabbit gamma globulin (RGG) and fractions 2 and 3 and the reaction of nonidentity between fractions 1 and 3. (From Putnam, F. W. et al.: The cleavage of rabbit γ-globulin by papain. J. Biol. Chem., *237*:717, 1962; courtesy of Dr. Shunsuke Migita.)

region of optimal proportion for the A–anti-A reaction may differ from that of the B–anti-B reaction. This may be due to differences in molecular weight or concentration, both of which can influence the rate of diffusion. With this technique, however, it is possible to determine whether two antigens are *identical, similar,* or *different* (Fig. 8–12) by juxtaposing the reactions between adjacent wells. For example, an antiserum reactive with both antigens is placed in a central well surrounded by wells containing the two suspected antigens. Diffusion is allowed to take place and bands of precipitate are formed. If the two antigens are identical, they will diffuse at the same rate and the zone of optimal proportions will be reached in the same location. Therefore, the two bands will coalesce, as shown in Figure 8–12, in the *reaction of identity*. With further diffusion of antigen or antibody, the formation of soluble complexes will occur. Coalescence will be maintained, however, since the bands continue to form and dissolve at the same rate. If, on the other hand, the two antigens are completely different, the bands will cross in the *reaction of nonidentity*, as shown in Figure 8–12. In this case, the concentration of one antigen has little influence on the behavior of the other, and the two bands that form will cross over each other. Sometimes two antigens may be similar and share a common determinant; this results in spur formation—the reaction of partial identity (Fig. 8–12).

Precipitation in agar gels is widely used in diagnostic immunology. It is most useful in the quantification of immunoglobulin concentrations and in immunoelectrophoresis (Chapter 21). In immunoquantification, the agar is impregnated by the antiserum and the material to be tested is placed in wells. The diameters of the concentric rings that form are directly proportional to the concentration of the antigen in question (Chapter 26). These techniques are useful in the quantification of immunoglobulins in many disease states such as the immunoproliferative diseases (Chapter 21) and the immunologic deficiency states (Chapter 22).

AGGLUTINATION REACTIONS

The same principles governing the antigen-antibody relationships seen in precipitin reactions also apply to agglutination reactions. The notable difference is that soluble complexes are not formed by the latter. Instead, in the region where antibody is in excess, visible agglutination may be inhibited. This is referred to as a *prozone phenomenon*. Owing to the particle size, electrostatic surface charge density, or immunochemical nature of the antibody, certain physicochemical conditions occur that affect agglutination reactions.

Any large particle, such as a red blood cell, suspended in solution contains a net surface electrostatic charge. This is due, in part, to cell surface chemical groupings that may be completely or partially ionized. Since red blood cell particles in any given reaction are similar, they carry an identical charge and therefore tend to repel each other. The net effect of this repulsion (zeta potential), as described below, tends to keep the particles at a given distance. In agglutination, the first stage of the initial antigen-antibody union takes place as in precipitation and is dependent upon ionic strength, pH, and temperature. The second stage, lattice formation, is dependent upon overcoming the electrostatic repulsion forces of the particles. In the agglutination of red blood cells, for example, in which antigenic receptor sites may be located in deep valleys on the cell surface, antibody is firmly bound to receptor sites on one cell. Lattice formation cannot occur until its free receptor valence attaches to antigen between adjacent cells. If the cells are held apart by repulsion forces, the free end of the antibody molecule will not approach the antigen closely enough to make a firm bond. The repulsion forces may be overcome by physical methods that force the cells into closer proximity, e.g., centrifugation or sedimentation. With some antigen-antibody systems, however, such measures have no effect and agglutination cannot occur.

Those antibodies capable of reacting with antigen in saline solution have been termed *saline* or *complete* antibodies and, for the most part, consist of IgM antibody. Those incapable of reacting in saline have been termed *incomplete* or *blocking* antibodies and include the IgG antibodies. *It should be pointed out, however, that the terms complete and incomplete are misnomers, since all antibodies are functionally complete.* Certain types of 7S IgG antibodies cannot agglutinate red cells in saline suspension even though firmly attached to antigens. In these cases, the size of the antibody molecule and its wide spatial arrangement prevent agglutination. Even high centrifugal forces cannot overcome these electrostatic repulsion effects and allow lattice formation to occur. Nevertheless, if these same antibodies are mixed with red blood cells in a colloidal medium such as albumin, agglutination will occur. This principle becomes important in the interpretation of various types of antibody associated with isoimmunization, e.g., hemolytic disease of the newborn or transfusion reactions (Chapter 20).

Zeta Potential

The distance between two particles in suspension is not solely dependent upon their net surface charge density. Ions in solution orient themselves around a particle so as to form a diffuse double layer or cloud. The difference in charge density between the inside and the outside of the ionic cloud creates an electrostatic potential known as the zeta potential. The zeta potential is the essential determining factor of the repulsion effects of two adjacent particles. By controlling this potential, it is possible to control the minimal distance two particles may achieve in suspension.

The zeta potential may be reduced by two methods: (1) pretreatment with enzymes, such as trypsin or neuraminidase, that alter chemical groupings on cell surfaces; and (2) the use of various colloidal diluents, e.g., serum albumin or Ficoll, that lower the zeta potential by changing the dielectric constant of the aqueous electrolyte solution. The net result is that the electrostatic repulsion effects are overcome and the cells or particles can approximate each other, permitting the firm coupling of antigen with antibody necessary for agglutination.

THE ANTIGLOBULIN (COOMBS) REACTION

In some cases, a short antibody molecule directed against a deeply located antigenic determinant cannot agglutinate, even when these various manipulations are employed. In such situations, a third type of serologic technique such as the antiglobulin (Coombs) reaction must be employed in order to demonstrate that antibody is present. The antiglobulin test consists of the addition of an antibody directed against gamma globulin, which provides a bridge between two antibody-coated cells (Fig. 8–13). Most commercially available Coombs reagents used in the clinical laboratory contain antihuman IgG in combination with some antihuman "non-gamma" antibody to detect bound complement components. These are the so-called broad-spectrum Coombs sera and contain broadly reactive antiglobulin activity. Additional sera are available, to detect class-specific antibody, e.g., IgG-, IgM-, IgA-associated antibody.

The Coombs test is performed in two ways: (1) the *direct* antiglobulin test, consisting of the detection of cell-bound antibody by the addi-

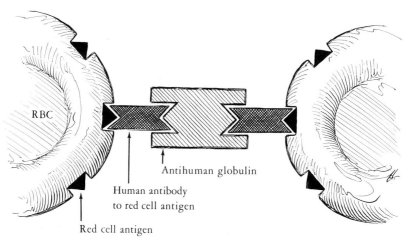

Figure 8–13. Schematic representation of the antiglobulin (Coombs) reaction.

tion of the antiglobulin reagent directly to the cell suspension; and (2) the *indirect* antiglobulin test, detecting the presence of circulating antibody that is adsorbed to the red cells to which is added the antiglobulin reagent. For example, the direct Coombs test would be useful for the detection of IgG-sensitized red cells in an infant suspected of having hemolytic disease of the newborn; the indirect Coombs would be useful for the detection of IgG-associated antibody in the serum of a mother suspected of being sensitized to the Rh antigen (Chapter 20).

PASSIVE AGGLUTINATION

Since agglutination tests are more sensitive indicators of antibody, it is sometimes desirable to convert systems that precipitate to those that agglutinate. This is referred to as *passive agglutination* and can be accomplished by coating a small soluble antigen onto a large insoluble particle, such as polystyrene, latex, bentonite, or red blood cells. Diagnostic tests employing this technique are in widespread use for the detection of a variety of antibodies, such as the rheumatoid factor (an IgM antibody directed against partially denatured IgG globulin) (Chapter 20).

Antigens may be coupled to erythrocytes by various techniques. Polysaccharide antigens readily adhere to the surface of unaltered red blood cells. Thus, specific polysaccharide antigens of certain bacteria adhere to erythrocytes and are used as test antigens for the detection of antibody. Protein substances may be attached to red cells that have been treated with tannic acid. The tanned-cell hemagglutination technique is valuable in detecting antibody to thyroglobulin in Hashimoto's disease (Chapter 20). Finally, certain antigens may be attached to red cells by means of a chemical linkage such as the bis-diazotized benzidine (BDB) coupling reaction. Thus, both precipitation and agglutination provide very specific and sensitive tests in current use in diagnostic immunology (Chapter 26).

COMPLEMENT-DEPENDENT REACTIONS

Complement has been described in detail in Chapter 6. Those complement-dependent effects useful in identifying antigen-antibody reactions include *lysis, phagocytosis, chemotaxis, opsonization, immune adherence, complement fixation,* and *altered permeability* (see Fig. 8–1).

LYSIS

Lysis represents destruction of the cell membrane through the action of the late-acting complement components (C8, C9) that are activated by the reaction of specific antibody to a surface antigen and mediated through the activation of the complete complement sequence. These reactions usually result in the destruction of red blood cells (hemolysis), white blood cells (lymphocytotoxicity), or certain gram-negative bacteria (bacteriolysis).

CHEMOTAXIS, OPSONIZATION, IMMUNE ADHERENCE, PHAGOCYTOSIS, AND ALTERED PERMEABILITY

The interaction of antigen with antibody together with complement can also affect the inflammatory response through chemotaxis, opsonization, immune adherence, phagocytosis, and altered permeability. This involves a multiphasic act including the generation of chemotactic factors (C3a, C5a, C$\overline{567}$), the activation of the phagocytosis-promoting factor (C3b), and the presence of complement receptors (C3b) and Fc receptors on the surface of phagocytic cells. The chemotactic and phagocytic factors can be initiated through the activation of either the classic or alternative complement pathway (Chapter 6). The antigen-antibody reaction usually leads to the activation of the classic pathway. Once initiated, these principles lead to the accumulation of phagocytic cells and to the enhancement of phagocytosis.

The activation of the complement cascade by the antigen-antibody interaction can also lead to the production of factors that alter the permeability of blood vessels. The action of these split products (C3a, C5a) is indirect and occurs through the release of vasoactive amines from mediator cells (Chapters 2 and 13).

COMPLEMENT-FIXATION

The sera of all animal species contain varying quantities of complement. For many years, normal guinea pig serum was used as the primary source of complement in most serologic systems, since this species of animal contains high levels of complement having very efficient lytic properties. Different sources of complement are used in various *in vitro* tests; for example, in cytotoxicity tests used in transplantation, rabbit complement is the ideal source.

Lytic antibodies are rarely used directly in *in vitro* tests. The reasons for this are the low sensitivity of the method and the unavailability of antigen in proper form. For example, although it is possible to detect lytic antibodies against *Bordetella pertussis*, it takes at least one molecule of IgM antibody or two molecules of IgG antibody to initiate the complement sequence for the lysis of a single cell. In order to produce a perceptible change by direct lysis, a huge number of bacterial cells would be required. The second limiting factor may be the type of antigen itself. There are certain organisms such as viruses, rickettsiae, fungi, and some spirochetes that are not susceptible to direct lysis.

For these reasons, the complement-fixation test capable of detecting the same antibody represents one of the most sensitive and frequently employed serologic tests in clinical medicine. The assay is based upon a two-stage reaction in which complement is consumed in the first stage of the antigen-antibody reaction. The binding of complement is assayed indirectly by a detection system consisting of antibody-coated erythrocytes that detect residual complement activity. In the first stage, the test antigen and the patient's heated serum (complement-inactivated) are incubated in the presence of a measured quantity of guinea pig complement. The amount of complement used is critical and represents a slight excess of that amount required to lyse a standard suspension of sheep red cells sensitized with rabbit antisheep red cell antibody (hemolysin or amboceptor). At the end of the primary incubation, the sensitized sheep red cells are added. If the patient's serum contains antibody directed against the test antigen, an antigen-antibody reaction occurs that consumes the complement. Therefore, little or no complement is available to lyse the sensitized sheep red cells. This is termed *complement-fixation* and represents the presence of antibody. If, on the other hand, the patient's serum is devoid of antibody, no antigen-antibody reaction takes place in the first stage, and complement remains in the system and is available for the lysis of the added sensitized sheep cells. This represents the lack of complement-fixation and implies the absence of the complement-fixing antibody. This technique is much more sensitive than the direct lysis of bacteria and provides a simple and quantitative method of antibody detection.

A special case of complement-dependent lysis is the *cytotoxicity test*. This assay employs a system in which the living cells are mixed with antibody and complement. When antibody to a cell-bound antigen is present, cell death will occur in the presence of complement. The endpoint or cell death can be ascertained by any of a number of methods, including supravital staining, gross appearance of cells, or enzymatic function. This assay has wide application in histocompatibility testing for organ transplantation and is also assuming importance in tests of cell-mediated immunity to viruses (Chapters 9 and 16) and tumor antigens (Chapter 19). A specialized example of the use of lytic techniques *in vitro* is the Jerne plaque technique. In this method, a suspension of presensitized immunocompetent lymphoid cells is incubated in agar in which red cells, antigen, and complement are also present. The *in vitro* production of antibody by these cells is detected by clear areas of lysis surrounding each of the antibody-producing cells.

CYTOTROPIC EFFECTS

Cytotropic effects are a property of some classes of antibody that can bind to a limited number of mediator cells of the body, such as mast cells and basophils, and in most mammalian species, including man, appear to be primarily associated with the IgE class of immuno-globulin. When involved in antigen-antibody interactions, this class of immunoglobulin has the capacity to release a number of vasoactive amines important in localized and generalized forms of anaphylaxis (Chapter 13). This class of antibody can be detected *in vitro* by means of the release of vasoactive amines from sensitized mediator cells (e.g., leukocyte histamine release) or by assays involving their effect on isolated target tissues (e.g., Schultz-Dale). In addition, these antibodies can be detected by radioimmunoassay tests (e.g., RAST).

SUMMARY

The manifestations of antigen-antibody interactions can be divided into three categories: the primary, the secondary, and the tertiary. The primary interaction of antigen with antibody is the basic event and may be demonstrated directly or through secondary manifestations, which include precipitation, agglutination, complement-dependent reactions, neutralization, and cytotropic effects. The secondary manifestations of antigen-antibody reactions encompass a number of physical and chemical interactions between antibody, antigen, complement, and the suspending media in which the antigen-antibody reaction occurs. The tertiary manifestations of the antigen-antibody interaction are biologic expressions, which may be either beneficial or harmful to the host.

SUGGESTIONS FOR FURTHER READING

Fudenberg, H. H., Stites, D. P., Caldwell, J. L., and Wells, J. V. (eds.): Basic and Clinical Immunology. Los Altos, Lange Medical Publications, 1976.
Haber, E., and Krause, R. M. (eds.): Antibodies in Human Diagnosis and Therapy. New York, Raven Press, 1977.
Henriksen, S. D. (ed.): Immunology. Baltimore, Williams & Wilkins Co., 1970.
Kabat, E. A. (ed.): Structural Concepts in Immunology and Immunochemistry. 2nd ed., New York, Holt, Rinehart and Winston, 1975.
Rose, N. R., and Friedman, H. (eds.): Manual of Clinical Immunology. Washington, D.C., American Society for Microbiology, 1976.
Voller, A., Bidwell, D. E., and Bartlett, A.: Enzyme immunoassays in diagnostic medicine. Bull. WHO, 53:55, 1976.

CELL-MEDIATED REACTIONS

Joseph A. Bellanti, M.D.,
and Ross E. Rocklin, M.D.

The previous chapter describes those manifestations of the specific immune response concerned with the reactions of antibody with antigen—the *antigen-antibody interactions.* This chapter is concerned with those expressions of the immune response that involve the interaction of cells of the immune system with antigen and are termed *cell-mediated immune* (CMI) reactions. Until recently, these reactions were considered to be mediated only by T-lymphocytes independent of antibody; it is becoming increasingly clear, however, that they may also be carried out by a variety of cell types, humoral substances, or combinations of both.

Although the term "delayed hypersensitivity" has been used previously to include both normal and pathologic expressions of cell-mediated immunity, its use here will be restricted to include only those *in vivo* manifestations of the cellular immune response that lead to tissue injury (Chapter 13). The more inclusive term cell-mediated or cellular immunity will be used to encompass both *normal* and *pathologic* events and will include both *in vitro* and *in vivo* expressions of specifically sensitized T-lymphocytes, as well as those activities carried out by other cellular and humoral components of the immune response.

The series of reactions involved in this type of immunity seems to be characteristically associated with effector–target cell interactions involved in (1) acquired microbial resistance, particularly that associated with intracellular parasitism (Chapters 14 through 18); (2) transplantation immunity (Chapter 20B); and (3) tumor rejection (Chapter 19). In each of these situations, antigen is either intracellular or architecturally inaccessible, and antigen-antibody reactions appear to be relatively inefficient. Cellular reactions, on the other hand, appear to be more effective in the elimination of such sterically inaccessible antigens.

HISTORICAL ASPECTS

The phenomenon of delayed hypersensitivity was first discovered by Edward Jenner in 1798, during the course of his studies with cowpox virus immunization, when he observed that an inflammatory lesion occurred within 24 to 48 hours at the site of revaccination of a previously immunized individual.

225

In the 19th century, during attempts at developing a vaccine for tuberculosis, Robert Koch observed a similar phenomenon. Following inoculation of culture broth of the tubercle bacillus into the skin of tuberculous guinea pigs, he observed a localized red lesion within 24 to 48 hours that occasionally became necrotic.

The characteristics and mechanisms of various types of tissue injury resulting from immunologic mechanisms, including delayed hypersensitivity reactions, will be described more fully in Chapter 13. The following biologic characteristics of the delayed hypersensitivity reaction in skin are presented briefly to illustrate the basic immunobiologic principles underlying these effects.

Following the intradermal injection of antigen into a sensitized host, a reaction occurs at the localized skin site within 24 to 48 hours, reaching a maximum at 72 hours. The lesion consists of a firm indurated "red bump," whose intensity is directly related to the degree of sensitization of the host. For years, this *in vivo* method of testing for cell-mediated responses was the only procedure available and by its nature was difficult to quantify.

It was subsequently shown that this dermal reactivity could be passively transferred from a sensitized individual to a normal host by the use of living lymphoid cells, e.g., blood lymphocytes, but not by serum. Cell extracts of human leukocytes were also shown to have the capacity to transfer this reactivity from sensitized donors to normal recipients.

The history of the dermal skin site reveals the presence of mononuclear cells and few neutrophils, in contrast to cellular reactions mediated by antibodies in which neutrophilic infiltration and edema predominate (Chapter 13). The early histologists were noncommittal in their descriptions of these cells and used the term "round-cell infiltration." Recently, the predominant type of leukocyte in cell-mediated reactions has been shown to be the macrophage. In experimental studies in guinea pigs in which radioactively labeled macrophages were employed to determine the source of these cells, it was demonstrated that the macrophages present in the reaction site were those of the recipient and not the donor. Furthermore, most of the cells in the cell-mediated lesion appeared to be derived from rapidly dividing populations of macrophages originating in the bone marrow. These cells arrive at the test site via the motile form of the macrophage, the monocyte (Chapter 2).

CELL TYPES AND EFFECTOR MECHANISMS

There are a variety of cell types and cellular mechanisms involved in the expressions or regulation of cell-mediated reactions. Shown in Table 9–1 are the cell types with their sites of origin, surface characteristics, and mechanisms of action. These cell types include (1) T-lymphocytes, (2) macrophages, (3) killer or K-cells, and (4) natural killer or NK-cells.

T-Lymphocytes

The first cell type to be described is the T-lymphocyte (Table 9–1). In addition to its collaborative role with B-lymphocytes in either a "helper" or "suppressor" function (Chapters 7 and 10), it is now recognized that the T-lymphocyte, either alone or in concert with other subsets of T-lymphocytes, is important in the expressions of cell-mediated

TABLE 9-1. Effector Cell Types Involved in Cell-Mediated Reactions

		Surface Markers or Receptors				
Cell Type	Precursor Cell or Site of Differ- entiation	mIg	Fc	C3b	T Anti- gen	Mechanisms of Action
T-lymphocytes	Thymus	−	−	−	+	Direct or elaboration of lymphokines
Macrophages	Monocyte precursor	±	+	+	−	Direct or armed with antibody; enhanced by MIF
K-cells	?	−	+	−	−	Armed with antibody (ADCC)
NK-cells	?	−	−	−	−	Direct

immunity. The clinically important reactions include the rejection of allografts, the rejection of tumors, and antimicrobial immunity.

The T-lymphocytes arise in the bone marrow and differentiate in the thymus; the mature forms contain characteristic markers (Table 9-1). Upon further differentiation these cells give rise to a population of cytotoxic T-cells that can destroy appropriate target cells either directly or through the elaboration of specific cell products, e.g., lymphokines. These cytotoxic lymphocytes can be generated *in vitro* in a mixed lymphocyte (MLC) reaction, *in vivo* during a graft-versus-host (GVH) reaction, or during the rejection of an allograft, tumor cell, or virally transformed or chemically modified target cell. Such cytotoxic cells can be demonstrated *in vitro* by the lysis of appropriate target cells.

Recently, cytotoxicity experiments in the murine system have suggested that certain genetic restrictions are involved in the recognition and destruction of virally infected or chemically modified target cells by T-lymphocytes. A requirement for identity at the H-2K or D locus has been demonstrated for both the sensitized T-lymphocyte and the target cell (Chapter 3). Although a similar relationship has not yet been demonstrated for the human, the biologic implications of these findings are very important with respect to antiviral immunity, autoimmunity, and malignancy. Furthermore, based upon these findings, the ability to differentiate between "self" and "nonself" appears to be intimately related to histocompatibility and immune responsiveness. From an evolutionary standpoint, it has been suggested that minor alterations of these strong immunogenic histocompatibility antigens by viruses or chemicals will immediately stimulate the immunologic system. Very recently, a genetic requirement for T-helper function in antibody synthesis by B-cells has also been demonstrated (Chapter 7).

MONONUCLEAR PHAGOCYTES

The mononuclear phagocytes make up a second set of cell types active in cellular immunity. These cells not only are important in the "processing" or "presentation" of antigen for the initiating events of antibody production by B-cells but also may perform an accessory function in the expressions of cell-mediated immunity by T-lymphocytes. Moreover, they may take part directly in the destruction of foreign substances by *phagocytosis* or by direct cytotoxic effects on target cells. In addition, some of the products of T-lymphocytes, e.g., migration inhibitory factor (MIF), may influence macrophage function by affecting cell movement or cellular metabolism. The enhancement of these macrophage functions by agents, e.g., immunopotentiators, is receiving widespread attention in cancer immunotherapy (Chapter 10).

The presence of an Fc receptor and a receptor for C3b may facilitate the uptake of complexes of antigen and antibody or antigen-antibody and complement, respectively. In addition, the presence of the Fc receptor may allow the cell type to participate in antibody-dependent cellular cytotoxic (ADCC) reactions, as described for the killer (K) cell.

KILLER CELLS

Another cellular type important in cell-mediated reactions is the killer or K-cells (Table 9–1). Although their precise identity and site of origin are unknown, these cells are morphologically indistinguishable from small lymphocytes, are Fc receptor–positive, surface immunoglobulin–negative (mIG–), and C3b receptor–negative (i.e., null cells). These cells have been shown to have cytotoxic activity with target cells coated with specific IgG antibody in an antibody-dependent cellular cytotoxic (ADCC) reaction, in which an antibody molecule appears to form a bridge between the target cell and the effector cell. This presumably occurs through a binding of the Fab region of the immunoglobulin molecule with the antigenic determinants on the target cell and the Fc portion of the antibody with the Fc receptor on the surface of the lymphocyte. Complement does not appear to participate in these reactions and, unlike the situation with T-lymphocytes, these reactions can occur with nonsensitized K-cells.

NATURAL KILLER CELLS

A fourth cell type has very recently been described that appears to be a natural killer or NK-cell. The identity of these cells is also unknown; they contain no known T- or B-cell markers and do not require prior sensitization for their generation. These cells occur naturally and are found in increased quantity in mice lacking thymuses (nude mice). This finding may explain the apparent discrepancy in the immune surveillance theory, which would predict an increased incidence of tumors in such animals. The apparent increase in NK-cells may offer an explanation for the lack of increased tumorigenicity in these animals. These cells are thought to be involved in nonspecific killing of virally trans-formed target cells, allografts, and tumor rejection. Although their role in man is as yet undefined, these cells may be of profound biologic significance in immune surveillance of malignant diseases in the human.

EFFECT OF ANTIBODY ON CELL-MEDIATED REACTIONS

In addition to its role in facilitating cell-mediated immunity through an ADCC mechanism, antibody may also exert a direct cyto-toxic effect on a target cell through a complement-dependent reaction (Table 9–1) (Chapter 6). Alternatively, antibody directed against a target cell can "block" the cytotoxic effect of T-lymphocytes, macro-phages, K-cells, or NK-cells, presumably by binding with antigenic de-terminants on the target cell surface. This interference by antibody or antigen-antibody complexes may have relevance for host immunologic reactions against certain tumors, and such "blocking antibody" may re-sult in intensified tumor growth, a phenomenon referred to as *enhance-ment*. Other species of antibody formed in the tumor-bearing host can "unblock" this blocking antibody and lead to the destruction of the tumor. Whether this unblocking effect is related to direct complement-depend-ent effects of antibody or is favored by an ADCC effect is unknown.

COMPONENTS OF THE CELL-MEDIATED REACTION

Like the antigen-antibody reactions, the T-lymphocyte-antigen re-actions may be divided into three stages: the *primary* stage, the *secondary* stage, and the *tertiary* stage (Figure 9–1).

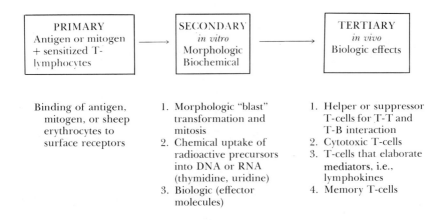

Figure 9–1. Schematic representation of cell-mediated events.

THE PRIMARY STAGE: COMBINATION OF ANTIGEN WITH SPECIFICALLY SENSITIZED T-LYMPHOCYTES

The cell-mediated reaction is initiated by the binding of antigen with an antigen receptor on the surface of a sensitized T-lymphocyte (Chapter 7). This may occur directly or may be mediated by macrophage-bound antigen. There are a number of other substances that can attach to the surface of the T-lymphocyte and either activate it, e.g., mitogens, or provide a basis for its identification, e.g., sheep erythrocyte binding in an E-rosette reaction (Chapter 7). Following the reaction of antigen with a sensitized T-lymphocyte, a sequence of morphologic and biochemical events occurs that forms the secondary stage.

THE SECONDARY STAGE: MORPHOLOGIC AND BIOCHEMICAL REACTIONS

The second stage of the antigen-T-lymphocyte interaction is made up of the *in vitro* manifestations of cell-mediated immunity that presumably result from the membrane perturbations established following the primary interaction of the T-lymphocyte with antigen or mitogen, and are detected indirectly through morphologic or biochemical events. The morphologic changes of lymphocytes in tissue culture consist of blast cell transformation with subsequent mitosis. Some investigators suggest that the macrophage is essential for this reaction to proceed and that cell populations depleted of these cells may be deficient in lymphoproliferative activity. The biochemical events that occur during the secondary stage are revealed by *de novo* DNA, RNA, or protein synthesis, detected by use of radiolabeled precursors. Collectively, these morphologic and biochemical changes have proved to be of considerable clinical importance, since they are used in *in vitro* measurements to assess the functional reactivity of blood lymphocytes in patients suspected of having impaired thymic-dependent immunity (Chapters 22 and 26).

THE TERTIARY STAGE: BIOLOGIC EXPRESSIONS

The tertiary effects of cell-mediated immunity are the biologic expressions of these earlier events (Figure 9–1). They consist of the following steps: (1) the generation of helper or suppressor T-cells for T-T and T-B interactions; (2) the generation of cytotoxic T-cells; (3) the generation of T-cells that elaborate the effector molecules (mediators) of CMI; and (4) the generation of memory T-cells.

For ease of discussion the cellular events that make up the tertiary stage of CMI in a murine system following interaction of antigen with T-lymphocytes are shown in Figure 9–2.

Thymocytes and thymus-derived lymphocytes (T-cells) are a heter-

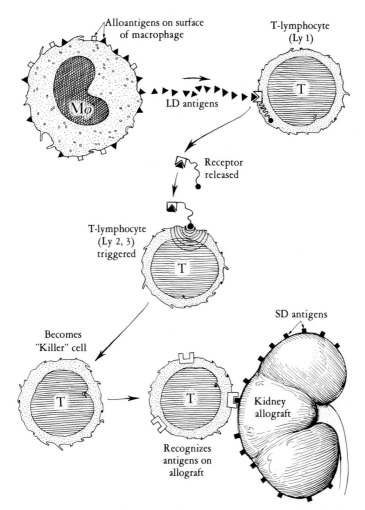

Figure 9-2. Cellular events that make up the tertiary stage of CMI in a murine system, soliciting interaction of antigen with T-lymphocytes.

ogeneous population of cells. This heterogeneity is reflected in differences in organ localization, surface antigen properties, recirculation potential, and function.

T-lymphocyte development depends on the presence of a thymus. Immunocompetent cells migrate from the thymus to T-dependent areas in peripheral lymphoid tissue—the periarteriolar areas of the spleen and the deep cortical areas of the lymph nodes.

Cell-mediated immune reactions are found to involve the sequential interactions of at least two types of thymus-derived lymphocytes (T-lymphocytes). T-lymphocytes in the mouse have been characterized by both Thy-1 (θ) antigen and a series of alloantigens termed Ly. One T-lymphocyte subpopulation bearing the Ly-1 marker responds to antigenic stimulation by proliferation and is responsible for T-lymphocyte proliferation in a mixed lymphocyte culture. A factor may then be elaborated (putatively Ia, see Chapter 3) that triggers a population of Ly-2,3-bearing T-lymphocytes. These cells mediate what has been termed cell-mediated lympholysis (CML) through a number of proposed mechanisms (i.e., lymphotoxin, for example). T-lymphocytes bearing Ly-1 markers may also produce factors such as MIF, which allows macrophages to provide additional help during an immune response against a tumor or tissue graft.

Human T-lymphocytes have been shown to interact in a similar manner. One population appears to recognize lymphocyte-stimulating determinants (Ld) on alloantigens and responds with a burst of DNA synthesis like the Ly-1 cell in the mouse. Members of this population have been termed proliferating helper cells (PHC). Another cell receives the signal from the PHC and differentiates into the cell that mediates CML through a killing mechanism similar to that of the Ly-2,3 cell described in the mouse. This cell recognizes serologically defined determinants (Sd) such as H-2 and HLA antigens. PHC or Ly-1-bearing T-lymphocytes may be the same subset that triggers B-lymphocyte responses during antibody production. Another subpopulation of Ly-bearing cells, the Ly-1,2,3 cells, may be the precursors for these two populations. Other subpopulations of T-lymphocytes and their precursors may be involved in killing neoplastic cells either through a similar response of cellular cooperation or through a response that is more nonspecific because of a phenomenon that allows killing without prior sensitization. It has been suggested that this latter phenomenon is mediated by the cells termed "natural killer" cells, which may be pre-T-lymphocytes. Other T-lymphocytes exist that regulate immune responses and are Ly-2,3-positive, like the killer cells. These have been termed suppressor T-lymphocytes and are discussed in Chapters 7 and 10.

In the response to antigen there is first a proliferation of helper cells bearing the Ly-1 marker. These cells, through the elaboration of soluble factors, can facilitate the differentiation of appropriate precursor cells to cytotoxic cells (Ly-2,3). The cytotoxic T-cells may then function directly in the destruction of target cells. Alternatively, the Ly-1 helper T-cells can also facilitate the production of antibody by B-cells. This antibody, also through the elaboration of antigen-specific factors, can participate directly in complement-dependent reactions to destroy target cells or may facilitate the action of macrophages or K-cells in ADCC reactions as described before. In addition, a subset of T-lymphocytes may be generated that elaborates the effector molecules of CMI (mediators). Whether these in fact represent the same or different subsets of T-lymphocytes involved in cytotoxic reactions is yet unknown. Another function ascribed to the T-cells is suppressor activity. Ly-2,3 lymphocytes appear to perform an immunoregulatory function, are involved in the termination of antibody synthesis, and may also suppress T-cell function. The final event is the generation of memory T-cells, which function in the anamnestic response upon subsequent encounter with antigen. Thus, the interaction of antigen with specifically sensitized T-lymphocytes is brought about by a complex set of interrelated and interdependent processes that ultimately form the common final pathway for the expression of both T- and B-lymphocytes.

EFFECTOR MOLECULES OF CELL-MEDIATED REACTIONS

Following the interaction of a sensitized lymphocyte with antigen, the lymphocyte is capable of elaborating an array of diverse substances. These factors have recently been shown to possess a variety of biologic activities that are thought to be the *in vitro* correlates of cell-mediated immunity. The physical and biologic activities of these effector molecules are shown in Tables 9–2 and 9–3. The knowledge of these effector molecules "has liberated immunologists from the firm,

TABLE 9–2.   Products of Activated Lymphocytes

   I. Mediators Affecting Macrophages
     (a) migration inhibitory factor (MIF)
     (b) macrophage activating factor (indistinguishable from MIF)
     (c) macrophage aggregation factor (MAF) (? same as MIF)
     (d) factor causing disappearance of macrophage from peritoneum (? same as MIF)
     (e) chemotactic factor for macrophages
     (f) antigen-dependent MIF
  II. Mediators Affecting Neutrophil Leukocytes
     (a) chemotactic factor
     (b) leukocyte inhibitory factor (LIF)
 III. Mediators Affecting Lymphocytes
     (a) mitogenic factors
     (b) antibody enhancing factors
     (c) antibody suppressing factors
     (d) ? chemotactic factor
 IV. Mediators Affecting Eosinophils
     (a) chemotactic factor*
     (b) migration stimulation factor
  V. Mediators Affecting Basophils
     (a) chemotactic augmentation factor
 VI. Other Cells
     (a) cytotoxic factors—lymphotoxin
     (b) growth inhibitory factors
       (1) clonal inhibitory factor
       (2) proliferation inhibitory factor
     (c) osteoclast activating factor (OAF)
 VII. Skin Reactive Factor
VIII. Interferon
  IX. Immunoglobulin

---

*Requires antigen-antibody complexes.

TABLE 9–3. Physical and Biologic Properties of Effector Molecules of Cell-Mediated Immunity*

	MOLECULAR WEIGHT	PHYSICAL PROPERTIES	ACTIVITIES	
			In vitro	*In vivo*
Transfer factor(s)	<10,000 ?	Heat labile; (a) dialyzable polypeptide (b) nondialyzable	Mediator production Lymphocyte transformation	Transfer of reactivity to uncommitted lymphocytes
MIF (macrophage activating factor)	25,000–55,000	Heat stable; nondialyzable protein	Prevents random migration of macrophages; may activate macrophages	May lead to accumulation of macrophages; may increase phagocytosis and killing
Leukocyte inhibitory factor	68,000	Protein	Prevents migration of PMN's	Untested
Lymphotoxin(s)	80,000–150,000	Heat labile; nondialyzable protein	Target cell injury	May destroy target cells
Skin-reactive factor(s)	70,000	Heat stable; nondialyzable protein		Localized cutaneous reaction
Chemotactic factors	35,000–55,000	Heat stable; nondialyzable protein	Attracts macrophages; attracts PMN's	Untested
Mitogenic factors	25,000	Heat stable; nondialyzable protein	Nonspecific lymphocyte transformation	Untested
Interferon	25,000	Heat stable; nondialyzable	Inhibits viral replication	Inhibits viral replication
Antibody	160,000	Heat stable; nondialyzable	Reactive with antigen	Varied

——— Involving thymic-dependent (T) lymphocytes.
– – – Involving thymic-independent (B) lymphocytes.
*Additional factors with undefined physical-chemical properties are listed in Table 9–2.

red bump" and allowed a better understanding of the dynamics of the *in vivo* reaction.

TRANSFER FACTOR

Following the *in vitro* interaction of the sensitized lymphocyte with its specific antigen, a substance is released that has the capacity to transfer delayed hypersensitivity to another nonreactive individual. This substance is referred to as transfer factor and has been described in the human and in primates. Lysates containing transfer factor are produced by freezing and thawing blood leukocytes. Both a dialyzable and nondialyzable transfer factor have been identified. The dialyzable transfer factor has a molecular weight of less than 10,000, is stable at 37°C, and is resistant to treatment with DNase, RNase, and trypsin. The nondialyzable factor has not been well characterized. Transfer factor is immunologically specific; i.e., it will confer reactivity only toward the antigen that caused the factor to be generated initially. For example, transfer factor produced from the interaction of tuberculin, with tuberculin-positive cells, will confer the ability to react only with tuberculin, not with any other antigen. Transfer factor also has been shown to be capable of mediating homograft (skin) immunity.

MIGRATION INHIBITORY FACTOR

Migration inhibitory factor (MIF) inhibits the migration of normal macrophages *in vitro*. When cells from a peritoneal exudate of animals are put into a capillary tube, the macrophages migrate peripherally from the end of the tube. If one adds to the medium small quantities of antigen to which the animal exhibits CMI, the macrophages fail to migrate from the tube. This phenomenon, referred to as migration inhibition, is the *in vitro* assay for the substance migration inhibitory factor. This phenomenon has also been observed in humans; it is not species-specific and can be produced by nonspecific mitogens. The MIF generated by human lymphocytes, for example, can inhibit the migration of guinea pig macrophages (Figure 9–3). MIF has a molecular weight estimated to range from 25,000 to 55,000; is destroyed by trypsin and neuraminidase, but not by DNase or RNase; and is stable when heated to 56°C for 30 minutes. Guinea pig MIF has properties of an acidic glycoprotein, whereas human MIF appears to be a protein.

MIF may be important *in vivo* as a substance that contains macrophages to the area of injury. It might also be involved in the formation of granulomatous lesions and those infectious diseases in which cell-mediated immunity and mononuclear infiltration are prominent features, e.g., the tuberculoma or tubercle granuloma. There is also evidence that MIF-rich fluids may alter morphology of macrophages,

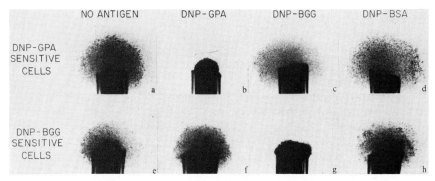

Figure 9–3. Inhibition of macrophage migration. *a–d,* Peritoneal exudate cells (macrophages and lymphocytes) from a guinea pig exhibiting delayed hypersensitivity to DNP coupled to guinea pig albumin (DNP-GPA). Migration of macrophages from the capillary tube has been inhibited (*b*) only by the immunizing antigen, not by DNP coupled to BSA (bovine serum albumin) or BGG (bovine gamma globulin). *e–h,* Cells from an animal exhibiting delayed hypersensitivity to DNP coupled to BGG. Again, this is the only antigen that inhibits migration. The experiment demonstrates the role of the carrier protein in determining the specificity of this *in vitro* correlate of delayed hypersensitivity. (From David, J. R., Lawrence, H. S., and Thomas, L.: J. Immunol., *93*:280, 1964.)

increase their ability to stick to glass surfaces, and augment their capacity to kill certain bacteria (Chapter 15). Therefore, MIF, or some similar factor, may profoundly alter the functional capacity of macrophages, the net outcome of which has been termed "macrophage activation."

LYMPHOTOXIN

Lymphotoxin (LT) is the term for a series of molecules liberated from specifically sensitized lymphocytes or nonspecific stimulants such as phytohemagglutinin (PHA). Lymphotoxin seems to be associated with target-cell injury and inhibits the capacity of cells to divide (Figure 9–4). It has a molecular weight of 80,000 to 150,000; is heat stable; and resists RNase, DNase, and trypsin but is destroyed by chymotrypsin. The biologic role of this mediator is unknown, but the obvious possibility exists that it destroys cells directly.

SKIN-REACTIVE FACTOR

This material is also produced by the interaction of specifically sensitized lymphocytes with antigen and mitogens. When introduced into the skin of normal guinea pigs skin reactive factor or factors produce an indurated and erythematous lesion within three hours. The lesion reaches its peak at 10 hours and disappears by 30 hours. The histologic picture of the lesion is similar to that produced in the delayed-type cutaneous lesion. Its biologic activity may well be the sum of the factors described above.

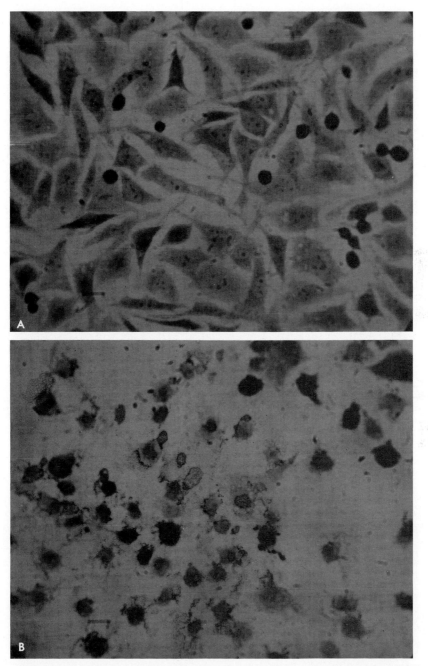

Figure 9–4.   The effect of lymphotoxin on target cells. *A*, Control monolayer of L strain fibroblasts. *B*, A similar monolayer after 24 hours of reaction with the supernatant from activated human lymphocytes that contained lymphotoxin. Extensive cell death is apparent. (Courtesy of Dr. G. A. Granger.)

CHEMOTACTIC FACTORS

Several chemotactic factors have been described that are released from the reaction of specific antigen with sensitized lymphocytes and can also be generated by nonspecific mitogens. One factor induces chemotactic migration of monocytes; other factors are selectively chemotactic for neutrophils, eosinophils, and basophils. These substances have molecular weights ranging from 40,000 to 60,000.

MITOGENIC FACTOR (BLASTOGENIC FACTOR)

When sensitized lymphocytes are stimulated with specific antigen, a substance is released with the capacity to cause blast cell transformation and increase tritiated thymidine uptake. This factor has a molecular weight of 25,000 and, together with transfer factor, may be important in augmenting or amplifying the cell-mediated response by recruiting uncommitted lymphocytes.

INTERFERON

Interferon is a substance of approximately 25,000 molecular weight that is released from infected cells following viral infection (Chapter 16). It is also released from sensitized lymphocytes upon interaction with specific antigens and nonspecific stimulators such as PHA. This factor is known to be an important effector molecule, significant in the recovery mechanisms of viral infections (Chapter 16). The substance is particularly well suited to cell-mediated responses involving viral interactions *in vivo*.

ANTIBODY

Antibody may also be released following interaction of antigen with specifically sensitized B-lymphocytes; however, it is not known whether antibody is produced by the same cells that elaborate MIF and other mediators. The role of antibody has been presented in previous chapters. Its function may be to augment the cell-mediated responses in a variety of ways, e.g., ADCC reactions.

CELL TYPES ELABORATING MEDIATORS

Studies in animals indicate that thymus-derived (T) lymphocytes are responsible for producing soluble mediators. The recent availability of methods to purify lymphocyte subpopulations with almost complete recovery of cells has permitted further investigation into the basis for antigen-induced lymphocyte activation. By use of purified populations, it has been shown that both T- and B-cells proliferate in response to mitogens such as PHA, Con-A, and pokeweed, but only T-cells proliferate directly in response to antigen. Both T- and B-cells produce MIF, chemotactic factor, and interferon in response to specific antigen or mitogens. However, only T-cells produce lymphocyte mitogenic factor to which both T- and B-cells are activated. Although the production of lymphocyte mediators may correlate with the presence of cell-mediated immunity, it is clear that these factors are not solely products of activated T-cells.

LYMPHOCYTE-MACROPHAGE INTERACTIONS

A surprising number of lymphocyte functions appear to be based upon low molecular weight substances. A small number of sensitized lymphocytes (effector cells) could amplify the total response by the recruitment of larger numbers of uncommitted cells (transfer factor, mitogenic factor). The elaboration of lymphotoxin could destroy unwanted foreign cells; the attraction of macrophages and polymorphonuclear leukocytes could be accomplished through the action of chemotactic factors; and interferon could be of particular value in inhibiting the replication of viruses. Finally, the role of antibody could participate in several of the antigen-antibody reactions or in ADCC reactions.

SUMMARY

Cell-mediated immunity includes those manifestations of the specific immune response expressed by a variety of cells and cell products. The hallmarks of these reactions, which differentiate them from humoral antigen-antibody reactions, are their delayed onset, the requirement for living lymphocytes or their products to elicit the response, and the recently discovered effector molecules with relatively low molecular weights, which appear to be the *in vitro* correlates of the *in vivo* response. This type of immunologic mechanism appears to be particularly well suited to antigens that are cell-bound or in other ways inaccessible to the antibody mechanism.

IN VIVO EXPRESSIONS

The *in vivo* manifestations of the immune response are a continuum consisting of the interactions of the host with all foreign macromolecular substances (immunogens) and include all the possible expressions of the immune response appropriate for the type of stimulus. The separation of these responses into "harmful" and "helpful" expressions of the immune response is artificial, since the total ar-

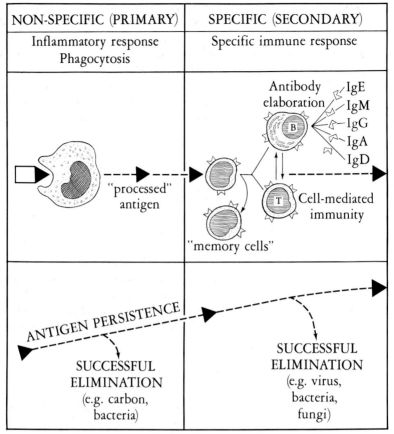

NON-SPECIFIC (PRIMARY)	SPECIFIC (SECONDARY)
Inflammatory response Phagocytosis	Specific immune response

Figure 9–5. Schematic representation of the *in vivo* expressions of the immune responses.

mamentarium of the immune response is available for the disposal of a foreign substance. The types of *in vivo* expressions that are available are shown in Figure 9–5. They consist of phagocytosis, the inflammatory response, and those responses mediated by products of the specific immune response, antibody and cell-mediated immunity. The host response depends on whether the encounter is *initial* or a *repeat.*

THE BODY'S FIRST ENCOUNTER WITH ANTIGEN

If a material is a particulate substance, such as a bacterium or a virus, the body will attempt to eliminate it by phagocytosis. Since this is the first encounter, there is no pre-existing antibody (opsonins) to facilitate engulfment. The fate of the disposal is decided by the efficiency of the unenhanced phagocytic process. If processing is successful, the material is eliminated and disease symptoms are not seen or are minimal. This is represented schematically in Figure 9–5. The specific immune response is induced to elaborate cells capable of antibody production or cell-mediated events (Figure 9–5). Subsequent encounter with the same material will result in an enhanced efficiency of this process (see below). This is shown schematically in Figure 9–5 and represents the elimination of all exogenous antigens (bacterial organisms, viruses, particulate matter), as well as altered or dead self components (effete red blood cells).

Phagocytosis may be unsuccessful because of the quantity or physical characteristics of the material or the general condition (health) of the host. For example, many encapsulated bacterial organisms (pneumococcus) escape engulfment because of the smoothness of the capsule. Other organisms may be engulfed but survive within the phagocyte (e.g., tubercle bacillus). In either event, active disease or death can occur (Figure 9–5). The outcome of the disease is then determined by the efficiency of the specific immune response, both antibody production and cell-mediated immunity. After the appearance of antibody, which with complement facilitates the uptake of an encapsulated organism, the phagocytes successfully destroy the disease-producing organism. Further, with the appearance of cell-mediated immunity and the elaboration of the effector molecules (MIF, mitogenic factor, and so on), phagocytosis by macrophages is enhanced, with elimination of organisms in this fashion. These events are described more fully in Chapter 15.

Subsequent Encounters

All subsequent encounters of the host with a foreign substance lead to the same events described previously, except that the responses are greatly enhanced. Because of rapid recall, there is an increased number of cells involved in antibody production or in cell-mediated events resulting in products of the specific immune response. These processes, either alone or in concert with phagocytosis, expedite the elimination of the unwanted material (Figure 9–5). However, even a subsequent encounter may be unsuccessful because of the general condition of the host, e.g., underlying disease, immunosuppressive therapy, or an overwhelming dose of challenge inoculum. The efficiency with which the immune response can dispose of foreign antigens determines whether the outcome will be beneficial or harmful. If antigen is successfully removed or eliminated by the more primitive responses of phagocytosis and inflammatory response, with or without enhancement by the specific immune response, then the outcome will be beneficial. If antigen cannot be eliminated, the more deleterious, devastating effects of the immune response (tertiary immune response) occur, manifested as the immunologically mediated diseases of man (Chapter 20).

Summary

The *in vivo* manifestations of the immune response may be viewed as the total capacity of the host recognition system to dispose of foreign substances (antigens). These include the primitive responses of phagocytosis and inflammatory responses, which can dispose of most foreign substances. In the case of pathogens that have assumed virulent characteristics to evade these responses, a more sophisticated secondary system, the specific immune response, can lead to products that facilitate or enhance these primitive responses. The products include the elaboration of antibody or cell-mediated events that can effect disposal of the antigen, either alone or in concert with the more primitive responses. The outcome of this encounter of the host with a foreign configuration will be either beneficial or harmful, depending upon the efficiency with which the foreign substance can be eliminated.

SUGGESTIONS FOR FURTHER READING

Bloom, B. R., and Glade, P. R. (eds.): In Vitro Methods in Cell-Mediated Immunity. New York, Academic Press, 1971.

David, J. R., and David, R. R.: Cellular hypersensitivity and immunity: inhibition of macrophage migration and the lymphocyte mediators. Progr. Allergy, *16*:300, 1972.

Edelman, G. M. (ed.): Cellular Selection and Regulation in the Immune Response. New York, Raven Press, 1974.

Lawrence, H. S.: Transfer factor. Adv. Immunol., *11*:195, 1969.

Rocklin, R. E.: Clinical applications of in-vitro lymphocyte tests. Progr. Clin. Immunol., 2:21, 1974.

Rose, N. R., and Friedman, H. (eds.): Manual of Clinical Immunology, Washington, D.C. American Society for Microbiology, 1976.

Williams, R. C., Jr., (ed.): Lymphocytes and Their Interactions. Kroc Foundation Series, Vol. 4. New York, Raven Press, 1975.

IMMUNOMODULATION: IMMUNOPOTENTIATION, TOLERANCE, AND IMMUNOSUPPRESSION

Samuel Waksal, Ph.D.

The immune system is a very complex homeostatic system consisting of a network of interacting cells. It allows the organism to exist within itself and maintain a surveillance mechanism to recognize certain components that are considered "nonself." In certain states, such as intrusions from the outside by foreign organisms or during somatic mutations, the immune system functions to recognize and destroy components that might harm the integrity of the organism. In some instances, however, disturbances of the system do not allow optimal function, and, therefore, malignant disease or infection overcomes the mammalian organism. In such cases it is necesssary to try to potentiate immune function in order to help the host with cancer or another disease control the invasion of the foreign intruder.

But, as in most biologic systems, immunity presents us with a two-edged sword. Since it protects the organism from outside invaders, it also inhibits organ and bone marrow grafts from saving the patient in life-threatening clinical situations. In these cases, the immune system must be suppressed to allow the grafts to become a part of the organism (Chapter 25).

IMMUNOPOTENTIATION

One of the newest and most exciting of the therapeutic modalities in the armamentarium of clinical immunology is *immunopotentiation*. Immunopotentiation may be defined as the augmentation of the host's nonspecific or specific immune responses through the use of a wide variety of biologically active substances. Discoveries in basic immunology that have permitted us to distinguish systems operating via either T-lymphocytes or B-lymphocytes, in addition to a variety of clinical observations, have led to the basic concepts of enhancing the ability of immunologically depressed hosts to respond to tumor antigens or to the

243

antigens of other infectious agents. This process may act to augment or totally restore the compromised immunologic system. It includes both specific and nonspecific mechanisms and may use both active and passive immunization. Current emphasis is on the use of immunopotentiation and the stimulation of the host's immune system to his own neoplasm (Chapter 19).

SPECIFIC IMMUNOPOTENTIATION

Utilizing the knowledge that the cell types involved in immunologic responses to foreign antigens act in a very specific manner and are mediated by receptor molecules on their surface that bind to restricted forms of antigen (Chapter 7), methods are now being tried that may transfer or confer immune specificity to the host to be used against his own tumor (Chapter 19).

Although a number of methods are being employed, all are in the experimental and clinical trial stages. Among the materials being used are transfer factor and immune RNA (Chapters 7 and 9). These substances have an advantage over the adoptive transfer of cells from a host to the tumor-bearing patient, since the chances of graft-versus-host disease due to immunocompetent lymphocytes are eliminated.

Transfer factor is a cell-free extract, produced from lymphocytes by freeze thawing, found to transfer delayed-type hypersensitivity (DTH) and cell-mediated immunity (CMI) from human subjects who could respond to certain antigens, e.g., PPD (tuberculin-sensitive) to subjects who could not (Chapter 9). This transfer was found to be specific to certain antigens and not an immunoadjuvant effect. Transfer factor, which was originally discovered by Lawrence in 1950, was found to be a DNase-resistant, heat-labile, and dializable material. It is now thought that it is derived from T-lymphocytes and acts on T-lymphocytes to effect its specific action. The most promising clinical trials with transfer factor have been in the restoration of immunocompetence in such immune deficiency diseases as Wiskott-Aldrich syndrome and in cases of systemic candidiasis (Chapter 22). The use of transfer factor in tumor immunology has not shown any real success. The clinical experiments that suggested that transfer factor may be promising involved making transfer factor from a healthy identical twin who responded to sarcoma tumor antigens on tumor cells of the twin with a malignant tumor. The transfer factor, given to the twin with the tumor, enabled his cells to make MIF to the tumor cells *in vitro* after three doses, although he had earlier been unresponsive to the tumor. However, there was no evidence of tumor regression with transfer factor treatment, and the subject remains poorly understood and needs continued research.

Another specific mediator is a hot phenolic extract of immune lymphocytes known as immune RNA (Chapter 7). Because of work suggesting that RNA may transfer immunologic specificity, studies were carried out in animal models in which allogeneic or xenogeneic lymphocytes were immunized to tumor cells, after which RNA was extracted from these lymphocytes. These studies suggested that tumor regression occurred in those animals receiving immune RNA. Studies utilizing immune RNA from patients with malignant tumors have also been promising. Immune RNA has been made from the lymphocytes from animals immunized with tumor; the patients' lymphocytes showed an increased ability to specifically kill the tumor cells that were used as the original immunogen. The immune RNA is susceptible to RNase but not DNase or protease.

Studies with both transfer factor and immune RNA are still in the preliminary stages, and, although the approaches seem hopeful, there is still no definitive evidence of success.

ADJUVANTS AND NONSPECIFIC STIMULATION OF THE IMMUNE SYSTEM

Utilization of the specificity of immunologic mechanisms has offered an apparently valuable approach to the problems concerning disease and neoplasia. Recently, there has been intensive research concerning materials that confer on the recipient an ability to respond in a heightened manner to noncross-reacting antigens, e.g., tumor antigens, and function as nonspecific stimulators (Table 10–1). Although much remains to be understood, nonspecific stimulators or adjuvants appear to induce their effects in a number of ways, including the following: (1)

TABLE 10–1.   Nonspecific Stimulators of the Immune System

Microorganisms and subcellular fractions
1. Mycobacteria
   Human and animal strains of mycobacteria (e.g., BCG, MER)
2. Gram-negative bacilli
   (e.g., Salmonella, *Haemophilus influenzae, Bordetella pertussis,*
   endotoxin moieties)
3. Gram-positive bacilli
   (e.g., *Corynebacterium parvum, Corynebacterium granulosum,* Listeria)
4. Gram-positive cocci
   (e.g., staphylococci, streptococci)
5. Others
   (e.g., zymosan, lactic dehydrogenase virus)

Nonbacterial materials
1. Macromolecules
   (e.g., nucleic acids, DNA, RNA; synthetic complementary homopolymers, double-stranded polyinosinic acid • polycytidylic acid
   (poly(I) • poly(C)), polyadenylic acid • polyuridylic acid (poly(A)•
   poly(U)); antilymphocyte serum
2. Small molecules
   (a) organic (e.g., vitamin A, fatty acids, and lipids)
   (b) inorganic (e.g., beryllium, betonite, alum, silica)
3. Pharmacologic agents
   (e.g., levamisole)

Prolongation of the release of antigen. Antigen injected subcutaneously in water in oil emulsions (e.g., incomplete Freund's adjuvant) markedly increases the half-life of the antigen, (2) *Antigen denaturation.* Certain antigens, especially serum proteins like gamma globulin, are to-lerogenic in their native forms but immunogenic if denatured or made particulate, (3) *Recruitment of antigen-reactive cells.* Granulomas develop at the site of injection of complete Freund's adjuvant (water in oil emulsion containing mycobacteria) and expose macrophages and lymphoid cells to a high concentration of antigen, (4) *Proliferation and differentiation of immunologically competent cells.* Lipopolysaccharide, for example (Table 10–1), a selective B-cell mitogen, vitamin A, which induces proliferation of cells in the T-dependent areas of draining lymph nodes, and other adjuvants probably provide a general immune stimulus through their ability to induce proliferation and differentiation of lymphocytes, (5) *Stimulation of cell-mediated immunity in addition to antibody formation.* Although most adjuvants do not increase delayed hypersensitivity to protein antigens, Freund's complete adjuvant, in contrast to Freund's incomplete adjuvant, facilitates the development of such responses against serum proteins (Fig. 10–1).

ADJUVANTS AND IMMUNOTHERAPY

In the early 1900's it was noted that patients with active or quiescent tuberculosis appeared to be less susceptible to pneumonic plague.

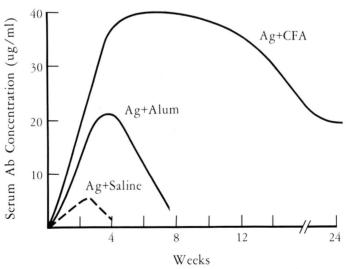

Figure 10–1. Effect of adjuvant on antibody production to a soluble protein antigen. A single injection of bovine-gamma globulin (BGG) in rabbits illustrates the effects of adjuvants on the induction of antibody formation. CFA = complete Freund's adjuvant.

Since that time, adjuvants have been found to be effective manipulators of the immune system, and their potential as a possible source of immunotherapeutic agents has come under intensive investigation. Although large numbers of adjuvants are being examined in experimental animal studies, and more recently in clinical studies, the most clinically significant data accumulated to date involve the adjuvant BCG. Developed by Calmette and Guérin as a vaccine against tuberculosis, BCG, an attenuated strain of *Mycobacterium bovis,* has been investigated as an agent that may heighten resistance to several types of cancer, including both solid tumors and leukemias.

Utilizing a chemically induced transplantable guinea pig hepatoma, it has been shown in experiments that BCG injected directly into a skin nodule can induce a higher number of complete regressions followed by resistance to challenge with the same tumor. The following points should be noted: (1) the tumor must not be too large—a larger tumor burden reduced or eliminated the effectiveness of BCG treatment; (2) the BCG must contain live organisms and must be injected directly into the nodule; and (3) the host must be capable of generating an immune response to the BCG.

BCG has also been studied in clinical trials, a number of which involved patients with malignant melanoma. As in the studies reported above, BCG injected directly into intradermal melanoma lesions resulted in the disappearance of more than 90 per cent of the nodules. A low percentage of noninjected lesions in these patients also disappeared, many of them in close proximity to the injected nodules. Again, it should be noted that (1) this approach is ineffective if the disease is subcutaneous or involves the body viscera; (2) the BCG must be injected directly into the lesion, and (3) the patient must be capable of generating an immune response against BCG.

In addition to these effects resulting from direct injection of BCG into tumor nodules, animal and, more recently, clinical studies have indicated that adjuvants can elicit a heightened systemic cell-mediated resistance to tumor when administered under certain conditions. Initially, animal studies indicated that adjuvants inoculated before tumor injection significantly prolonged survival time or prevented tumor-induced mortality. As a result of these studies, investigations were performed on the effects of adjuvants administered after tumor injections. Using a murine leukemia system, G. Mathé demonstrated that BCG given intraperitoneally one day after a lethal dose of tumor significantly inhibited tumor growth. More recently, investigators have carried out clinical studies examining the efficacy of BCG as a "systemic" stimulator of the immune system of tumor patients. Although much of the data are not complete and a number of "uncontrollable" variables admittedly persist, the findings can be summarized as follows: (1) Following remission, acute lymphoblastic leukemia patients were given various immunotherapeutic regimens. Significantly prolonged remission occurred when BCG together with allogeneic tumor cells was administered, as opposed to BCG alone or no treatment at all. (2) Acute myelogenous leukemia patients, following chemically induced remission, were found to have significantly increased median survival when a combination of chemotherapy and immunotherapy (BCG plus allogeneic tumor cells), as opposed to chemotherapy alone, was administered. (3) Acute myeloblastic leukemia patients were found to have significantly longer remissions (as well as estimated survival times) following a therapeutic protocol consisting of BCG and chemotherapy, as opposed to chemotherapeutic treatment alone. It must be noted that, to date, there is no direct evidence that the adjuvant administered was solely responsible for the increase in remission or survival time.

How BCG exerts its effect on the host's immune system remains a major question. There are a number of possible mechanisms, including the following: (1) The "innocent bystander" effect. Tumor cells are killed nonspecifically by activated macrophages, lymphocytes, and cytotoxic lymphokines attracted to the tumor site by the adjuvant-initiated granuloma reaction. (2) Enhancement of the ongoing immune responses. This necessitates that the host be capable of recognizing the tumor cell and generating a specific immunologic response against it. The adjuvant would simply amplify the specific responses. (3) Cross-reaction between BCG and tumor antigens. Recent findings have indicated that BCG and the guinea pig hepatoma of Rapp and Zbar share antigenic determinants. Similar cross-reactivity has been reported between BCG and some human melanomas. (4) Nonimmunologic mechanisms. In blood disorders BCG may stimulate stem cell proliferation, repopulating the hematopoietic system being depleted by tumor or chemotherapeutic drugs.

Another immunopotentiating agent that has recently come under increased observation is a gram-positive bacillus, *Corynebacterium parvum* (Table 10–1). *C. parvum* is one of the several anerobic corynebacteria (*C. granulosum, C. diphtheroides*) that have a marked affinity for the reticuloendothelial system (RES) and are of low pathogenicity in man. Halpern and others demonstrated that *C. parvum* heightens protection against bacterial infection and resistance against tumors in animals and man. It has been shown that within 24 hours after intravenous injection of *C. parvum* into mice, a gradual increase occurs in the weight of the liver and spleen as a result of marked cellular hyperplasia. In addition, the phagocytic capacity of these RES organs is increased (Fig. 10–2). The treatment of mice with *C. parvum* before immunization with BSA, for example, resulted in markedly increased levels of antibody production in the primary and secondary responses. Treatment with *C. parvum* before infections with bacteria, e.g., Brucella (the RES is the major site of this bacterium), markedly inhibits bacterial proliferation. *C. parvum* has also been demonstrated to protect against certain viral infections

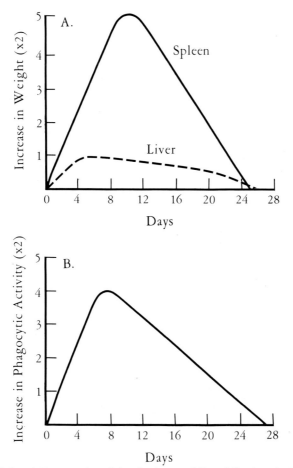

Figure 10–2.   *A*, Increase in weight of spleen and liver following single intravenous injection of *C. parvum. B*, Increase in phagocytic activity following single intravenous injection of *C. parvum.*

(e.g., Mengo virus), and unconfirmed reports suggest that interferon production may also be important.

The study of two tumor systems has also illustrated the capacity of *C. parvum* to enhance host resistance to neoplasia. C3H and Swiss mice were implanted subcutaneously with the β sarcoma J, and one half of each group was injected intravenously the same day with *C. parvum.* Six to seven weeks later, there were 50 per cent more survivors in the group given *C. parvum.* It is noteworthy that no such protection was afforded in the BALB strain, in which the sarcoma J is highly virulent. A single intraperitoneal injection (500 μg) of *C. parvum* or *C. granulosum*, administered the same day as 50,000 Ehrlich's ascites tumor cells, in Swiss mice, markedly increased the survival time of the recipient mice (Fig. 10–3).

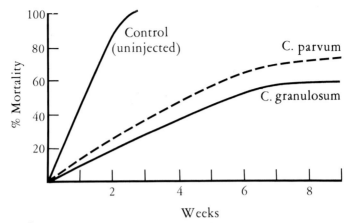

Figure 10–3. A typical experiment illustrating the immunopotentiative effect of *C. parvum* or *C. granulosum* in protection to tumor challenge when 50,000 Ehrlich's ascites tumor cells were inoculated intraperitoneally into Swiss mice. The same day 500 μg of *C. parvum* or *C. granulosum* were injected intraperitoneally into the experimental groups. The experimental groups showed a decreased mortality and an increased survival time.

Additional experiments demonstrated that the route of inoculation of *C. parvum* was critical. When the adjuvant was injected intravenously and not intraperitoneally, no increased resistance was elicited against the Ehrlich's ascites cells inoculated intraperitoneally the same day. These studies indicate that this immunopotentiator must be anatomically close to the tumor to exert its effect.

INTERACTION OF ADJUVANTS WITH CELLS INVOLVED IN IMMUNE RESPONSES

Macrophages

It has already been mentioned that *Corynebacterium parvum* strikingly enhances the phagocytic activity and intracellular killing power of macrophages. Some adjuvants, owing to their particulate nature (e.g., *Bordetella pertussis* and mycobacteria in complete Freund's adjuvant), are readily ingested by macrophages. Other adjuvants form complexes with serum proteins (e.g., beryllium plus serum phosphate) that are also readily taken up by macrophages. These findings suggest that at least some of the effects of adjuvants might be brought about by macrophages.

Studies in a number of laboratories have demonstrated the significance of pertussis-treated macrophages in the enhanced level of antibody response to the antigen MSH (*Maia squinado* hemocyanin). After noting that the injection of pertussis organisms *in vivo* enhanced the ensuing antibody response to MSH, the antigen-containing macrophages *in vitro*, when treated with pertussis and injected into syngeneic mice, elicited a greater antibody response than antigen-containing macrophages that were not incubated with the adjuvant. When lymph node cells were used instead of peritoneal macrophages, no increase or decrease in antibody levels was observed. Additional experiments illustrated that the adjuvant effect could also be induced if separate populations of macrophages, one pulsed with antigen, the other with pertussis organisms, were simultaneously injected into mice. Experiments using BSA as the antigen yielded similar results. Macrophages also appear to be involved in some of the effects of the double-stranded polyribonucleotide adjuvants, e.g., poly I:C. Peritoneal macrophages incubated with BCG and poly A:U and injected into syngeneic mice induced markedly higher antibody levels as compared to mice injected with antigen-incubated macrophages (Table 10–1).

Two additional mechanisms may be important in affecting the relationship between adjuvants, macrophages, and the resultant immunologic responses: (1) trapping and (2) chemotaxis. A number of adjuvants have been shown to induce lymphocyte trapping, including complete and incomplete Freund's adjuvant, *C. parvum*, vitamin A, alcohol and vitamin A palmitate, and pertussis and alum particles. The trapping induced by these adjuvants differs from that induced by normal antigens in that the trapping extends over a longer period at high levels. Since adjuvants have been shown to boost the antibody responses to a number of weak immunogens (weak immunogens, as opposed to strong immunogens, do not initiate trapping), Lance and others have suggested that adjuvant action may be explained on the basis of the adjuvants' ability to initiate a trap on behalf of the weak immunogen, thereby effecting a good response. Since depletion of lymphocytes does not affect the ability of an animal to trap, and circumstantial evidence indicates that the macrophage could be the relevant cell, adjuvanticity may again be linked to a macrophage-affiliated mechanism.

A number of anerobic corynebacteria including *C. parvum, granulosum*, and *diphtheroides* have been shown to produce a chemotactic factor specific for macrophages (several strains of mycobacteria show chemotactic activity, but neutrophils are also attracted). Although no direct relationship between macrophage activity and adjuvant activity could be demonstrated in these studies, it is noteworthy that the same group of organisms enhanced both functions.

T- and B-Lymphocytes

It is not surprising that adjuvants can affect the function of T- and B-lymphocyte populations, although the data are not as direct as those concerning macrophages. Indeed, adjuvant-stimulated macrophages are believed to affect the activity of T- and B-cells. Poly A:U has been demonstrated to increase the incorporation of thymidine in lymphocytes from sensitized subjects exposed to tuberculin *in vitro,* as well as in mixed lymphocyte reactions (MLR). Studies by Halpern and coworkers have demonstrated that lymph node lymphocytes from both normal and tumor-bearing mice injected intraperitoneally with *C. parvum* have increased cytolytic activity as assayed against lymphoma target cells. Endotoxin, or its lipopolysaccharide (LPS) moiety, has a direct mitogenic effect on B-cells, and therefore, some of the adjuvant effects of LPS may be attributable to this action (Chapter 7).

C. parvum has also been found to inhibit a number of T-cell-dependent responses when administered in a systemic manner. There is a marked inhibition in the ability of spleen cells from *C. parvum*–injected animals to (1) mount a graft-versus-host reaction; (2) respond in MLR cultures; and (3) proliferate in response to PHA stimulation. The removal of a glass adherent cell population or a population sensitive to carbonyl-iron treatment (i.e, macrophages) restored the ability of spleen cells from *C. parvum*–injected animals to respond to PHA. In addition, spleen cells from such animals, when mixed with syngeneic normal spleen cells, inhibit the latter's ability to respond to PHA. These data suggest that *C. parvum*–activated macrophages can influence T-lymphocyte function. In contrast, splenic B-cells from *C. parvum*–treated animals respond normally to the mitogen LPS. There is, however, an adjuvant effect on the IgM response to higher immunizing doses of the T-independent antigen pneumococcal polysaccharide (S-III) (Chapters 4 and 7). Notably, the reactivity of spleen cells to S-III is suppressed when they are transferred to animals irradiated with 900 R or injected with silica (an antimacrophage reagent) and pretreated with *C. parvum.* It is therefore suggested that the mechanism of action of *C. parvum* is to inhibit T-cell-mediated mechanisms while enhancing B-cell activity. In turn, it is likely that both of these influences are in some fashion mediated by the macrophage.

Other specific mediators of the immune response have been utilized in both animals and clinical trials. These include the polynucleotides such as poly I:C and poly A:U and drugs such as levamisole. Both function as immunoadjuvants and appear to act nonspecifically on many of the cell types involved in the immune response.

Polynucleotides have been shown to greatly enhance antibody responses to a wide variety of antigens, as well as affecting T-lymphocyte and macrophage function. Levamisole, an anthelmintic drug $(-)$-2,3,5,6-Tetrahydro-6-phenylimidazo[2,1-*b*]thialzole monohydrochloride), is also a nonspecific stimulator of the immune response and affects both humoral and cell-mediated immunity. Treatment of tumor-bearing patients with this drug has been shown to restore delayed-type hypersensitivity dermal responses. It has also been shown to affect monocyte function, increasing all functional activities. Thus, levamisole has all the hallmarks of a good immunopotentiator.

SUPPRESSION OF IMMUNE RESPONSIVENESS

Just as it is necessary to potentiate the immune response in some instances, it becomes necessary at other times to benefit the host by manipulating the immunologic system in a negative way so that it cannot respond to the presence of a foreign configuration or, at best, will have a diminished response to it. As in the case of immunopotentiation, negative manipulation can affect both specific and nonspecific responses, and collectively comes under the general heading of *unresponsiveness*. *Immunologic tolerance* is a form of specific unresponsiveness and may be defined as the inability to respond to a specific antigenic stimulation, based upon an immature or incompetent immunologic system, the genetic constitution of the host, or the properties of the antigen. *Immunosuppression* comes under the heading of nonspecific unresponsiveness, refers to the artificial prevention or diminution of expression of immune response, and involves a more generalized form of unresponsiveness (Chapter 25).

IMMUNOLOGIC TOLERANCE

Implicit in all previous discussions of immunity is the fundamental ability of the immunologic system to differentiate "self" from "nonself." The idea that the body should never react with its own tissues was clearly enunciated by Ehrlich in his dogma "horror autotoxicus." One of the first challenges to this dogma came from the brilliant observations of Owen, who in 1945 demonstrated that nonidentical twin calves derived from two separate ova commonly shared two sets of red cells in their circulation, one set of its own, the other from its twin. This state is referred to as *mosaicism* or *chimerism*. Owen correctly assumed that this state of chimerism resulted from the well-known finding in such twin cattle of a common placental circulation that allowed the exchange of hematopoietic elements from one twin to another early in fetal life. Paradoxically, if these same cells were introduced into the calf at a later time, they would lead to an immunologic response and their prompt rejection and destruction.

The second set of observations that challenged the classic dogmas of immunology were made in the late 1940's by Medawar, who used specifically inbred strains of mice. If, for example, one obtains two strains of mice, A and B (A with white skin, B with black), A will accept skin grafts from another A mouse but not from a mouse of the B strain; similarly, a B mouse will accept a graft from another B mouse but not from a mouse of the A strain (Fig. 10–4). However, when lymphoreticular cells of strain B were introduced into mice of strain A, the recipients treated were capable of accepting skin grafts from mice of strain B (Fig. 10–4). Medawar termed this effect "specific immune tolerance."

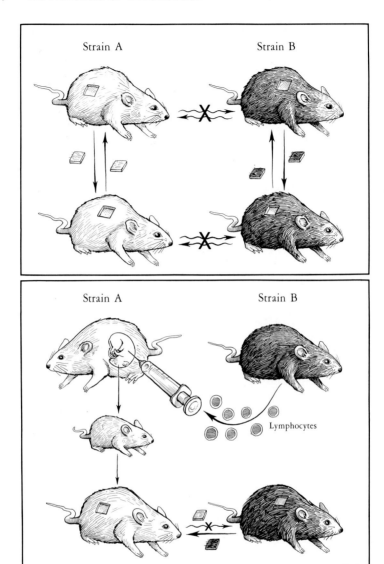

Figure 10–4. Representation of Medawar's experiment illustrating the fetal induction of tolerance in the mouse.

Once these observations were connected, further studies showed other ways to induce tolerance. The inoculation of embryos or young animals with antigens, for example, failed to elicit an immune response. Additional experiments showed that these animals actually became tolerant to the antigen with which the immature immune system had come in contact. In older animals, moreover, repeated high doses of certain antigens appeared to have a similar effect.

THE ROLE OF ANTIGEN IN TOLERANCE

The introduction of an antigen into a host can result in either immunologic responsiveness or unresponsiveness, depending on the nature of the antigen. Broadly speaking, an *antigen* may be defined as an *immunogen*, if it is capable of eliciting an immune response, i.e., it is said to be immunogenic; or a *tolerogen*, if an immune response does not ensue, i.e., it is said to be tolerogenic (Chapter 4). Recent observations emphasize two important factors controlling immune tolerance: (1) Immunologic unresponsiveness is an active phenomenon—not merely the lack of a response. Burnet initially proposed that tolerance to self antigens was the result of the destruction or elimination of "forbidden clones" of T-lymphocytes, i.e., T-cells that had contacted self antigens, during the developmental periods of the host's immune system. However, sufficient data have now been accumulated to demonstrate that clones of host lymphoid cells do "recognize" self antigens, but that an immune response does not ensue, because of either the nature of the interaction or the host mechanisms, which prevent the necessary events for a successful immune response. (2) Immunologic unresponsiveness is specific for the inducing tolerogen, just as an immune response is specific for the inducing immunogen. For example, an animal rendered unresponsive to bovine serum albumin (BSA) will respond in a normal fashion to horse serum albumin (HSA) or any other serum protein.

The events associated with the *induction, maintenance,* and *termination* of unresponsiveness are complex and varied. The following descriptions will emphasize the best-documented factors known to influence each of these phases.

INDUCTION

Nature of Antigen

The nature of the antigen is significant in determining whether or not it may act as a tolerogen. The form of heterologous serum proteins (e.g., gamma globulin) has been shown to be critical in influencing the ensuing response. Aggregated gamma globulins (e.g., HGG and BGG) have been found to be excellent immunogens, as contrasted with deaggregated globulins, which result in tolerance (Fig. 10–5). The polymeric nature of the former (i.e., repeating determinants), in contrast to the monomeric state of the latter, is believed to be a key factor responsible for these effects.

The nature of the antigen is also important because it determines the *in vivo* fate of the antigen, i.e., its tissue distribution (Chapter 7).

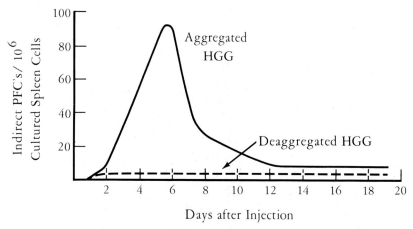

Figure 10–5. Plaque-forming capability of spleen cells from mice injected with either aggregated or deaggregated human gamma globulin (HGG).

It is thought that the greater the number of antigen-reactive cells the tolerogen may contact, the greater the resultant unresponsive state will be; i.e., those antigens that persist for a longer duration are generally more potent tolerogens. The most widely studied group, soluble substances, e.g., serum proteins, have a relatively simple molecular structure and low antigenicity and are easily obtainable in pure and large quantity. These proteins equilibrate extremely well between the intravascular and extravascular spaces following intravenous injection and are potent tolerogens. In contrast, bacterial and viral antigens, as well as heterologous red blood cells, are complex and highly antigenic and neither persist for long periods of time nor equilibrate to any extent. They are therefore not as effective at inducing unresponsiveness, although they generally can induce a hyporesponsive condition. Synthetic polypeptides and haptens, which appear to form conjugates with circulating proteins *in vivo*, e.g., dinitrophenol (DNP), plus isogeneic serum proteins, lead to unresponsiveness against DNP and exemplify another group of effective tolerogens.

Species and Genetic Factors

Several conclusions can be drawn from data reported on unresponsiveness in different species following the introduction of serum proteins in the production of neonatal induction of tolerance. Rabbits and mice appear to be more effectively tolerized (i.e., the tolerant condition persists for longer periods of time) than guinea pigs and chickens. Within a species, the genetic background also influences the induction of tolerance. Following the injection of deaggregated HGG as a tolerogen, C57BL/C mice (H-2^b) are rendered tolerant with a single injection of 0.1 mg; in contrast, Balb/C (H-2^d) animals do not become unresponsive even with a dose of up to 10 mg.

Immunocompetence of the Host

As a general rule, the greater the degree of host immunocompetence, the greater the difficulty in inducing unresponsiveness. It is not surprising therefore that embryonic and neonatal animals are susceptible to tolerization. Billingham, Brent, and Medawar made neonatal animals tolerant to alloantigen by injecting viable cells, and therefore exposing potential (but incompetent) antibody-forming cells to the antigen. The use of replicating viable cells, moreover, provides a continuing source of antigen, which provides yet another basis for the development of tolerance, as will be described below. Rabbits can be made tolerant to BSA when antigen is administered prior to day 9, since the neonatal rabbit develops immune capacity to respond to BSA between 8 and 21 days after birth.

Adult animals can also be made tolerant by treating them with various immunosuppressive techniques, including irradiation, antilymphocyte globulin (ALG), or thoracic duct drainage, followed by antigen administration. For example, rabbits subjected to 800 R whole-body irradiation and a single dose of aqueous BSA are rendered unresponsive for up to nine months, at which time 80 per cent of these animals become unresponsive. Chemical immunosuppressives, i.e., 6-mercaptopurine and cyclophosphamide, administered over a period of time preceding antigen injection can also produce an unresponsive state.

A number of investigators have shown that when two forms of an antigen, e.g., bovine gamma globulin (BGG), are available, the deaggregated (monomeric) form can induce unresponsiveness in mice up to nine months following a single injection. Deaggregated BGG administered to adult rabbits induced a tolerant condition in a majority of attempts. It was also demonstrated that deaggregated BSA given to adult mice or aqueous BSA or HSA injected into guinea pigs also results in an unresponsive state.

Since memory cells are also present in sensitized adults, unresponsiveness is difficult to induce. Sequential injection of the tolerogen may lead to a gradual decrease in the antibody response and "exhaustively differentiating" the relevant cell populations, resulting in an unresponsive state. Immunosuppressives have also been used to aid in the induction of tolerance in sensitized adults, as will be described below.

The Route of Antigen Injection

This parameter depends to some extent on both the antigen and the recipient. The route of inoculation does not appear to be as critical in neonatal animals as in the adult. In the latter, the nature of the antigen is also important. As described previously, the deaggregated form of a number of serum proteins is tolerogenic. The injection of aggregated BGG into the mesenteric, but not the jugular, vein led to the development of tolerance. The explanation for this finding was believed to be deaggregation of the protein in the liver following inoculation via the mesenteric route.

The route of inoculation of haptens appears to be critical in determining the resultant response. Intravenous injection of large doses inhibits later attempts at sensitization, whereas inoculation by the intradermal route leads to the production of antibody as well as a delayed-hypersensitivity response. The fate of the hapten, i.e., the nature of its binding to various proteins, and the eventual distribution of these conjugates may also account for the differential responses observed following the various routes of inoculation. Data supporting this theory can be interpreted from observations employing DNP coupled to isologous serum proteins. When this hapten carrier conjugate was administered prior to the injection of antigen, the coupling resulted in an unresponsive condition that was specific for the hapten.

Dose of Antigen

As a general rule, the greater the dose of antigen, the greater the resultant unresponsive state. It should be emphasized, however, that numerous small injections of serum proteins are more effective in inducing tolerance than a single large one. Following three injections of BSA weekly into adult mice, Mitchison observed that low and high doses of the antigens induced tolerance referred to as *low-dose tolerance*

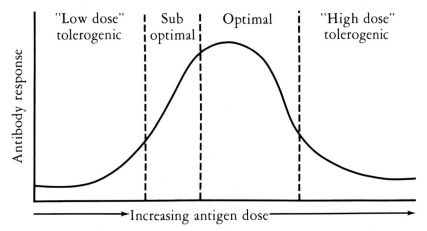

Figure 10–6. Schematic representation of the dose-response relationship between antigen concentration and the resultant immune response.

and *high-dose tolerance*; an intermediate level of antigen resulted in immunity. These events are represented schematically in Figure 10–6. The high-low zone tolerance has been found to be an unusual occurrence. Most other antigens tested have been found to fall only in the high-zone classification. It is thought that in order for high-low zone tolerance to occur, both forms of antigen (immunogen and tolerogen) must be present in the preparation, since the two-zone phenomenon does not occur when only the tolerogenic form is present or when the animal is unable to respond to the immunogenic form.

Cellular Interactions in the Induction of Unresponsiveness

Initial experiments designed to investigate the cell populations affected following the induction of unresponsiveness in an animal indicated that T-lymphocytes appeared to be the "target" cells. Thymectomized irradiated adult rats, reconstituted with bone marrow, responded normally to BGG when T-cells from normal syngeneic mice were administered (Table 10–2) but did not respond to this antigen (in its immunogenic form) when the T-cell source was from unresponsive animals. Additional evidence for T-cell involvement was demonstrated by use of mice made tolerant to BSA. Twenty-four hours after the injection of the tolerogen, host T-cells examined were unresponsive to the antigen, whereas host B-cells responded in a normal manner. Similar results were obtained with these cell populations 48 hours after the induction of tolerance to SRBC. In 1970, Chiller and Weigle demonstrated that both T- and B-lymphocytes could be rendered unresponsive to deaggregated HGG. Bone marrow and thymus were removed from adult mice 21 days after a tolerizing injection of deaggregated HGG. Using these cell populations in transfer experiments together with either normal thymocytes or normal bone marrow, it was shown that both the T-lymphocyte and the B-lymphocyte populations were rendered unresponsive in the tolerized animals, and that unresponsiveness in only one of these populations was sufficient to induce a state of overall unresponsiveness in an otherwise normal animal (Table 10–3). The specificity of the induced unresponsiveness was clearly indicated by the normal response to the unrelated antigen, turkey gamma globulin (TGG).

TABLE 10–2.   Donor Effects of T-Cell Sources in Immunologic Unresponsiveness

Thymectomized and X-Irradiated Recipient Rats	Normal Bone Marrow	Syngeneic T-Lymphocyte Source *Normal*	*Unresponsive*	BGG Response
Group I	Yes	Yes	—	+
Group II	Yes	—	Yes	—

TABLE 10-3. Effects of T- and B-Lymphocytes in Tolerance

Source of T-Cell		Source of B-Cell		Response to	
				HGG	TGG
Unresponsive	Normal	Unresponsive	Normal		
	+		+	+	+
+			+	−	+
	+	+		−	+
+		+		−	+

Although both T-cells and B-cells can be rendered tolerant to an antigen, there is a marked difference between the two populations in the induction and duration of their unresponsiveness. Chiller and Weigle removed thymus and bone marrow from unresponsive animals up to 150 days following a single tolerizing dose (2.5 mg) of deaggregated HGG, and examined their ability to respond to aggregated HGG in the transfer system described in the preceding paragraph. As shown in Figure 10–7, T-cells became 100 per cent unresponsive much more rapidly than B-cells (i.e., three to five days for T-cells versus 19 to 22 days for B-cells). In addition, the duration of unresponsiveness of the B-cells is much shorter than that of the T-cell population (40 to 45 versus 120 to 130 days for T-cells). Figure 10–7 also illustrates that the termination of unresponsiveness in the B-cell population is much more rapid than that of the T-cells.

There is also a pronounced difference in the dose of antigen required to make T- and B-lymphocytes tolerant. When low doses of deaggregated HGG were injected, only T-cells were rendered unresponsive. Although significant differences between the two populations have recently been defined regarding the kinetics of induction and

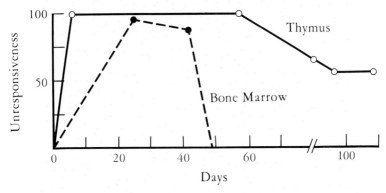

Figure 10–7. Comparison of the induction and duration of unresponsiveness in thymus and bone marrow populations following a single injection of 2.5 mg deaggregated HGG.

maintenance of unresponsiveness, the mechanisms responsible for these differences remain poorly understood.

TERMINATION OF TOLERANCE

The tolerant state is usually ended in one of two ways: either spontaneously (probably related to persistence of antigen) or specifically, following the injection of some cross-reactive antigen.

Several reports have noted that accompanying the spontaneous loss of unresponsiveness to an antigen is the appearance of an antibody response to that antigen. This could be the result of the loss of the high levels of antigen required to maintain tolerance but persistence of enough to stimulate an antibody response. If the critical level of antigen needed to maintain tolerance in some manner constantly inhibits the development or differentiation of new T-lymphocyte clones with specificity for the antigen, the spontaneous loss of tolerance may be accompanied by the appearance of newly specific T-cells that will provoke an antibody response from B-cells, which some time earlier returned to normal competency.

Tolerance can be intentionally abrogated by the injection of a chemically altered preparation of the original antigen, or some cross-reacting material. For example, if rabbits tolerant to BSA are injected with a cross-reacting albumin, the resultant antibody will react with BSA and the albumin. Several weeks later, the injection of BSA will stimulate antibody production that is directed only against the determinants on the BSA that cross-react with those on the albumin used to terminate the unresponsive state. It is notable that since the injection of the cross-reactive antigen raised antibody with BSA determinants, precursor cells for antibody production against the tolerogen do exist in an unresponsive animal. This would suggest that the level of control in the tolerant condition is directed at a more peripheral mode of the normal response.

SUPPRESSION OF IMMUNE RESPONSIVENESS

Recent studies in many laboratories have shown that active suppression by cellular components can be involved in the development of immunologic tolerance. As in many instances involving the immune response, suppression can be either *specific* or *nonspecific*. All of the major cellular components involved in the positive regulation of the immune response have also been shown to have suppressive capabilities. Studies by Gershon and coworkers have demonstrated that thymectomized mice that had been irradiated and reconstituted with bone marrow and thymocytes and then pretreated with sheep red blood cells were tolerant to subsequent challenge by this antigen even if more thymocytes were given. Mice that did not receive thymocytes after irradiation could not develop tolerance. It was also shown that the tolerant state could be transferred from spleen cells derived from these animals to normal mice, and that this was a function of T-lymphocytes. T-lymphocytes have been shown to play a suppressive or regulatory role in nearly all types of tolerance systems studied. These cells carry the same Ly phenotype as cytotoxic T-lymphocytes (see Chapter 2) and may exert their effect by cytolysis of specific helper T-lymphocytes or B-lymphocytes. Suppression may be antigen-specific, suppressing responsiveness to one antigen while leaving immune responses to other antigens intact, or it may suppress the cellular or humoral response to all antigens. Suppression may also be specific for a class of antibody, IgG rather than IgM, or for a subclass of IgG, such as has been shown in allotype suppression.

Macrophages have also been implicated in suppression of immune responsiveness in a number of systems, including progressive tumor growth.

Suppressor cells may play an important role in disease states. There is an abnormal activation of suppressor cells in such diseases as agammaglobulinemia. Suppressor cells have been shown to play a role in the immunologic enhancement of tumor growth, and loss of normal suppressor cell activity has been shown to be involved in certain autoimmune disease states. The NZB mouse, which has been studied as a model of systemic lupus erythematosus in man, shows a loss of suppressor activity due to thymic dysfunction as early as four weeks of age. This loss of suppressor activity precedes the onset of the autoimmune manifestations, e.g., autoantibody to DNA.

Much of the earlier work on tolerance can now be correlated to involvement of suppressor cells. For example, it has been shown that the generation of suppressive activity in response to erythrocyte antigens is directly correlated to the amount of immunizing antigen. Helper T-lymphocyte activity from hyperimmune animals was significantly lower than that from optimally immunized mice. These experiments also showed that immune suppression due to antigen dose effects may depend on the proportion of helper and suppressor T-lymphocytes involved in the response.

The role of suppressor cells in the genetics of the immune response has been under intense investigation (Chapter 7). Induction of suppression has been linked to the responder or nonresponder status of certain animal strains and has also been linked to the I region of the MHC in the mouse. This involvement is discussed in more detail in Chapter 3.

Since the T-lymphocyte has been shown to have the most important suppressive and regulatory role in both normal and induced tolerance, it has been postulated that most suppression involves T-lympho-

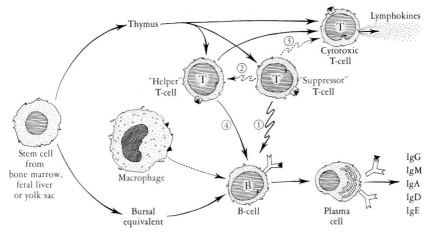

Figure 10–8. Schematic representation of the central immunoregulatory role of the T-lymphocyte acting in T-B interactions to suppress (1) or help (4) antibody-forming B-cell precursors or in T-T interactions to suppress helper T-lymphocytes (2) or cytotoxic lymphocytes (3).

cytes acting on either helper or cytotoxic T-lymphocytes and on antibody-forming cell precursors (Fig. 10–8).

IMMUNOSUPPRESSION

Nonspecific immune suppression has been used in both organ transplantation and bone marrow transplantation in leukemia. Among the agents used are radiation, corticosteroids, cytotoxic chemicals, and antisera to lymphocyte populations.

Radiation. Radiation has been used to rid the body of neoplastic leukemic cells in conjunction with bone marrow grafts. Extracorporeal irradiation of blood may eventually be of some value as an adjunctive modality in some clinical situations.

Corticosteroids. In many species it has been shown that corticosteroids (i.e., prednisone) can wipe out subpopulations of small lymphocytes. In mice, administration of cortisone destroys cortical thymocytes while having no effect on medullary thymocytes. Corticosteroids in man have been shown to facilitate homograft acceptance. The mechanisms may include anti-inflammatory activity, disruption of phagocytosis, and inhibition of lysozyme release from granulocytes.

Cytotoxic Chemicals. There are many chemicals that have been used as both antitumor agents and immunosuppressants. These include alkylating agents such as nitrogen mustards, antimetabolites such as azathioprine (Imuran), and folic acid antagonists such as methotrexate, which has been useful in treating such autoimmune diseases as systemic lupus erythematosis.

Antilymphocyte Serum (ALS).   ALS is probably the most widely studied of the general immunosuppressive agents. It has three properties that set it apart from all the other agents: (1) it has selective activity against the cellular limb of the immune response but not the humoral limb; (2) it wipes out immunologic memory and greatly weakens second-set rejection; and (3) it has insensitivity to antigenic differences. Although most conventional immunosuppressives fail when histocompatibility differences are strong, with ALS even xenografts have been shown to be possible for a certain period of time. The problems occur when ALS suppresses the T-lymphocyte limb of the immune response, thus weakening the immune surveillance system and allowing maligant disease to arise.

Drug-induced Tolerance.   Experiments have shown that activation of clones of lymphocytes by specific antigen, along with simultaneous treatment by immunosuppressive drugs, can induce specific tolerance for many months. Presumably, antigen activates a specific clone of lymphocytes that has a receptor for that antigen; following this, a cytotoxic chemical, e.g., cyclophosphamide, is administered and selectively destroys this activated clone. If after this procedure antigens C and D are administered, the population with receptors for antigen D will

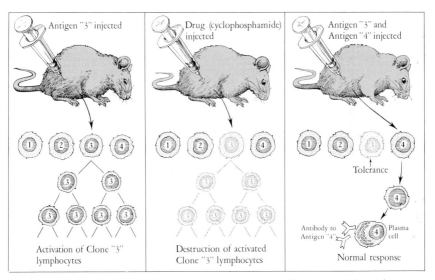

Figure 10–9.   Schematic representation of drug-induced tolerance. (After Schwartz, R. S.: Immunosuppressive drugs. Progr. Allergy, *9*:246, 1965.)

be capable of expansion and will give rise to cells capable of forming antibody to D; since clone C is depleted, antigen C will not elicit an immune response and therefore the tolerant state is maintained. For example, animals given sheep red blood cells plus one dose of cyclophosphamide can induce tolerance specific for SRBC's but not horse red blood cells. SRBC's are then injected many times to maintain the tolerant state (Fig. 10–9).

SUGGESTIONS FOR FURTHER READING

Amery, W. K., Spreafico, F., Rojas, A. F., Denissen, E., and Chirigos, M. A.: Adjuvant treatment with levamisole in cancer. Cancer Treatment Reviews (in press), 1977.

Cantor, H., Shen, F. W., and Boyse, E. A.: Separation of helper T cells from suppressor T cells expressing different LY components. II. Activation by antigen: after immunization, antigen-specific suppressor and helper activities are mediated by distinct T-cell subclasses. J. Exp. Med., *143*:1391, 1976.

Chiller, J. M., Louis, J. A., Skidmore, B. J., et al.: Manipulation of the Tolerant State: Cells and Signals. *In* E. E. Sercarz, A. R. Williamson, and C. F. Fox (eds.) The Immune System: Genes, Receptors, Signals. New York, Academic Press, 1974.

Chirigos, M. A. (ed.): Control of Neoplasia by Modulation of the Immune System. New York, Raven Press, 1977.

Gershon, R.: T-cell control of antibody production. *In* M. D. Cooper and N. L. Warner (eds.): Contemporary Topics in Immunobiology. Vol. 3. New York, Plenum Press, 1974.

Immunopotentiation. Ciba Foundation Symposium 18. Amsterdam, Associated Scientific Publishers, 1973.

Moller, G.: Suppressor T-lymphocytes. Transplant. Rev., 76, 1975.

Schwartz, R. S.: Immunosuppressive drugs. Progr. Allergy, *9*:246, 1965.

Terry, W. (ed.): Immunotherapy in Malignant Disease. Med. Clin. North Am., *60*:387–648, 1976

Waldmann, T. A., and Broder, S.: Suppressor cells in the regulation of the immune response. Progr. Clin. Immunol., *3*:155, 1977.

Weigle, W. O., Sieckman, D. G., Doyle, M. V., et al.: Possible roles of suppressor cells in immunological tolerance. Transplant. Rev., *26*:186, 1975.

A UNIFYING MODEL FOR IMMUNOLOGIC PROCESSES

Joseph A. Bellanti, M.D.

It may now be possible to construct a unifying model for immunologic processes based upon the various principles of the immunologic system described in Section One. The model, which is an adaptation of one suggested by Talmage, will also serve as a framework for further descriptions of immunologic mechanisms (Section Two) and the clinical applications of immunology (Section Three). For ease of discussion, we may speak of five components of the host's encounter with foreignness: (1) *the environment,* (2) *the target cell,* (3) *the phagocytic cells,* (4) *the mediator cells* and mediator products, and (5) *the specific antigen-recognition cells* (B-lymphocytes and T-lymphocytes) and their products.

THE ENVIRONMENT

Since most substances that confront, and ultimately activate, the host's immunologic system arise from the exterior world, the place to begin in any discussion of the immunologic system is with the external environment (Fig. 11–1). Included within the external environment are the myriad foreign substances that range from the simplest of low molecular weight chemicals to the most complex microbial agents. It should also be emphasized that the immunologic system may be activated not only by foreign substances that arise from the external environment, but also by those that present from the internal environment, e.g., transplanted cells or altered self-components (virally transformed or malignant cells). Those substances that have the capacity to evoke immunologic responses are referred to as *immunogens* or *antigens* and all share the common characteristic of being recognized as *foreign* by the host (Chapter 4). Occasionally, the encounter with a foreign configuration may lead to an inability to respond, a state that is referred to as *immunologic tolerance;* such configurations are referred to as *tolerogens* (Chapter 10). Allergens are a specialized class of immunogen and take

266

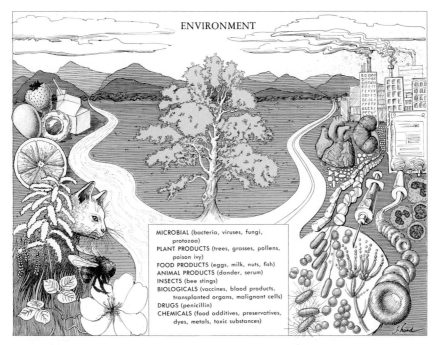

ENVIRONMENT

MICROBIAL (bacteria, viruses, fungi,
    protozoa)
PLANT PRODUCTS (trees, grasses, pollens,
    poison ivy)
FOOD PRODUCTS (eggs, milk, nuts, fish)
ANIMAL PRODUCTS (dander, serum)
INSECTS (bee stings)
BIOLOGICALS (vaccines, blood products,
    transplanted organs, malignant cells)
DRUGS (penicillin)
CHEMICALS (food additives, preservatives,
    dyes, metals, toxic substances)

Figure 11–1. Examples of environmental agents.

part in hypersensitivity (allergic) reactions (Chapter 20). Antigens may be complete and lead to an immune response *per se* (immunogens), or they may be incomplete (haptens) and require prior attachment to a carrier protein to become fully immunogenic (e.g., penicillin). As our environment becomes more complex, not only does the number of antigens increase but also the potential number of allergens to which we are exposed (Fig. 11–1). Thus, the physician must be constantly aware of the many types and varied routes of exposure to immunogens and allergens that comprise our complex environment not only to prevent and treat certain diseases (e.g., vaccines), but also to be able to recognize the possibility of immunologically mediated diseases that may take unexpected forms or masquerade as other entities.

TARGET CELLS

The introduction of an environmental agent into a host may have an adverse effect on a target cell (Fig. 11–2, Table 11–1). There are a variety of target cells upon which an environmental agent may impact. They vary according to their type and location and the portal of entry of the foreign substance. It is important to emphasize that the target cells

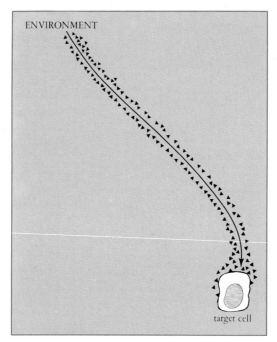

Figure 11–2. Effects of environmental agents on target cells.

TABLE 11–1. Effects of the Environment on Target Cells

LOCATION OF TARGET CELL	EXAMPLE OF EFFECT	RESULT
Skin	Disruption of epidermal cells	Dermatitis
Gastrointestinal tract		
Mucosal cell	Destruction	Gastrointestinal bleeding
Smooth muscle	Increased contractility	Diarrhea, vomiting
Glandular cell	Increased secretion	Increased mucus production
Respiratory tract		
Smooth muscle	Increased contraction	Bronchospasm
Glandular cell	Increased secretion	Increased mucus production
Circulatory system		
Endothelial cell	Increased intercellular pore size	Edema
Formed elements	Destruction of erythrocytes	Anemia

may be normal host cells that become the adventitious targets of injury by the environmental agent or immunologic processes, or they may represent altered host cells that have become modified through the interaction with the environmental substance (e.g., chemical), by infection (e.g., virus), or by malignant transformation (e.g., tumor cells); alternatively, the target cell may be a foreign cell introduced by transplantation (Chapter 20). The target cell may thus sustain direct injury from the environmental agent or indirect injury through immunologic processes (Chapter 20). The net effect leads to disruption of cell function or cell death. Some of the more common target cells are shown in Table 11–1. Included are cells of the skin, gastrointestinal tract, respiratory tract, and the circulatory system. For example, disruption of epidermal cells following contact with an environmental agent, e.g., poison ivy, could lead to dermatitis; destruction of mucosal cells of the gastrointestinal tract secondary to ingestion of an environmental agent, e.g., an offending food substance, may result in gastrointestinal bleeding. If the target cells are smooth muscle and glandular cells of the respiratory tract, the impact of the environmental agent may lead to increased contractility with bronchospasm and increased secretion of mucus characteristic of bronchial asthma. Alternatively, endothelial target cells of blood vessels might respond by showing an increase in intercellular pore size with resultant loss of fluids and the production of edema. The impact of the foreign substance on the formed elements of the blood, such as red cells, might lead to their destruction and the development of anemia.

During the course of evolution, a number of *nonspecific* and *specific* immunologic mechanisms have appeared within the vertebrates (Chapter 2). This collection of cellular elements, referred to as the lymphoreticular system, is distributed strategically throughout the body and lines the lymphatic and vascular channels. Their function may be considered the protection of the target cell from injury. *Phagocytosis* and the *inflammatory response* are the body's first line of defense and represent the most primitive of the nonspecific immune responses (Chapters 2, 12, and 13).

THE PHAGOCYTIC CELLS

The phagocytic cells are those elements that are involved in the process of engulfment and uptake of particles from the external environment; subsequent digestion of these substances may lead to their elimination (Chapter 2). The phagocyte may be considered then as a barrier between the environment and the target cell, protecting the target cell from subsequent injury (Fig. 11–3, Table 11–2). In the human, phagocytosis is carried out primarily by mononuclear phagocytes (macrophages), neutrophils, and eosinophils (Chapter 2). These

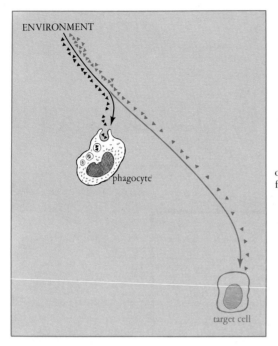

ENVIRONMENT

phagocyte

target cell

Figure 11–3. Phagocytic cells: Mobilization factors and functions.

phagocytic cells, together with the effector mechanisms triggered by or involved in their mobilization, are shown in Table 11–2. There are a variety of chemotactic factors — generated from the complement system (Chapter 6) or derived from specific lymphocytes, e.g., the lymphokines (Chapter 9) or from the phagocytic cells themselves — that can lead to the accumulation of phagocytic cells in an area of inflammation. The net effect of these processes is the mobilization of phagocytic cells into areas in which their action is required for the protection of target cells from injury.

TABLE 11–2. Mobilization Factors and Functions of Phagocytic Cells

Phagocytic Cell	Agents Responsible for Mobilization of Cells	Cell Product or Function
Macrophages (monocytes)	Chemotactic factors, e.g., migration inhibitory factor (MIF), lymphokines	Processed immunogen, removal of environmental agent
Neutrophils	Chemotactic factors (complement-associated and bacterial factors), lymphokines	Kallikreins (producing kinins), SRS-A, basic peptides, ECF-A
Eosinophils	Identical with neutrophils, specific chemotactic factors, lymphokines	Ingestion of immune complexes, antagonize effects of mediators, e.g., SRS-A

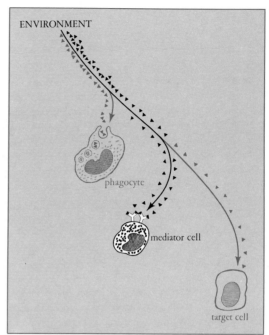

Figure 11–4. Mediator cells: Products (mediators) and functions.

MEDIATOR CELLS

Certain cells of the body contain macromolecular and low molecular weight substances that have biologic properties that can amplify the effects of the phagocytic cells or that may have a direct effect on the target cells. These cells are referred to as mediator cells. Following their interaction with the environmental agent, they perform their function by the release of chemical substances having a variety of biologic activities, e.g., the increase of vascular permeability or the enhancement of the inflammatory response (Fig. 11–4, Table 11–3). The mediator cells, like the target cells, represent a heterogeneous collection of

TABLE 11–3. Products and Functions of Mediator Cells

Mediator Cell	Product	Action
Mast cells	Histamine, SRS-A, prostaglandins, ECF-A	Increased vascular permeability, bronchoconstriction, eosinophilotaxis
Basophils, platelets	Vasoactive amines (histamine, serotonin)	Increased vascular permeability, smooth muscle constriction
Enterochromaffin cells	Serotonin	Vasodilation
Neutrophils	SRS, ECF	Contractility of smooth muscle, eosinophilotaxis

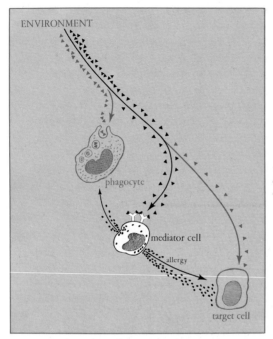

Figure 11–5. Mediator products and their effects on target cells (e.g., allergy) or phagocytic cells.

morphologic types that includes mast cells, basophils, platelets, entero-chromaffin cells, and neutrophils (Table 11–3). The best studied of these are the mast cells and basophils, which are important in certain immediate hypersensitivity diseases of man (Chapter 20).

The term "mediators" encompasses a group of substances that are formed and released by mediator cells in response to an environmental agent (Fig. 11–5, Table 11–4). The best studied of these substances include histamine, serotonin, kinins, slow reactive substance of anaphylaxis (SRS-A), prostaglandins, eosinophilic chemotactic factors of ana-

TABLE 11–4. Mediators Released in Response to Environmental Agents

Low molecular weight mediators (<1000)
    Histamine
    Serotonin
    Kinins
    Slow reactive substance of anaphylaxis (SRS-A)
    Prostaglandins
    Eosinophilic chemotactic factors of anaphylaxis (ECF-A)
    Platelet-activating factor (PAF)
Macromolecular mediators (>1000)
    Lysosomal enzymes
    Cationic proteins of polymorphonuclear leukocytes
    Complement and coagulation components

phylaxis (ECF-A), and platelet-activating factor (PAF). Other macro-molecular substances are derived from the phagocytic cells, e.g., lyso-somal enzymes. Although most of these substances are synthesized in the mediator cells, some mediators, e.g., the complement and coagu-lation components, are synthesized in other cells and are found pre-dominantly as serum components (Chapter 6).

Once they are released or generated, the mediators have a twofold effect on the nonspecific immunologic responses and act with (1) the target cell, e.g., allergy, or (2) the phagocytic cells, e.g., promotion of chemotaxis (Fig. 11–5, Table 11–4).

CELLS OF THE SPECIFIC IMMUNOLOGIC SYSTEM: THE SPECIFIC ANTIGEN-RECOGNITION CELLS

These cells, in contrast to those of the nonspecific immunologic system, interact with the environmental agent in a highly specific way. The responses display *specificity, memory,* and *heterogeneity* and are basi-cally carried out by two universes of lymphocytes: (1) the bone marrow or bursal-dependent B-lymphocytes, which provide humoral immunity; and (2) the thymus-dependent or T-lymphocytes, which participate in cell-mediated immunity (Chapter 2).

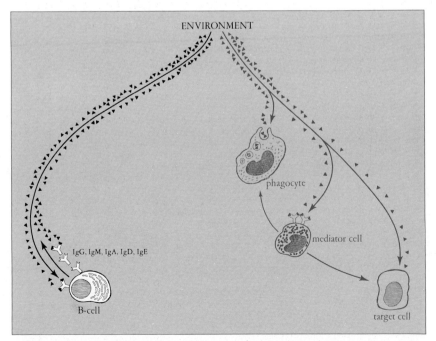

Figure 11–6. Reaction of B-lymphocyte to environmental agent through its surface receptor, with resultant antibody production.

The B-lymphocytes are those cells that ultimately respond to the environmental agent, either through immunization or infection (Fig. 11–6). The exquisite specificity for the recognition of antigen by the B-cell is a function of immunoglobulin on the surface of these cells. As a consequence of the binding of antigen with the surface receptor, the cell differentiates into clones of antibody-secreting plasma cells, each of which secretes a single class of immunoglobulin that is specific for the antigen. There are five classes of immunoglobulins, IgG, IgM, IgA, IgD, and IgE, each differing in physical, chemical, and biologic properties (Chapter 5). The primary effect of antibody is its direct binding with the environmental agent (Fig. 11–6). In addition, antibody may interact with the phagocytic cells, the mediator cells, or the target cells. The effect of antibody on phagocytic cells is shown in Figure 11–7. Three types of interactions are seen: (1) the direct binding of antibody to the surface of the phagocytic cells (cytophilic antibody), (2) the uptake of antigen-antibody (Ag-Ab) complexes through the Fc receptor, and (3) the uptake of antigen-antibody-complement (Ag-Ab-C) complexes through the C3b receptor (Fig. 11–7 insert). The effect of antibody on mediator cells is shown in Figure 11–8. Certain classes of gamma globulin, e.g., IgE, can attach to the mediator cells by virtue of their Fc fragments. Following the interaction of at least two of these membrane-bound molecules with antigen, the release of mediators occurs (Fig. 11–

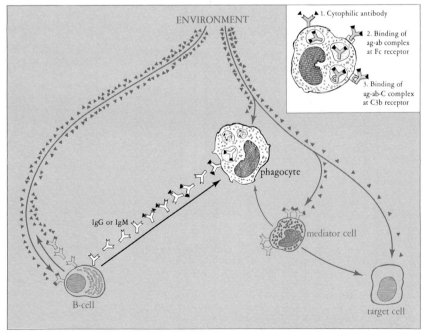

Figure 11–7. Responses of antibody with phagocytic cells.

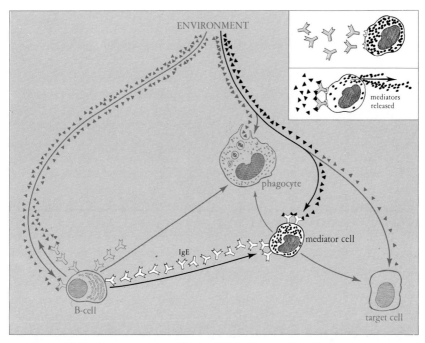

Figure 11-8. Responses of antibody with mediator cells with resultant release of mediators (insert).

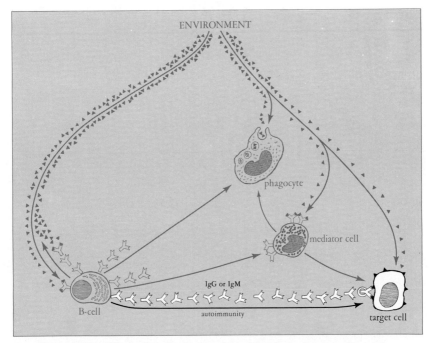

Figure 11-9. Effects of antibody on target cells with resultant autoimmunity.

8 insert). Occasionally, under abnormal circumstances, antibody may be directed against the target cells (Fig. 11–9). This is a totally anomalous situation but is seen in some of the immunologically mediated diseases of man—the autoimmune diseases (Chapter 20C).

The T-lymphocytes are those cells responsible for cell-mediated immunity (Chapter 9). These cells respond to the environmental agent through surface receptors (Fig. 11–10). Although not intact immunoglobulin, these receptors are analogous to the antigen-binding receptors on the B-cells.

Following the interaction of the environmental agent with the T-cell, a series of morphologic, biologic, and biochemical events occurs in which the cell may function either directly or through the elaboration of certain products, the lymphokines (Chapter 9). The best studied of the lymphokines is migration inhibitory factor (MIF), which not only inhibits the migration of macrophages but also can activate the cell metabolically (Fig. 11–11). In addition, the T-lymphocyte can participate in the recognition of antigen on the surface of foreign target cells in any of three ways (Fig. 11–12). The cell may participate in direct lymphocyte-dependent cytotoxicity; or the elaboration of cytotoxin may lead to target-cell destruction; or certain subsets of lymphocytes, the killer or K-cells, may lead to target-cell destruction through antibody-dependent cytotoxicity (ADCC) reactions (Fig. 11–12 insert).

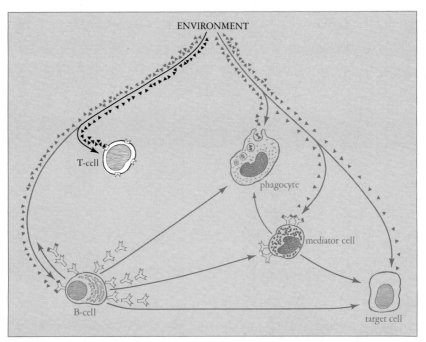

Figure 11–10. Reaction of T-lymphocyte to environmental agent through its surface receptor.

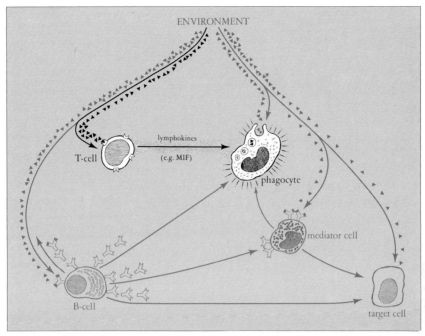

Figure 11-11.   Responses of lymphokines (e.g., elaborated from T-lymphocytes) on phagocytic cells (e.g., macrophages).

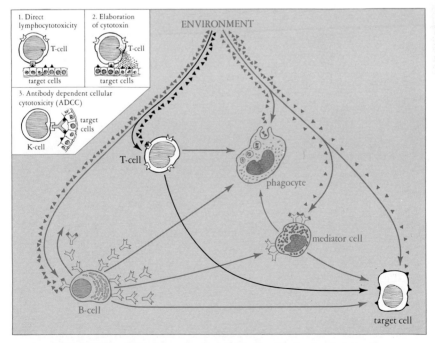

Figure 11-12.   Responses of activated T-cells with foreign target cells.

The T-lymphocytes may also interact with the B-cells in two ways: (1) a subset of T-cells (the helper cells) can interact with B-cells to facilitate the production of antibody, and (2) another subset of T-cells (the suppressor cells) can inhibit the production of antibody by B-cells (Fig. 11–13).

The macrophage may also interact with the T- or B-lymphocytes through antigen presentation or processing of antigen or by the elaboration of lymphocyte activating factors (Fig. 11–14). The macrophage is known to interact with these T- and B- lymphocytes in facilitating the production of antibody.

Thus, the immunologic system may be viewed as a multicellular system involving the interaction of foreign substances with a wide variety of cell types (Fig. 11–15). The immunologic responses concerned with the recognition and disposal of foreignness are termed "immunity" when they lead to a beneficial response; when the interaction of the immunologic components and the environmental agent leads to injury of target cells, the responses are referred to as hypersensitivity or allergy; when the target cells of the host are injured directly by immunologic mechanisms, these responses are referred to as autoimmunity (Chapter 20). Occasionally, when the immunologic surveillance of a foreign target cell, e.g., tumor cell, is evaded, the manifestations of malignant disease may be manifested (Chapter 19). The total array of these responses is shown in Figure 11–15.

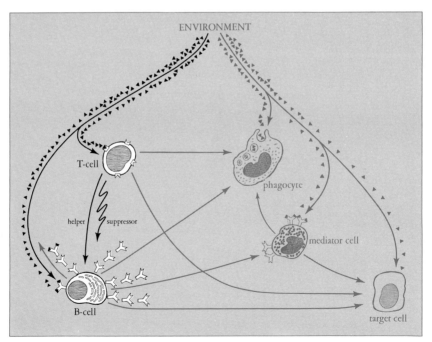

Figure 11–13. Helper and suppressor effects of T-lymphocytes on B-lymphocytes.

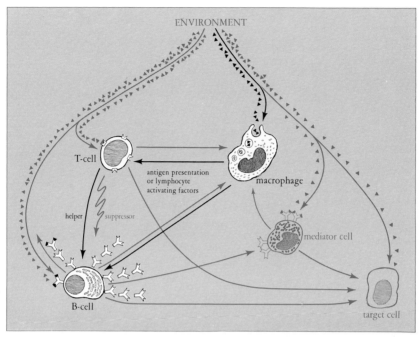

Figure 11–14. Responses of macrophages with T- and B-lymphocytes.

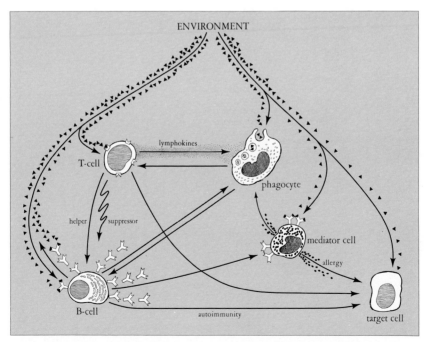

Figure 11–15. Total array of immunologic responses to the environment.

Section Two

MECHANISMS OF RESPONSE

Part 1

MECHANISMS OF TISSUE INJURY

Chapter 12

INFLAMMATION

Peter A. Ward, M.D.

Inflammation can be considered as that complex series of events that develops when the body is injured either by mechanical or chemical agents or by self-destructive (autoimmune) processes. Although there is a tendency in clinical medicine to consider the inflammatory response in terms of reactions harmful to the body, a more balanced view is that inflammation is essentially a *protective* response in which the body attempts either to return to the preinjury condition or to repair itself after inflicted injury. The inflammatory response sets apart living bodies from machines, since, in the latter case, there is no intrinsic capacity for restoration of a damaged or broken part. Thus, the inflammatory response is an essentially protective and restorative reaction of the body since it attempts to maintain homeostasis under adverse environmental influences.

The classic signs of inflammation are well known. They include *swelling, redness, heat, pain,* and *altered function.* The inflammatory response is critically dependent upon both intact blood vessels and the circulating cells and fluids within these channels. Generally, three states of inflammation are recognized: *acute, subacute,* and *chronic,* each being defined by typical histologic criteria. The *acute inflammatory* response is heralded by dilatation of blood vessels and the outpouring of leukocytes and fluids. Grossly, the result is *redness* (erythema) due to blood vessel dilatation, *swelling* (edema) due to escape of fluids into soft tissues, and *firmness* (induration) due to accumulation of fluids and cells. The result of these processes leads to a loss of the normal capacity of

283

blood vessels to retain fluids and cells within the vasculature; however, such changes do not necessarily reflect structural impairment of the vessel. Leukocytes may be responding to chemical attractants that are diffusing toward the vessel from an extravascular site. Moreover, it is known that the release of certain factors, e.g., histamine from tissue mast cells, may subsequently render the vessel more permeable to plasma fluids (Chapter 13). In most cases, the acute inflammatory response reflects the effects of mediators acting on the blood vessel, rather than a nonspecific injury to the vessel, resulting in the selective release of fluids and cells. Following mechanical trauma or thermal injury, vasopermeability changes may appear early in the acute inflammatory response. In fact, histamine-dependent permeability appears within minutes after thermal injury, probably owing to the release of granular contents of tissue mast cells. This phase of permeability is brief, however, lasting only a few minutes. Within 30 minutes, a more prolonged phase of permeability begins. The mediators responsible for this delayed phase of increased permeability are not known but are believed to consist of several factors, including complement products, kinins, and prostaglandins.

Within 30 to 60 minutes of injury, neutrophilic granulocytes make their appearance. They are first seen clustering along endothelial cells of vessels in the injured area. This remarkable accumulation of neutrophils, still within lumina of vessels, is referred to as *margination.* Soon thereafter, the leukocytes thread their way out of the vessel by squeezing through junctions between endothelial cells (see Fig. 2–14). Within minutes, the granulocytes are extravascular and begin to accumulate in the area of injury (Fig. 12–1). Once out of the confines of vessels, neutrophils represent the first line of defense against invading microorganisms. The prime function of neutrophils is to ingest (phagocytose) and destroy potentially dangerous agents, such as bacteria. Within four to five hours, if the acute inflammatory response progresses, mononuclear cells (including lymphocytes and monocytes) will appear at the inflammatory site, after leaving the vessels through mechanisms similar to that of the neutrophils. The arrival of these cells augments the protective barrier between foreign agents and the lymphatic channels, blood vessels, and neighboring tissues. Monocytes augment the defense by adding their own phagocytic function to the area, while lymphocytes convey the immunologic capacity to respond to foreign agents by specific *humoral* and *cell-mediated* phenomena, described in Chapter 2.

The description so far has stressed the protective function of the inflammatory process. It should be understood, however, that if the inflammatory response is aberrant, serious consequences may occur. The outpouring of too much fluid from the vasculature into an area such as the brain may lead to a serious rise in intracranial pressure. The accumulation of fluid due to inflammation in the pleural or pericardial cavities may seriously compromise organ function. Likewise, the arrival of excessive numbers of neutrophils and the subsequent discharge of

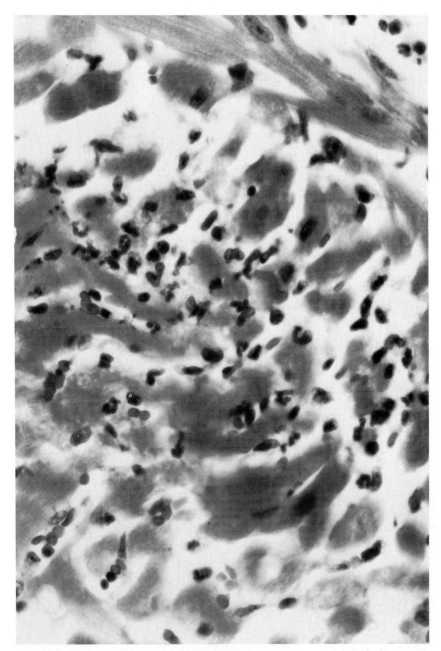

Figure 12-1. Accumulation of neutrophilic granulocytes in myocardium five hours after damage or destruction of tissue due to anoxia. Hematoxylin and eosin stain, ×530. (Armed Forces Institute of Pathology photograph.)

their enzymatic contents may result in serious structural damage. This is well illustrated in cases of immunologic vasculitis or nephritis, in which dissolution of basement membrane occurs as a consequence of enzymatic hydrolysis, sometimes with catastrophic results (Chapters 13 and 20). Many diseases confronting the clinician are due to an uncontrolled inflammatory response. The joint damage in rheumatoid arthritis, the functional and structural damage in glomerulonephritis, and the demyelinating diseases of the central nervous system are examples of excessive or uncontrolled inflammatory responses. The treatment of these entities (since we lack information about the causative agents) is anti-inflammatory therapy (Chapters 10 and 25). Some of the most active areas under investigation at the present time are involved with the identification and characterization of mediators of the acute inflammatory response and the mechanisms by which homeostasis or immunologic balance can be maintained (Chapter 2).

Mediators of the acute inflammatory response can be separated into the *vasopermeability factors* (including the kinins, vasoactive amines, leukokines, anaphylatoxins from complement, and, perhaps, the prostaglandins) and the *leukotactic factors*. The former induce a reversible opening of the junctional zones between endothelial cells. The leukotactic factors operate independently of vasoactive factors, are, for the most part, peptide in nature, and are derived from the complement system or from lymphocytes. (Other sources of leukotactic factors include bacterial products and fibrin split products.) The specificity of leukotactic factors varies; some are restricted to a single cell type such as the neutrophil, the eosinophil, the basophil, or the monocyte, while other factors are more broadly reactive. Defects in the leukotactic system, whether due to abnormal humoral or cellular elements, are usually associated with the inability to cope with bacterial infections or the inability to respond to stimuli that usually incite delayed hypersensitivity reactions.

The *subacute inflammatory response* is, by definition, a somewhat delayed phase of the acute inflammatory response and is characterized by the accumulation of lymphocytes and monocytes and the formation of *granulation tissue*. For example, one to three days following a skin laceration, there occurs a dramatic proliferation of endothelial cells and fibroblasts. Collectively, these cells form a lush forest of fine capillaries that grow into the area of injury (Figs. 12–2 and 12–3). The capillaries deliver a greatly increased supply of blood to the area and provide nutrients for the accelerated metabolic requirements of inflamed tissues. Fibroblasts are actively synthesizing proteins and mucopolysaccharides, and their main function seems to be the deposition of collagen in the injured area. As this protein accumulates, its tensile strength gradually increases and reaches its maximum within five days, at which time there is a bridge of connective tissue across a previously open and exposed area. For the wound to heal properly, there must be adequate nutrition following surgery. Concomitant with the appearance of gran-

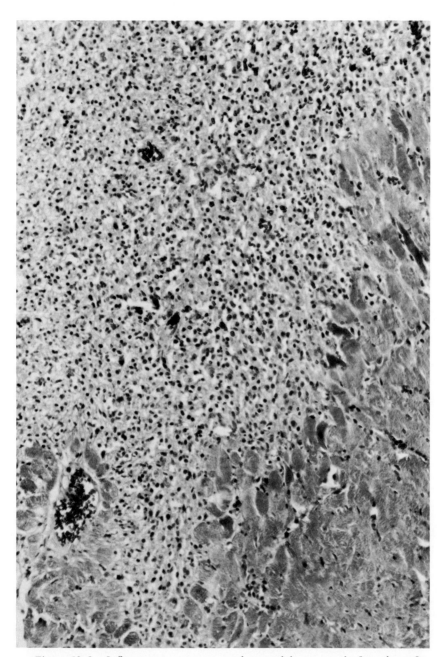

Figure 12–2. Inflammatory response to destroyed heart muscle four days after anoxic injury. The surviving myocardium (*lower right*) gives way to dense granulation tissue that replaces the destroyed muscle. Hematoxylin and eosin, ×100. (Armed Forces Institute of Pathology photograph.)

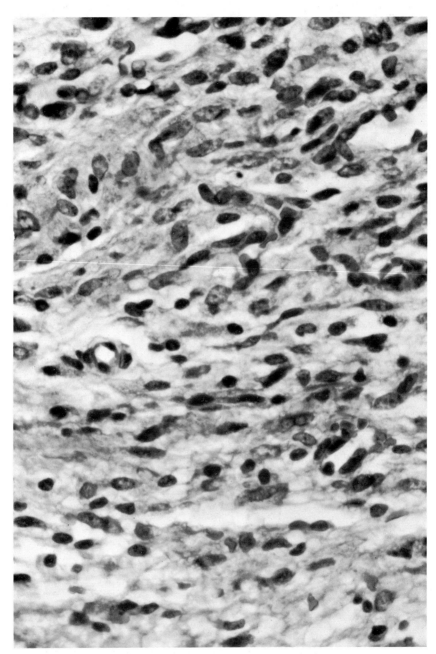

Figure 12-3. Higher magnification of granulation tissue in Figure 12–2. A lush network of fibroblastic and angioblastic elements is present. Between elongated nuclei, collagen fibrils are being laid down. Eventually these will form a dense collagenous scar. This is one outcome of the inflammatory response. Hematoxylin and eosin, ×530. (Armed Forces Institute of Pathology photograph.)

ulation tissue is the proliferation of epithelial cells, which provide a protective structure for the exposed and injured area.

If the inflammatory response is not completely successful in restoring the injured tissue to its original state (e.g., failure of elimination of foreign substance) or if repair of tissue cannot be accomplished, the events may progress to a state of *chronic inflammation.* This is characterized by the continued presence of lymphocytes, monocytes, and plasma cells. The explanation for such a progression of events to this stage may be persistence of foreign material, either living or dead, that mobilizes immunologic reactions. For example, in viral hepatitis, replicating virus may persist within the liver. Plasma cells and lymphocytes accumulate in large numbers, probably conveying immunologic defenses to the local area in the form of specific antibody-synthesizing B-cells or sensitized T-lymphocytes. The persistence of these inflammatory cells could result in functional impairment of the tissue, either because of the direct action of mediators elaborated by lymphoid cells, e.g., lymphotoxin (Chapter 9), or because of unremitting deposition of collagen by fibroblasts. If this happens in the liver, dense fibrous scar tissue results in cirrhosis. In the heart, the outcome may be a fibrous scar that replaces muscle.

It should be stressed that although a given inflammatory response may follow the progression of events as described, this is not always the case. In pneumococcal pneumonia, an acute inflammatory response may be seen with massive exudate of neutrophils and fibrin deposition in an entire lobe of lung (lobar pneumonia). Yet, if the outcome is favorable, particularly with antibiotic therapy, the entire exudate disappears dramatically within 48 hours. Under unusual circumstances, the inflammatory response progresses to the subacute stage, and the individual is under duress as the exudate is invaded by granulation tissue. In this case, the only result can be massive fibrosis with functional loss of a large area of lung. In other situations, such as rejection of a solid homograft, chronic inflammatory (lymphoid) cells are seen in the inflammatory reaction. Very little is known about factors that govern the initiation of the inflammatory response or the manner in which it is modulated or controlled. The lack of such an understanding represents one of the deficient areas of knowledge in medicine. Successful treatment for a large number of diseases awaits the accumulation of this knowledge.

A special type of chronic inflammation is *granulomatous inflammation.* This condition was first appreciated in tuberculosis when it was noted that in certain patients dying of the disease there were peculiar white granules (granulomas) scattered throughout the body. It was found that these small bodies, also referred to as tubercles, consisted of characteristic spheric accumulations of large phagocytic or histiocytic cells (unfortunately termed "epithelioid cells"). A prominent feature of the granuloma is the formation of giant cells (Fig. 12–4) containing a peripheral zone of lymphocytes, with or without plasma cells. Granulo-

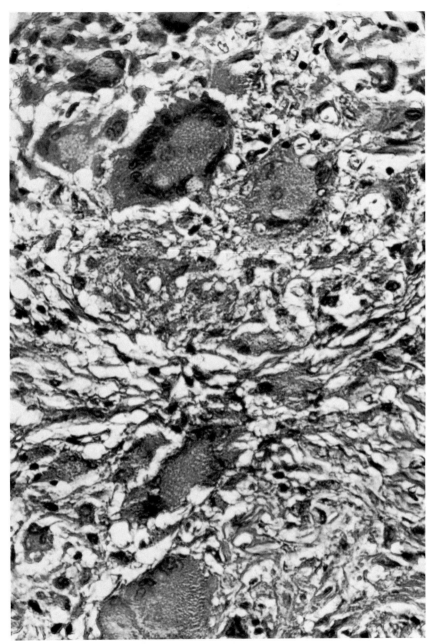

Figure 12–4. Granulomatous inflammation with eliptical macrophages ("epithelioid cells") and giant cells. From a patient with pulmonary sarcoidosis. Hematoxylin and eosin, ×350. (Armed Forces Institute of Pathology photograph.)

matous inflammation is now known to occur in other disease states in which there is persistence of foreign agents, either infectious (e.g., fungal infections) or noninfectious (e.g., silica). Generally speaking, granulomatous inflammation is an undesirable outcome of the inflammatory response, since, as in syphilis, tuberculosis, or helminthic infections, there may be extensive destruction of tissue with cavitation (necrosis) or scarring (fibrosis).

It is now known that granulomatous inflammation may reflect either *immunologic* or *nonimmunologic* mechanisms. The pioneering studies of Warren indicate that in experimental schistosomiasis intact immunologic responsiveness is a prerequisite to the formation of granulomas. In that disease, a variety of immunosuppressive measures precludes granuloma formation and the extensive pulmonary scarring is prevented. On the other hand, Warren has also shown that another system of granuloma formation, induced by the injection of talc (a trisilicate), is unaffected by immunosuppressive therapy but significantly retarded by drugs that interfere with activation of the kinin-generating (kallikrein) system (Chapters 2 and 13). It thus appears that granulomatous inflammation may result from two separate mechanisms: (1) an immunologically determined pathway (as in granulomatous inflammation of tuberculosis, with extensive tissue destruction due perhaps to the release of factors from lymphocytes, see Chapter 9), and (2) a nonimmunologic pathway requiring an intact kinin-forming system.

Tissue injury due to immunologic reactions has its origin in the inflammatory response, which is initiated by the reactions to antigen in tissues (Chapter 13). The initiating event may be either a mediator such as a leukotactic factor generated from the complement system or a factor produced by bacteria. Once the leukocyte has arrived from the bloodstream, the inflammatory process is initiated and the tissue will recover if adequate leukocyte defense is marshaled. Conversely, if too many leukocytes arrive, or if control mechanisms fail to function adequately, the tissue may become the adventitious target of damage. When the factors that determine these differences are understood, therapeutic measures may be more effectively applied in the prevention of these aberrancies rather than in the symptomatic treatment of disease manifestations.

SUGGESTIONS FOR FURTHER READING

Epstein, W. L.: Granulomatous hypersensitivity. Prog. Allergy, *11*:36, 1967.
Florey, H. W.: General Pathology. 4th ed. Philadelphia, W. B. Saunders Company, 1970.
Warren, K. S., Domingo, E. O., and Cowan, R. B. T.: Granuloma formation around schistosome eggs as a manifestation of delayed hypersensitivity. Am. J. Pathol., *51*:735, 1967.

MECHANISMS OF TISSUE INJURY PRODUCED BY IMMUNOLOGIC REACTIONS

Peter M. Henson, Ph.D., B.V.M.&S., M.R.C.V.S.

The encounter between a foreign substance and a host is followed by the induction of an immune response; the host is then in an immunologically primed state. Upon subsequent contact with the same antigen, the immune response will occur more rapidly and with greater vigor (secondary or anamnestic response) (Chapter 7). This subsequent reaction, which has exquisite immunologic specificity, can have either a *protective* function, forming the basis of host resistance to infectious diseases (Chapters 14 to 18) and malignant diseases (Chapter 19), or a *deleterious* function, the outcome causing *tissue injury* (Chapter 20). This chapter is concerned with the mechanisms of tissue injury due to immunologic responses.

The term allergy was originally coined by von Pirquet to include both facets of the altered state: the beneficial was termed *immunity* and the harmful, *hypersensitivity*. Today, however, despite the advantages of this nomenclature, the term allergy has become synonymous with the deleterious effects of hypersensitivity, and the broader responses to antigens are encompassed by the term immunity (Chapter 2). Allergy, or hypersensitivity, may therefore be defined as the altered reactivity to an antigen that can result in pathologic reactions upon the exposure of a sensitized host to that particular antigen (Chapter 20A).

Originally, the pathologic effects of immunologic processes were separated into two hypersensitivity reactions, *immediate* and *delayed*, that referred to the time required for the reaction to appear after challenge with antigen. With the increase of knowledge in many areas of immunobiology, Gell and Coombs have further classified these reactions as Types I, II, III, and IV allergic reactions. These include immediate hypersensitivity reactions (Type I), toxic effects of anticell and antitissue antibodies (Type II), toxic effects of complexes between antibody and antigen (Type III), and delayed hypersensitivity (cell-mediated) reactions (Type IV), which are listed in Table 13–1.

292

TABLE 13–1. Immunologic Mechanisms of Tissue Injury

Type	Manifestation	Mechanism
I	Immediate hypersensitivity reactions	IgE and other immunoglobulins
II	Cytotoxic antibody	IgG and IgM
III	Antigen-antibody complexes	IgG mainly
IV	Delayed hypersensitivity (cell-mediated)	Sensitized T-lymphocytes

It is important at the outset to emphasize that any given pathologic process (e.g., the production of an autoimmune disease) may comprise mechanisms belonging to several or all of these groups of reactions. The clinical applications of these overlapping reactions will be described more fully in Chapter 20.

PATHOGENESIS OF IMMUNOLOGIC INJURY

IMMEDIATE HYPERSENSITIVITY

Administration of a soluble antigen to a previously sensitized host can, under appropriate conditions, produce a reaction within minutes of the challenge. This reaction has been termed "immediate" in order to distinguish it from those of slower onset that are called "delayed." The most rapid hypersensitivity reaction of the immediate type is known as *anaphylaxis*. It is characterized by an explosive response that occurs within minutes of the challenging dose, and it can be either *systemic* (generalized) or *localized* (cutaneous). In immediate-type reactions, a variety of immunologic mechanisms may be operative but most have a mediation pathway that involves the release of pharmacologically active substances from mediator cells. The primary effect of these mediators is interaction with target cells, producing a functional alteration, e.g., contraction of smooth muscle, increase of vascular permeability, or increased secretion. These reactions are all characteristic features of Type I immediate hypersensitivity reactions.

Generalized Anaphylaxis

In the laboratory, generalized anaphylaxis is usually produced by injecting a small dose of antigen (sensitizing dose) into an animal followed within several days by an intravenous dose of antigen (challenging dose). The manifestations of generalized anaphylaxis vary with different species, in which different shock organs may be affected. The guinea pig, a few minutes after challenge with antigen, will scratch, sneeze, and cough, may convulse, and can collapse and die. This is primarily the result of respiratory impairment due to constriction of smooth muscle in the bronchioles and to bronchial edema. A sharp drop in blood pressure and a generalized increase in vascular permeability may also accompany the reaction. The lungs at postmortem examination are characteristically overinflated. In the rabbit, on the other hand, the shock organ is the heart, and right-sided heart failure is the main cause of death. In the human, generalized anaphylaxis presents with itching, erythema, vomiting, abdominal cramps, diarrhea, and respiratory distress. In severe cases, laryngeal edema and vascular collapse may result in death.

Passive Transfer of Anaphylaxis.   Since the reaction is antibody-mediated, anaphylactic sensitivity can be transferred to a normal recipient by means of serum. The source of antibody may be the same species *(homocytotropic)* or a different species *(heterocytotropic)*, as described below. For example, a guinea pig sensitized by an intravenous injection of rabbit antibody to ovalbumin and challenged with ovalbumin 48 hours later will suffer a fatal anaphylactic shock. A similar reaction can occur following the use of homologous (i.e., guinea pig) antiserum.

Types of Anaphylaxis

There are three different types of anaphylaxis: (1) *cytotropic*, (2) *aggregate*, and (3) *cytotoxic*.

Cytotropic Anaphylaxis.   In cytotropic anaphylaxis, the antibodies become fixed to mediator cells in the tissues of the recipient after a two-day latent period between injection of antiserum and antigen challenge. These antibodies with the property of binding are called cytotropic; those derived from the same species are call *homocytotropic*, and those from a different species are called *heterocytotropic*. Challenge with small amounts of antigen can produce cytotropic anaphylaxis. The antigen combines with antibody bound to mediator cells, e.g., mast cells, containing a variety of mediator substances including vasoactive amines, and the reaction results in the release of mediators from the cells.

Aggregate Anaphylaxis.   A second type of anaphylactic reaction occurs following the release of mediators that is triggered by antigen-antibody complexes. In this type, referred to as aggregate anaphylaxis, a latent period is not required. Antigen may be injected immediately after the injection of antiserum. After the antigen-antibody interaction in the blood, a secondary effect may be exerted on target cells through the release of mediators. The injection of soluble immune complexes may be used to induce a similar anaphylactic response, although not strictly caused by "aggregates." Aggregate anaphylaxis, therefore, is an example of tissue injury mediated through antigen-antibody complexes (Type III reaction) and is considered here because the final common pathway is similar to that of cytotropic anaphylaxis.

Cytotropic and aggregate anaphylactic reactions can occur simultaneously. For example, if antigen is rapidly injected into a sensitized animal containing both tissue-bound and circulating antibody, a massive release of mediators will result in anaphylaxis. Anaphylaxis can be avoided by injecting the antigen *slowly* or in divided doses, or by employing the subcutaneous or intraperitoneal routes. These observations assume clinical importance in the administration of antigen in the human. Intravenous routes, in contrast to other routes, are generally more likely to be associated with severe anaphylactic reactions.

Cytotoxic Anaphylaxis.   Cytotoxic anaphylaxis is caused by the injection of antibodies directed against antigens present on cells and represents a Type II reaction. For example, the intravenous injection of rabbit anti-Forssman antiserum into a guinea pig will produce anaphylaxis. Since all guinea pigs have this heterophil antigen on their cell surfaces, extensive cytotoxic damage can lead to an anaphylactic reaction in the presence of complement. In man, some transfusion reactions may be of this type (Chapter 20B). Cytotoxic anaphylaxis is therefore due to antitissue antibodies. These effects are described in greater detail below.

It is apparent that generalized anaphylaxis may be induced by different immunologic reactions, including Type I, II, and III mechanisms. However, the pathogenesis in each involves a common final pathway—the release of pharmacologically active substances (mediators) from mediator cells.

Cutaneous Anaphylaxis

Active Cutaneous Anaphylaxis.   Upon injection of antigen into the skin of a sensitized animal, a local anaphylactic reaction will occur within a few minutes. It consists of localized swelling and redness—a wheal and flare reaction. Skin tests in man for allergy to a wide variety of antigens (allergens) are characteristic of this phenomenon (Chapter 20A).

In animals, the cutaneous reaction is similar to that in man but is less readily visible. The local increase in vascular permeability that is characteristic of this reaction may be demonstrated by the use of tracer dyes (such as Evans blue dye), which leak out of vessels at the reaction site and stain the tissues. The anaphylactic reactions are mediated by substances such as histamine and serotonin, which have only a transient effect, since they are quickly inactivated by tissue and plasma enzymes, e.g., histaminases. Consequently, the true immediate hypersensitivity reaction is short-lived and recovery occurs within hours.

Passive Cutaneous Anaphylaxis.   Localized anaphylaxis can also be passively transferred and, in some cases, may be the only satisfactory way in which antibodies responsible for immediate hypersensitivity can be studied. In animals, the reaction in the skin is called *passive cutaneous* *anaphylaxis (PCA)*. Sensitizing antibody is injected intradermally and, after an obligatory latent period (usually 24 to 72 hours), antigen is given intravenously with Evans blue dye. The local permeability reaction, as evidenced by bluing of the skin, appears within minutes (Fig. 13–1). The requirement for a latent period in the skin is not fully understood but presumably represents the time required for cytotropic antibodies to diffuse and become fixed to mediator cells in the tissues, particularly the mast cells.

The PCA reaction is especially useful for study, since it provides a model for a purely cytotropic reaction. Although initial histologic examination of the skin usually reveals minimal cell infiltration in most species, including man, a leukocytic infiltration with a predominance of eosinophils is noted 2 to 24 hours after a challenge with antigen. In *active cutaneous anaphylaxis*, on the other hand, the animal has formed circulating antibodies, and the reaction evoked by intradermal antigen is often complex, with an Arthus lesion superimposed on the anaphylaxis.

Human Atopy and the Prausnitz–Küstner (P-K) reaction. A proportion of humans are peculiarly susceptible to natural sensitization by a variety of environmental antigens, including pollens, spores, animal danders, house dusts, and foods. These individuals appear to be genetically predisposed or susceptible (Chapters 3 and 20). This susceptibility is known as *atopy* (from *atopia*: Gr., strange disease); however, the term allergy is often used synonymously. Subsequent contact of these individuals with the antigens by inhalation or ingestion produces

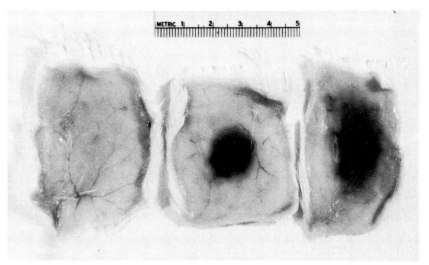

Figure 13–1. Passive cutaneous anaphylaxis (PCA) in guinea pigs. The two skins on the right come from animals injected intradermally with cytotropic antibody and, after a latent period, intravenously with antigen and Evans blue dye. The skin on the left is a control, injected with saline only. The leakage of the dye out of vessels with increased permeability is apparent.

such conditions as allergic rhinitis, asthma, and allergic urticaria (Chapter 20A).

These hyperactivities in man can also be passively transferred to unreactive subjects by the injection of serum antibodies. In order to avoid generalized reactions and sensitization, a completely localized transfer may be performed. This procedure is referred to as the Prausnitz–Küstner, or P-K, reaction. Serum from a sensitized individual is injected intradermally into a normal recipient. After a latent period of one or more days, antigen is injected into the same site and a localized wheal and flare reaction occurs within minutes. The P-K test, the human counterpart of the PCA reaction, has proved to be of importance in the study of immediate hypersensitivity in man and is sometimes used clinically to detect the presence of these antibodies (Chapter 20A).

Homocytotropic Antibodies Responsible for Immediate Hypersensitivity

In man, the term *reagin* or skin-sensitizing antibody has been used interchangeably for cytotropic antibody. However, in spite of the ability to passively transfer the reaction with serum, identification of the particular immunoglobulin class responsible for this activity had been difficult owing to its extremely low levels in serum.

In recent years, however, the bulk of antibodies responsible for immediate hypersensitivity in man has been shown to belong to the newest immunoglobulin class, IgE. Purified normal IgE, injected with reaginic antibody, can inhibit the P-K reaction by competing for receptor sites on mediator cells, e.g., mast cells. Moreover, as an indication that IgE is present in the skin of atopic as well as nonatopic individuals, intradermal injection of a specific rabbit antibody to IgE will induce a typical wheal and flare reaction. The salient properties of IgE globulins are shown in Table 13–2. IgE antibody (8S) is slightly larger than IgG (7S) and does not fix complement through the classic pathway; aggregated IgE, however, is able to initiate the complement cascade through the alternative pathway (Chapter 6). There is no good evidence, however, for complement requirement in immediate hypersen-

TABLE 13–2. Comparison of Properties of IgE and IgG Antibodies

IgE Antibody	IgG Antibody
8S	7S
Noncomplement fixing	Complement requirement in many reactions
Heat labile	Heat stable
Present in trace amounts in serum	Highest concentrations in serum
Biologic activity seen in both atopic and nonatopic individuals; higher in atopic	Biologic activity seen in both atopic and nonatopic individuals

sitivity reactions mediated by homocytotropic antibody. Another property of the antibody that has been used for characterization is its heat lability. Heating antibody at 56°C for two to four hours results in alteration of the Fc fragment of the IgE molecule and loss of its ability to fix to receptors on mediator cells. IgE is present in only nanogram quantities in human serum and is also present in individuals who show no evidence of atopy, suggesting that other factors in addition to the mere ability to synthesize IgE are involved in the induction of the atopic state.

Guinea Pig.   In the guinea pig, PCA reactions are produced by antibodies of the IgG1a and IgG1b, as well as IgE (Table 13–3). These IgG1 antibodies exhibit some clear differences from the IgE antibodies. They are less heat labile and persist in the skin for relatively shorter periods of time. In addition, shorter latent periods are required for detection of the IgG1 than for the IgE homocytotropic antibody by the PCA reaction.

Other Species.   As shown in Table 13–3, in the rat, rabbit, and dog, homocytotropic antibody of a type similar to human reagin (IgE) can be detected. Mice, on the other hand, have antibody similar to both reagin and that antibody found in guinea pigs. Recent reports suggest that more than one type of homocytotropic antibody can be found in other species, including man. For example, a short-acting IgG reaginic antibody has been implicated in anaphylaxis in the human; although not definitively proved, it has been suggested that this could be IgG4. In addition, a late cutaneous anaphylactic reaction (LCAR) of IgE has been described at four to six hours (Chapter 20A).

Stimulation of Homocytotropic Antibodies.   In the experimental animal (e.g., the rabbit), homocytotropic antibodies analogous to human IgE have been difficult to demonstrate after immunization. This is presumably due to the minute amounts of antibody produced rather than a lack of IgE production. When detected, the antibody is only found early in the process of immunization. Many animals can be induced to synthesize more homocytotropic antibody by the simultaneous injection of materials (adjuvants) such as alum, pertussis vaccine, or lipopolysaccharide.

Certain humans readily respond to antigen by synthesis of reagins. If an individual reacts in a skin test to one pollen allergen, he is likely to show some sensitivity to a great variety of other allergens. Further, it has been shown that the injection of nonatopic individuals with ragweed antigen incorporated in adjuvant may lead to the production of IgE reaginic antibody. Such antibodies, however, tend to be transient, and sensitization is often short-lived.

Of particular interest is the observation that infestation with parasites, especially helminths, leads to the production of homocytotropic antibody (Chapter 17). It is not known what properties of helminthic antigens predispose the host toward synthesis of these antibodies; how-

TABLE 13–3. Characteristics of Mammalian Homocytotrophic Antibodies*

	GUINEA PIG			MOUSE		RAT		RABBIT	DOG
	Type I	Type I	Type II	Type I	Type II	Type I	Type II	Type II	Type II
Optimal latent period for PCA	4–6 h	16h	7–8 d	1–2 h	72 h	2–6 h	24–72 h	72 h	36 h
Persistence at passively sensitized skin site	>2–<4 d	7–8 d	28 d	<1 d	10 or >d	<1 d	31 or >d	long	long
Amount of antibody present in serum after immunization	++++	++++	trace	++++	trace	++++	trace	trace	trace
Heat lability	−	+	+	±	+	−	+	+	+
Sedimentation coefficient	6.5S	6.5S	8S	7S	sl. > 7S	7S	8S	>7S	?
Immunoglobulin class	IgG1a	IgG1b	IgE	IgG	IgE	IgGa	IgE	IgE	IgE

*(After Bloch, K. J.: The antibody in anaphylaxis. *In* H. Z. Movat, (ed.): International Symposium of the Canadian Society of Immunology. Cellular and Humoral Mechanisms in Anaphylaxis and Allergy. New York, S. Karger, 1969, p. 1.)

ever, the phenomenon has been observed in a variety of species. For example, humans infected with ascaris have elevated levels of IgE globulins, and their serum can be used to induce PCA reactions in baboons, with ascaris antigens. (PCA activity in primates is a known property of human IgE antibody.) There is some evidence that a homocytotropic, antibody-mediated, local anaphylactic reaction in the gut of rats is involved in the ridding of infestation by the intestinal worm *Nippostrongylus braziliensis*. Furthermore, this reaction seems to be dependent on the presence of eosinophilic leukocytes.

Fixation to Tissues. One of the most common properties of homocytotropic antibodies is their ability to become attached to mediator cells in the tissues, e.g., mast cells. The skin-fixing properties of the antibody molecule appear to reside in the Fc fragment, since its removal by enzymatic digestion or its alteration by heating leads to a loss of its biologic activity, e.g., cutaneous anaphylaxis. Once antibody is fixed to mediator cells, a combination of antibody with the Fab fragments can occur. This leads to the release of mediators from these cells. Alternatively, intradermal injection of preformed complexes of antigen with IgE antibody will cause a wheal and flare reaction. The fixation of homocytotropic antibody to mediator cells appears to be due to a particularly firm, but not irreversible, bond. IgE antibody will remain at the site of intradermal injection in man for up to two months and will still be capable of reacting with a subsequent injection of antigen.

In addition to their skin-fixing ability *in vivo*, homocytotropic antibodies will bind to isolated mast cells and basophils *in vitro*. Since mast cells are important reservoirs of pharmacologically active mediators such as histamine, it has been postulated that homocytotropic antibody becomes bound to these cells *in vivo*. Such antibody fixed to mast cells has been demonstrated in humans, monkeys, and guinea pigs by the use of a wide variety of immunohistochemical techniques, e.g., immunofluorescent, autoradiographic, and ferritin-labeled antibody techniques.

The receptor on basophils for the Fc fragment of homocytotropic antibody seems to be quite specific, since passive sensitization of cells can be performed by incubation with whole serum from a sensitive animal. The low levels of homocytotropic antibody compete successfully with large amounts of other immunoglobulins present in the serum. After a suitable incubation with antibody, the basophils may be washed and will release contained histamine upon incubation with specific antigen. This forms the basis of an *in vitro* measurement of IgE antibody in the human through the release of histamine—the leukocyte histamine release assay (Chapter 26).

Nonhomocytotropic Antibodies. Release of mediators from cell reservoirs can also be induced by immune complexes of antigen combined with antibody that is not homocytotropic, as described previously. Thus, aggregate anaphylaxis in rabbits can result from rabbit

IgG antibody reacting with antigen, but the pathogenesis is more closely related to that of the Arthus reaction than that of immediate hypersensitivity. The reaction involves many cell types, including platelets and neutrophils. *Heterocytotropic antibodies* are another example of cytotropic antibodies that are usually IgG in nature. Rabbit IgG antibodies, injected into the skin of guinea pigs, will allow the induction of a strong PCA reaction after intravenous challenge with antigen. Whether or not binding sites for these heterologous antibodies are the same as those for homologous antibody, however, is at present unknown.

Blocking Antibodies and Desensitization (Immunotherapy). Immediate hypersensitivity reactions do not occur in the presence of large amounts of so-called *blocking antibodies.* A blocking antibody presumably competes locally or in the circulation for the antigen and prevents the reaction with homocytotropic antibody fixed to mediator cells. In serum, these antibodies are predominantly IgG and may be induced in man by repeated injections of antigen.

This observation forms the basis for an approach to desensitization or hyposensitization (immunotherapy) of allergic individuals (Chapter 20A). Minute quantities of the allergen to which the patient is sensitive are injected in increasing doses over a prolonged period. There seems to be a therapeutic benefit from this procedure in some individuals, but it is not certain whether the production of blocking antibodies is the sole mechanism involved.

Pharmacologically Active Mediators of Immediate Hypersensitivity

Early in the study of anaphylaxis, it was found that histamine injected into normal guinea pigs could mimic the immediate reaction. Since that time, many pharmacologically active substances have been implicated in immediate hypersensitivity reactions (Fig. 13–2), including histamine, serotonin, kinins, prostaglandins, prostaglandin intermediates, platelet-activating factors (PAF), and slow-reacting substances (SRS). There is no direct evidence that any one of these agents actually causes anaphylaxis. The presence of some mediators during an anaphylactic reaction *in vivo* or *in vitro* is the only available information. Specific antagonists of mediators, such as histamine and serotonin, prevent some manifestations of the hypersensitivity reactions. Additional evidence for the involvement of such mediators comes from the reproduction of actual hypersensitivity reactions when a substance such as histamine is injected in pure form.

Much of the information concerning mediators has been obtained from *in vitro* studies using isolated perfused organs or suspensions of organs, such as the lung and skin, as well as suspensions of mast cells and basophilic leukocytes. Antigen added to chopped lung tissue from

Histamine

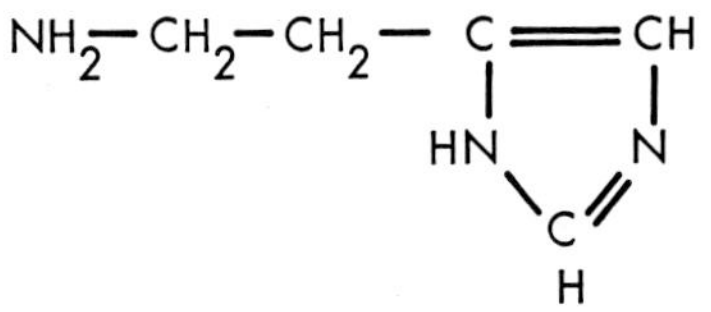

$$NH_2-CH_2-CH_2-C=CH$$

Serotonin
(5 Hydroxytryptamine)

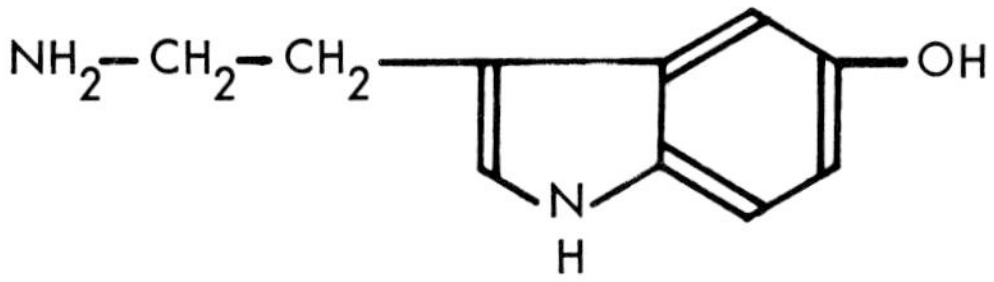

$$NH_2-CH_2-CH_2$$ OH

Bradykinin   Arg. pro. pro. gly. phe. ser. pro. phe. arg.

Lysylbradykinin   Lys. arg. pro. pro. gly. phe. ser. pro. phe. arg.

SRS-A   acid sulfate ester (<500 MW)

PAF (platelet activating factor)   ?phospholipid

ECF-A (eosinophil chemotactic   mixture of two tetrapeptides (<500 MW)
        factor of anaphylaxis)   Ala·gly·ser·glu and Val·gly·ser·glu

Prostaglandins and   (endoperoxides and
Prostaglandin intermediates   thromboxanes)   COOH

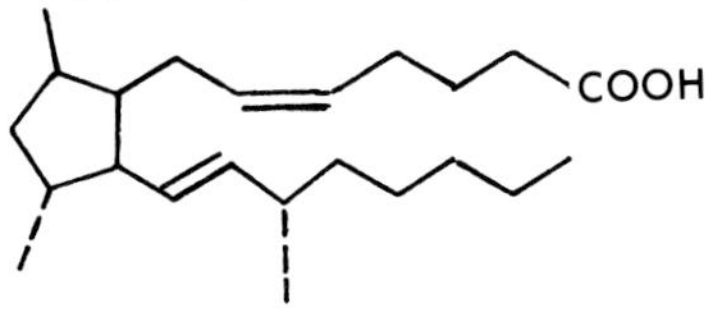

Figure 13-2.   The structure of some pharmacologic mediators of immediate hypersensitivity.

a guinea pig sensitized to that antigen will induce the release of up to 30 per cent of the total histamine in the tissue. In addition, other mediators, including SRS-A, PAF and eosinophil chemotactic factor of anaphylaxis (ECF-A), may be detected in the supernatant after the reaction. Lung tissue can also be passively sensitized when incubated with serum containing homocytotropic antibody, and it has provided a useful tool for the study of the anaphylactic reaction. Today, however, studies are concentrated upon individual cells that cause the release of these mediators.

Histamine.   Histamine is found in many tissues and is particularly localized in the granules of mast cells and basophils. Some species (e.g., the rabbit) also store large quantities of histamine in granules within platelets. Mast cell and basophil granules also contain heparin, which gives them their characteristic metachromatic staining with toluidine blue, but there is little evidence that this plays a direct role in anaphylaxis. The reaction of antigen with mast cells from sensitized animals results in extrusion of the granules (degranulation) and the release of histamine. Degranulation of mast cells may be seen *in vivo*, as well as *in vitro*, in tissue sections that have undergone anaphylactic reaction.

Histamine is formed by decarboxylation of histidine, which is stored in the mast cell granules. Once released, histamine can exert its many pharmacologic effects, including smooth muscle contraction, increased vascular permeability, and increased mucus secretion. The effects of histamine are transient, however, since the amine is rapidly broken down in the plasma and tissues by histaminases. The bioassay for histamine makes use of its effect on smooth muscle and measures the contraction of the guinea pig ileum by the Schultz-Dale reaction. Histamine can also be assayed by chemical, enzymatic, and radioactive techniques (Chapter 26).

Recent evidence indicates the existence of two types of histamine receptors: the H1 receptors, inhibited by standard antihistamines, and the H2 receptors, affected only by specific antihistamines such as burimamide and metiamide. Acting through H1 receptors, histamine contracts smooth muscles, increases vascular permeability and increases mucus secretion of goblet cells. Interaction of histamine with H2-type receptors results in increased gastric secretion and a decrease of mediator release from anaphylactically reacting mediator cells (e.g., mast cells and basophils). Another important biologic action of histamine that relates to immediate hypersensitivity reactions is its chemotactic potential for eosinophilic leukocytes. Not only can histamine attract eosinophils into sites of allergic reactions, but it can also deactivate and arrest these cells from further outward migration. The latter two properties, characteristic also for ECF-A, may have important biologic implications in the modulation of allergic inflammation through eosinophil-derived products, as described below.

Just as histamine can mimic some of the effects of anaphylaxis in the guinea pig, so can antagonists of histamine, the antihistamines, prevent anaphylactic reactions. This indicates that histamine is an important mediator of immediate hypersensitivity in both man and animals. However, the inability of these useful therapeutic substances to completely abolish the reactions *in vivo* indicates that other mediators participate. In rats and in mice, mast cells contain serotonin as well as histamine, and both mediators may participate in these species.

Serotonin (5-Hydroxytryptamine). This vasoactive amine is found in mast cells in rats and mice and in the platelets of most species. It is also present in the brain and the gastric mucosa. The role of serotonin in human anaphylaxis is questionable, but it may be important in other species. Although it does not directly induce increased vascular permeability in rabbit skin, as it does in rats and mice, it may participate in immune complex disease in the rabbit. The amine produces increased vascular permeability, capillary dilatation, and contraction of smooth muscle.

Kinins. Kinins are basic peptides with vasoactive properties that are found in plasma and in tissues. They are split by kininogenases (kallikreins) from certain precursor plasma proteins, the kininogens. Kininogenases may be activated in the plasma but are also present in organs such as the pancreas. The kinins produced include bradykinin, a nonopeptide, and lysylbradykinin, a decapeptide (Fig. 13–2). These peptides increase vascular permeability and cause a lowering of blood pressure and a contraction of smooth muscle. They are bioassayed by their ability to contract the uterus from a rat in estrus. Although kinin levels in the blood do increase slightly in some species during anaphylaxis, there is little evidence that they play a major role in the reaction. As with other mediators, they are rapidly degraded by enzymes in the plasma (kininases).

Slow-Reactive Substance of Anaphylaxis. Substances that can produce a relatively slow contraction of an isolated smooth muscle preparation have been termed slow-reactive substances (SRS). Slow-reactive substance of anaphylaxis (SRS-A) is found in the perfusate from sensitized guinea pig lungs perfused with antigens and is released from chopped sensitized human lung fragment by antigen. The molecule is an acidic sulfated ester with a molecular weight of less than 500. Its action on smooth muscle is not inhibited by antihistamines. In the human, SRS-A may be partly responsible for the prolonged bronchospasm seen in asthma and may account for the inability of antihistamines to completely alleviate the reaction. Recent experimental evidence suggests that SRS-A is elaborated by mast cells, basophils, and perhaps neutrophils.

Eosinophil Chemotactic Factor of Anaphylaxis (ECF-A). Following the reaction of antigen with cell-bound IgE, there is the release of a mediator that is selectively chemotactic for eosinophils, ECF-A. Stored as a preformed moiety in mast cells and basophils, the molecule is a mixture of at least two tetrapeptides that have an overall molecular weight of less than 500 (see Fig. 13–2). It is noteworthy that eosinophilic leukocytes are commonly found at sites of allergic reactions, although their function is at present unknown. It has recently been suggested that they may function to modulate the extent of allergic inflammation by affecting the metabolism of the mediators, as described below, e.g., the neutralization of SRS-A by aryl sulfatase.

Platelet-Activating Factor. PAF is a low molecular weight lipid, probably a phospholipid, that induces platelet aggregation and secretion. It has been found in man, rabbit, and rat and may serve as a potent amplifying agent for acute allergic and anaphylactic reactions.

Prostaglandins. A variety of C_{20} unsaturated hydroxy aliphatic acids with potent biologic properties have been termed prostaglandins. They are widely distributed in tissues and depending on their nature can contract (e.g., $F_{2\alpha}$) or relax (e.g., E_1 and E_2) smooth muscle. Prostaglandins are released from tissues undergoing anaphylaxis. An exciting new development in this area has been the demonstration that intermediates of prostaglandin synthesis, the prostaglandin endoperoxides or perhaps even more likely the thromboxanes, for example, appear to be the key mediators of platelet aggregation and smooth muscle contraction (see Fig. 13–2). These highly labile compounds are released from lungs undergoing anaphylaxis and may mediate some of the anaphylactic processes. They may also be responsible for mediation of other effects, including perhaps the muscle-contracting action of kinins. Endoperoxides and thromboxanes are produced during the synthesis of prostaglandins from arachidonic acid. The fact that their generation is inhibited by aspirin and indomethacin provides a biochemical rationale for the potent anti-inflammatory effects of these drugs.

Injury Produced by Antitissue Antibody (Cytotoxic Antibody)

The second type of immunologic injury occurs as a result of antibodies directed to tissue antigens. This has been referred to as a *cytotoxic or Type II reaction*. Previously, antitissue antibodies were considered important contributors to immunologic disease. Now their role appears more limited compared to injury mediated by antigen-antibody complexes. Nevertheless, such antibodies are involved in human disease and have been shown to induce experimental tissue damage in animals. There are two main mechanisms for such injury. The first is the reaction of antibody with tissue cells. The antibody can induce direct cytolysis and killing by activation of all nine components of complement (Chapter 6). The cytotoxic anaphylaxis described earlier may be the result of this type of process. In the human, certain hemolytic reactions may be of this type. The second mechanism of injury by cytotoxic antibody involves the participation of cells, such as the neutrophil and macrophage. When the antitissue antibody reacts with its antigen, whether on a tissue cell or basement membrane, the antigen-antibody complex so formed can interact with phagocytic cells. These cells adhere to the bound immunoglobulin itself, but the adherence is greatly enhanced by the fixation of complement through C3b, a split product of the third component of complement, C3 (Chapter 6). Reaction of antibody with circulating cells such as the erythrocyte, therefore, can cause not only cytolysis but also phagocytosis by cells of the reticuloendothelial system. In tissues, the fixation of antibody and complement can cause accumulation of cells, such as neutrophils, that release injurious constituents when they react with antibody or complement. This process is identical with that for immune complexes, the only difference being that antigen is itself part of the target tissue. In addition to these effects, antibody can also facilitate the cytotoxic action of lymphocytes and perhaps macrophages, e.g., killer (K-) cells, in the so-called antibody-dependent cellular cytotoxic (ADCC) reactions (Chapters 9 and 11) described below.

These processes may occur together, as in autoimmune hemolytic anemia in which both hemolysis and increased clearance contribute to the destruction of erythrocytes. In addition, there may be other mechanisms of damage induced by direct reaction of antibody with tissues that are not yet understood. An example of the damage produced by antitissue antibody is *nephrotoxic nephritis*, produced experimentally by the injection of heterologous antiglomerular basement membrane (a-GBM) antiserum.

Nephrotoxic Nephritis

This classic model, first described by Masugi, is produced in a variety of animals, including the rat and the rabbit. Antikidney antibody is produced by injecting an animal, such as a sheep, with a preparation of rabbit glomerular basement membrane (GBM); the a-GBM antibody is then injected back into a normal rabbit with the production of a nephritis. The a-GBM antibodies are injected intravenously and, if radiolabeled, can be shown to bind to basement membranes in various organs of the body that cross-react with the glomerular basement membrane. A larger amount of antibody binds to the kidney, however, and it is here that injury is produced.

The so-called heterologous phase of nephrotoxic nephritis follows the injection of antiserum by only a few hours. Upon reaction of antiserum with antigen (glomerular basement membrane), the antibodies fix complement and neutrophil accumulation results. In the absence of C3, or if pepsin-treated antibody (which does not fix complement) is used, neutrophils are not found in the glomeruli, and damage is reduced. In a similar way, neutrophil depletion alone will also diminish these lesions. The pathologic changes within glomeruli vary with the species but generally involve some proliferation and basement membrane thickening. The degree of damage is directly related to the amount of antibody fixed in the glomeruli, and thus to the amount injected. Large quantities of antiserum also produce fibrin deposition and necrosis, common findings in severe, neutrophil-mediated tissue damage. Immunoglobulin and complement (C3) may be demonstrated by immunofluorescence in a linear pattern along the glomerular basement membrane (Fig. 13–3). This is in contrast to the granular pattern observed in immune-complex glomerulonephritis (See Fig. 13–9A).

When studied with the electron microscope, neutrophils may be seen along the basement membrane and have pushed aside the covering endothelial cells (Fig. 13–4). Adherence of the neutrophils to the antibody, or the C3, or both along the basement membrane stimulates release of injurious enzymes from the neutrophils, which then cause much of the resultant damage. Indeed, specific neutrophil enzymes can

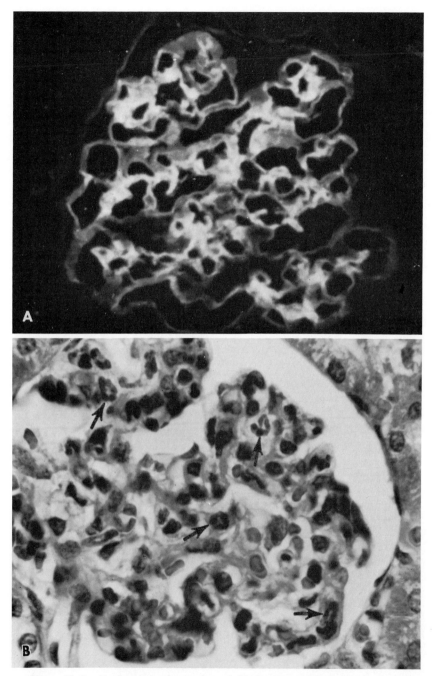

Figure 13–3.   Nephrotoxic glomerulonephritis in the rat. The sections were taken two hours after injection of rabbit antirat glomerular basement membrane antiserum. *A*, Section stained for the presence of rabbit IgG with fluorescent antibody. The IgG can be seen lying in a *linear* fashion along the glomerular basement membrane. Staining for rat C3 revealed a similar pattern of fluorescence. × 850. *B*, Section stained with hematoxylin and eosin. Neutrophils are filling the capillary loops (*arrows*). × 1000.

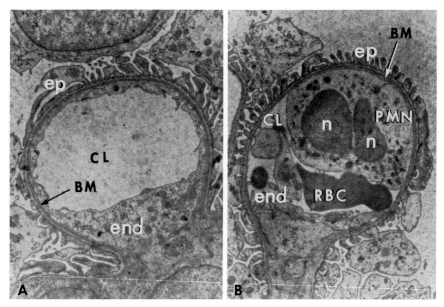

Figure 13-4. Electron photomicrograph of glomerular capillary loops in nephrotoxic nephritis. *A*, Neutrophil infiltration has not occurred and the endothelial cell (end) is spread normally over the basement membrane (BM). *B*, A neutrophil has pushed aside the endothelial cell and is closely adherent to the denuded basement membrane. CL: Capillary lumen; ep: epithelial cell. × 7000. (From Cochrane, C. G., Unanue, E. L., and Dixon, F. J.: A role of polymorphonuclear leukocytes and complement in nephrotoxic nephritis. J. Exp. Med., *122*:99, 1965.)

be detected in the urine during this type of glomerulonephritis, along with fragments of glomerular basement membrane. This relatively simple neutrophil-mediated mechanism may not be the only pathogenetic process occurring in nephrotoxic nephritis. Administration of high levels of sheep antirabbit GBM to rabbits depleted of complement or neutrophils may still result in proteinuria. This damage seems to involve a different type of antibody and in larger amounts than is required for the neutrophil-mediated injury. Its mechanism of action has not yet been elucidated.

In this experimental system, heterologous antiserum is used, and this is itself antigenic to the recipient. Consequently, antibodies formed against the foreign proteins after about a week react with the a-GBM antibodies along the glomerular basement membrane and produce an exacerbation of the glomerular damage. This is known as the autologous phase of the disease. Such antibodies are not autoantibodies, and the process described before does not occur naturally, except perhaps when antilymphocyte sera contain anti-basement membrane antibodies. However, injection of heterologous, and sometimes homologous, kidney extracts has been used to induce autoimmune nephrotoxic nephritis in experimental systems; i.e., antibodies are produced that can react with the recipient's own basement membrane. It has also been possible to produce an immune-complex nephritis this way, when the antibody that is induced forms complexes with low levels of circulating kidney antigens.

Glomerulonephritis in man is sometimes associated with synthesis of anti-GBM antibodies, although their pathogenetic role is not certain. Some evidence of binding of immunoglobulins to human glomeruli *in vivo* has been obtained, for example, in patients with Goodpasture's syndrome and chronic glomerulonephritis (Chapter 20C). Sections of kidneys from patients with these diseases often show a linear fluorescence along the basement membrane. Moreover, the fact that antihuman GBM can be eluted from such kidneys and can induce nephritis if transferred to monkeys suggests that this antibody may have a possible pathogenetic role. Patients with this type of antibody in their glomeruli who are given kidney homografts often develop glomerulonephritis in the transplanted kidney as well.

Autoimmune Antitissue Antibodies

Antibodies against various tissues have been described in human autoimmune diseases (Chapter 20C). Indeed, their detection by immunofluorescence has generally been the only indication that the disease is related to autoimmunity. Unfortunately, there is little evidence available in man to determine whether the antibodies actually cause the damage or are the result of it. Where complement-fixing antibodies that can react with the surface of cells in the body are present, destruction of cells can occur. This may be most clearly seen in autoimmune hemolytic anemia. Activation of the entire cytolytic sequence of complement components results in lysis of the erythrocytes, and in addition, they may be engulfed by phagocytes reacting with the $C3b$ fixed to their surfaces. In a similar way, idiopathic thrombocytopenic purpura may result from the presence of antiplatelet antibodies. The possible nature of the abnormality that leads to the production of these antibodies is described in Chapter 20C.

INJURY PRODUCED BY ANTIGEN-ANTIBODY COMPLEXES

After antibody has combined with antigen within the body, certain effector mechanisms, such as phagocytosis, eventually result in the elimination of the immune complexes. In some cases, however, the process is accompanied by a variety of inflammatory reactions, known collectively as the *Type III reaction*. Since these pathogenic effects of immune complexes are important contributors to a number of human disease conditions, a considerable amount of experimentation has been directed toward elucidation of the mechanisms involved.

In general, the pathogenesis of injury produced by immune complexes can be divided into four phases: (1) the combination of antibody with antigen to produce the complexes; (2) the localization of these complexes at particular sites in the body; (3) the accumulation of humoral and cellular factors; and (4) the production of tissue injury. The process can be best understood by first considering the local effects of immune complexes in the skin, the Arthus reaction, and then considering the more complicated systemic immune-complex disease that is characteristic of serum sickness.

The Arthus Reaction

Injection of antigen into the skin of a sensitized animal results in an edematous, hemorrhagic, and eventually, necrotic lesion, which was first described by Maurice Arthus in 1903. This reaction, known as the Arthus phenomenon, is produced by the combination of precipitating antibody with antigen in the skin and may be elicited in four ways. The *active Arthus reaction* is that originally described, whereby antigen is injected into a previously immunized animal possessing circulating antibodies. The *direct passive Arthus reaction* is identical, except that circulating antibody is supplied passively to a normal recipient by an intravenous injection of antiserum. If the administration is reversed so that antiserum is injected intradermally and antigen intravenously, a *reversed passive Arthus reaction* is produced. Finally, both antibody and antigen can be injected at the same site and, in fact, may even be combined together *in vitro* prior to injection.

Specificity and Type of Antibody. Since the reaction is produced by antigen-antibody combination, its specificity is that of the antibodies produced (active) or administered (passive). A wide variety of antigens and species of animal exhibit the reaction. From 50 to 100 μg of antibody nitrogen is generally required for the reversed passive lesion, and similarly large amounts of circulating antibody are necessary for the direct reaction. The process thus requires an appreciable quantity of immune complexes. The antibodies must also be of a precipitating, complement-fixing type, but for the passive reaction they need not come from the same species of animal.

Morphology. The typical lesion develops rapidly. Local swelling, erythema, and edema appear within an hour, and the lesions become hemorrhagic and increase in intensity over the next few hours (Fig. 13–5). The severity is dependent upon the quantity of antigen and antibody available, and, with large amounts of antigen-antibody complex, necrosis may result. Over the next two days, the reaction gradually diminishes and eventually disappears.

Microscopically, an acute inflammatory reaction is seen. Retarded blood flow in small vessels is accompanied by leukocyte clumping and diapedesis, with occasional microaggregates of platelets and leukocytes. The strikingly characteristic feature of this lesion, however, is the

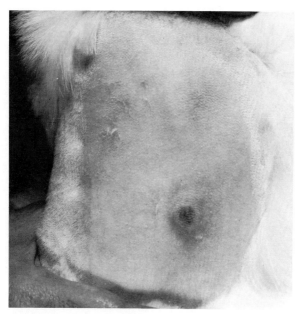

Figure 13-5.   Active Arthus reaction in an immunized rabbit eight hours after the intradermal injection of antigen (60 μg N and bovine serum albumin). The edema and central hemorrhagic area are apparent. A control site injected with saline is above the lesion. No reaction can be seen.

marked accumulation of neutrophils within capillary and venule walls (Fig. 13-6*A*). After about eight hours, there is a gradual infiltration of mononuclear cells, such as lymphocytes, macrophages, endothelial cells, and fibroblasts. By 24 hours, mononuclear elements predominate, and after three to six days plasma cells are seen in islands of lymphoid cells in the perivascular spaces.

Pathogenesis.   In the active Arthus reaction, antigen such as bovine serum albumin (BSA) is injected into the skin. Circulating antibody meets this antigen at the local blood vessel wall and precipitates with it. In the reversed passive reaction, the process is similar, except that it is the antigen that is circulating. The antigen-antibody complexes have ample opportunity to fix complement, and immunofluorescent techniques show that BSA, antibody (gamma globulin), and complement (C3) are localized within the blood vessel wall at the site of antigen injection (Fig. 13-6*B*, *C*, and *D*).

The formation and localization of the immune complexes do not themselves induce tissue damage. From the characteristic observation of neutrophil infiltration it might be expected that these cells are also involved in the reaction, and indeed, this seems to be the case. Thus, if the reaction is performed by administering nitrogen mustard or antineutrophil antiserum to rabbits depleted of circulating neutrophils,

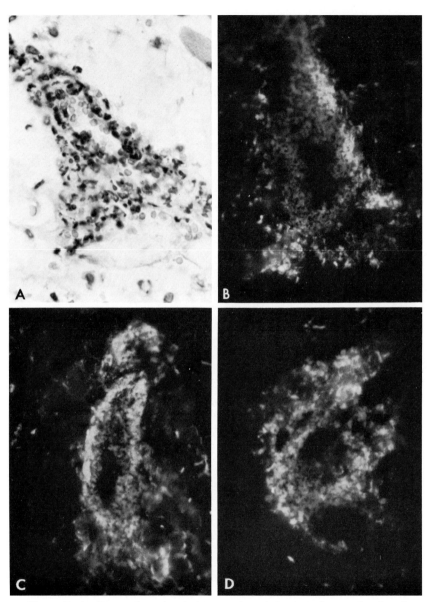

Figure 13–6. Reversed passive Arthus reaction. *A*, Section of a venule taken three hours after the injection of antigen (bovine serum albumin [BSA]) intravenously and antibody (rabbit anti-BSA) intradermally. Large numbers of neutrophils have accumulated in the vessel wall. Edema and extravasated red cells may also be seen. ×250. A section of a similar venule was stained with fluorescent-anti-BSA (*B*), antirabbit IgG (*C*), and antirabbit C3 (*D*). Antigen, antibody, and complement may be seen in the vessel walls.

immune complexes can be seen within blood vessel walls, but no inflammatory reaction ensues.

The process whereby neutrophils accumulate at the site of immune-complex deposition requires activation of the complement sequence. This conclusion follows the observation that the Arthus reaction may be largely prevented or reduced by depletion of circulating complement components. This has been achieved in a number of ways, but most successfully by the use of a factor from the venom of the cobra, *Naja naja*, which inactivates C3 and later-acting components. A possible mechanism for the action of complement in the induction of neutrophil accumulation involves the release of chemotactic factors C5a and $\overline{C567}$ during complement fixation by the immune complexes (Chapter 6). Neutrophils might migrate from the blood vessels up the concentration gradient of chemotactic materials toward their source, the immune complexes. This process would be augmented by local hemostasis, since the factors would not be carried away by blood flow. It has been difficult, however, to determine whether this is the only mechanism involved. For example, Arthus reactions may be elicited in rabbits genetically deficient in C6, animals that cannot produce the $\overline{C567}$ chemotactic factor, although C5 factors may be generated normally.

Another property of neutrophils, which may be of importance in their accumulation at sites where antigen-antibody complexes are localized, is their ability to adhere to immune reactants. Neutrophils will adhere both to antibody that has combined with antigen and to complement fixed to antigen-antibody complexes. The name immune adherence has been given to the latter reaction (Chapter 6), and it is the third component of complement (C3) that is primarily involved (C3 immune adherence). The immune adherence bond is a strong one, and there are many available sites for adherence on the neutrophil. When such cells pass immune complexes in or on a blood vessel wall, they may become adherent and thus localized at this site. Moreover, adherence would be the end result of chemotaxis after the cell has reached the immune complex that is generating the chemotactic factor. Adherence of neutrophils is generally followed by phagocytosis of the immune complexes, and, in the lesions of the Arthus reaction, the neutrophils have engulfed the immune complexes they encounter (Fig. 13–7).

The process described so far has still not accounted for the tissue damage that ensues. However, neutrophils contain a variety of hydrolytic enzymes and other active materials that, if released, could produce the observed effects. Studies of these cells *in vitro* have revealed that they do release some of these lysosomal materials into the extracellular environment during the process of phagocytosis. Within the neutrophil may be found proteolytic enzymes capable of hydrolyzing collagen, elastic tissue, and cartilage; thus they are capable of destroying base-

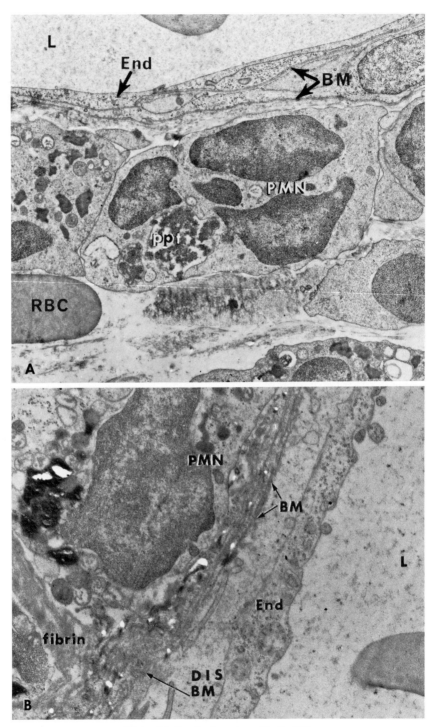

Figure 13-7. *See legend on opposite page.*

ment membrane and other supporting structures. At least some of these enzymes are known to be released and may be implicated in the damage to blood vessel walls, hemorrhage, and necrosis of the Arthus reaction.

Another feature of the lesion is the increased vascular permeability and edema. This may be clearly demonstrated by intravenous injection of Evans blue dye with the antigen or antibody. The dye binds to albumin, and when plasma proteins leak from the more permeable vessels at the Arthus site, a blue area is produced in the skin. The increased permeability is also mainly dependent upon the neutrophil accumulation, since depletion of these cells largely prevents it. In the search for the mediators of this effect, neutrophils were found to contain a variety of permeability-increasing factors, in addition to the proteolytic enzymes. Four small basic proteins have been described that are localized intracellularly in the granules and are probably released along with the lysosomal enzymes. Three of these induce vascular permeability by an as yet unknown process, and the fourth causes mast cells to release the vasoactive amine histamine. Since the increase in vascular permeability in the Arthus reaction is largely unaffected by antihistaminics, the factor acting on mast cells probably plays only a supportive role in the process. Release of vasoactive amines from mast cells, basophils, or platelets does not appear to play a major role in the permeability increase.

An influx of neutrophils in the Arthus reaction is thus the primary factor responsible for the observed tissue damage. However, not all the results of the accumulation are harmful. The cells phagocytose and digest the immune complexes that induced the reaction. Later, there is a change in cell population from granulocytes to mononuclear cells (macrophages) in the lesion. These mononuclear cells presumably help to clear up the debris and thus aid the healing process. Neutrophils are known to contain a potent chemotactic factor for monocytes that may be instrumental in bringing this latter type of cell into the lesion.

This relatively simple neutrophil-mediated injury, which constitutes the classic Arthus reaction, may, at times, be confused with superimposed processes of different pathogeneses. Thus, the presence of homocytotropic antibody in the skin may contribute to an immediate histamine-mediated increase in vascular permeability. Such antibody usually requires a latent period in the skin for maximal activity when

Figure 13–7. Electron photomicrograph of Arthus reactions in the rabbit bladder wall. *A,* Ferritin was used as the antigen. Immune complexes of this electron-opaque material and antibody (ppt) may be seen in the vessel wall and within phagocytic vacuoles of neutrophils that have accumulated at this site. This is an early lesion and little basement membrane damage is apparent, although an extravasated red cell is present. *B,* At a slightly later stage, dissolution of the basement membrane (dis BM) can be seen and fibrin has been deposited. PMN: neutrophil; BM: basement membrane; L: vessel lumen; End: endothelial cell. ×10,500.

given passively, but may be present in an actively immunized animal. The characteristic feature of this immediate hypersensitivity reaction is its onset within minutes of intravenous antigen administration, as compared to the Arthus reaction, which develops more slowly. After the Arthus reaction has occurred in suitably sensitized animals, a delayed hypersensitivity lesion may follow. This reaction is characterized by its delay in onset and by the type of cells (mononuclear) involved.

Serum Sickness (Immune-Complex Disease)

Following the injection of foreign serum to humans, a number of unpleasant side-effects are known to occur. The disease, which came to be known as serum sickness, can result in vascular, cardiac, renal, cutaneous, and joint lesions. Evidence has accumulated that the immune complexes formed when antibodies are produced against the foreign serum proteins are the cause of the tissue damage. Other antigens may induce disease by a similar process, i.e., following combination with specific antibody in the bloodstream. Such antigens include bacterial, viral, and even autologous materials, which may for a variety of reasons be recognized as foreign.

The Arthus reaction follows the formation of antigen-antibody complexes locally. Immune complexes formed in the bloodstream produce a more generalized effect and can induce tissue injury in a variety of target organs, depending upon where they become localized. The pathogenesis of these lesions therefore includes mechanisms of deposition of immune complexes, as well as their subsequent effect on the tissues.

A considerable amount of information about the mechanisms involved has come from two experimental forms of the disease that may be induced in rabbits. *Acute serum sickness* (immune-complex disease) results from immune complexes formed when the animal first makes antibody to an antigen that is still present in the bloodstream. *Chronic immune-complex disease* involves repeated administration of antigen to immune animals with continuous formation of antigen-antibody complexes over a prolonged period. Counterparts of both variants of these pathogenic processes have been implicated in human disease.

Acute Immune-Complex Disease. A description of the pathogenesis of experimentally induced acute serum sickness in rabbits will serve to indicate some of the factors and mechanisms involved in the production of tissue injury by circulating immune complexes. The course of the disease is shown in Figure 13–8. The antigen, bovine serum albumin (BSA), is given as a single large intravenous injection (250 mg per kilogram). The clearance of this antigen from the circulation may be monitored if it is previously labeled with radioactive iodine (^{131}I) (Fig. 13–8). Following an initial equilibration with the extravascular space, the BSA is for a time catabolized at the same rate as rabbit al-

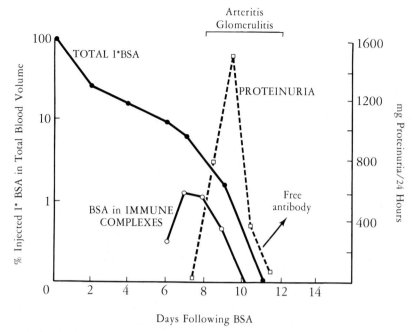

Figure 13–8. The course of acute experimental immune-complex disease in the rabbit. The antigen used is radiolabeled bovine serum albumin (I* BSA).

bumin. Production of antibody to the BSA then causes an increased clearance rate and, at this time, complexes between antigen and antibody can be detected in the blood.

Concurrent with the formation and circulation of the immune complexes is the appearance of the characteristic lesions. Glomerulonephritis is most easily detected, since damage to the glomeruli results in proteinuria. Sections of the kidney (Fig. 13–9) reveal that the capillaries in the glomeruli have been almost completely occluded, mainly because of proliferation of the endothelial cells (proliferative glomerulonephritis). Neutrophil accumulation is not a characteristic feature of this acute immune-complex disease nephritis. Other lesions include endocarditis and vasculitis. Figure 13–10 shows a section of a coronary artery, which is a common site for this lesion. Endothelial proliferation or accumulation of mononuclear cells, or both, is apparent. In addition, and in contrast to the glomerular lesions, neutrophil accumulation is marked. Damage to the internal elastic lamina, penetration of neutrophils into the media, and medial necrosis are seen.

Pathogenesis. One of the most important contributions to a knowledge of the causation of this disease comes from the demonstration that the immune complexes may be deposited in the blood vessels at the site of the lesions. Immunofluorescent techniques demonstrate this

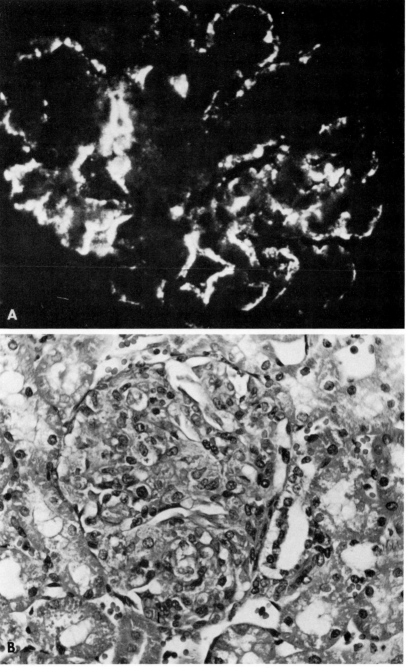

Figure 13–9. Kidney sections from a rabbit with acute immune-complex disease. *A*, Glomerulus showing staining with fluorescent antirabbit IgG in *granular* deposits along the basement membrane. Fluorescent antisera against the antigen (BSA) and rabbit C3 give a similar pattern of fluorescence. *B*, Hematoxylin- and eosin-stained section. There is great proliferation of cells in the glomerulus, and the capillary lumina have been occluded. Neutrophils cannot be seen. ×300.

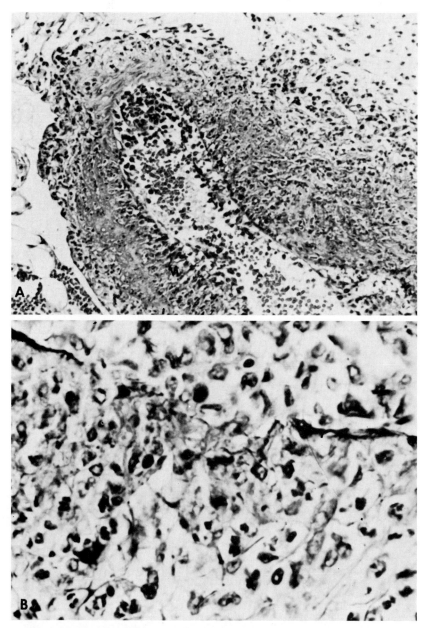

Figure 13–10. Arteritis in acute immune-complex disease in rabbits. *A,* Neutrophil accumulation, intimal proliferation, and early medial necrosis are present. ×200. *B,* Higher power showing breaks in the internal elastic lamina and penetration of neutrophils into the media. The lumen is toward the top.

clearly in the kidney, where by use of suitable antisera, BSA, rabbit immunoglobulin, and rabbit complement can be detected in a characteristically granular pattern (Fig. 13–9A). Deposited complexes have also been demonstrated in the arteries, although the presence of neutrophils soon results in their phagocytosis and digestion.

Deposition of Circulating Immune Complexes in Blood Vessel Walls. An increase in vascular permeability is involved in the deposition of the antigen-antibody complexes. Injection of carbon particles in rabbits developing serum sickness showed that the carbon was trapped along filtering basement membranes or internal elastic lamina and suggested a similar mechanism for immune complex deposition; i.e., the increased flow through the vessel walls might trap large complexes. Consequent upon this hypothesis was a lower limit to the size of immune complexes capable of being deposited. Experiments with increased vascular permeability induced in guinea pigs demonstrated that materials having a sedimentation rate greater than 19S were required for deposition. In rabbits, density-gradient ultracentrifugation of serum, taken at the time when complexes were circulating, enabled determination of the size of the circulating complexes. The fact that rabbits with complexes less than 19S did not develop the disease indicates a requirement for complexes above this size.

The mechanism of increased vascular permeability and the nature of its mediators are not completely known. Vasoactive amines appear to be the most likely candidate for this. If antagonists of histamine and serotonin are administered during the induction of serum sickness, both immune deposition and subsequent disease are inhibited; this suggests a pathogenetic role for these two amines (Table 13–4). Similarly, platelets (which contain a large amount of histamine and serotonin) appear to be reservoirs for the vasoactive amines. The fact that depletion of circulating platelets with antiplatelet antiserum leads to the prevention of these lesions indicates that the release of vasoactive amines from platelets may be involved.

A number of immunologic reactions can cause release of histamine and serotonin from rabbit platelets *in vitro* and may account for the

TABLE 13–4. Effect of Antagonists of Vasoactive Amines and of Platelet Depletion on Acute Immune-Complex Disease

	GLOMERULITIS		ARTERITIS
	Immune-Complex Deposition	*Proteinuria (mg/day)*	*Per cent Rabbits with Lesions*
Antagonists of histamine and serotonin	±	5	9
Platelet depletion	±	86	18
Control	++	513	80

release *in vivo.* Most of the reactions require complement activation and probably involve immune adherence of platelets to the immune complexes. Only one mechanism is clearly independent of complement action, the reaction of blood basophils, antigen, and platelets. A basophil sensitized with IgE antibody reacts with antigen and causes the release of its contents of histamine, the low molecular weight mediator, and the platelet-activating factor (PAF). This in turn stimulates aggregation of platelets and secretion of their histamine and serotonin. It is this leukocyte-dependent reaction that appears to be involved in producing increased vascular permeability in serum sickness of rabbits. Since dep-

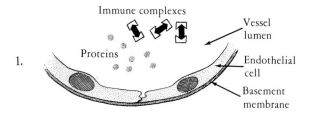

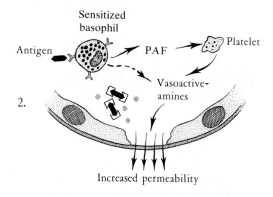

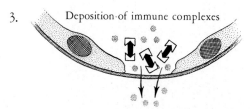

Figure 13–11. Hypothetical scheme for deposition of immune complexes in acute immune-complex disease. (*1*) Constituents of the deposition process. (*2*) The reaction of antigen with a basophil sensitized with IgE antibody leads to the release of vasoactive amines and platelet-activating factor (PAF), which also can cause platelets to release vasoactive amines with a subsequent increase in vascular permeability. (*3*) With the outflux of fluid, the larger immune complexes become trapped by the filtering basement membrane.

osition of complexes occurs in animals depleted of complement (C3–C9) with the cobra venom factor, complement does not appear to be involved in this reaction. A possible scheme for the vascular deposition of immune complexes in rabbits is shown in Figure 13–11.

Areas of greater blood turbulence where complexes and platelets may be impacted against vessel walls with more force, are predilection sites for these vasculitis lesions. It is of interest that similar sites are involved in atherosclerosis; indeed, atherosclerotic lesions may be experimentally produced with greater facility in rabbits undergoing acute serum sickness. It is possible, therefore, that immune-complex deposition may participate in the initiation of this disease.

Production of Tissue Injury. For reasons that are not clear, the glomerular lesions in acute immune complex disease are relatively free of neutrophils. Unlike the case in nephrotoxic nephritis, depletion of neutrophils or complement does not prevent the glomerulonephritis. The mechanism by which deposited immune complexes induce endothelial cell proliferation, increased glomerular permeability, and subsequent proteinuria is unknown.

The arteritis lesions, on the other hand, appear to be neutrophil-mediated. As with the Arthus reaction, neutrophil or C3 depletion prevents neutrophil accumulation and tissue damage, although complexes are still deposited and some endothelial changes occur. In this type of lesion, immune adherence of neutrophils to antigen-antibody-complement complexes on the blood vessel walls may be of considerable importance in bringing these cells to the site of injury. Following neutrophil accumulation, damage to the internal elastic lamina occurs, probably the result of released neutrophil constituents. The cells may then penetrate into the media and perpetuate their injurious action there. Similarities to the Arthus reaction are apparent. The lesions gen-

TABLE 13–5. A Comparison of the Glomerulonephritis in Immune-Complex Disease and Nephrotoxic Nephritis

	GLOMERULONEPHRITIS	
	Nephrotoxic Nephritis	*Acute Immune-Complex Disease*
Antibodies	Directed against the glomerular basement membrane	Directed against circulating antigens (immune complexes are deposited in glomeruli secondarily)
Fluorescence	Linear (IgG, complement)	Granular (antigen, IgG, complement)
Histology	Neutrophil accumulation	Proliferative glomerulonephritis
Complement and Neutrophils	Generally required for injury	Not required for injury (in contrast to the vasculitis of this disease)

erally heal within a few days after disappearance of the immune complexes. Table 13–5 compares glomerulonephritis induced by anti-glomerular basement membrane antiserum with that caused by circulating immune complexes.

Systemic Immune-Complex Disease (Serum Sickness) in Man. Administration of large amounts of foreign serum to humans results in a disease process identical to that in rabbits. At the time when antibodies are first formed, they complex with circulating antigen and produce the serum sickness syndrome. Manifestations of this immune-complex disease include fever, enlarged lymph nodes, erythematous rashes, painful joints, and vascular inflammatory reactions. The clinical details of serum sickness in man will be described in Chapter 20A. Evidence for a similar pathogenesis of deposition of immune complexes in blood vessels in man comes from studies of leukocytoclastic angiitis. Injection of histamine into normal areas of skin in an individual with an attack of this disease results in localization of gamma globulin and complement and the development of tissue injury (Chapter 20).

Chronic Immune-Complex Disease. The acute immune-complex disease is transient and disappears when no more complexes circulate. However, some diseases of man that may be mediated by immune complexes are chronic and persistent, including lupus erythematosus and possibly rheumatoid arthritis. Consequently, an experimental model has been established in rabbits in which immune complexes repeatedly subject the main target organ (the kidney) to injury.

In this model, the animal receives daily injections of antigen over a period of several weeks. When antibody is produced, the antigen dose is adjusted to maintain circulating complexes. This is because injection of small amounts of antigen into a rabbit producing large quantities of antibodies results in large complexes that are cleared too rapidly by the reticuloendothelial system to induce damage. Disease is produced in rabbits when antigen-antibody complexes are formed in relative antigen excess (Chapter 8). In this situation, the antibody response is too small to cause immediate clearance of antigen but large enough to produce circulating complexes.

Glomerulonephritis develops after 1 to 14 weeks of continued insult by the circulating complexes. Moderate to severe proteinuria with some hypoproteinemia and elevated blood urea nitrogen are found. Histologically, the appearance is one of membranous glomerulonephritis (Fig. 13–12B). Basement membranes are thickened, but there is less endothelial cell swelling and proliferation found in the glomeruli in chronic serum sickness. After more prolonged insult, proliferation, crescent formation, adhesions, and scarring may occur.

Antigen, antibody, and complement may be detected by fluorescence in these glomeruli and are distributed in a lumpy, irregular fashion, indicating that immune complexes are again deposited in the kidney (Fig. 13–12A). Electron microscopic examination of sections of

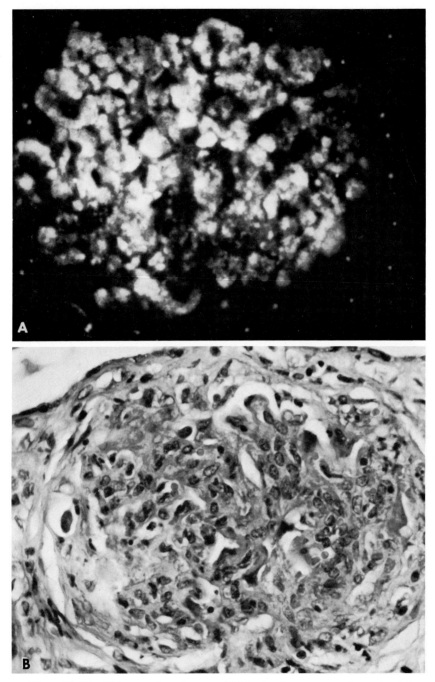

Figure 13–12. Kidney sections from a rabbit having immune complexes circulating for several months as a result of daily injections of antigen (chronic immune-complex disease). *A*, Coarsely granular fluorescent staining of the glomerulus due to deposited antigen (or rabbit IgG or C3) demonstrated with fluorescent anti-BSA antiserum. *B*, The glomerulus shows proliferation of cells, obliteration of capillaries with crescent, and adhesion formation.

glomeruli reveals electron-dense masses on the epithelial side of the basement membrane. These have been shown to be immune complexes, although it is not yet known how they reach this location from the capillary lumen.

Pathogenesis. The pathogenesis of chronic immune-complex disease is less well understood than that of the acute form. Complex localization may initially follow processes similar to those seen in the acute disease, but once initial deposition has occurred it is self-perpetuating. For reasons that are not clear, vascular and joint lesions are an uncommon finding. The high rate of blood flow through the glomerulus and its filtering action may predispose this structure to injury by continuously circulating complexes.

Glomerulonephritis Produced by Immune Complexes in Man and in Animals. Considerable emphasis has recently been placed on immune complexes as being responsible for a large number of immunologically mediated diseases in man (Chapter 20). In few cases is the antigen within the complex known. Nevertheless, when the characteristic granular deposits of immunoglobulin and complement are found in sections of glomeruli of patients, an etiology involving immune complexes is suggested. In some cases, however, a knowledge of the antigen is available. A number of groups of possible antigens involved in these processes are listed below.

Autoantigens. In systemic lupus erythematosus in man and in the autoimmune disease of New Zealand black (NZB) and New Zealand white (NZW) hybrid mice, antinuclear antibodies are found in the serum. Glomerulonephritis in these conditions has been shown to be related to immune complexes of DNA and anti-DNA. Immunoglobulin and complement can be detected in the glomeruli by immunofluorescent techniques. Moreover, elution of the kidneys reveals the presence of nuclear antigens and antibody in the eluates.

Viral Antigens. Chronic infection with certain viruses results in a situation in which virus persists in an animal for a long period of time. Antibodies to the virus that are produced can thus precipitate with it and induce a chronic glomerulonephritis. Examples in animal systems include lymphocytic choriomeningitis (LCM) virus in mice and Aleutian disease in mink. There have been preliminary reports of virus-like particles observed in the kidney biopsies of patients with lupus erythematosus.

Bacterial Antigens. Poststreptococcal glomerulonephritis in man may be an example of deposition of complexes with bacterial antigens inducing immune complex nephritis (Fig. 13–13).

Cross-Reacting Antigens. Body constituents that normally circulate in small amounts in the blood may be involved in immune-complex nephritis. Experimentally, rats injected with rat-kidney homogenates produce an antibody that cross-reacts with normal kidney tubular antigens circulating in low levels. The immune complexes thus formed

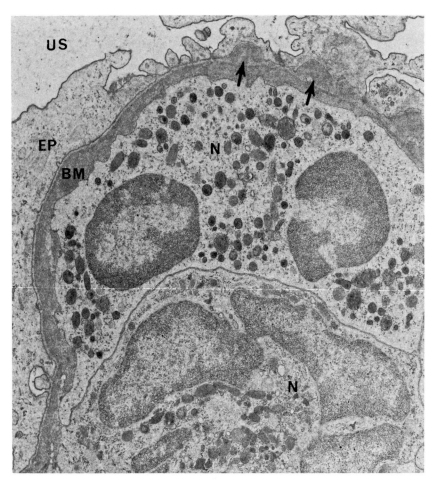

Figure 13–13. Electron photomicrograph of a glomerulus from a case of poststrep-tococcal glomerulonephritis in man. Neutrophils (N) fill the capillary lumen and push the endothelial cell away from the basement membrane (BM). Deposits (*arrows*) can be seen along the basement membrane and human IgG and C3 could be detected in a granular distribution along the basement membrane with fluorescent antisera. EP: epithelial cell; US: urinary space. (Courtesy of Dr. J. D. Feldman.)

become deposited in the kidneys and induce a glomerulonephritis that is due to the complexes and is quite unrelated to the source of the antigen. It is possible that exposure to environmental (e.g., bacterial) antigens cross-reacting with antigens within the body may produce a similar type of disease.

DELAYED HYPERSENSITIVITY

Delayed hypersensitivity is a manifestation of what has come to be called cellular or cell-mediated immunity. The principles underlying this phenomenon have been described in a previous chapter (Chapter 9). Delayed hypersensitivity may be defined as an increased reactivity to specific antigens mediated not by antibodies but by T-cells. This phenomenon was first observed in 1801 by Jenner in connection with cowpox reinoculation and was later developed by Koch and von Pirquet into a test for tuberculosis. The reaction in the skin that follows intradermal injection of antigen into a suitably sensitized animal was called "delayed" hypersensitivity because of its slow onset, taking 24 hours to reach maximal intensity. The phenomenon, which is exemplified by the tuberculin reaction, was thus distinguished from immediate hypersensitivity and the Arthus reaction. Differences underlying the pathogenesis of these immunologic reactions became apparent later.

Cell-mediated immunity is more difficult to define or quantify than humoral immunity (Chapter 9). The reaction of antibody with its antigen can be detected directly or indirectly in a number of ways. Until recently, the reaction of a specifically sensitized lymphocyte with its antigen could be ascertained only by *in vivo* reactions of the delayed type (Chapter 9). One of the characteristics of the delayed response is that it can be transferred to an unreactive recipient by cells but not by serum. This procedure was first described by Landsteiner and Chase in the 1940's and has assisted considerably the study of the phenomenon. Even now, however, despite a vast quantity of accumulated literature, our understanding of delayed hypersensitivity is relatively superficial.

Interest in this phenomenon lies in its involvement in such problems as graft rejection, tumor rejection, autoimmune disease, and contact sensitivity and its role in antimicrobial immunity. The benefit to the animal from the presence of a cellular reactivity to antigens has long been debated and may be related not only to resistance to bacterial and viral infection but also to recognition of abnormalities of self, as in autoimmune disease and neoplasia. Unfortunately, as with humoral immunity, the manifestation of the cellular response to antigen sometimes involves tissue damage and disease.

A discussion of the cutaneous delayed reaction will serve to illustrate some characteristics of the phenomenon. Its involvement in graft rejection and autoimmunity are considered in Chapter 20.

Induction of Delayed Hypersensitivity

Classically, delayed hypersensitivity was found after infection with bacteria such as *Mycobacterium tuberculosis*. In addition, it may be produced experimentally by the injection of a variety of protein antigens, usually in low doses and accompanied by killed tubercle bacilli. Antigen incorporated into an oil-in-water emulsion containing tubercle bacilli (Freund's complete adjuvant) is generally used to induce delayed hypersensitivity. The component of the bacteria responsible for the increased sensitizing effect is a lipopolysaccharide—Wax D. The route of sensitization is important, the intradermal route being the most efficacious (Chapter 10).

Although they may be produced in all animals, including man, delayed hypersensitivity reactions have been studied most productively in the guinea pig. The sensitivity generally appears early, e.g., four to seven days after antigen injection. In some situations, delayed hypersensitivity is the only immunologic reaction evoked by the sensitization. However, since complete Freund's adjuvant also increases antibody production, the early onset of delayed hypersensitivity is often followed by a humoral immune response. Testing an animal at this time for delayed reactivity may be complicated by superimposed immediate hypersensitivity and Arthus reactions. Since larger quantities of antigen induce antibody formation, small sensitizing doses (1 to 50 μg) are generally more effective.

The Cutaneous Reaction

The tuberculin test in man is an example of this process. To test for delayed hypersensitivity *in vivo*, a small quantity of antigen (often less than 1 μg) is injected intradermally. In detecting sensitivity to *Mycobacterium tuberculosis*, the antigen employed for skin testing is tuberculin, a purified protein derivative (PPD) of the organism. Characteristically, the onset of the skin reaction is slow, and nothing may be seen for 6 to 12 hours. Erythema and nonedematous, indurated swelling gradually develop, reach maximal intensity after 24 to 72 hours, and then slowly regress. In severe reactions, hemorrhage and necrosis may be seen. With protein antigens, a milder but similar reaction occurs. The reaction is sometimes considered qualitatively different and called a Jones-Mote reaction.

Histology

The delayed hypersensitivity lesion is characterized by mononuclear cell infiltration, although some neutrophils may appear in the early (six hour) lesion. Nests of macrophages and lymphocytes may be seen around blood vessels and nerves (Fig. 13–14). Macrophages are found invading tissues such as the dermis. A previously ignored cell, the basophil, has recently been found to accumulate quite commonly in these lesions, and although its effect is unknown, it is seen in the Jones-Mote reaction. Occasionally in tuberculin sensitivity, a lesion is seen with fibrin, neutrophils, and central necrosis. In addition, where antibody production has begun, a superimposed Arthus reaction may contribute to the overall picture. With protein antigens the mononuclear cell invasion is characteristic and is usually accompanied by some disruption in the surrounding tissues. This type of lesion is also found in all the reactions

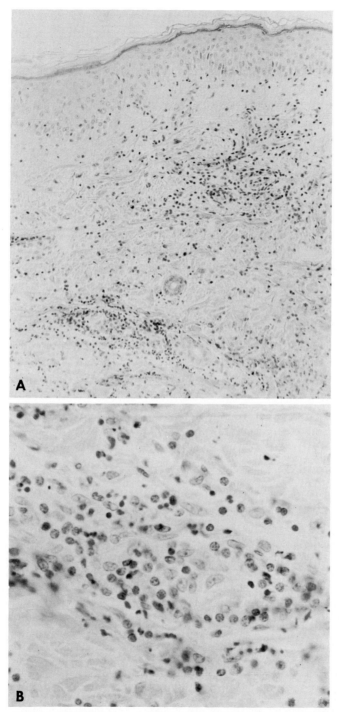

Figure 13–14. Delayed hypersensitivity in man. *A*, Biopsy of a skin reaction in a sensitized individual 48 hours after the intradermal injection of tuberculin. The extensive infiltration of mononuclear cells (macrophages and lymphocytes) is apparent. ×200. *B*, Higher magnification. ×430. Sections stained with hematoxylin and eosin.

involving delayed activity, such as graft rejection, and in many of the autoimmune diseases.

Other Forms of Delayed Hypersensitivity

A systemic reaction can be elicited in a hypersensitive animal following intravenous administration of antigen, e.g., tuberculin. The generalized reaction is initially a febrile one, and tuberculin has been shown to release endogenous pyrogen in sensitive animals (Chapter 14). This tuberculin shock reaction can result in lymphocytopenia, shock, and even death. In animals with tuberculosis, absorption of tuberculin into the bloodstream can result in reactions around the tuberculous lesions anywhere in the body.

Contact Hypersensitivity

A delayed inflammatory reaction can be produced by application of certain low molecular-weight materials to the skin. The response has been best studied in the human and in the guinea pig. Sensitization follows the same general pattern as the usual delayed hypersensitivity reaction. A week after the percutaneous application of a low molecular weight sensitizer, such as picric acid or dinitrochlorobenzene (DNCB), a delayed skin reaction may be elicited by a second application of a challenging dose of antigen to the skin. In man, this is sometimes applied as a patch test (a piece of filter paper soaked in a solution of the substance applied to the skin).

The cutaneous inflammation is similar to that described for classical delayed hypersensitivity lesions. The onset is slow and erythema and swelling are observed. Histologically, there is a mononuclear cell infiltration more closely concentrated in the upper layers of the skin and around hair follicles because of the route of antigen administration (Fig. 13–15).

The unique feature of this reaction is the size of the antigen employed (less than 1000 molecular weight). Such materials are not usually immunogenic and act only as haptens, i.e., require a carrier protein (Chapter 4). In contact sensitivity, the low molecular weight sensitizer is bound to protein in the skin itself. To induce the sensitivity, it has been shown that the antigen (hapten) must be able to bind covalently to proteins. Thus, 2,4 dinitrobenzene requires a Cl, F, Br, or SO_3H group for activity; H, CH_3, or NH_2 groups, which do not bind to proteins, are incapable of causing this hypersensitivity.

Interestingly, administration of preformed hapten-protein complexes (e.g., picrylated bovine gamma globulin) will elicit only weak contact sensitivity skin reactions when the guinea pig is later tested with the hapten itself. This is due to the nature of the specificity of the reaction, which is directed not only to the hapten but also to the carrier

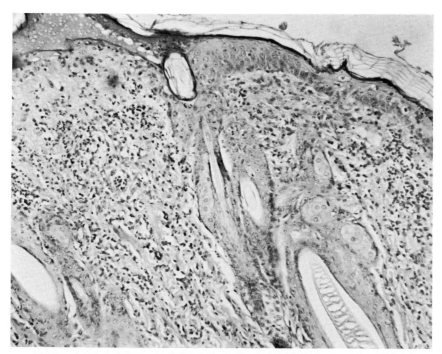

Figure 13-15. Contact sensitivity in a guinea pig. Section of a skin reaction in a sensitized animal 24 hours after the percutaneous application of dinitrofluorobenzene (DNFB). The mononuclear cell infiltration is similar to that in Figure 13-14 but is more superficial and is seen surrounding the hair follicles (reflecting the route of administration of antigen). (Courtesy of Dr. J. D. Feldman.)

protein (Chapters 4 and 7). In the skin test, when the hapten enters the skin it combines with proteins different from those to which it was bound in the initial inoculum, and no reaction ensues. In support of this conclusion is the observation that testing with the original hapten-protein conjugate will produce a delayed hypersensitivity reaction. Moreover, if the initial sensitization was performed with hapten bound to homologous skin proteins, later skin testing with hapten alone will result in positive reactions.

Contact Sensitivity in Man

One of the best-known examples of contact sensitization is the allergic contact dermatitis resulting from exposure to poison ivy. The sensitizer in this instance is a plant catechol, urushiol, that acts in the same way as the synthetic chemicals described earlier. Skin reactions to industrial chemicals, cosmetics, and drugs (such as penicillin) are often manifestations of contact hypersensitivity. Sensitization requires penetration of the chemical into the skin, which is generally easier for hydrophobic materials; however, the sweat glands in humans do provide a penetration route for hydrophilic substances. Sensitization of an individual persists, and, even though the reaction is weaker, a skin test can elicit a response after many years. In man, the histologic picture is similar to that in animals and that of classic delayed hypersensitivity; however, damage to the epidermis often results in vesicle and blister formation.

Transfer of Delayed Hypersensitivity

Characteristically, delayed hypersensitivity is a cellular phenomenon and the reactivity to a given antigen can be transferred passively to a normal recipient by sensitized T-lymphocytes from a sensitized donor. Serum is ineffective. Delayed hypersensitivity is thus clearly differentiated from immediate hypersensitivity, which is transferred by serum. However, it must be noted that transfer of antibody-forming cells (B-cells) will also elaborate antibody in the host, perhaps resulting in cellular transfer of immediate hypersensitivity and Arthus reactions. In spite of the requirement for transfer by cells, however, one mechanism of delayed hypersensitivity has postulated the presence of minute amounts of high-affinity antibody in the circulation. This possibility does not seem likely, since passive transfer of large amounts of high-affinity antibody has not been effective; but it cannot be completely excluded until the true mechanism is known.

Cells from the spleen, lymph nodes, or peritoneal exudates have usually been used for transfer. The lymphocyte responsible is the T-cell or thymus-derived lymphocyte, and there is increasing evidence that this cell belongs to a different population from that responsible for "helper" function in antibody synthesis (Chapter 7). The cells in species other than man must be viable. It has also been shown that active metabolism of the transferred cells is required. Twenty-four hours after transfer of cells from a sensitized donor to a normal guinea pig, for example, delayed reactions may be detected in the recipient. In inbred strains, the sensitivity persists. Where the donor cells are incompatible with the recipient, reactivity will disappear after a week, when the host mounts an immune attack against the foreign cells. The transient nature of the transfer in outbred animals suggests that the sensitized cell itself is involved in the reaction and is not merely passing "information" to host cells.

Cell transfer has been an important tool in the study of delayed hypersensitivity and its possible involvement in experimental diseases. By using this technique, it has been possible to show that labeled donor cells (i.e., sensitized cells) constitute only a small proportion of the cells in a lesion; the majority are of host origin. A more difficult problem has been whether there is a specific accumulation of sensitized T-cells at a site of antigen injection as compared to a control site. Experiments from different laboratories have yielded conflicting results. What specific accumulation there is seems to be small. The cells that do make up the cell infiltrate (i.e., predominantly unsensitized host cells) are dividing cells. Of interest is that transfer of cells to irradiated recipients fails to support delayed hypersensitivity, again showing the importance of dividing host cells.

Transfer Factor in Man

In man, the situation is somewhat different. Delayed hypersensitivity can be transferred with cells such as peripheral leukocytes. What is unique, however, is that extracts of the leukocytes will also transfer the specific sensitivity. The material responsible has been called "transfer factor," is dialyzable, and appears to have a molecular weight below 10,000 (Chapter 9). It is resistant to trypsin, ribonuclease, and heat. Its character and mechanism of action remain unknown, and it is possible that more than one factor is involved. The factor is released from sensitized leukocytes upon incubation with antigen *in vitro;* and, upon injection into a human recipient, it can sensitize him within a matter of hours. Following the injection of transfer factor into skin test–negative recipients, the previously negative skin sites become positive within six hours, but "conversion" can last years. This short latent period provides evidence that the phenomenon is not due to antigen transfer resulting in sensitization of the host. Moreover, transfer has been achieved with sensitization to synthetic antigens that the recipient could not have experienced, so that stimulus by transferred antigen of a pre-existing sensitivity cannot be the explanation. Attempts to detect antibody in the transfer factor have always been negative, and since its small molecular weight became known, this possibility has been excluded. The nature of this factor is an important question and its answer may help to elucidate the mechanisms of delayed hypersensitivity. Recently, transfer factor prepared from normal donors has been used in the immunologic reconstitution of individuals with impaired cellular immunity, e.g., Wiskott-Aldrich syndrome, and chronic mucocutaneous candidiasis. The uses of transfer factor will be described more fully in Chapter 22.

Specificity of Delayed Hypersensitivity

Cellular immunity, like humoral immunity, is exquisitely specific. There are, however, some clear and interesting differences between the two responses. Antiserum to a hapten-carrier complex will usually contain antibodies to the hapten itself, which will react with it free in solution or attached to another carrier. Delayed hypersensitivity, on the other hand, tends to be directed toward the carrier proteins as well as to the hapten. Guinea pigs sensitized to dinitrophenol–guinea pig albumin (DNP-GPA) conjugates will give delayed reactions to DNP-GPA but not to DNP or GPA separately or to dinitrophenol–bovine gamma-globulin (DNP-BGG). An *in vitro* model for delayed hypersensitivity, the inhibition of macrophage migration, exhibits exactly the same type of specificity. As we have seen earlier, contact sensitivity involving haptenic groups also exhibits this carrier specificity. In this case, the carriers are proteins in the skin to which the chemical (e.g., DNCB) is administered topically or intradermally. It appears, therefore, that delayed hypersensitivity requires a larger antigenic determinant, i.e., the hapten and a portion of the carrier.

An indication of the necessity for the antigen to be degraded in the animal prior to the induction of delayed hypersensitivity has been obtained by the use of polymers of the nondegradable D-amino acids as carriers. In this case, delayed hypersensitivity could not be produced, in contrast with the effectiveness of haptens coupled to L-amino acid polymers. It is also extremely difficult to induce delayed hypersensitivity to polysaccharides, which are known to be difficult to degrade; however, since polysaccharides can induce humoral antibody, degradation does not appear to be the only explanation.

Desensitization and Tolerance

Administration of large doses of antigen can specifically desensitize animals that had previously exhibited delayed hypersensitivity, so that a subsequent skin test with antigen is negative. Desensitization is considerably easier for proteins than for bacterial antigens such as tuberculin. Thus, 1 to 2 mg of ovalbumin given intravenously or intradermally can effectively prevent a delayed reaction, even if the desensitizing injection is given up to two hours after the intradermal challenge. This emphasizes that the interaction of antigen and cells in the skin is relatively slow, probably because of the reduced rate of accumulation of specific cells. Flooding the system with excess antigen can prevent the local lesion, even though the initial reaction has already started.

Animals may be made tolerant or unresponsive to specific antigens so that it is not possible to stimulate an antibody response to that antigen (Chapter 10). In the same way, tolerance usually results in the inability to induce delayed hypersensitivity. Injections of large quantities of antigens to neonates appear to be the most effective method of induction of unresponsiveness. Tolerance to homografts can also be produced in this way. The feeding of contact allergens, such as DNCB, to guinea pigs can cause a state of unresponsiveness to a subsequent application of the chemical to the skin. However, these animals are not tolerant to the hapten if it is conjugated to a non-guinea pig protein, such as egg albumin. Such experiments indicate once again the critical role of the carrier in delayed hypersensitivity and show that immunologic unresponsiveness in this type of reaction has similar specificity.

Pathogenesis of Tissue Damage in Delayed Hypersensitivity

It is generally thought that the specifically sensitized T-lymphocyte is responsible for recognition of the antigen in lesions of delayed hypersensitivity. When the antigen is injected there are two possibilities for contact with lymphocytes—either antigen leaks out into the bloodstream to react with passing lymphocytes, or lymphocytes that are constantly migrating through tissues by chance encounter the locally deposited antigen. Lymphocytes have been observed to accumulate and migrate out of blood vessels in the lesions; however, the mechanisms involved in the accumulation are still to be determined.

The sensitized lymphocyte, after encounter with antigen, becomes a metabolically activated cell and may release a variety of factors. These have been described in Chapter 9. The release of these factors has been observed *in vitro* but is only surmised *in vivo*. One of these substances is chemotactic for macrophages. Macrophages are known to accumulate with lymphocytes at the delayed hypersensitivity site. The migration inhibition factor (MIF) capable of inhibiting the macrophages' migration *in vitro* may possibly be involved in keeping the macrophages in the lesion once they have arrived. Other factors may "activate" the macrophage, inducing increased metabolism and increased synthesis and perhaps secretion of its constituents. Some of these constituents may be injurious to the tissues, e.g., elastase. The reciprocal reaction, macrophage-mediated or catalyzed activation of lymphocytes may also be operative in this phenomenon through lymphocyte-activating factors (Chapters 7 and 11). In addition, nonsensitized lymphocytes make up most of the accumulated cell population, and their localization may be related to a mitogenic factor (Chapter 9).

The most likely cause of the actual tissue damage would be soluble agents released from the participating cells. Candidates for these are lysosomal enzymes and cytotoxic factors from macrophages and toxic factors (lymphotoxin liberated from lymphocytes). Macrophage lysosomes contain the usual array of hydrolytic enzymes, and some of these can be released to the external environment during phagocytosis. Cytotoxic factors are released from lymphocytes *in vitro* when they react with antigen. The release from lymphocytes is fairly slow, taking 24 hours to yield appreciable levels. Moreover, injection of these supernatants into the skin produces a reaction that, to some extent, mimics the delayed hypersensitivity reaction (skin-reactive factor). The characteristic mononuclear cell infiltrate is, in this case, greatly enhanced and the reaction becomes intense within four to six hours. These recent observations support the idea that lymphocyte factors play some role in the lesion, although the actual tissue damage could still result from macrophage infiltration with release of harmful factors.

It will be clear from this brief consideration that the pathogenesis of delayed hypersensitivity is not fully understood and only now are techniques becoming available that may eventually answer this vitally important question.

CELL REACTIONS INVOLVED IN IMMUNOLOGIC INJURY

Damage to tissues by immunologic reactions *in vivo* involves a variety of cellular and humoral interactions. Study of these cells and their activities *in vitro* has increased our knowledge of their *in vivo* function and may ultimately yield the means to control the injurious processes while retaining those that are beneficial. In this section, reactions of the immunologically important cells will be described, together with their interaction with plasma mediation systems, such as the complement, coagulation, and kinin systems (biologic amplification systems). Some *in vitro* models of the delayed hypersensitivity phenomena that have gained prominence recently will also be considered.

MAST CELLS AND BASOPHILS

The main cell reservoirs of the vasoactive amines, particularly histamine, have been extensively studied because of their importance in immediate hypersensitivity reactions. In most species, histamine resides primarily in mast cells and basophils, but in the rabbit high levels are also found in platelets (Chapter 2). Many earlier experimental studies of anaphylaxis involved perfused or chopped sensitized lungs and measured the release of histamine and other pharmacologic mediators following challenges with antigen. More recently, histamine release from preparations of peritoneal mast cells (rat, mouse) or blood leukocytes containing basophils (man, rabbit) have provided a more defined system. However, the possibility of other sources of histamine and the relative importance of other mediators, such as serotonin, slow-reactive substance of anaphylaxis (SRS-A), kinins, and prostaglandins, must be taken into account.

Mast Cells

Some of the mechanisms that result in release of histamine from cells such as rat peritoneal mast cells are indicated in Figure 13–16. Probably the most important mechanism is that mediated by homocytotropic antibody, the analog in the rat of human IgE globulin. Mast cells may be actively sensitized with this type of antibody if they are taken from an animal producing the antibody *in vivo*. Alternatively, passive sensitization can be achieved by incubating the normal mast cells with homocytotropic antibody *in vitro*. Upon subsequent reaction of specific antigen with at least two IgE antibodies on the mast cell surface, the cell is stimulated to release its contained chemical mediators (Chapter 20).

MAST CELL

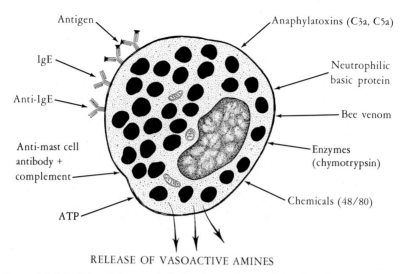

RELEASE OF VASOACTIVE AMINES

Figure 13–16. Stimuli that can induce release of vasoactive amines from mast cells.

Factors produced by immunologic reactions unrelated to mast cells may also induce release of histamine. Fixation of complement to antigen-antibody complexes results in the liberation of C3a and C5a (fragments of C3 and C5), which are known to have anaphylatoxin activity. These contract the guinea pig ileum, possibly by releasing histamine from mast cells within the gut fragment, and at least one of them (C3a) will cause isolated rat peritoneal mast cells to release histamine. A basic protein contained in neutrophil granules can act in a similar manner and cause degranulation of mast cells. Since this protein is liberated from neutrophils during their interaction with immune complexes, its participation in the increase of vascular permeability seen in neutrophil-mediated reactions must be considered. A synthetic material, compound 48/80, and certain bee and snake venoms have also been used in studies of mast cell reactions. They, too, induce release of histamine.

The complete mechanism of release is not yet understood. Stimulation of the mast cell membranes by these various agents activates cell enzymes (esterases), and, by a process that requires mast cell energy metabolism, histamine is released into the extracellular environment. Additional changes accompanying histamine release include a fall in intracellular cAMP paralleled by an increase in cGMP (Chapter 20A). The histamine is contained in characteristic mast cell granules, and, in some of these reactions, there is an overt extrusion of granules to the

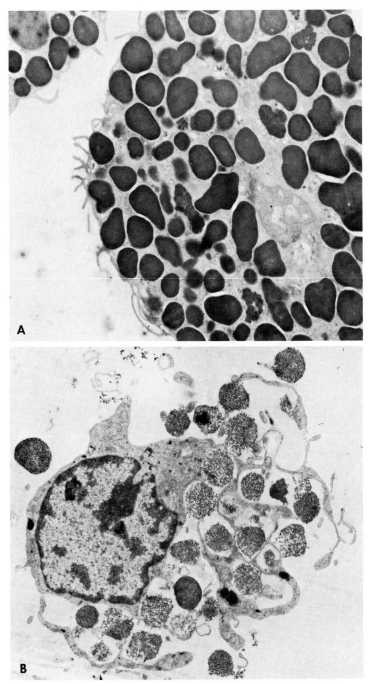

Figure 13–17. Degranulation of rat peritoneal mast cells. *A*, Electron photomicrograph of a control mast cell. Note dense granules filling the cytoplasm. ×9200. *B*, Cell treated with C3a anaphylatoxin (Chapter 6). The granules are being extruded from the cell and are apparently disintegrating. The cell itself is not lysed by this process. ×7500. (Courtesy of Dr. C. G. Cochrane.)

outside (Fig. 13–17). Interestingly, the cells are not killed and do not release potassium or the cytoplasmic enzyme lactic dehydrogenase. A completely different mechanism of release follows the reaction of anti-mast cell antibodies with mast cells in the presence of complement. This is a cytotoxic reaction and involves a breakdown of the cell with liberation of all its constituents.

Blood Leukocytes and Basophils

Blood leukocytes enriched in basophil content release histamine by reactions similar to those described for mast cells. These cells have been shown to contain IgE on their surfaces (approximately 20,000 to 80,000 molecues per cell) and will release their histamine if reacted with an antigen to which the individual is sensitive, e.g., ragweed. In addition, the reaction of anti-IgE with leukocytes from an atopic individual will release histamine. The stimulus to the cell membrane in both cases is probably the same and involves the participation of the cyclic nucleotide system (Chapters 7 and 20A). Basophils that are morphologically different from the tissue mast cells are also stimulated to secrete their content of vasoactive amines by C5a anaphylatoxin. Other mediators released from basophils (and mast cells) include SRS-A, ECF-A, a basophil kallikrein of anaphylaxis, and PAF. Recent studies have also concentrated on the control mechanisms that are operative on the secretion process, and a number of therapeutically effective drugs (e.g., isoproterenol, disodium cromoglycate) have been shown to inhibit particular steps in the secretory processes of mast cells and basophils. More precisely, β-adrenergic agents, e.g., isoproterenol, stimulate adenylate cyclase for increased cAMP accumulation; methylxanthines, e.g., theophylline, lead to an accumulation of cAMP by inhibiting the enzyme phosphodiesterase (Chapter 20A). Other agents, such as sodium cromolyn, seem to impair the influx of calcium, an ion necessary for mediator release.

Eosinophils

Eosinophilia is considered to be the "hallmark of the allergic disease," but the exact function of eosinophils in allergic reactions is yet to be fully understood. Tissue eosinophilia is marked at the sites where immunologic reactions involving reaginic antibodies occur. The initial blood eosinopenia accompanying acute anaphylaxis results from the migration of these cells to the tissue sites involved in the allergic inflammation where at least two chemotactic factors are released from reacting cells. These events are shown schematically in Figure 13–18. The first factor, ECF-A, generated from mediator cells, e.g., mast cells, during the allergic reaction, is involved in the unidirectional migration of eosinophils against a concentration gradient. Once at the reaction

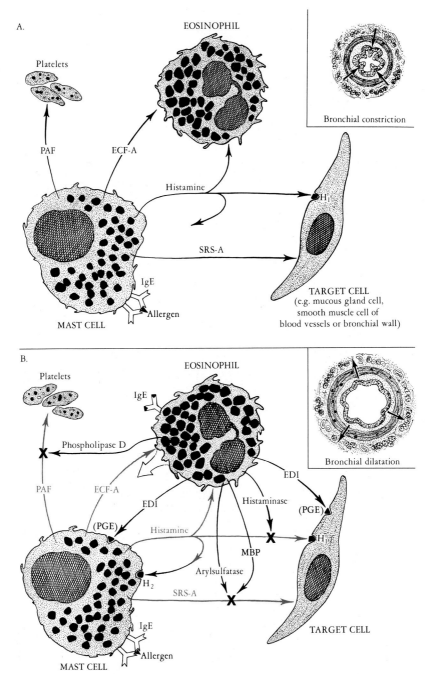

Figure 13–18. *A*, Schematic representation of the release of mediators from a mast cell and their effects on a target cell, causing bronchial constriction (insert) or on the eosinophil, causing movement, e.g., ECF-A. *B*, After the postulated interaction of eosinophil-bound IgE with antigen or the phagocytosis of antigen-antibody (IgE) complexes, the subsequent release of eosinophil-derived factors causes the neutralization or feedback inhibition of mediator release that results in a reversal of the target cell effect, e.g., bronchial dilatation (insert). (Adapted from Hubscher, T. T.: Ann. Allergy, *38*:83, 1977.)

sites, ECF-A deactivates and arrests the eosinophils from further outward migration. The second chemotactic factor is histamine, which has been shown to exert a selective chemotactic action on the eosinophils. The chemotactic activity of the histamine is concentration-dependent. At concentrations between 3×10^{-7} and 1.25×10^{-6} molar, for example, histamine is selectively chemotactic for eosinophils. Higher concentrations inactivate and inhibit eosinophil migration, effects similar to that observed for ECF-A. That the chemotactic activation of histamine is not inhibited by either H-1- or H-2-type antagonists suggests the existence of a different histamine receptor on the eosinophils.

A number of enzymes have been identified recently that are in and released by eosinophils that appear to affect the synthesis, the metabolism, or the release of specific mediators from mediator cells or that inactivate or destroy the mediators in extracellular fluids.

These enzymes include the following: a histaminase that destroys histamine, an arylsulfatase and a myelobasic protein (MBP) that detoxify SRS-A, a phospholipase D that inactivates PAF, and an eosinophil-derived inhibitor (EDI) that inhibits histamine release from mediator cells (Fig. 13–18). These *in vitro* findings, which have been observed in both the human and the experimental animal, have prompted the postulate that the eosinophil may be an important cell in the modulation of allergic inflammation. Although attractive, the theory will require further *in vivo* confirmation.

PLATELETS

The importance of the circulating platelets in hemostasis is well known; however, platelets also contain pharmacologic mediators that are involved in immunologic reactions. Rabbit platelets store large quantities of histamine and serotonin, and most of the histamine in the blood is found in these cells. Other platelet constituents that are potentially injurious include lysosomal enzymes, permeability factors unrelated to the vasoactive amines, epinephrine, and clotting factors.

Platelets may be involved in the deposition of circulating immune complexes in the rabbit by releasing vasoactive amines and thus increasing vascular permeability. Other permeability reactions may also result from the reactions of these cells. Aggregates of platelets and leukocytes are common findings in the blood vessels of patients with acute inflammatory reactions (e.g., Arthus reaction) and may also be seen in kidney homografts that are being rejected (Chapter 20B).

Release of Constituents from Platelets by Immune Complexes

A number of immunologic mechanisms for release of histamine from rabbit platelets are shown in Figure 13–19. Rabbit platelets have the property of adhering to immune complexes that have fixed complement through C3. This is prominently seen with particulate an-

PLATELET

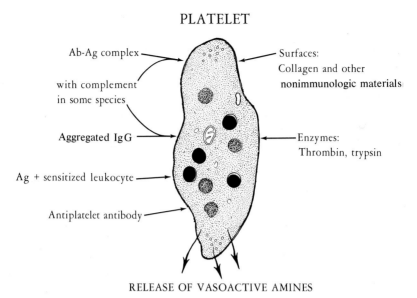

Ab-Ag complex

with complement
in some species

Aggregated IgG

Ag + sensitized leukocyte

Antiplatelet antibody

Surfaces:
Collagen and other
nonimmunologic materials

Enzymes:
Thrombin, trypsin

RELEASE OF VASOACTIVE AMINES

Figure 13–19.   Some stimuli that can induce release of vasoactive amines from platelets.

tigens. The ability to undergo C3 immune adherence is shared by neutrophils, eosinophils, and macrophages. Following adherence, the platelet may be stimulated to release histamine, serotonin, and nucleotides (ATP, ADP, and AMP). Since ADP is a potent platelet-aggregating agent, its release causes additional platelet clumping. Most of these reactions of platelets may thus be divided into two phases — an initial adherence and then aggregation that leads to an amplification of the effect by bringing more platelets into the reaction, i.e.:

Immune complexes → Adherence of platelets → Release of ADP →
Aggregation of more platelets

This effect is also true of reactions of platelets with nonimmune materials, such as collagen, or inert surfaces. The release of histamine from rabbit platelets following immune adherence may be augmented by the presence of neutrophils that can also react with immune complexes. It may be significant that *in vivo*, both cell types are often found together.

The vasoactive amines within the platelet are contained within specialized granules, distinct from the lysosomes. Their release requires platelet energy metabolism, platelet esterases, and environmental calcium. Since platelet lysis is minimal, an active release process is thought to be involved. It is of interest that the active release of substances from many different cell types appears to involve similar mechanisms, although the initiating events for release may be different.

Another reaction of rabbit platelets is with soluble immune complexes in antibody excess, with activation of the total complement sequence. This results in the complete lysis of platelets, the liberation of lysosomal and cytoplasmic enzymes, and the release of vasoactive amines and nucleotides. Immune adherence brings together platelets and complexes that have fixed complement up to the C3 stage. Then, the fixation of complement to complexes closely adherent to the platelet surface leads to lysis of the platelet. The platelet in this type of reaction has been termed an "innocent bystander."

In man, platelets cannot be shown to undergo C3 immune adherence. By contrast, in the human, erythrocytes can adhere to fixed C3b (Chapter 6). Platelets from other species, e.g., ruminants and pigs, also fail to react with C3; however, such platelets, including those from the human, will react with immune complexes, in this case adhering to the gamma globulin. Since the adherence results in the release of vasoactive amines (serotonin) and ADP, the end result is similar to that in the rabbit, although the mechanism is different. Allergy in man to certain drugs also involves platelets. Thus, drug reactions to quinidine and apronalide (Sedormid) sometimes result in thrombocytopenia. It has been suggested that antibody-drug complexes adhere to the platelets, which in the presence of complement result in platelet lysis by the innocent bystander mechanism. However, since only certain antigens (drugs) do this, another more likely possibility is that the Sedormid combines with the platelet surface, providing a new antigen with which specific antibody can react and cause cytolysis (Chapter 20A).

An Immunologic Reaction of Platelets Involving Basophilic Leukocytes

An interesting reaction of rabbit platelets that apparently does not involve complement or immune complexes has recently been described. Basophils from the blood of an immunized rabbit have IgE antibody on their surface, react with specific antigen, and then cause platelets to release their contained vasoactive amines. The action of the antigen on the sensitized cell probably induces the immediate release of the soluble factor PAF, which then stimulates an active, energy-requiring release of histamine and serotonin from platelets (Fig. 13–11). The reaction is of some interest because of its involvement in the deposition of immune complexes in immune complex disease and in IgE-mediated anaphylaxis in the rabbit. Recent evidence of similar reactions in man and rat has been presented.

NEUTROPHILS

Polymorphonuclear neutrophilic leukocytes have a number of properties that are important in the mediation of tissue damage. As described earlier, these typical inflammatory cells are essential for the pathogenesis of acute necrotic reactions, such as the Arthus reaction, vasculitis of immune-complex disease, severe glomerulonephitis of nephrotoxic nephritis, and many others. Neutrophils are also involved in inflammatory reactions of nonimmunologic origin and are instrumental in the defense of the body against bacterial infection (Chapter 15). The reactions of neutrophils that will be briefly described here are chemotaxis, adherence, phagocytosis, and the release of constituents (Fig. 13–20).

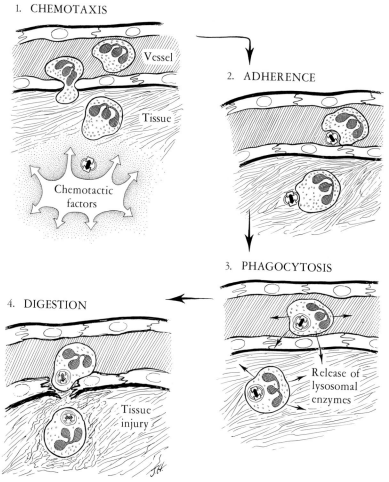

Figure 13–20. Sequence of reactions leading to tissue injury associated with PMN influx. Note that in addition to chemotaxis, adherence, phagocytosis, and digestion processes that normally result in particle inactivation, there may also be the release of neutrophilic constituents (lysosomal enzymes) that result in tissue injury.

Chemotaxis

For years it has been known that neutrophils migrate actively toward certain stimuli by a process referred to as chemotaxis (Fig. 13–20). This, of course, is a property of many phagocytic cells, including unicellular organisms such as amebae. The phenomenon in regard to neutrophils has recently been studied by a technique in which neutrophils migrate through a micropore filter with pores of a specified size toward a chemotactic stimulus (Chapters 2 and 26). Neutrophils are placed in an upper chamber, separated from the source of chemotactic factors by the micropore filter. The number of neutrophils that negotiate the narrow pores of the filter and emerge on the lower surface is an indication of the strength of the chemotactic stimulus.

Activation of the complement sequence by antigen-antibody complexes leads to the liberation of factors that are chemotactic to neutrophils (Chapter 6). The small fragments of C5 (C5a) and the activated trimolecular complex $\overline{C567}$ can cause neutrophils to migrate through the filter, when placed in the lower chamber. The cells move up the concentration gradient of the chemotactic factor, and the migration may be prevented if the factor is mixed with the neutrophils in the upper chamber.

The stimulus for chemotaxis apparently involves activation of a proesterase on the neutrophil surface and at least one other activated esterase. Neutrophil energy metabolism, primarily through glycolysis, is also a requirement for chemotaxis (Chapter 2).

When antibody combines with antigen in the tissues and the complex fixes complement, the chemotactic factors generated will diffuse away from the complex and set up concentration gradients. Neutrophils contacting the factors and stimulated by them can migrate toward their source until they reach the immune complexes. In the Arthus reaction, this accumulation takes but a few hours. A wide variety of bacteria also liberate a peptide during growth that is chemotactic for neutrophils and may account for the early accumulation of neutrophils at sites of local infection in the absence of an immunologic reaction. It is also of interest that tissue damage (e.g., infarction) can liberate proteolytic enzymes capable of splitting chemotactic fragments from complement components. Other chemotactic materials include a number of denatured proteins, small peptides containing formylated methionine, a factor derived from neutrophils themselves, and the important enzyme of the coagulation and kinin-forming systems, kallikrein.

Neutrophil Adherence

Neutrophils have the ability to adhere to antigen-antibody-complement complexes (Figs. 13–20 and 13–21). The reactions may be

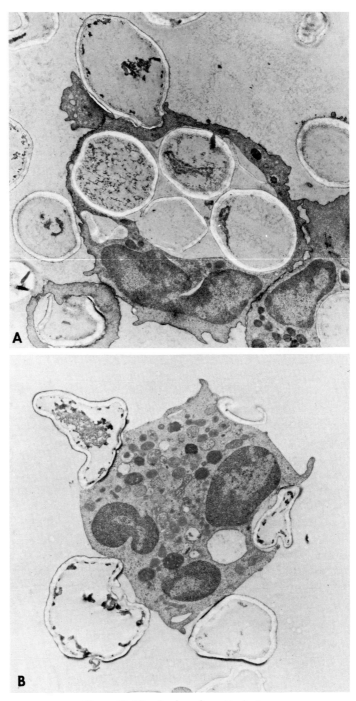

Figure 13-21. *See legend on opposite page.*

easily demonstrated by reacting antibody with particulate antigens, such as erythrocytes, and then observing the ability of the antibody-coated particle to bind to neutrophils. In this way it has been shown that neutrophils adhere to immunoglobulin either as specific antibody bound to antigen or to previously aggregated gamma globulin. This reactivity is dependent upon the presence of the Fc fragment of the immunoglobulin. Since this process results in phagocytosis of the complexes under suitable conditions, it represents one form of what was originally called opsonization.

Neutrophil adherence can also be induced by C3 fixation (Fig. 13–21*B*). This can be shown by using IgM antibody to erythrocytes in relatively low quantity and by fixing complement as far as the C3 step. Since a large number of C3 molecules are fixed for every antibody molecule, the C3 acts as an amplification of the adherence reactivity of the immune complex. The receptors on the neutrophil for the C3 adherence are different from those for gamma globulin. It is not known, however, what the relationship is between C3b receptors on the neutrophils, macrophages, platelets from some species, and primate erythrocytes.

Phagocytosis

Following adherence of the neutrophil surface to the immune complex, the cell is stimulated to phagocytose the complex (Fig. 13–20). An esterase in the cell is involved, energy metabolism is stimulated, and by an invagination process the complex is taken into the cell within a phagocytic vacuole (Chapter 2). The increase in the surface area of membrane produced by the presence of membrane-bounded vacuoles or phagosomes is provided by increased lipid synthesis.

Once inside the cell, the complex, bacteria, or other foreign material has to be degraded. The neutrophil contains at least two, and possibly three, types of granules, each bounded by a membrane and containing degradative enzymes separated from the cell cytoplasm. Following phagocytosis, the granule membranes fuse with those of the phagocytic vacuole and thus liberate the granule contents into the vacuole where they can digest the phagocytosed materials. The pH within the vacuole falls, probably because of the lactic acid production, and, since many of the granule enzymes work best in an acid medium,

---

Figure 13–21. Adherence and phagocytosis by rabbit neutrophils. *A*, Electron photomicrograph of a neutrophil that has phagocytosed zymosan particles (yeast cell walls) that have fixed complement. Four particles are seen within a large vacuole, and the cell is adherent to a fifth. Note the paucity of granules in the cytoplasm. × 7500. *B*, A similar cell adherent to zymosan particles with fixed complement. The cell's metabolic pathways have been inhibited to prevent ingestion of the particles and to demonstrate the adherence process. If the zymosan has no fixed complement, neither adherence nor phagocytosis occurs. × 9300.

conditions are ideal for the digestive process. By employing radiolabeled antibody in the phagocytosed immune complex, the degradation of proteins to small peptides in the neutrophil can easily be demonstrated. A variety of other reactions are also initiated in the neutrophil that are instrumental in the killing of phagocytosed bacteria, e.g., the generation of peroxide and superoxide, the release of bactericidal proteins, and the initiation of peroxidase-mediated bacterial halogenation. These events are described in detail in Chapter 2.

Release of Neutrophil Constituents

If all these neutrophil constituents were carefully contained within the phagocytic vacuoles it would be difficult to see how these cells could be responsible for the tissue damage attributed to them. There is a release, however, of constituents to the extracellular environment during the phagocytic process (Fig. 13–20). This can be shown *in vitro* by feeding immune complexes or particles coated with antibody or complement, or both, to neutrophils and measuring materials in the supernatant afterwards. There are many potentially harmful neutrophil constituents (Table 13–6). In recent studies, many of these have been shown to be released. Proteolytic enzymes (cathepsins, collagenase, elastase, and so forth) are of particular importance, since they could be instrumental in the damage to basement membranes and connective tissue.

Another group of materials released include basic protein materials of low molecular weight that have bactericidal activity and also induce increased vascular permeability. The production of SRS-A has been attributed to neutrophils and could contribute to the wealth of the pharmacologically active mediators mentioned. Likewise, kinins can be generated by neutrophil kininogenase. Neutrophil proteases can cleave

TABLE 13–6. Injurious Constituents of Neutrophils

Constituent	Activity
Proteases Collagenase Elastase	Hydrolysis of basement membranes, internal elastic laminae, and connective tissue
Basic proteins (3)	Increased vascular permeability
Basic protein (1)	Activation of mast cells, release of vasoactive amines
Slow-reactive substance(?)	Increased vascular permeability, contraction of smooth muscle
Kininogenase	Hydrolysis of kininogen with release of vasoactive kinin
Procoagulant activity	(?) Generation of fibrin, activation of platelets

C5 to generate C5a, which itself can stimulate neutrophil secretion, as well as functioning as a potent chemotactic agent. In addition, neutrophils contain substances that interact with the coagulation system and may initiate the fibrin deposition, which is a common consequence of neutrophil accumulation. Neutrophils also produce endogenous pryogen after phagocytosis and their involvement can lead to fever as well.

The mechanisms involved in the release processes are yet to be determined. It is of interest, however, that neutrophils adherent to immune reactants along a surface too large to be phagocytosed, such as is found along the glomerular basement membrane in nephrotoxic nephritis, will also release some of their lysosomal enzymes. Other contributions to severe tissue damage arise from neutrophil death and disintegration, possibly resulting from such factors as anoxia, lowered pH, and the large amounts of degradative enzymes present at a site of such severe inflammation. Finally, neutrophils contain a factor that is chemotactic for macrophages and that may be instrumental in the gradual change-over from neutrophils to mononuclear elements in, for example, an Arthus reaction.

MONOCYTES AND MACROPHAGES

Monocytes and macrophages (monocytes that have undergone the phagocytic process and thus have vacuoles and secondary lysosomes) are cells characteristic of delayed hypersensitivity. They are also found in many inflammatory reactions, particularly later in the course of the inflammation, i.e., after the neutrophil-dependent reaction.

Like neutrophils, these cells also respond to chemotactic stimuli *in vitro*. The factor in neutrophils chemotactic for macrophages has already been mentioned. Another such factor is produced by lymphocytes (as described below). C5a is also chemotactic for macrophages. Monocytes are phagocytic cells, and they will adhere to immune complexes, both to the fixed immunoglobulins and to the C3b. Following the adherence, phagocytosis, granule discharge into the phagocytic vacuole, and digestion of the complexes occur. Recent experiments also show liberation of lysosomal enzymes to the external medium. A difference from neutrophils is that macrophages are more versatile. They can actively synthesize and secrete new enzymes, make more granules, and can also undergo mitosis and divide.

The release of macrophage enzymes may play an important role in the tissue damage of delayed hypersensitivity, since in the reaction these are the cells that invade the tissues and are considered to be the chief mediators of delayed hypersensitivity reactions. Various *in vitro* models of delayed hypersensitivity involve the macrophage and use its migration, aggregation, or disappearance as end points. Factors released from lymphocytes (e.g., MIF) have been implicated in the retention of macrophages at a site of delayed hypersensitivity once they have arrived there.

The possibility that, after immunization, macrophages may gain the property of specifically reacting with antigen has long been controversial. This has been particularly evident with regard to bacteria as antigens, in which immunity to certain bacteria, such as those that multiply intracellularly (e.g., *Brucella*), has seemed to be associated with the increased killing by macrophages. It is now apparent that at least two phenomena have contributed to this controversy, which is by no means completely settled. One of these phenomena is that when an animal has experienced certain bacterial infections, such as tuberculosis, its reticuloendothelial system and macrophages appear more capable of destroying the tubercle bacillus; however, this heightened bactericidal response is not specific for the tubercle bacillus alone and applies to other nonrelated bacteria. This phenomenon can also be elicited by other factors, such as endotoxin. An "activated" macrophage is produced that exhibits a number of changes, including morphologic alterations, increased metabolism, increased secretion of enzymes, and increased ability to inhibit target cell growth. Although the factors responsible for macrophage activation, i.e., lymphokines, are quite specific in their action, the macrophage, once activated, exhibits many of its effects in a nonspecific way, e.g., phagocytic killing, inhibition and destruction of intracellular microorganisms, and destruction of tissue target cells, e.g., tumor cells (Chapters 14, 15 and 19).

The ability of certain types of antibody to adhere to macrophage membranes in a fashion that still allows them to react with antigen may

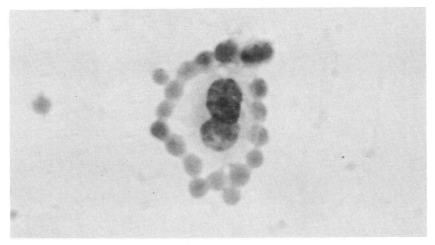

Figure 13–22. Macrophage cytophilic antibody. The mouse peritoneal macrophages have been preincubated with mouse cytophilic antibody against sheep erythrocytes. After the macrophages have been washed, sheep erythrocytes, reacting with antibody that has been bound to the cells, give the rosette appearance shown. Leishman stain. (Courtesy of Dr. I. R. Tizard.)

also be involved in macrophage-mediated protection against infection. This type of antibody has been termed cytophilic and requires its Fc fragment for the adherence. Macrophages can be passively sensitized with this type of antibody *in vitro*, washed, and then tested by addition of the antigen (e.g., erythrocytes) that will combine with the antibody and, in becoming thus attached to the cell, will yield a rosette appearance (Fig. 13–22). Under suitable conditions phagocytosis will follow.

The possible role of the macrophage in antigen uptake and processing has been described in Chapters 2 and 7.

LYMPHOCYTES

The lymphocyte is now regarded as the keystone of immunology. Upon reaction with specific antigen, B-cells can differentiate into plasma cells and produce antibody. This simplified statement, however, covers a multitude of steps, a number of which, at the moment, are purely hypothetical. These processes are described more fully in Chapters 2 and 7. The T-lymphocytes are also instrumental in the production of cell-mediated immunity or delayed hypersensitivity (Chapter 9). It is thought that this type of cell reacts with antigen by means of a receptor on its surface. The nature of the receptor is not known, but its great specificity argues for an antibody-like molecule incorporated into or on the cell membrane (Chapter 7). Knowledge of the importance of the specifically sensitized lymphocyte in the mediation of delayed hypersensitivity comes from cell transfer studies. The consequences of its reaction with antigen in the tissue include macrophage emigration, further lymphocyte accumulation, and tissue injury. A number of *in vitro* studies of lymphocytes have revealed properties that may be involved in these processes.

Release of Lymphocyte Factors

It has recently become apparent that lymphocytes can also release a battery of materials, the lymphokines, when they react with antigen *in*

TABLE 13–7.   Factors (Lymphokines) Released from Lymphocytes

Macrophage migration inhibition factor (MIF)
Macrophage aggregation factor (MAF)
Macrophage-spreading inhibitory factor
Factors chemotactic for macrophages and PMN's
Mitogenic factor
Lymphotoxin
Inhibitors of proliferation, DNA synthesis, and so forth
Skin reactive factor
Interferon
(Lymph node permeability factor)

vitro (Chapter 9). Although not fully characterized, these effector molecules of relatively low molecular weight are thought to represent the *in vitro* correlates of delayed hypersensitivity (cell-mediated) reactions *in vivo*. A list of some of these factors is shown in Table 13–7. Their known physical and biologic properties are given in Chapter 9 (Table 9–3).

Direct Cytotoxic Activity of Lymphocytes

The reaction of cellular elements with target cells has been described in Chapter 9 and is composed of a heterogeneous set of reactions involving many subclasses of lymphocytes, e.g., killer (K-) and natural killer (NK-) cells, and reactions mediated by macrophages. The reaction of sensitized T-lymphocytes with target cells bearing foreign antigens may lead to direct cytotoxic effects of the lymphocytes. The first step in this reaction involves the clustering of lymphocytes around target cells after which killing occurs by mechanisms that involve close contact between these cells. It is not yet clear whether locally produced cytotoxic factors might be causing the cell death. Nonsensitized lymphocytes may be induced to kill target cells by nonspecific mitogens, e.g., phytohemagglutinin, that bring the lymphocyte and target cells together and may also activate the lymphocytes to release lymphokines. Consequently, contact appears to play an important role in lymphocyte cytotoxicity.

This phenomenon of T-cell cytotoxicity may be distinguished from two other forms of lymphocyte-mediated cytotoxicity (Chapter 9): (1) T-lymphocytes that produce soluble cytotoxic factors, e.g., lymphotoxin, and (2) a subpopulation of lymphocytes that has not yet been fully identified—the killer or K-lymphocytes that react with antibody on a target cell and kill the cell in the so-called antibody-dependent cellular cytotoxic (ADCC) reactions. As mentioned previously, macrophages can also exhibit cytotoxic properties, as can neutrophils, under certain circumstances, particularly when the target cells are coated with antibody.

HUMORAL SYSTEMS

Three major systems that do not require cells may also contribute to immunologic injury. Complement is the one most closely involved and has been discussed in Chapter 6. However, a brief mention of the coagulation and kinin systems will serve to indicate how cells and humoral factors may interact.

Fibrin formation is an extremely common finding in reactions mediated by neutrophils, although it is not completely clear how the activation occurs. Of interest in this respect is that neutrophils and monocytes have some procoagulant activity themselves.

In addition to the primary role of B-cells in elaborating antibody that can facilitate these reactions, B-cells also have C3b and IgG receptors (Chapter 7) and thus can react with immune complexes. Recent experiments have demonstrated the release of chemotactic factors from such B-cells so that they may participate directly in the inflammatory process, as well as indirectly by the production of antibody.

Kinins are small peptides with very potent pharmacologic activities that result in lowered blood pressure and increased vascular permeability. They are formed as an end result of a sequence of enzymatic steps in the plasma similar to those found in the complement and coagulation systems. Hageman factor, the first component of the intrinsic coagulation pathway, initiates the sequence, and antigen-antibody complexes may activate the plasma kinin system. Neutrophils also contain enzymes capable of interacting with the sequence, and these are known to be released during phagocytosis of antigen-antibody complexes. Activated macrophages secrete plasminogen activator, activation of which initiates the fibrinolytic system leading to the generation of biologically active fragments of fibrinogen and fibrin.

SUMMARY

Immunologic tissue injury may result from four main types of reaction. (1) Reaction of antigen with certain types of homocytotropic antibody fixed to mast cells and basophils results in the release of some of the pharmacologic mediators of immediate hypersensitivity reactions (Type I reaction). (2) Humoral antibody can initiate damage either by reacting with tissue antigens directly (Type II reaction) or (3) as a result of the inflammatory properties of antigen-antibody complexes (Type III reaction). The damage is generally a consequence of cellular interaction with the complexes, and the neutrophil is the cell most clearly implicated. (4) In delayed hypersensitivity, the recognition of antigen occurs at the cellular level, and the small T-lymphocyte appears responsible (Type IV reaction). Tissue damage results from an accumulation of lymphocytes and macrophages at the site of antigen localization, but the exact mechanism involved remains to be elucidated.

SUGGESTIONS FOR FURTHER READING

Austen, K. F., and Orange, R. P.: Bronchial asthma: The possible role of chemical mediators of immediate hypersensitivity in the pathogenesis of subacute chronic disease. Am. Rev. Resp. Dis., *112*:423, 1975.

Becker, E. L., and Austen, K. F. (eds.): Second International Symposium on Biochemistry of the Acute Allergic Reactions. Oxford, Blackwell Scientific Publications, 1971.

Becker, E. L., and Henson, P. M.: In vitro studies of immunologically induced secretion of mediators from cells, and related phenomena. Adv. Immunol., *17*:93, 1973.

Cerrottini, J-C., and Brunner, K. T.: Cell-mediated cytotoxicity, allograft rejection and tumor rejection. Adv. Immunol., *18*:67, 1974.

Cochrane, C. G.: Immunologic tissue injury mediated by neutrophilic leukocytes. Adv. Immunol., *9*:97, 1967.

Cochrane, C. G., and Koffler, D.: Immune complex diseases in experimental animals and man. Adv. Immunol., *16*:186, 1972.

David, J. R.: Lymphocyte mediators and cellular hypersensitivity. N. Engl. J. Med., *288*: 143, 1973.

Hubscher, T. T.: Immune and biochemical mechanisms in the allergic disease of the upper respiratory tract; role of antibodies, target cells, mediators and eosinophils. Ann. Allergy, *38*:83, 1977.

Rocklin, R. E.: Clinical applications of in vitro lymphocyte tests. Prog. Clin. Immunol., *2*: 21, 1974.

Weissmann, G. (ed.): Mediators of Inflammation. New York, Plenum Publishing Corp., 1974.

Part 2

PROTECTIVE MECHANISMS INVOLVED IN THE IMMUNE RESPONSE TO INFECTIOUS AGENTS

Chapter 14

HOST-PARASITE RELATIONSHIPS

Joseph A. Bellanti, M.D.

Two factors are implicit in the term host-parasite relationship: (1) the properties of the infecting microorganisms, and (2) the host's total response to the infecting agents. The eventual outcome of the host-parasite struggle will be the net result of the interaction of both.

Immunity is a condition that exists in the host, not in the parasite. The immunity with which the host responds may be influenced by an alteration of the microorganism or deleterious changes in the environment that predispose the host to parasitic invasion. Changes in age, nutrition, environmental pollution, and underlying disease processes, for example, may have profound effects on the host-parasite relationship. Thus, the host-parasite relationship must be viewed from the standpoint of the host, the parasite, and the environment in which the interaction occurs.

DEFINITIONS

Infections versus Infectious Disease

The process of *colonization* of organisms in or on the host is termed *infection*. An infection may or may not result in an illness; e.g., the colonization of the intestinal flora of the newborn is an infection. The term *infectious disease* refers to the signs and symptoms of frank illness caused by the infection of tissues normally free of significant numbers of organisms.

Pathogenicity versus Virulence; Opportunistic Infections

Microbes that are usually incapable of penetrating natural defenses and therefore normally fail to produce disease are referred to as *non-pathogenic* organisms. Conversely, those that are capable of overwhelming these defenses and producing disease are termed *pathogenic*. Some microbes are so highly pathogenic that whenever they infect they are capable of producing disease; these are referred to as *virulent* organisms. From a practical point of view, the terms pathogenic and virulent are often used synonymously. It is becoming increasingly apparent, however, that many microorganisms that are not ordinarily considered pathogenic or virulent may, under certain circumstances, become so when the immunologic capacity of the host is impaired. These infections are referred to as *opportunistic infections* (e.g., candidiasis) and are assuming increasing clinical importance as the number of patients with compromised defense mechanisms continues to increase. Shown in Table 14–1 are some examples of opportunistic infections and their predisposing factors. Virulence thus represents the interaction between the properties of the host and the pathogen that permits expression of the pathogenic properties of a parasite to the detriment of the host.

TABLE 14–1.   Opportunistic Infections in Patients with Compromised Defense Mechanisms

Agents	Predisposing Factor	Mechanism
Staphylococcus epidermidis, *Escherichia coli*	Indwelling catheter or prosthesis	Foreign body
Staphylococcus aureus, *Pseudomonas aeruginosa*	Extensive burns	Breach in body perimeter, diminished cell-mediated immunity (?)
Cytomegalovirus, *Pneumocystis carinii*	Allograft recipients, patients with malignant disease receiving chemotherapy	Diminished cell-mediated immunity
Candida albicans	Newborn	Diminished cell-mediated immunity, (?) diminished macrophage function
Streptococcus (Diplococcus) *pneumoniae,* *Salmonella paratyphi*	Absence or malfunction of the spleen (splenectomy, sickle cell anemia)	Diminished IgM (opsonic) antibody synthesis, diminished clearance

Organotropism

Organotropism refers to the high degree of selectivity of infection for certain tissues that organisms display. For example, certain viruses are neurotropic and infect primarily the central nervous system, e.g., rabies. Other viruses have a predilection for the respiratory tract, e.g., influenza. The mechanism for tropism is poorly understood but may be explained by metabolic requirements of certain organisms, the protective characteristics that certain tissues afford, or the availability of essential receptor sites on host cells.

Patterns of Disease: Clinical, Subclinical, or Latent Infections

Infectious disease may be considered a state in which an infection has become sufficiently active to involve normally uninfected tissues, thus giving rise to signs and symptoms of the illness. There are conditions, however, in which infection is present but not sufficiently active to give rise to recognizable signs and symptoms. These types of infection are referred to as *inapparent* or *subclinical infections.* Inapparent or subclinical infections are exemplified by viral illnesses such as type A hepatitis, rubella, and mumps. In such cases, infection may be so mild that it does not give rise to recognizable signs or symptoms of disease. An alternative explanation for infection being only subclinical is a preexistent immunity in the host. For example, the passive administration of gamma globulin to individuals exposed to type A hepatitis will prevent the overt clinical disease as manifested by an absence of jaundice, but may not prevent a subclinical infection, shown by a characteristic rise in serum liver enzymes. Subclinical infections are of great medical importance, since they may induce immunity without the overt morbidity of the disease. Furthermore, they may pose a problem for the physician by obfuscating the problems associated with the disease. For example, administration of gamma globulin to a pregnant female exposed to rubella may convert a clinical case of rubella to a subclinical case. In this instance, a viremia may still occur, with spread to the unborn fetus and resultant production of the congenital rubella syndrome in the absence of overt clinical disease in the mother.

A special case of subclinical infection is the *carrier state.* This refers to the excretion of an organism, ordinarily considered to be a pathogen, following recovery from a clinical disease. For example, a patient recovering from streptococcal pharyngotonsillitis may excrete the organism for several weeks after recovery. In the case of typhoid fever, most individuals stop excreting the organism in the stool by two months, but some continue to excrete the organism for many years and are therefore contagious. These individuals are referred to as typhoid carriers and are important reservoirs of infection.

Latent infections are persistent inapparent infections in which the presence of the microbe cannot readily be detected by any of the methods currently available. This type of infection is known to flare up from time to time under various conditions. Herpes labialis (cold sores) caused by herpes hominis (simplex) viruses is a good example of a latent-type infection that may be exacerbated by such factors as excessive sunlight, menstruation, stress, or infection. During the interim, the virus cannot be readily detected. Recent evidence suggests that a diminution of specific cell-mediated immunity may be associated with exacerbations of these latent infections.

Communicability

Communicability refers to the ease with which an infection is transmitted from one individual to another. Although communicability may be exhibited by nonpathogenic organisms, it is a prerequisite for the important pathogenic organisms of man.

The efficiency of transmission depends upon four factors: (1) an adequate source, (2) a large enough inoculum, (3) a method of survival for the organism in transit, and (4) a susceptible host (Fig. 14–1).

The communicability of a disease is an important consideration for the physician. It provides both a basis for the containment of disease and a rationale for vaccine prophylaxis. In the case of rubella, for example, the concern is largely with the individual's immunity; in the case of poliomyelitis, the production of population immunity (herd immunity) is of greater importance.

It should be emphasized that the hands of medical-care personnel

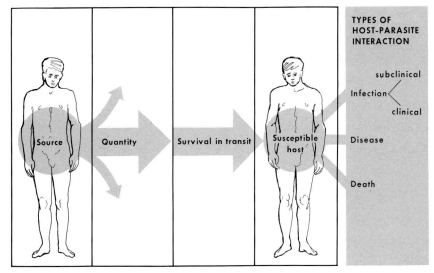

Figure 14–1. Requirements for parasitism.

remain an important vehicle for the transmission of infectious diseases. Ironically, hand washing represents the best and most often neglected preventive measure in the control of infectious diseases. Recently, intimate forms of contact such as kissing and sexual intercourse have been recognized as important vehicles for the transmission of a wide variety of infectious agents, e.g., EB virus and herpes hominis viruses (Chapter 16).

PROPERTIES OF THE PARASITE

MODES OF INFECTION

Generally speaking, the pathogenic microorganisms that give rise to disease may be divided into two groups: (1) the *extracellular parasites* and (2) the *intracellular parasites* (Table 14–2). This arbitrary classification is based upon the site of replication of the organism relative to certain cellular elements of the immune system, e.g., phagocytes.

The *extracellular parasites* are those that establish infection by replicating outside of phagocytic cells and that generally produce an acute, fulminating type of infection of relatively short duration. These organisms are, for the most part, bacteria, such as the staphylococcus and the streptococcus. For destruction of these organisms, phagocytosis, particularly by the polymorphonuclear leukocytes, followed by intracellular killing is a critical event. The subsequent production of opsonizing antibody together with complement may enhance these processes.

The second group of parasites are those that establish an *intracellular* domicile within phagocytes (Table 14–2). These can be subdivided further into: (1) the *facultative intracellular parasites* and (2) the *obligate intracellular parasites*. The facultative intracellular parasites are those organisms that, although readily taken up by phagocytic cells, particularly the macrophages, are relatively resistant to subsequent intracellular

TABLE 14–2.   Classification of Pathogenic Microorganisms

TYPE	CHARACTERISTICS	EXAMPLE OF CAUSATIVE ORGANISM
Extracellular parasites	Acute, fulminating, of short duration	*Staphylococcus aureus*
Intracellular parasites		
Facultative intracellular	Chronic, taken up by phagocytes but not killed	*Mycobacterium tuberculosis* *Histoplasma capsulatum* *Toxoplasma gondii*
Obligative intracellular	Chronic, require intracellular parasitism for their replication	*Mycobacterium leprae* *Rickettsia rickettsiae* viruses

digestion. These organisms include many bacteria (e.g., *Mycobacterium tuberculosis*), fungi (*Histoplasma capsulatum*), and protozoa (e.g., *Toxoplasma gondii*) that establish chronic infections. Once these organisms have been phagocytosed, the macrophage shows a heightened metabolic state with increased reactivity, not only toward the infecting organism but also against nonrelated organisms and tumor cells. Knowledge of this heightened state of macrophage activity, "cellular immunity," toward tumor cells has been utilized in cancer immunotherapy, e.g., use of BCG (Chapter 10).

The obligate intracellular organisms are those that show an absolute requirement for intracellular parasitism for their replication. These include some bacteria (e.g., *Mycobacterium leprae*), rickettsiae, (e.g., *Rickettsia ricksettsii*), chlamydia (e.g., *Chlamydia psittaci*), and all viruses. Many of these organisms show a tropism for cells of the reticuloendothelial system, and cellular immunity and cell-mediated immunity (delayed hypersensitivity) are prominent features of these interactions.

A third type of interaction representative of certain viruses, including the oncogenic viruses, leads to the incorporation of part of the viral genome with host nucleic acid. These segments encode for the production of proteins or fully infectious viral particles. The oncogenic viruses are believed to play a role in the malignant transformation (Chapter 19). Cell-mediated immunity is also a prominent feature of these complex interactions.

VIRULENCE

The basic mechanisms through which pathogens cause disease are the following (1) attachment to and penetration of epithelial surfaces, (2) invasiveness of tissues, (3) production of toxic materials (toxins), and (4) capacity for genetic alteration.

Attachment to Epithelial Cells

In order for a microorganism to establish infection it must first breach the primary line of defense provided by the intact skin and mucous membranes and become attached to an epithelial surface such as the skin, respiratory tract, gastrointestinal tract, the genitourinary tract, or the eye. These sites have primary importance as attachment sites for most pathogenic organisms. There are a number of mechanisms by which organisms have been shown to attach to these epithelial cells. These include certain surface proteins of a bacterium, e.g., M protein of *Streptococcus pyogenes*, or certain structures, e.g., pili (fimbriae) of *Neisseria gonorrhoeae* and *Shigella*. Other organisms such as the *Streptococcus mutans* elaborate certain products, e.g., glucans and fructans, which can attach to the enamel surface of teeth and have been implicated in the causation of dental caries. Following attachment, the organism can either replicate locally and produce localized infection or penetrate the epithelial cell with systemic spread and produce more generalized disease.

There are a number of host factors that are directed against this phase of host virulence. The integrity of the body perimeter, e.g., skin and mucous membranes, can protect against attachment. The normal microbial flora and the acidity of the gastrointestinal tract may also prevent attachment of these organisms. The defense provided by local IgA immunoglobulins in restricting the spread of organisms in the respiratory tract, gastrointestinal tract, and possibly the genitourinary tract may provide a highly efficient localized type of defense (Chapter 5). The mechanisms by which secretory IgA functions are not entirely clear but several possibilities exist: (1) direct neutralization, (2) direct lysis of organisms, (3) their opsonic effect, or (4) the direct coating of mucosal cells, preventing surface attachment.

Invasiveness

Following the encounter of a pathogen with a susceptible host, invasiveness is a requirement for the production of disease. The factors that contribute to virulence vary with different organisms. In the case of acute bacterial infections, these factors consist of the elaboration of *capsules* and the production of *enzymes* that facilitate invasion.

Encapsulated microorganisms, such as *Streptococcus (Diplococcus) pneumoniae* and *Haemophilus influenzae,* and also certain fungi are protected from the effects of phagocytosis. In contrast, unencapsulated organisms are readily phagocytosed. The mechanism for this phenomenon is not well understood but may be due to the inability of binding at the capsule-phagocytic interface owing to characteristics related to hydrophobicity and surface tension properties of the capsule. Of interest is the finding that when the capsule is removed or when the organism is treated with specific antibody (opsonins), the organisms are rendered susceptible to phagocytosis and subsequent intracellular digestion.

A number of bacteria elaborate enzymes that may enhance their invasive properties. For example, certain of the gram-positive bacteria produce hyaluronidase, which is capable of hydrolyzing the hyaluronic acid material of the ground substance of cells, and this may be important as a "spreading factor." Coagulases, which clot plasma, are produced by staphylococci; streptokinases, which catalyze the lysis of fibrin, are produced by certain strains of streptococci. Clostridia and anaerobic gas-producing organisms elaborate collagenases, which destroy the collagen matrix of muscle and are believed to be important in the spread of these organisms. Illustrative enzymes, their actions, and their bacterial sources are listed in Table 14–3. Other enzymes elab-

TABLE 14–3. Examples of Enzymes Elaborated by Microorganisms Contributing to Virulence

ENZYME	BACTERIA	ACTION	POTENTIAL EFFECT
Hyaluronidase	Gram-positive (e.g., *Streptococcus pyogenes*)	Depolymerizes hyaluronic acid	"Spreading factor"
Coagulases	Gram-positive (e.g., *Staphylococcus aureus*)	Clots plasma	Builds up a fibrin network
Streptokinase	Gram-positive (e.g., *Streptococcus pyogenes*)	Lyses fibrin	Allows the streptococci to spread
Collagenases	Gram-positive (e.g., *Clostridium perfringens*)	Destroys collagen	Allows proliferation of the clostridia with production of gas gangrene
Hemolysins	Gram-positive (e.g., *Streptococcus pyogenes*)	Lyses red blood cells	Anemia

orated by pathogens play a detrimental role for the host, such as the hemolysins, which can cause transient hemolytic anemias in patients with infectious disease. Paradoxically, certain enzymes produced by microorganisms may facilitate their own destruction. For example, children with the inborn deficiency of neutrophils, chronic granulomatous disease, are predisposed to infections with peroxide-negative organisms (Chapter 22). Bacteria deficient in catalase (peroxide-positive) appear to provide bacterial sources of peroxide, replacing the defect found in these leukocytes.

Toxin Production

Once the organism has successfully invaded the host, toxic materials may be elaborated by the organism. There are two types: (1) exotoxins and (2) endotoxins.

Exotoxins are proteins elaborated by bacteria as extracellular products that have the capacity of acting as cell poisons. Examples of exotoxins are the diphtheria and the tetanus toxins. *Endotoxins* are composed of a lipid-polysaccharide complex.

The biologic effects of exotoxins are of clinical importance. Exotoxin activities are revealed by such diverse effects as cytotoxic effects, inhibition of protein synthesis (diphtheria toxin), interference with neuronal transmission (botulinus toxin), and transport of ions and water across cell membranes (possible mechanism of cholera toxin). Exotoxins do not induce an inflammatory response, although the organisms that produce them are phlogistic (inflammation-producing). Exotoxins are soluble proteins that bind to tissue and, once bound, cannot be neutralized readily by circulating antibody. These proteins are capable of producing an antibody response (antitoxin). Moreover, they can be altered (denatured) to form substances that retain their immunogenicity but lose their toxicity. These denatured forms of toxins are referred to as *toxoids* and are important sources for bacterial vaccines (Chapter 23). Antitoxin may be assayed by *in vitro* techniques, e.g., toxin neutralization, or by *in vivo* techniques, e.g., Schick and Dick tests (Chapter 8).

The biologic effects of endotoxins are equally important. Their toxicity resides in the phospholipid fraction and their immunogenicity in the polysaccharide fraction. When used in large quantity, endotoxin produces the biologic effects of shock, fever, leukopenia, hyperglycemia, and intravascular coagulation. They are also capable of eliciting the Sanarelli-Shwartzman reaction.

If two small subcutaneous doses of endotoxin are given 24 hours apart, the second injection results in a localized vasculitis and a hemorrhagic necrosis (localized Shwartzman reaction); however, if the injections are given intravenously, the animal dies within 24 hours and bilateral cortical necrosis of the kidneys is seen (generalized Shwartzman reaction).

The clinical counterpart of this phenomenon is seen in septicemias due to gram-negative organisms such as the meningococcus and in the hemolytic-uremic syndrome. Autopsy findings show similar bilateral cortical necrosis of the adrenals or kidneys, respectively. Disseminated intravascular coagulation, seen in many overwhelming septicemias, is also believed to be related to effects of endotoxin. The presence of minute quantities of endotoxin in body fluids may be detected by the Limulus lysate assay.

Capacity for Genetic Change

A factor that contributes to the maintenance of the virulence of an organism in a population is the ability of certain pathogens to undergo mutation periodically. The influenza virus represents the pathogen *par excellence* that manifests this phenomenon and has caused the most frequent epidemics. Influenza can be maintained in nature only within a susceptible population. Following an epidemic, a population that has developed immunity to any given serotype is no longer susceptible. Many variants of influenza, e.g., A2 Victoria, are known to occur, however, and these are responsible for new waves of epidemics, since the population is again susceptible. Similar mutations among other pathogens permit maintenance of virulent strains in nature.

One genetic relationship of potential importance for future vaccine development is the recognition that certain organisms show cross-reacting antigens. For example, asymptomatic carriage of *Escherichia coli* K100 leads to the production of a protective antibody to *Haemophilus influenzae* type b. Similarly, the K1 antigen of *E. coli,* an important pathogen of the newborn, has been shown to cross-react with the capsular polysaccharide of the meningococcus.

PROPERTIES OF THE HOST

From the vantage point of the physician, the protective mechanism of the host involves his ability to maintain *homeostasis.* This homeostasis or immunologic balance must be as variable as the mechanisms expressed by the organisms that establish the infections. The homeostasis of man's immunologic system is different from that seen in other metabolic processes of the body, however. In the latter, e.g., normoglycemia, the maintenance of blood sugar is achieved through complex metabolic processes that regulate the quantity of one product, sugar. In the case of the immune response, one type of parasitic invasion affects many immune mechanisms that involve the interplay between a variety of cell types and a multitude of structurally unrelated products differing in quantity and function (heterogeneity). The pathogens against which the immunologic surveillance is directed are constantly undergoing changes in virulence. These changes therefore must be countered swiftly and efficiently by the recognition system of the host so as to reinstate immunologic homeostasis, or balance.

The physician must evaluate the many factors that affect the responses of the host to infectious agents. These include age, genetic predisposition to infection, nutrition, the psychological state of the host, and the environment (Chapter 1).

AGE

The maturation of man, from fetal life to senescence, is accompanied by a corresponding development of the immunologic responses. With regard to the protective mechanisms against infecting agents, the fetus is a unique host. It is now recognized that the fetus is not immunologically incompetent; it is immunologically pristine. If the fetus is exposed to an infectious agent *in utero,* it is capable of a limited but specific immunologic response. Specific antibody synthesis to agents such as those that produce toxoplasmosis, rubella, cytomegalovirus, herpes, and syphilis (TORCHS syndrome) have all been demonstrated early in gestation. All immunoglobulins can be synthesized as early as the twelfth week of fetal life; however, the mature lymphoid tissues are not fully developed and, as a result, the full expression of cell-mediated immunity is not optimal in the fetus and neonate. Consequently, convalescence from infections, recovery from which is dependent upon this mechanism, e.g., infections of cytomegalovirus or rubella virus, may be delayed and lead to devastating effects in the infant. These infants are known to excrete virus for prolonged periods of time after birth and become silent reservoirs of virus, capable of infecting susceptible individuals.

The polymorphonuclear responses are likewise less efficient in the newborn and young infant. Passive transfer of IgG-associated antibodies to many viruses and bacteria occurs, so that the infant is protected from many of the common pathogenic organisms; however, there is no transfer of IgM-associated antibodies, such as those to the gram-negative bacteria. These findings may explain in part the well-known susceptibility of the newborn infant to infection with gram-negative organisms. In older infancy and childhood the spectrum of disease changes. With a changing maturation, additional immunologic responses are available to the older child. The susceptibility to gram-negative enteric organisms disappears after the first month of life. This is associated with the increased synthesis of IgM immunoglobulin. Concomitant with the disappearance of maternal IgG immunoglobulin during the first six months of life, there is a susceptibility to infection with organisms such as the *Haemophilus influenzae, Streptococcus (Diplococcus) pneumoniae,* and beta hemolytic streptococci and other common respiratory viruses.

It has been suggested by several workers that the presence of this passively acquired IgG-associated antibody may at times be harmful to the host. It has been considered that bronchiolitis in the young infant may be due in part to the viral antigen-antibody complexes formed during the course of viral infection. The complexes, formed between the maternally derived antibody and viral antigen within the respiratory tract, may contribute to immunologic injury of the lungs during bronchiolitis. Alternatively, the cell-mediated immunity and IgE antibody have been suggested to participate in the pathogenesis of the bronchiolitis syndrome. The changing spectrum of infection with age is seen with other organisms, such as the group A beta hemolytic streptococci (streptococcosis). In the newborn infant, group A streptococcal infection may be restricted to the skin; in children two to three years old, it may be restricted to the nasopharynx; and in the five- to six-year-old child, the classic pharyngotonsillitis is seen. Another possible factor contributing to localized infection seen in the developing child is the delayed development of the IgA immunoglobulins, which do not assume adult capability until adolescence (Chapter 3).

Within a wide range of normality, the mature adult expresses full immunologic competence that is due to previous immunizing exposure to an immense variety of infectious and noninfectious stimuli. As a consequence, re-exposure to a previously encountered pathogen usually results in an anamnestic stimulation of the immunologic response with minimal or no sequelae.

Finally, in later adult life, reinfection occurs in spite of prior infection. For example, herpes zoster is known to occur in patients who have recovered from varicella infection. In fact it has been stated that "whooping cough is a disease of infants and grandmothers." It has been reported that there is a measurable diminution in serum gamma globulins in persons over the age of 50. Finally, the increase in autoimmunity and malignancy known to occur in the elderly may reflect a waning immunity or an increase in errors of the immunologic mechanisms.

GENETIC PREDISPOSITION TO INFECTION

Several genetic factors affect host susceptibility to infection in man and other species. The defects may or may not involve the immunologic system. Recently, a relationship has been demonstrated between histocompatibility types and susceptibility to certain infectious diseases (Chapter 3).

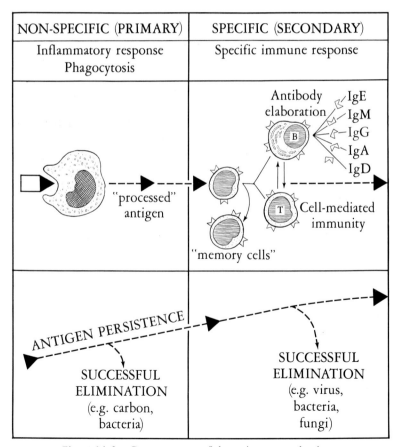

Figure 14–2. Compartments of the resistance mechanisms.

Within the immunologic defects, there are two compartments of resistance: those concerned with nonspecific immune responses and those concerned with specific immune responses (Fig. 14–2). The genetic predisposition to infection in a normal population is expressed by the wide variations in both types of resistance mechanisms. The extreme aberrations of this variation are best exemplified in the immune deficiency diseases (Chapter 22).

The genetic defects unrelated to the immune response that affect the susceptibility or resistance to infection include such entities as sickle cell anemia, glucose-6-phosphate dehydrogenase deficiency, and many hemoglobinopathies. In areas of the world where malaria is endemic, individuals who possess these defects have less severe malaria than individuals without these defects. In the case of sickle cell disease, the homozygote is at a disadvantage from the primary disease. Individuals with the sickle cell trait, however, appear to have a survival advantage when living in malaria-infested areas; the trait confers a disadvantage in nonmalarious areas and in adverse environments, e.g., high altitudes. Thus, environmental differences can affect the expression of a single hereditary factor in infectious disease susceptibility. Another aspect is that of the deficiency of pneumococcal opsonins, which have been demonstrated in individuals with sickle cell disease.

Genetic susceptibility, correlated with racial factors and sex factors, is seen in the increased incidence of tuberculosis in nonwhites. Furthermore, a greater proportion of male infants than female infants is known to be victims of serious bacterial infections.

Thus, genetic susceptibility to infectious disease appears to be under the control of many genes (polygenic). The effect of defects in specific immunologic and nonimmunologic systems and the role of the environment must be evaluated in the total expression of genetic predisposition to infection.

NUTRITION

The nutritional status of the host plays an important role in the prevalence and severity of infectious diseases, particularly among those suffering from nutritional deficiency. Although malnutrition does not depress antibody formation or phagocytosis in the adult, such a nutritional deficit can lead to a profound deficiency in cell-mediated reactivity in the developing infant and child. For example, in patients with marasmus and kwashiorkor there is a high susceptibility to viral, bacterial, and parasitic diseases as a consequence of protein malnutrition.

Malnutrition may also interfere with recovery from infectious diseases. For example, the walling-off processes initiated by an infecting agent require the synthesis of fibrin, polysaccharides, and collagen. During malnutrition, these responses are retarded because of an inadequate intake of essential precursors, including protein. The rate of healing of wounds, for example, is markedly retarded by dietary deficiencies.

PSYCHOLOGIC STATUS OF THE HOST

The psychologic status of the patient with infectious disease can markedly affect the course of the disease. In those diseases that are not readily treated by antibiotic therapy, the psychologic state of the host assumes a major factor in the recovery of the individual. In addition, the effect of stress in such disease states can be associated with a more prolonged convalescent course through physiologic alterations. For example, in recruits in basic training who are known to be susceptible to acute respiratory disease (ARD), hormonal levels of 17-hydroxy-corticosteroid increase markedly during the early weeks of basic training. The timing of this event coincides with the period of increased susceptibility to many of the ARD agents.

PREGNANCY

Pregnancy represents a special category of an altered metabolic state. Pregnant women are more prone to certain infections than nonpregnant women for a variety of causes, including anatomic and metabolic ones. For example, the compression of ureters with obstruction due to fetal positioning predisposes the patient to urinary tract infections. The reasons for the susceptibility to other infectious diseases, e.g., influenza and poliomyelitis, are not apparent. Recently, a diminution in cell-mediated immunity has been demonstrated during pregnancy that provides yet another basis for susceptibility to certain infectious diseases, e.g., viral diseases, during this period. The precise basis for this transient diminution is unknown, but several hormones, e.g., α fetoprotein, human gonadotropin, and progesterone, have been shown to exert an immunosuppressive effect on lymphocytes.

ENVIRONMENT OF THE HOST AND PARASITE

The host-parasite relationship is influenced directly by the external environment. In the case of the parasite, the environment affects the type of parasite, its rate of mutation, its geographic distribution, and its transmissibility. Man-made alterations in the external environment result in a disturbed ecologic balance in the natural flora and fauna; for example, the widespread use of fertilizers and insecticides produces changes in parasitic forms and the clustering of disease-causing parasites. In addition to this, the artificial and rather complete dissemination of parasites occurs in our modern world through modern transportation. Thus, one can easily see the potential for widespread epidemics of disease, e.g., smallpox and influenza. The indiscriminate use of antibiotics has added to the problems, because of the development of antibiotic-resistant strains of bacteria that present a very real therapeutic difficulty for the physician. Thus, the physician should be aware of these and other variables that can affect the host-parasite relationship in his patients.

The external environment of the host affects the host-parasite relationship to disadvantage, either by self-administered toxic substances such as drugs, alcohol, tobacco impurities, or a deficient diet (e.g., malnutrition) or from substances imposed upon him such as pollutants, insecticides, food additives, and toxic substances used in certain manufacturing industries.

Alterations of the external environment clearly affect both the host and the parasite. Thus, the physician is faced with expressions of disease that may take unexpected form or emerge as a new disease entity because of altered form and condition of the parasite.

SUMMARY

The host-parasite relationship represents the overall interplay between the factors controlling the changing virulence of an organism and the immense variability of the host's surveillance system, which must swiftly and efficiently counteract in order to maintain immunologic balance (homeostasis). The many factors that influence the host-parasite relationship include the age, genetic predisposition, nutrition, metabolic state, and psychologic state of the host, as well as the environment in which the host-parasite relationship occurs.

SUGGESTIONS FOR FURTHER READING

Davis, B. D., Dulbecco, R., Eisen, H. A., Ginsberg, H. S., and Wood, W. B., Jr.: Microbiology, 2nd ed. New York, Harper & Row, Publishers, 1973.
Mudd, S.: Infectious Agents and Host Reactions. Philadelphia, W. B. Saunders Company, 1970.

Chapter 15

MECHANISMS OF IMMUNITY TO BACTERIAL DISEASES

Joseph A. Bellanti, M.D.

Bacterial infections in man best illustrate the mechanisms involved in the host-parasite relationship, the outcome of which is determined by the genetic endowment of the host and the genetic capability of the bacteria. It has been firmly established that bacteria possess an extreme degree of variability owing to such factors as mutation, metabolic alterations induced by a changing environment, lysogenization with bacteriophage, production of toxins, and capability for prolonged survival (sporulation). Such complex responses from the bacterial pathogen are met with equally complex and diverse immune responses in man.

The field of immunology is a direct outgrowth of the study of host responses to bacterial infection, and, in fact, the early successes of bacteriology are the foundations upon which modern immunology rests. *Immunoprophylaxis*, the prevention of disease by vaccines, and *immunotherapy*, the prevention and treatment of disease through the use of immune sera or gamma globulin, are the tools of the physician in assisting the patient (i.e., the host) to enhance the natural immune responses to bacteria and other pathogens (Chapters 23 and 24).

In the early days of bacteriology, research emphasis was on humoral factors. This restriction of interest was due to a primary concern with the protective role of serum antibody, particularly as related to antitoxic immunity. It is now known, however, that cellular responses are also involved in the immune responses to bacteria and these play perhaps the most critical and decisive role in certain host-parasite interactions. Thus, immunity to bacterial diseases must include a very broad biologic view, encompassing the vast interplay of humoral and cellular factors that compose the total immunologic responses of the host.

CLASSIFICATION OF BACTERIAL INFECTIONS

Three broad categories of bacterial infections are recognized: (1) the *acute* or highly productive type of infection; (2) the *chronic* type, exhibiting the capacity of certain bacteria, e.g., intracellular parasites,

370

TABLE 15–1. Classification of Bacterial Infections

		IMMUNITY MECHANISMS				
		Nonspecific		_Specific_		
				Antibody		
TYPE	EXAMPLES	HISTOPATHOLOGY	Phagocytosis	Inflammatory Response	Serum	Local	Cell-mediated
Acute							
Localized	Staphylococcal abscess, streptococcal pharyngitis	Polymorphonuclear leukocytes ("abscess")	+	+	+	?	?
Generalized	Meningococcemia	Varied	+	+	+	0	?
Chronic	Tuberculosis, leprosy, brucellosis	Macrophage ("granuloma")	+	+	0	0	+
Toxigenic	Diphtheria, tetanus, cholera	Exotoxin – none	0	0	+	+	0
		Endotoxin – varied	?	0 to +	?	?	0

to establish intracellular parasitism (Chapter 14); and (3) the *toxigenic* or *toxin-producing* type of infection, usually seen in acute infections (Table 15–1).

ACUTE

The first type of infection is exemplified by bacteria, e.g., *Staphylococcus* or *Streptococcus*, that may gain access to the body through any of the natural portals of entry, including the gastrointestinal tract, the respiratory tract, or skin lesions. The bacteria may undergo a limited replication and cause a localized lesion, which may be accompanied by abscess formation (a collection of polymorphonuclear leukocytes). Some bacteria are effectively killed by polymorphonuclear leukocytes; others require the presence of antibody (opsonins) and complement (Chapters 5 and 6). If host defense mechanisms are sufficient to contain this pyogenic (pus-forming) response locally, resolution and healing will occur. If, on the other hand, host defense mechanisms are insufficient to restrain these bacteria locally, the infection could spread regionally or gain access into the systemic circulation, causing a fulminating sepsis. Other organs may be "seeded" as a result of the latter process. These organisms causing acute infection may be completely disposed of or may enter into chronic infection.

CHRONIC

The second type of bacteria-host interaction is that characterized by a protracted or chronic course of infection, in which bacteria enter into a mutualism with the host (Table 15–1). These types of infection are caused by such organisms as *Mycobacterium tuberculosis*, *Mycobacterium leprae*, and the *Brucellae* and may be protracted over long periods of time. Such infections establish a delicate balance with the host and evoke an inflammatory response characterized by macrophage and lymphoid accumulation with granuloma formation (Chapter 12). The infections are characterized by the intracellular residence of organisms within phagocytes (macrophages) for extended periods of time. An example of chronic infection of significance to the physician is the carrier state, which represents a specialized example of inapparent infection (Chapter 14). In this state, an infection exists (e.g., staphylococcus nasal carrier) in the absence of overt disease; hence, the pathogen is not deleterious to the host but can be transmitted to susceptible individuals. A carrier state can be seen as a further manifestation of acute infections such as typhoid fever and streptococcal and meningococcal infections. The mechanism for this phenomenon is unknown.

TOXIGENIC

A third type of bacteria-host interaction involves production of toxin, after a limited replication of the bacterium. The toxin may be one of two types: endotoxin or exotoxin (Chapter 14). The effects of exotoxin account for many of the consequences resulting from diseases such as the myocarditis of diphtheria and the paralysis of tetanus. Exotoxins may be elaborated after only limited bacterial replication but may have wide distribution through the circulation and exert highly specific effects. In general, the tissue response to exotoxins is minimal, while the response to endotoxin may be more prominent and include a variety of vascular changes and effects on the hematopoietic system (Chapter 14).

Thus, the antibacterial mechanisms of host defense vary according to the nature of the bacterial infection (Table 15–1). The relative roles of nonspecific factors (e.g., phagocytosis and the inflammatory response) and specific factors (e.g., antibody and cell-mediated events) will vary according to the nature of the infection.

ANTIBACTERIAL IMMUNITY MECHANISMS OF THE HOST

Antibacterial immunity mechanisms operative in man are directly influenced by the environment in which he lives. There are certain predisposing physical and emotional conditions that may alter the expression of the immune response. Noteworthy are the occupational hazards (e.g., pneumoconiosis, pollutants, drugs, chemical additives, and insecticides) that may overtax the immune response. Alcohol, for example, directly depresses the functional and metabolic activities of phagocytes, e.g., chemotaxis and microbicidal activities. In addition, malnutrition is known to adversely affect the immune response to bacterial agents.

Many bacteria found on the body surfaces are in a state of balance with the host and are restricted to superficial sites of the body. If these bacteria gain access to deeper tissues, symptoms and signs of disease will result. Thus, the defense function of the lymphoreticular tissues must be active in order to restrict these bacteria and maintain a state of health.

The mechanisms involved in a primary or immediate encounter of the host with a bacterial pathogen are termed *nonspecific immunologic mechanisms;* those involved in encounters subsequent to the primary encounter are the *specific immunologic responses.* It should be noted that both processes are stimulated in all infections and the expressions will vary.

NONSPECIFIC FACTORS

The intact skin and mucous membranes offer a mechanical barrier against invasion by bacteria. When the integrity of the skin is broken, e.g., because of burns or eczema, bacterial skin infections (pyoderma) may result. These infections are most often associated with organisms that normally colonize the skin, e.g., *Staphylococcus aureus.* Similarly, the well-known secondary staphylococcal pneumonia that occurs following influenza may be explained, in part, by loss of respiratory epithelium, which is a sequela of the viral infection and offers entry to the *Staphylococcus aureus.* There may also be direct effects of viral infection on the activity of phagocytes, which may be incriminated in staphylococcal pneumonia.

There are several other nonspecific factors important in antibacterial defense. The gastric juice, because of its acidity, may destroy many types of bacteria, whereas certain pathogenic bacteria, such as *Salmonella typhosa,* may survive this acid medium and produce gastrointestinal or systemic infections. Humoral factors important in antibacterial defense include the unsaturated fatty acids of the skin, which kill many surface bacteria. Also, lysozyme, an enzyme found in tears, saliva, and nasal secretions, is capable of degrading the mucopeptide layer of cell walls of many bacteria. This appears to be an important nonspecific defense mechanism of the host, which cleanses the normal mucous membranes of the upper respiratory passages.

Microbial antagonism is a factor important in maintaining an ecologic balance of microorganisms on the body surface. The balance may be upset by disease or by treatment. For example, the overgrowth of pathogenic *Staphylococcus aureus* following the use of the broad-spectrum antibiotics is an example of the type of interaction in which homeostasis is altered.

Phagocytosis and the Inflammatory Response

If bacteria overcome the initial barriers, primitive responses of the host are stimulated, i.e., phagocytosis and the inflammatory response (Chapters 2 and 12). After invading deeper tissues, bacteria may be engulfed by wandering tissue macrophages (histiocytes), a random encounter that is not an efficient process (Fig. 15–1). More commonly, the organisms undergo limited replication and then trigger the inflammatory response with mobilization and emigration of neutrophils toward the infection site (Fig. 15–1). These cellular elements confront the microorganisms and, in the case of many acute pyogenic infections, the microorganisms are engulfed and digested efficiently. The capsules of some bacteria, e.g., pneumococcus, resist phagocytosis and contribute to increased pathogenicity; however, with the subsequent development of antibody (opsonin), the bacteria are coated and phagocytosis is facilitated (Fig. 15–4). The familiar abscess or furuncle, which is a collection of polymorphonuclear leukocytes, is an example of this type of phagocytic mechanism important in antibacterial defense. In addition, a number of other factors are triggered by the inflammatory response, such as activation of the complement sequence and the coagulation sys-

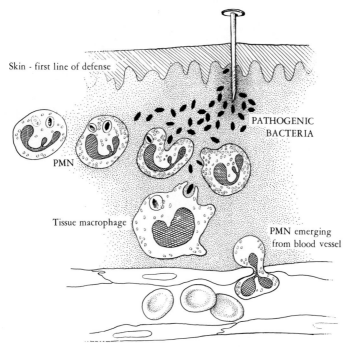

Figure 15–1. Schematic representation of phagocytosis by polymorphonuclear leukocytes (PMN) and tissue macrophages following penetration of the skin and introduction of pathogenic bacteria into deeper tissues. The PMN's are more efficient in phagocytosis than the macrophages. Note that the PMN's are mobilized into tissues from blood vessels during the inflammatory response.

tem, with deposition of fibrin. These factors may also facilitate phagocytosis and the repair processes.

If bacteria are not successfully killed at the local sites, they may continue to replicate locally or further invade the host by way of the lymphatics to the regional lymph nodes (Fig. 15–2). The well-known "red streaks" that extend up the arm (lymphangitis) with enlarged epitrochlear or axillary lymph nodes are examples of this response. Within lymph nodes, the bacteria encounter elements of the phagocytic system (macrophages) that may be prerequisite for the initiation of specific immune responses (Fig. 15–3). Those organisms escaping phagocytosis may initiate an acute inflammatory response within the lymph node (lymphadenitis).

Bacteria may overcome the lymphatic-associated barriers and gain access directly into the bloodstream. Here they come into contact with circulating phagocytes (polymorphonuclear leukocytes and monocytes) or they may reach organs such as the liver and the spleen where they can interact with fixed phagocytic elements. Enlargement of the spleen (splenomegaly) is an important clinical finding in sepsis and reflects this

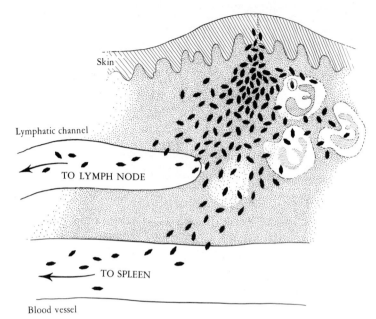

Figure 15-2. Schematic representation of the cellular events occurring if the PMN leukocytes are unsuccessful in killing the bacteria. The organisms are shown replicating in the tissues and entering a lymphatic channel and a blood vessel.

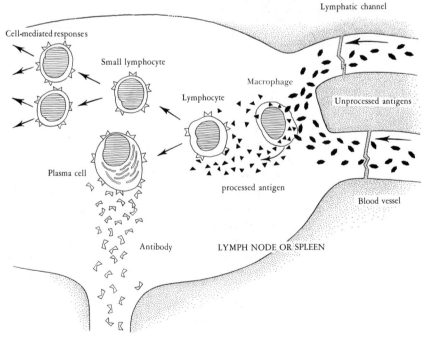

Figure 15-3. Schematic representation of the induction of a specific immune response in a lymph node or the spleen with elaboration of cell-mediated (delayed hypersensitivity) responses and antibody.

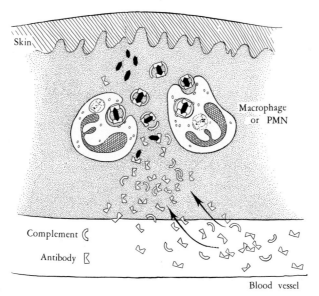

Skin

Macrophage
or PMN

Complement

Antibody

Blood vessel

Figure 15–4. Schematic representation of the enhancement of phagocytosis, occurring with the development of specific antibody, together with the participation of complement.

increased phagocytic function. Although a powerful defense system of the host, the final reticuloendothelial barrier may also be overcome with seeding of such organs as the bone (osteomyelitis), the brain (brain abscess), or the kidney (renal abscess), terminating in fatal septicemia. Thus, the first encounter of the host with a bacterial pathogen of the acute pyogenic type summons elements of the nonspecific defense system, with participation by the products of the specific immune system that may interact in bodily defense.

SPECIFIC ANTIBACTERIAL MECHANISMS

During the course of bacterial infection or immunization, elements of the specific immune response are activated via cells of the lymphoid tissues. Involvement of the following may occur: regional lymph nodes, in the case of localized infection (skin); specialized lymphoid nodules lining the respiratory, gastrointestinal, and genitourinary tracts, in the case of organisms that infect at these sites; or the spleen, in the case of organisms invading the bloodstream. Although all elements of the specific immune response may be activated in every type of infection, the relative roles vary with the type of invading organism. In the case of highly productive acute types of infection, antibody, primarily of the IgG variety, is stimulated. Certain bacteria, however, such as the gram-negative enteric bacteria, stimulate antibody that is primarily of the IgM class. Furthermore, in certain types of localized infections, particularly those of the respiratory and gastrointestinal tracts, there is evidence that local IgA antibody synthesis occurs. For example, in the case of cholera, local IgA antibody is produced within the gastrointestinal tract (coproantibody) that appears to be an important antibacterial mechanism at mucosal surfaces, as described below.

Antibody

The host response to infection by bacteria or to immunization leads to a sequential appearance of specific antibodies. The antibody appearing initially is usually of the high molecular weight IgM variety and is followed by IgG antibody. These differences, in order of appearance, however, may be laboratory artifacts and may reflect sensitivity of the antibody-detecting system. There is now evidence that on a molar basis, IgM antibodies have greater relative opsonizing, bactericidal, and agglutinating abilities than IgG; the IgG antibodies, on the other hand, possess greater relative precipitating abilities (Chapter 8).

From an operational standpoint, each of these antibodies seems to be well suited to perform specific functions. For example, IgM antibody, which is formed early in the immune response, appears to function best as an opsonin, facilitating and cooperating with the phagocytic events described earlier. Additionally, this class of antibody can immobilize bacteria by agglutination or, in the case of gram-negative bacteria, can lyse cell walls in the presence of complement (Chapters 5 and 6). Further, since IgM antibody is confined largely to the vascular compartment, it seems to be uniquely well suited to perform its function within the blood vascular system. IgG antibody, on the other hand, appears to diffuse quite readily between vascular and extravascular compartments. These IgG antibodies, which show good precipitating capacity, are effective in neutralizing toxins that might be found both in blood and the tissues. The IgA antibody in secretions appears to have a number of novel features that make it well suited to function at body surfaces. The secretory IgA antibody, with its additional secretory component, is endowed with a unique stability, allowing it to function within the milieu in which other immunoglobulins would be degraded, e.g., the gastrointestinal tract (Chapter 5). These IgA mucosal antibodies, therefore, appear to be an important "first line of defense" in body secretions.

Upon subsequent encounter between a host and a bacterial pathogen, there occurs a secondary or anamnestic response that results in elaboration of antibody in an enhanced fashion, i.e., markedly increased quantity. This rapid "recall" of immunity terminates the infection quite rapidly. There are infections, however, the nature of which makes them insusceptible to these host defenses. These include infections such as abscesses or other chronic infections that by their nature prevent the ready access of antibody into areas of infection.

Cell-Mediated Immunity (Delayed Hypersensitivity)

Those bacterial infections that overcome the nonspecific factors of the host induce a tissue response that is characterized by the production of cell-mediated events (delayed hypersensitivity). The reactivity is induced during a primary encounter with a bacterial pathogen and is seen in all subsequent encounters with the same pathogen. Although this response occurs in all bacterial infections, it is most prominent in infections of the chronic type, e.g., intracellular infection. The presence of reactivity is also useful in the diagnosis of certain chronic infections, e.g., tuberculosis.

In certain chronic infections, e.g., leprosy, a state of anergy is seen in which there is a loss of delayed hypersensitivity skin testing. The diminished reactivity is proportional to the progression of disease. A loss of primary bacterial delayed hypersensitivity is also seen when there are concurrent infections such as measles. These findings indicate a possible explanation for the aggravation effect of concurrent viral infection on the course of a pre-existing bacterial infection. For example, influenza is known to exacerbate an old quiescent tuberculosis into an active form.

INTERRELATIONSHIPS BETWEEN THE COMPARTMENTS OF THE IMMUNE RESPONSE DURING THE PATHOGENESIS OF BACTERIAL INFECTIONS

The compartments of the immunologic system work in concert so that, when the primitive defense mechanisms of the host have been surmounted and the specific immunologic responses are stimulated, the products of the latter will enhance the former (Fig. 15–4). In stimulating the specific immune response, the resultant production of opsonins and simultaneous stimulation of cell-mediated events (delayed hypersensitivity) result in products that can enhance phagocytosis by macrophages or polymorphonuclear (PMN) leukocytes (Chapters 8 and 9). Both responses are stimulated in all infections. It must be emphasized that although there is a predominant expression of one or the other mechanism, depending upon the type of infection, there is a quantitative relationship between the mechanism expressed and the infective characteristics of the pathogen. The three types of bacterial infection in man exemplify these relationships: (1) the acute bacterial infection, (2) the chronic infection, and (3) the toxigenic infection.

ACUTE INFECTION

In Figure 15–5 it can be seen that in an acute infection a nonencapsulated organism will be readily phagocytosed. In contrast, in the

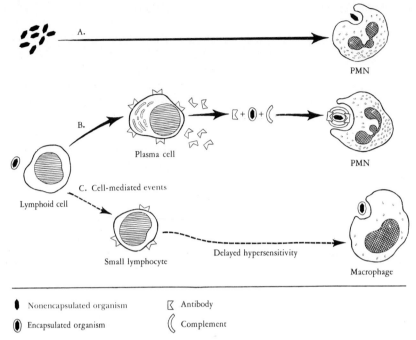

Figure 15–5. Schematic representation of relative roles of antibody and cell-mediated events in enhancement of phagocytosis in *acute* bacterial infections. *A*, Phagocytosis of an unencapsulated organism through an unenhanced process; *B*, the enhanced process of phagocytosis through antibody and complement; and *C*, the relatively lesser importance of cell-mediated events during acute infection. Note the interrelationship of antibody and phagocytosis by PMN leukocytes and its relatively greater importance than cell-mediated events during acute infections.

case of the encapsulated organism following the subsequent production of antibody (opsonins) and the initiation of the complement cascade, phagocytosis by PMN leukocytes will be greatly enhanced. Simultaneously, there is stimulation of cell-mediated immunity, which enhances phagocytosis by macrophages. Since such organisms are not regularly phagocytosed by macrophages, this scheme normally appears to be of relatively lesser importance (Fig. 15–5).

However, in clinical situations in which the PMN leukocytes are deficient, as in the newborn or in CGD (chronic granulomatous disease), a prominent but low-efficiency macrophage interaction is seen, indicating that this mechanism can be utilized (Chapter 22).

CHRONIC INFECTION

The chronic type of infection is best exemplified by tuberculosis in man (Fig. 15–6). In the initial encounter between tubercle bacillus and polymorphonuclear leukocytes, a paradoxical situation arises. This cell can ingest the organism but cannot degrade the lipid capsule. Thus the invading microorganism has an advantage, since transport is provided to deeper tissues along with nutriment for necessary life processes and protection from the extracellular effects of antibody. The short-lived cells (PMN) provide only a limited period of intracellular parasitism, however. The major cellular response in the infection is subsequent phagocytosis by macrophages, in which the organisms survive for an even longer period of time. In addition, upon ingestion, there is a simultaneous stimulation of cell-mediated events (delayed hypersensitivity), with the elaboration of products such as the macrophage inhibitory factor (MIF) and chemotactic factors (Chapters 9 and 13) (Fig. 15–6) that can further enhance the activity of macrophages. If these pathogens remain viable, further response of the host is manifested through granuloma formation, which serves to wall off or localize the infected area. Any breakdown in bodily defense, such as concurrent viral infection, is known to permit dissemination of the tubercle bacillus with exacerbation of the disease. Some individuals can terminate infection successfully during macrophage phagocytosis and show no granuloma formation. Evidence indicates that termination of intracellular parasitism is coincident with the development of increased macrophage efficiency ("activated macrophages"), which seems to be under the control of the effector molecules released from sensitized lymphocytes, e.g., MIF. Such increased efficiency also confers an increased ability of the macrophage to kill nonrelated organisms.

Of importance in the host-parasite relationship is the recognition that the expressions of certain bacterial diseases may reflect the relative

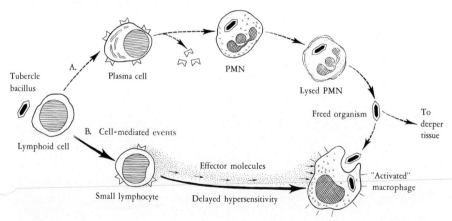

Figure 15–6. Schematic representation of relative roles of antibody and cell-mediated events in enhancement of phagocytosis during *chronic* bacterial infections. *A* shows limited activity of the polymorphonuclear leukocytes and *B*, the major cellular response in chronic infection, carried out through macrophages with simultaneous stimulation of cell-mediated events, further enhancing immunity. Note the interrelationship between the cell-mediated immunity effector molecules with phagocytosis by macrophages and its relatively greater importance than antibody enhanced phagocytosis by PMN leukocytes in chronic infection.

status of cell-mediated immunity. For example, in lepromatous leprosy, a diminution of cell-mediated immunity is known to exist, whereas in the tuberculid form a heightened cell-mediated immunity is found.

TOXIGENIC INFECTION

A third type of bacterial infection involves toxin production (Fig. 15–7). Exotoxins are proteins elaborated as extracellular products of microorganisms. The extracellular metabolites may be produced in toxic quantities after even minimal infection of the host or may be produced outside the host and enter via ingestion, e.g., botulism. The prime defense of the host against toxins is through neutralization by production of specific antibody (antitoxin). This detoxification process leads to the production of toxin-antitoxin complexes that are usually removed by phagocytic degradation (Fig. 15–7). However, under conditions of antigen excess, these complexes can be injurious to the host (Chapter 13) and lead to IMD (immunologically mediated disease) (Chapter 20). The endotoxins exhibit a more generalized effect on the host, including pyrogen release by polymorphonuclear leukocytes re-

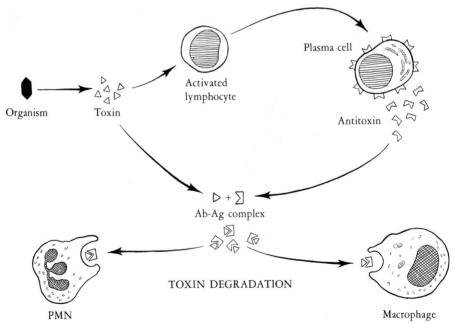

Figure 15–7. Schematic representation of the immunologic mechanism of toxin neutralization by antibody. The neutralized toxin-antitoxin complexes are shown being taken up and degraded within both types of phagocytic cells.

sulting in fever, leukopenia by destruction of PMN leukocytes, and the initiation of the coagulation sequence resulting in intravascular coagulation and sometimes shock (Chapter 14). Obviously, the host is placed at great risk, since many of these effects, e.g., leukopenia, lead to impaired phagocytic defense. In addition, although they are formed against endotoxins, antibodies do not appear to be as protective as those against exotoxins. Furthermore, the mechanisms of response to endotoxins appear to be as varied as the generalized effect of the endotoxins themselves.

IMMUNOLOGIC INJURY SECONDARY TO BACTERIAL INFECTION

If the response of the host to any of the types of microorganisms is inappropriate, inadequate, or aberrant, the pathogen is placed at distinct advantage with respect to the host. Factors altering host responsiveness, such as age, pre-existing disease, nutrition, and concurrent infections, obviously will have a significant effect on the outcome of the host-bacteria interaction.

When the host response is aberrant, products of the immune response may result in immunologically mediated tissue injury (Chapters 13 and 20). For example, following group A beta hemolytic streptococcal infection, rheumatic heart disease can result, presumably through cross-reactions of cardiac tissue with the organism (Chapter 20). Similarly, acute glomerulonephritis may occur following infection with these organisms owing to injury mediated by antigen-antibody complexes. The physician must be aware of these potential tertiary manifestations of the immune response when assessing the course of a bacterial infection.

SUMMARY

The immune mechanisms displayed by the host in bacterial defense are best viewed according to the type of host-parasite interaction — *acute, chronic,* or *toxigenic* types of infection. Bacterial pathogens as a group evoke in the host all the known types of immune effector mechanisms. Some of the processes are poorly understood, and others are completely unknown. In general, the participation of both nonspecific and specific immune mechanisms occurs in all bacterial infections in man. The relative roles of each, however, vary with the type of infection. At times, the products of the immune response can be harmful and are manifested as immunologically mediated diseases of man.

SUGGESTIONS FOR FURTHER READING

Davis, B. D., Dulbecco, R., Eisen, H. A., Ginsberg, H. S., and Wood, W. B., Jr.: Microbiology. 2nd ed., New York, Harper & Row, Publishers, 1973.

Mackaness, G. B., and Blanden, R. V.: Cellular immunity. Progr. Allergy, *11*:89, 1967.

Mudd, S.: Infectious Agents and Host Reactions. Philadelphia, W. B. Saunders Company, 1970.

Suter, E., and Ramseier, H.: Cellular reactions in infection. Adv. Immunol., *4*:117, 1964.

MECHANISMS OF IMMUNITY TO VIRAL DISEASES

Joseph A. Bellanti, M.D.

Viruses are a unique class of infectious agents that are obligate intracellular parasites. They differ from all other types of microorganisms in their organization, composition, and mechanism of replication. A complete viral particle, or virion, may be regarded as a basic block of genetic material, consisting of either DNA or RNA and surrounded by a protective coat of protein that may also serve as a vehicle for its transmission from one host cell to another. In addition, some viruses have lipid in an outside envelope that is derived from the host cell (Fig. 16–1). The increased awareness during the past 50 years of the prevalence of viruses and their frequency as etiologic agents of human infectious diseases has stimulated widespread interst in their pathogenicity and immunogenicity. The spectrum of diseases produced ranges from acute viral infections, in which the interaction of virus and host immune response leads to virus clearing and immunity or dissemination, infection, and death, to more chronic forms of viral infection, in which a prolonged viral replication, in concert with the immune response, may lead to tissue injury and result in disease. Moreover, the

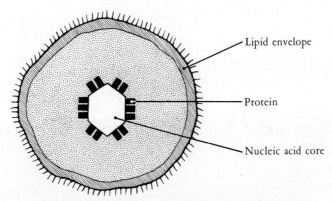

Figure 16–1. Schematic representation of a viral particle.

385

discovery of an association between viruses and tumors has initiated areas of intensive research (Chapter 19).

The eradication of many of the viral infections has been made possible through the use of effective vaccines that stimulate the specific immunologic responses (Chapter 23). Other types of agents that stimulate other components of the immunologic system, e.g., immunopotentiators (Chapter 10), may soon be available for therapy. Thus, it is important for the student of medicine to have a fundamental grasp of the immunologic mechanisms involved in viral immunity. A knowledge of these mechanisms is also essential for a clear understanding of some atypical responses seen in patients during viral infection, or after immunization.

CLASSIFICATION OF VIRAL INFECTIONS

The outcome of an encounter between a virus and an appropriate host cell will depend upon the properties of the *virus*, the *cell*, and the *environment* in which the virus–host cell interaction occurs. In general, the properties of the virus that are of prime importance are (1) the ability of virus produced in one cell to invade another, producing a spreading infection and (2) the ability of the virus to produce functional alterations within infected cells.

For ease of discussion, the responses seen following viral infection may be divided into the following: (1) *cytolytic*, (2) *steady-state*, and (3) *integrated*. Rapid viral replication leads to early cell death (cytolytic effect), with release of virus into the extracellular fluid. (No maturation occurs at cell surfaces.) Steady-state infections are characterized by slow intracellular replication during which the cell may or may not die. In this interaction, most of the virus is intracellular, and release occurs as a "budding" process at the cell surface (steady-state effect). The integrated effect is differentiated in that part of the viral nucleic acid that becomes assimilated into the DNA of the host cell. In the latter case, there is an initial brief interaction of virus with a cell, after which accelerated cell growth commences and persists indefinitely in the absence of fully infectious virus.

Examples of these events are given in Table 16–1 and are shown schematically in Figure 16–2.

CYTOLYTIC EFFECT

Perhaps the most common and best-studied virus–host cell interaction is the type in which a virus first infects a susceptible cell and then, after a brief intracellular phase of replication, destroys the cell (Fig. 16–2). This type of interaction leads to a highly productive type of acute infection with high release of fully infectious virus into the extracellular fluid following cell death. There are two important points in

TABLE 16–1.   Virus–Host Cell Interactions

Host-cell Response	Target Organ	Examples
Cytolytic		
Localized	Skin	Warts
	Respiratory tract	Rhinoviruses
	Gastrointestinal tract	Enteroviruses
	Genitourinary tract	Enteroviruses
Generalized	Multisystemic	Poliomyelitis
		Smallpox
Steady-State Effect		
Localized	Skin	Herpes simplex
	Mucous membranes	Varicella-zoster
Generalized	Multisystemic	Rubella, rubeola
		Varicella
Integrated Effect		
	Seen in experimental animals; humans	DNA viruses, Papova (adenovirus, SV 40)
		Herpes viruses

this type of interaction: (1) infection leads to cell death and release of infectious virus and (2) the assembly and maturation of viral particles occurs intracellularly with extracellular release of virus occurring only following cell death (cytolysis).

If cell death occurs on a sufficient scale, the results of tissue damage become obvious and symptoms of disease result. If damage is restricted to the portal of entry, localized symptoms are seen, such as with common respiratory tract infection (Table 16–1). On the other hand, if virus is disseminated and damage is more widespread, the symptoms of disease are of a more generalized nature, e.g., smallpox or poliomyelitis.

STEADY-STATE INFECTIONS

A second type of virus–host cell interaction is the type in which there may or may not be cell death. In either case, however, extracellular release of virus occurs as a membrane-associated event, and virus is released into the extracellular fluids through a "budding" process at cell surfaces (Fig. 16–2). Many viruses enter into this type of interaction, including the RNA viruses, e.g., influenza, and certain DNA viruses, e.g., herpes (simplex) hominis. Both of these virus types are rich in lipid in their outer envelope. They lead to cell death in some cases; in others, they persist in a steady-state interaction in which infected cells synthesize and release new virus while the host cell continues to survive. Moreover, under certain conditions, the cells may divide, with transmission of virus to daughter cells (Fig. 16–2). In that case, the

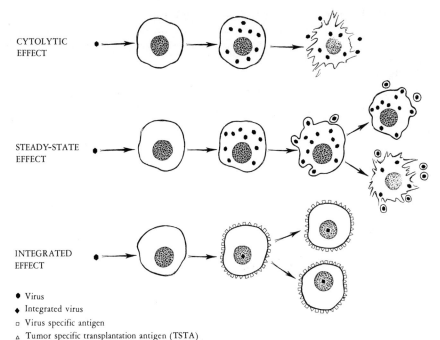

CYTOLYTIC
EFFECT

STEADY-STATE
EFFECT

INTEGRATED
EFFECT

● Virus
◆ Integrated virus
□ Virus specific antigen
△ Tumor specific transplantation antigen (TSTA)

Figure 16–2. Schematic representation of three types of virus-host cell interactions.

cells go on multiplying or carrying out their normal functions without apparent disturbance, although fairly large quantities of virus are produced. In steady-state infections, cell death does not appear to be prerequisite to the release of fully infectious virus. Dissemination of certain of these viruses is by contiguous spread from cell to cell. This may explain how such viruses, e.g., herpes (simplex) hominis, can persist in the presence of circulating antibody.

Other types of viruses that display these characteristics are those that produce congenital infections, e.g., lymphocytic choriomeningitis (LCM) in mice and avian leukemia in chickens. Mice infected *in utero* with LCM virus sustain a high level of viremia throughout life and excrete virus in all their secretions. Most of their tissues contain large amounts of infectious virus, since every cell type appears to be infected from the time of conception. The mouse infected congenitally is able to maintain viral antigen in all somatic cells without detectable antiviral antibody, i.e., they are "immunologically tolerant" (Chapter 10). More recent evidence, however, suggests that antibody is formed but is not detectable because it is complexed. Infection of adult mice, on the other hand, produces a rapidly fatal disease. A similar situation obtains in chickens infected congenitally with leukemia virus. However, unlike mice infected with LCM, these congenitally infected chickens suffer other consequences from their infection. Although infection is not cytocidal, certain infected cells become transformed and the bird may develop leukemia or other types of solid tumors. Certain congenital infections of mice with murine leukemia virus also appear to follow a similar course (Chapter 19).

Infection of the human fetus with rubella virus exemplifies the generalized steady-state, noncytocidal type of infection. Cells are not destroyed but instead are infected and pass on large quantities of virus to daughter cells in the presence of circulating antibody. Since this type of infection occurs *in utero* at a time when the immunologic system is incompletely developed, it may explain the anomalous relationship between virus and host cells in a steady-state infection. Moreover, it may explain the rare cases of agammaglobulinemia seen in early infancy that appear to result from an intrauterine viral infection, e.g., rubella, that occurred when the immunologic system was developing (Chapter 22).

Infections with herpes (simplex) hominis or varicella-zoster (V-Z) viruses may be considered examples of latent steady-state infections of a localized nature that are reactivated by certain stimuli. During this reactivation, the presence of viral antigen stimulates antibody formation. Apparently, both classes of virus, which belong to the same general family (the herpes group), may remain latent in nerve cells of sensory ganglia for months or years. Although the mechanism by which

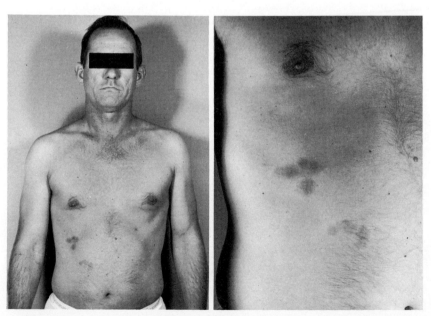

Figure 16–3. Lesions of herpes zoster in a patient with lymphoma. (Courtesy of Dr. S. Gerald Sandler.)

reactivation occurs is poorly understood, it seems that the virus travels down Schwann cells by contiguous growth from cell to cell until it reaches the skin, where vesicular eruptions appear (Fig. 16–3). Herpes zoster infections are believed to represent a reactivation of varicella virus infections that have occurred previously and remained latent in sensory ganglia. The pathogenesis of recurrent herpes simplex follows a course similar to that of the varicella-zoster group. In both activated zoster and herpes (simplex) hominis infections, virus replicates success-fully and produces disease despite the presence of high levels of serum antibody. Protection of virus owing to its intracellular location may explain this phenomenon. Of particular importance in immunity to this type of infection are the cell-mediated responses.

INTEGRATED INFECTIONS

The third type of virus-host interaction is referred to as an in-tegrated virus infection (Table 16–1; Fig. 16–2). The viral DNA, or part of it, appears to become integrated into the host cell DNA in a fashion analogous to lysogenic bacteriophage interactions with bacterial cells. This type of interaction differs from the previous two in that fully infectious virus is neither assembled nor released from the host cell. As described above, some steady-state viruses may enter into an integrated state, e.g., herpes viruses. Thus far, most integrated infections have been observed only in experimental animals and under specialized circum-stances, e.g., inoculation of virus into a host at birth or shortly thereafter. The host that is inoculated is not a natural host for the virus; for example, type 12 adenovirus may induce tumors in the hamster, a host that is normally not infected by adenovirus. Integrated infections have not been demonstrated with papovaviruses or adeno-viruses in natural hosts. In most integrated infections, the transformed cells do not release fully infectious virus; however, other stigmata of the presence of viral DNA can be detected, for example, the appear-ance of new antigens including viral-specific and tumor-specific trans-plantation antigens (TSTA) as described in Chapter 19.

PATTERNS OF DISEASE

Based upon this biologic classification, we may arbitrarily divide the types of infection due to viruses into the following classes, accord-ing to their clinical appearance: *localized, generalized, inapparent,* and *"slow" virus.*

LOCALIZED INFECTIONS

Localized infections are those in which viral multiplication and cell damage remain at the portal of entry. The virus may first infect and then spread from cell to cell either directly, in the case of cytolytic viruses, or by contiguity, as with some steady-state viruses. The virus may then exert its effect by forming a single lesion or a group of lesions at the portal of entry. For example, warts represent a type of localized infection of the skin, and the common cold is a type of localized infection of the respiratory tract (Table 16–1).

GENERALIZED INFECTIONS

Other viruses undergo a progression through a number of steps, including the following: (1) primary multiplication at the portal of

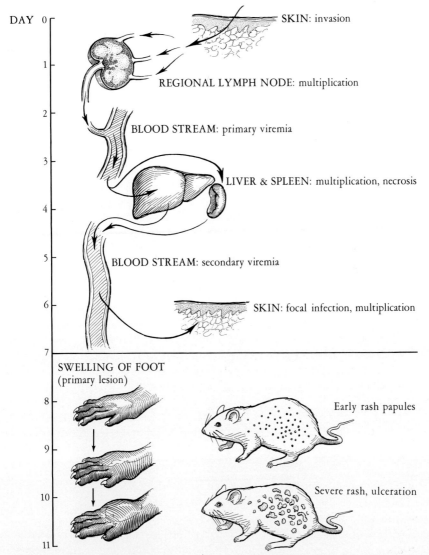

Figure 16–4. Sequential events in pathogenesis of viral infection. (After Fenner, F.: Pathogenesis of acute exanthems. Lancet, 2:915, 1948.)

entry and spread to regional lymph nodes; (2) spread of progeny virus through blood to internal organs (viremia); (3) replication at an internal site; and (4) secondary viremia with spread to target organs, causing cell damage, pathologic lesions, and clinical disease (Fig. 16–4).

Generalized infection may be seen with either the cytolytic infections (poliovirus) or with the steady-state viruses (measles). In the case of the cytolytic viruses, the effects of disease appear to be caused by the direct spread of virus and cell death. In the case of the membrane-associated steady-state viruses, the disease pattern appears to be related to the spread of virus and to cell death; additionally, some of the manifestations may be due to hypersensitivity, e.g., rash of measles. Still other manifestations of disease may be mediated by the effects of humoral antibody, e.g., renal injury mediated by viral-antiviral complexes in the mouse, or by the effects of cell-mediated immunity or meningeal infiltration in lymphocytic choriomeningitis. These will be described more fully later.

INAPPARENT INFECTIONS

Many infections of both cytolytic and steady-state varieties may occur without symptoms of disease. These appear to be of great importance in medicine because they confer immunity without overt clinical disease. This may be due to the nature of the virus or the status of host immunity.

For example, passive administration of gamma globulin can convert a clinical disease such as rubella or hepatitis type A into a subclinical disease. In the case of rubella, for example, administration of gamma globulin to a pregnant female may prevent the overt signs of disease but not the subclinical infection. The congenital rubella syndrome can occur in the fetus without overt disease in the mother (Chapter 24).

Failure of the virus to reach the target organ may be another cause of inapparent infection. In some cases of poliomyelitis in which limited replication of virus occurs in the gastrointestinal tract, the infection may not spread to the central nervous system. Instead, a localized infection may occur within the gastrointestinal tract that may be abortive or productive of few signs and symptoms within the infected host and yet capable of transmission to another susceptible individual with the production of overt paralytic disease.

SLOW VIRUS INFECTION

Slow virus infections may be defined as a group of entities putatively caused by viruses in which the incubation periods are very long and the clinical expressions of disease are relatively slow in progression. The hallmark of these infections is the persistence of a viral agent or genome in a host that ultimately sustains cellular and tissue injury from

TABLE 16–2.   Slow Virus Infections

	Target Organ	Cardinal Features
Man		
Kuru	CNS	Neurologic
Creutzfeldt-Jakob	CNS	Neurologic
Subacute sclerosing panen-cephalitis (SSPE)	CNS	Neurologic
Progressive multifocal leuko-encephalopathy (PML)	CNS	Neurologic
Multiple sclerosis	CNS	Neurologic
Animals		
Scrapie	CNS	
Visna	CNS	Neurologic
Mink encephalitis	CNS	
Aleutian mink disease	Generalized connective tissue	Generalized
Lactic acid dehydrogenase (LDH)	Liver	Liver failure
Lymphocytic choriomeningitis (LCM)	Generalized	Renal, CNS

the effects of the virus. Thus, the immunologic responses in the host that are normally efficient in eliminating conventional viruses are either not stimulated or rendered inoperable. Moreover, in some cases, cellular and tissue damage may actually develop as a result of the immune response itself. Such slow virus infections have been found both in man and in animals (Table 16–2).

TABLE 16–3.   Classification of Agents Associated with
Slow Virus Infections*

	Conventional Agents	Unconventional Agents
Examples	Subacute sclerosing panence-phalitis (SSPE), progressive multifocal leucoencephalop-athy, rabies, lymphocytic chori-omeningitis, visna, herpes, hepatitis type B	Scrapie, kuru, Creutzfeldt-Jakob disease, transmiss-ible mink encephalopathy
Morphologic properties	Definite evidence of viral struc-ture	No evidence of viral struc-ture
Biochemical properties	Have nucleic acid genomes, can be inhibited by inhibitors, some can be "rescued" (SSPE); usual lability	No evidence of nucleic acid; unusual stability
Immunologic properties	Immunogenic manner of other viruses; some may modify the immune response; the im-mune response may modify expression of disease	Nonimmunogenic
Tissue tropism	Many organs and tissues	Only CNS disease
Tissue pathology	Degenerative and/or inflamma-tory changes	Only degenerative changes

*After R. P. Hanson as modified by D. L. Walker: Behavior and properties of viruses associated with slow virus infections. *In* Slow Virus Infections, Sixty-Fourth Ross Confer-ence on Pediatric Research, Columbus, Ohio. Ross Laboratories, 1972, p. 3.

Agents associated with slow virus infections have been conveniently classified by Hanson into two major categories: (1) those that are fairly *conventional* in their behavior, and (2) those that are distinctly *unconventional* (Table 16–3).

The conventional viruses include such agents as those associated with subacute sclerosing panencephalitis (SSPE), progressive multifocal leukoencephalopathy, rabies, lymphocytic choriomeningitis (LCM), and visna. The herpes group of viruses, including herpes (simplex) hominis types 1 and 2, cytomegalovirus (CMV), the varicella-zoster (V-Z) virus, and the Epstein-Barr (E-B) virus, and the hepatitis viruses, particularly type B, should also be added to this list, since they, too, can produce a lingering persistent infection with a slow progression of disease. These agents all have in common morphologic evidence of either complete viral structure or substructure that can be inhibited by metabolic antagonists. In some cases, a complete virus can actually be rescued from its incomplete precursor form, e.g., rubeola or rubella viruses. The conventional viruses all elicit immune responses in the infected host. In some cases, the viruses may actually diminish the immune response; in others, the expression of disease may be modified by the state of the immunity of the host. These viruses induce either degenerative or inflammatory changes in a wide variety of tissues. Because of their capacity to exist in more than one set of conditions, these viruses are sometimes referred to as facultatively slow viruses.

In contrast, the "unconventional viruses," which include the agents of scrapie, kuru, Creutzfeldt-Jakob disease, and transmissible mink encephalopathy, present striking differences from the conventional viruses. Thus far, all attempts at demonstrating virion or viral nucleic acids in these diseases have been uniformly unsuccessful. The unconventional viruses appear to be nonimmunogenic, and no immune response has been detected thus far in the infected host. Moreover, these agents are unusually stable to a wide variety of physical and chemical agents, and they produce only degenerative changes that are confined primarily to the central nervous system. Thus, the evidence for consideration of these agents as true viruses is indirect at best and is based primarily on their transmissibility to other hosts.

The importance of these slow virus infections is in their possible application to other human diseases of unknown etiology that affect large segments of the population. Such neurologic diseases as multiple sclerosis, the leukodystrophies, and Parkinson's disease are being assessed for a possible slow virus pathogenesis. There are also implications for other diseases of unknown etiology such as malignant and autoimmune diseases (Chapters 19 and 20).

CLASSIFICATION OF IMMUNITY MECHANISMS

Immunity is defined as encompassing all those mechanisms that are concerned with the recognition of foreignness, and includes both

TABLE 16–4.   Mechanisms of Viral Immunity

Type of Encounter	Immunity Mechanisms	Effector Mechanisms
Primary	Nonspecific (recovery)	Skin, mucous membranes, fever, nonspecific inhibitors, interferon
Subsequent	Specific immunity (resistance)	Cell-mediated responses, antibody-mediated responses

the primary encounter of a host who is susceptible and nonimmune and the subsequent encounters of a host who is immune. Those mechanisms the host may employ upon initial encounter with a virus are the *recovery mechanisms*, or nonspecific immunity; those employed upon all subsequent encounters with the same virus are the *resistance mechanisms*, or the specific immunologic responses (Table 16–4).

MECHANISMS OF RECOVERY: NONSPECIFIC IMMUNITY

There are a number of nonspecific elements that the host has at its disposal for initial encounter with virus. The first line of defense against viral invasion is usually provided by the intact skin or mucous membranes. In addition to the passive barrier of the skin, other factors such as sweat (containing lactic acids), sebaceous secretions (fatty acids), lysozyme, ciliated epithelium, and mucous secretions play a significant role. The protective effect of these factors appears to be nonspecific except for the specific virus-inactivating properties of mucous secretions that are associated with the IgA globulins.

Blood contains a number of substances that act in a nonspecific manner. One such factor is properdin, a serum protein that in the presence of the third component of complement (C3 or $\beta_1 C$) and magnesium ions has been shown to have bactericidal and viricidal properties (Chapter 6). Although originally properdin was thought to be different from antibody and related to a natural mechanism of host resistance, it is now felt that the presence of minute amounts of antibody may account for the properdin effect.

Many tissues of the body, including brain, lung, and intestine, have receptors to which viruses attach during the first stage of infection. When cells have been treated with a receptor-destroying enzyme (RDE) from *Vibrio comma* prior to exposure to influenza virus, infection is prevented, since cellular receptors essential for virus attachment have been removed. The influenza virus itself contains neuraminidase, an enzyme that hydrolyzes the neuraminic acid linkages of many mucoproteins in the body, including those on cell surfaces. This enzyme, with the hemagglutinin, plays an important role in the genetic variability leading to new serotypes.

The influence of the inflammatory response on viral infection has been investigated. It would appear that such factors as acid metabolites, elevated temperature (fever), and lowered oxygen tension may adversely affect the multiplication of some viruses and thus be beneficial to the host in overcoming the infection. Phagocytosis, widely known to be an important defense mechanism in bacterial infections, may also be important in resistance to viral infections. Macrophages remove antibody-neutralized virus from the circulation and degrade the complexes to low molecular weight substances. In some cases, virus may enter a macrophage and be unable to replicate; in others, the macrophages may serve as potential vehicles for infection. In the case of herpes (simplex) hominis virus, it has been suggested that the macrophages from newborns are more susceptible to infection with this virus than those of the adult. It has been suggested that age-dependent resistance to certain viruses may be related to maturation processes.

Interferon

In recent years, a large body of evidence has been accumulated to suggest that certain phases of resistance to viral infection are mediated by nonantibody substances. Of prime importance in this regard is the factor called interferon, first discovered by Isaacs and Lindenmann in 1957. They showed that chick allantoic tissue exposed to inactivated influenza virus produced a soluble substance that rendered fresh chick membranes resistant to challenge by fully infectious virus. Since then interferon production has been demonstrated with many viruses.

TABLE 16–5. List of Substances That Can Induce the Production of Interferon*

I. MICROORGANISMS
Viruses
Rickettsiae
Bacteria
Protozoa
Chlamydia

II. MICROBIAL EXTRACTS
Bacterial extracts (endotoxins)
Viral extracts (double-stranded RNA)
Rickettsial extracts
Fungal extracts
Plant extracts (phytohemagglutinin, pokeweed)

III. SYNTHETIC POLYMERS
Polyphosphates (polyinosinic acid/polycytidylic acid)
Polysulfates
Polycarboxylates
Polythiophosphates

*After DeClercq, E., and Merigan, T. C.: Current concepts of interferon and interferon induction. Ann. Rev. Med., *21*:17, 1970.

However, interferon induction is not restricted to viruses but includes a markedly diverse collection of bacterial, rickettsial, and synthetic polymers (Table 16–5).

The term "interferon system" has been suggested to describe the antiviral mechanism, since it is now thought that the interferon effect is divisible into at least two components (Fig. 16–5). It is generally accepted that interferon is a protein produced or released by cells following viral infection or after exposure to certain inducers, shown in Table 16–5. Interferon is not directly antiviral but produces an antiviral effect in cells by reacting with them and inducing the formation of a second protein. The latter may be a polypeptide or a protein and is referred to as the antiviral protein (Fig. 16–5). Following infection of a cell, interferon production is thought to occur by derepression of the interferon cistron, leading to the formation of interferon mRNA, which then results in the production of interferon protein. Completed interferon is then rapidly released from the cells and reacts with surrounding cells that are uninfected. By some mechanism, the interferon reacts with the uninfected cells and produces the proposed antiviral protein by a derepression of another cistron and the formation of mRNA for this polypeptide. This second antiviral protein is thought to mediate the antiviral action of interferon by altering the cell's protein synthesis. In this way, the viral infection of the cell that is protected by interferon still leads to the release of viral genetic material, but new viruses remain unassembled.

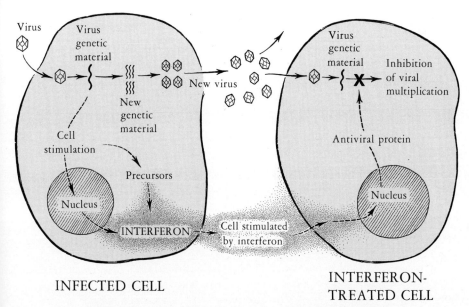

INFECTED CELL

INTERFERON-
TREATED CELL

Figure 16–5. Schematic representation of interferon activity.

TABLE 16–6.   Properties of Interferon

Nonglobulin protein
Molecular weight = 20,000–34,000
Destroyed by proteolytic enzymes (i.e., trypsin)
Not affected by amylase, lipase, deoxyribonuclease, or ribonuclease
Relatively insensitive to heat
Stable between pH 2 and pH 11
Only weakly antigenic
Nondialyzable

This type of two-component system has been compared with the effects of hormones. An important property of hormones is their effects on cells distant to the site of their production. It is believed that interferon may also be distributed throughout the body via the bloodstream and may exert its effects at sites distal to the site of production.

Early studies by a number of investigators documented the facts that interferon is a nonglobulin protein, relatively resistant to heat and acid, and only weakly antigenic. The important properties of interferon are given in Table 16–6.

Interferon appears to be species-specific to a great extent; that is, interferon produced by rabbit tissue culture is more effective when applied to other rabbit cells than to chick cells. Interferon produced in response to one virus, however, is just as effective against other viruses. For example, interferon produced by influenza virus type A is active against eastern equine encephalitis virus and vaccinia virus, as well as influenza type A.

Certain cells appear to be better producers of interferon than others. Embryonic tissues do not appear to produce interferon as well as adult tissues do. There is also some evidence that the attenuated viruses, such as vaccine strains, may induce infected cells to produce interferon in higher concentration than fully virulent strains. One explanation for the increased virulence of certain viruses is their relative resistance to the effects of interferon. Interferon differs from serum antibody in a number of respects, as indicated in Table 16–7.

Recently, a number of synthetic double-stranded RNA biopolymers have been shown to be effective in stimulating interferon in the experimental animal. These agents are now being tested for their

TABLE 16–7.   Comparison of Antibody and Interferon

ANTIBODY	INTERFERON
Globulin	Nonglobulin
Produced by B-lymphocytes	Produced by infected host cells
Specific—for one antigen	Nonspecific—for many viruses
Inactivates virus extracellularly	Acts on host cells to inhibit virus replication

therapeutic feasibility in the human. On the basis of experimental evidence of arrest of virally induced neoplasia in mice, similar trials are being conducted in humans with malignant disease. It has also been shown that interferon may be released from specifically sensitized lymphocytes themselves following interaction with specific antigen. Thus, interferon may be considered a part of both the recovery and the specific resistance mechanisms.

MECHANISMS OF RESISTANCE: SPECIFIC IMMUNITY

In contrast to the stereotyped responses that the host has at its disposal for a primary encounter with virus, all subsequent encounters with a viral agent call forth the specific immunologic responses, both antibody-mediated and cell-mediated. They are characterized by their exquisite specificity, heterogeneity, and memory (Chapter 1).

Cell-Mediated Immune Responses

The cell-mediated immune (CMI) responses are important in viral resistance and include cellular responses that may directly destroy virally infected cells or result in the elaboration of specific cell products that can enhance viral clearance (Chapter 9). Upon interaction with immunogen, specifically sensitized T-cells of the lymphoid series are capable of responding to the virally infected cell either directly or through the release of a number of effector molecules, including interferon, macrophage inhibitory factor (MIF), and lymphotoxin (Chapters 9 and 13). Moreover, activated macrophages, in addition to their role in phagocytic and viricidal activity, can participate directly in the destruction of virus-infected cells. Of importance in the cytotoxic effects of lymphocytes are the requirements for certain histocompatibility restrictions that appear to exist in cytotoxic activity (Chapter 9). In the mouse, these have been identified at the H-2 D or H-2 K locus and they require identity for both the effector lymphocyte and the target cell. Alternatively, the release of cytotoxin from sensitized T-lymphocytes may also facilitate the destruction of virus-infected cells. Recently, the recognition of antibody-dependent cytotoxicity (ADCC) mechanisms has been made in connection with cell-mediated immune responses. This presumably occurs through K-cells that have receptors for Fc fragments of immunoglobulins, which are attached to virus-specific antigens on infected target cells (Chapter 9). Alternatively, the coating of virus particles with antibody or the coating of macrophages with virus-specific cytophilic antibody (armed macrophages) could enhance the phagocytic processes.

The role of cell-mediated immunity is believed to be an important component of the specific immunologic response, particularly in the type of infection caused by noncytolytic agents, including both steady-state and integrated-type infections. Intracellular replication and cell-to-cell transfer of virus occur in spite of circulating antibody. The recurrence of herpes labialis (cold sores) in patients with circulating antibody illustrates this point. The overwhelming and devastating effects of vaccinia in infants with thymic-dependent immunologic deficiencies are also examples of the importance of this parameter in host resistance (Chapter 22).

The precise mechanism by which cell-mediated events are involved in viral immunity is not clear. It would appear that cell-mediated events are particularly well suited for infections in which viral antigens are produced at cell surfaces. This would allow greater cell-to-cell interaction with an increasingly efficient elimination of intracellular virus by the effector substances released by the interaction of lymphocyte and cell-bound antigen. In the case of cytolytic infections, cell-mediated events appear to be of lesser importance than antibody, although this remains to be shown.

Antibody-Mediated Immunity

As shown in Table 16–8, there exist in the human at least five major classes of immunoglobulin—the IgG, IgM, IgA, IgD, and IgE globulins (Chapter 5). All of these except IgD and IgE have known functions in virus-host interactions. The most thoroughly studied of the serum immunoglobulins are the IgG globulins, which contain most of the antiviral activity in serum. This class of immunoglobulin has many interesting properties such as the ability to fix complement, which is believed to be necessary for certain steps in viral neutralizaton. Perhaps one of the most important biologic functions in the human is the ability of IgG to be transported across the placenta, a property not shared by the other immunoglobulins. In this manner, the newborn infant is endowed with a vast variety of preformed antibody at birth, including practically all the maternal antiviral antibody. In addition, it is this type of passive transfer that may inhibit active immunization of the infant with live-virus vaccines. A knowledge of this must be taken

TABLE 16–8.   Human Serum Immunoglobulins

CLASS	SERUM CONCENTRATION* (mg/100 ml)	MW/S RATE	EXAMPLES
IgG	1240	150,000 (7S)	Most "late" viral antibodies
IgM	120	1,000,000 (19S)	Early "viral" antibodies, heterophil, cold agglutinin
IgA	280	170,000 (7S–14S)	Some serum antibody; local secretory antibody
IgD	3	150,000 (7S)	Unknown
IgE	0.03	196,000 (8S)	Reaginic-type antibody

*Normal adult values

into account when planning immunization schedules in the young infant (Chapter 23). The IgG class of immunoglobulins is also the type that is administered in immunotherapy against many of the viral infectious diseases (Chapter 24).

The serum IgA globulins have been studied somewhat less, mainly because of technical difficulties encountered in their characterization. Recently, however, it has been possible to demonstrate IgA viral antibody in the serum. One of the most important recent discoveries in immunology is that a unique form of IgA is found in the external secretions of the body, i.e., in the external secretory system (Chapters 2 and 5). These secretory antibodies have been shown to be an important part of the protection of the host against viruses, particularly those that produce localized infections.

The secretory IgA globulins are found in relatively large quantities in the external secretions of the body that bathe organs and tissues in continuity with the external environment. These globulins have structural and functional properties significantly different from those of the serum IgA globulins (Chapter 5). The relevant properties of the secretory IgA globulins compared to those of serum are summarized in Table 16–9.

Many types of antiviral activity have been described in various external secretions, including those from the respiratory, gastrointestinal, and genitourinary tracts. These immunoglobulins are believed to be synthesized locally. As a prerequisite to immunoglobulin production, an immunogen must gain access to local cells in continuity with the external environment. The production of secretory IgA globulins is favored after natural infection and immunization with live attenuated vacccines. In the normal respiratory tract, the IgA globulins have been shown to be the prime mediators of antiviral activity. Under experimental conditions, IgA antibody in secretions appears to correlate better with immunity than circulating antibody, particularly in infections whose pathogenesis is localized. This class of immunoglobulin has also been produced after administration of attenuated vaccines, such as measles vaccine and live oral poliovirus vaccine. Although inactivated vaccines appear to be effective in producing serum antibody, they are less effective in producing local IgA antibody when administered parenterally. This compartmentalization of serum and local antibody

TABLE 16–9. Properties of Serum and Secretory IgA Globulins

Property	Serum IgA	Secretory IgA
Sedimentation rate	7S	11.4S
Molecular weight	170,000	390,000
Presence of secretory component	None	Present
Effect of proteolytic enzymes	Destroyed	Resistance
Sites of production	Systemic, local	Local

may lead to tertiary manifestations of hypersensitivity that are responsible for adverse immunologic reactions, as described later.

Various new approaches have been suggested for the production of this IgA antibody for immunoprophylaxis in the human, such as the local application of viral antigen directly into the respiratory tract. This enhanced antibody production has been demonstrated in the case of influenza vaccines (Chapter 23).

The IgM globulins are the largest of the immunoglobulins and include antiviral antibodies produced early in the immune response. These globulins have also been shown to be phylogenetically and ontogenetically primitive forms of antibody that are characteristic of the fetal or newborn antibody response in man (Chapter 2). Other viral antibodies of this type include the cold agglutinins found in viral pneumonia and the heterophile antibody seen in infectious mononucleosis (Table 16–8).

Following immunization or infection with viruses, there appears to be a sequential appearance of the molecular varieties of antibody. Initial antibody is usually associated with the IgM class and is followed later by IgG antibody. The precise timing of the IgA antibody is unknown but it appears within a few days or several weeks after the appearance of IgM and IgG antibody. Macroglobulin is more pronounced in the fetal or newborn response than in that of the adult. Elevated levels of IgM globulins as seen in intrauterine infections, such as rubella, and cytomegalovirus (CMV) syndromes have been suggested as an aid in diagnosing intrauterine infection (Chapter 26).

WORKING HYPOTHESIS OF THE ROLES OF VARIOUS ELEMENTS OF THE IMMUNE RESPONSE DURING THE PATHOGENESIS OF VIRAL INFECTIONS

It may now be possible to construct a hypothesis of the interactions of the factors of immunity that may be involved in the host-parasite defense against viral agents. For a nonimmune and susceptible host, primary encounter with a virus of any type may be countered by the nonspecific defense mechanisms. If these are successful, infection will be prevented; if not, the virus may establish a *localized* infection, or it may become disseminated as a consequence of viremia and seed a number of target organs, producing a *generalized* infection. Prevention of local dissemination or viremia may be accomplished by the interferon system, which is activated by any of the cells invaded by virus, especially the phagocytes. The effect of interferon in the bloodstream and of interferon-producing leukocytes may be amplified, since these cellular elements are continuously circulating; i.e., the interferon effect may be transmitted to noninfected cells in advance of actual virus spread.

Within 24 to 48 hours after infection, the stage is set for the development of specific immunologic events that consist of antibody- and cell-mediated immunity. In cytolytic and noncytolytic interactions, it appears that both humoral and cell-mediated events are stimulated upon release of sufficient virus from infected cells. The induction of the specific immune response occurs with the subsequent appearance of *antibody*. In serum, the predominant antibody is associated with IgG, and in secretions it is associated with the secretory IgA immunoglobulins. Thus it would appear that following natural infection, both compartments of the antibody response — circulating and local — are stimulated. The same dual response is seen following immunization with live vaccine. The duration of IgA antibodies in secretions is much shorter than the duration of IgG antibody in serum. The role of the IgE immunoglobulins in secretions is unknown, but it may be to amplify the immune response during infection. Another role of antibody is in ADCC reactions, as described above.

The development of cell-mediated immunity may precede antibody production. It is associated with many of the signs and symptoms of the disease itself. For example, the rash of many childhood exanthems (e.g., measles) is thought to represent a cell-mediated attack on virus localized within cells of the skin. Here again, it should be pointed out that the term "cell-mediated immunity" is more appropriate than the term "delayed

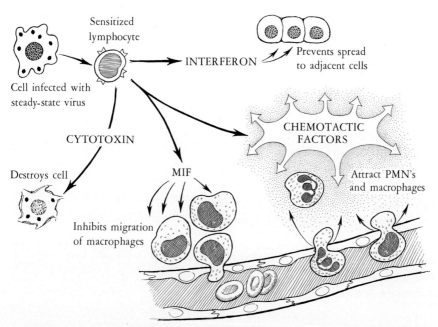

Figure 16–6. Schematic representation of cell-mediated events in viral infections. MIF: migration inhibitory factor.

hypersensitivity," which implies that the event is something undesirable. It would appear that infections that lead to noncytolytic relationships with host cells, i.e., steady-state or integrated infections, stimulate cell-mediated events to a much greater degree than cytolytic types of infection, since all steady-state viruses mature at cell surfaces and, therefore, have sites with which the effector mechanism of cell-mediated immunity can interact (Fig. 16–6).

The interaction between the cellular elements of the immune system and the virus-infected target cell includes any or all of the mechanisms described in Chapters 9 and 11, including: (1) direct lymphocytotoxicity by T-cells; (2) elaboration of lymphotoxin; (3) participation of K-cells in antibody-dependent cellular cytotoxic (ADCC) reactions; (4) action of macrophages; and (5) natural killer (NK) cells. In addition, the lymphocytes generate chemotactic factors that recruit phagocytes to remove debris and may release interferon to prevent a spread of virus to adjacent cells (Fig. 16–6).

Since it is known, for example, that there is an increased risk of malignant disease and autoimmune events in individuals with depressed cell-mediated immunity (Chapter 22), the importance of cell-mediated immunity in man is becoming more prominent. Thus, there appears to be an interaction of the various components of immunity, conferring an advantage to the host. (The relative roles of specific immunologic mechanisms are summarized in Table 16–10.) It seems clear that serum antibody confers protection in the generalized types of cytolytic or steady-state infections such as measles, poliomyelitis, and hepatitis type A; when relatively small quantities of antibody contained in gamma globulin are inoculated into susceptible individuals, temporary resistance is provided against these three viral diseases. It should be pointed out that although clinical disease is prevented, subclinical disease may occur. These events indicate that serum antibody provides resistance to infection or, if infection occurs, resistance to overt illness. The explanation for this protection is that virus must pass once or twice through the blood. Antibody in serum is therefore extremely effective in neutralizing or in inactivating viruses that have a blood-borne phase.

TABLE 16–10. Relative Roles of Specific Immunologic Mechanisms in Viral Infection

| | CYTOLYTIC TYPE | | STEADY-STATE TYPE | |
	Localized	*Generalized*	*Localized*	*Generalized*
Virus released	+	+	0 or +	0 or +
Cell death	+	+	0 or +	0 or +
Humoral	+	++++	+	+++
Local IgA	++++	+	+++	+
Cell-mediated	+	+	++++	++++

In localized infections, however, protection from infection does not correlate with serum antibody, but it does correlate with the presence of local IgA antibody. For example, studies of experimental infection in volunteers, using parainfluenza Type I, clearly demonstrated that protection against challenge with this virus correlated much better with the presence of local IgA in secretions than the presence of circulating IgG antibody. This has been shown in a number of other localized types of infections that are restricted to the respiratory tract (e.g., respiratory syncytial virus and influenza) or to the gastrointestinal tract (e.g., poliomyelitis). At times, the presence of serum antibody, in the absence of local IgA, may lead to an aberration of the immune response, resulting in hypersensitivity rather than in protective immunity.

In steady-state types of infection, too, such as varicella-zoster and recurrent herpes (simplex) hominis, it is clear that serum antibody may fail to provide protection. In these instances, however, the virus may be protected by virtue of its intracellular residence. As mentioned before, cell-mediated events may be of greater importance in immunity to these kinds of viral disease.

There is evidence that in certain types of steady-state infections, antibody itself may lead to undesirable effects. For example, in some of the slow virus infections, such as LCM in mice and leukemia virus in birds, minute amounts of antibody that are too small to be detected may be produced in serum. However, these serum antibodies form a complex with virus, and the resulting antigen-antibody complexes may localize in the kidney, leading to immune-complex disease (Chapter 8). There is accumulating evidence that a similar pathogenesis for non-streptococcal nephritis may occur in the human during the course of certain viral infections.

In summary, serum antibody seems to be effective in preventing infections of a generalized nature in both cytolytic and steady-state types of interaction; however, in localized infection of both varieties, the presence of local IgA antibody appears to correlate much better with protection than circulating IgG antibody. In steady-state infections, serum antibody may restrict virus replication but does not abolish the steady state. Indeed, serum antibody may be responsible for certain of the long-term adverse sequelae of these infections.

ABERRATIONS OF THE IMMUNE RESPONSE SEEN IN VIRAL IMMUNITY: IMMUNOLOGIC IMBALANCE

The definition of immunologic imbalance presented in Chapter 1 included aberrations of the immune response that may occur when the nature of either the immunogenic stimulus (virus) or the immunologic response is inappropriate to the other.

ABERRATIONS DUE TO IMMATURITY OF THE IMMUNE RESPONSE: CONGENITAL INFECTIONS

The first to be considered concerns cases in which the immunologic stimulus is greater than the response of the host, on the basis of developmental immaturity. It is now clear that certain intrauterine infections due to viruses such as rubella and cytomegalic inclusion disease virus (cytomegalovirus) lead to a progressive chronic infection of the host in which large amounts of virus are disseminated in many tissues. These infections occur early in embryogenesis when the immunologic system is incompletely developed. In the case of congenital rubella, maternal disease during the first trimester leads to a clinical state in which multiple congenital defects occur involving virtually every system of the body, including the lymphoreticular system. Infection can occur unimpeded by any of the specific immunologic components. Later, a steady state is established in which large amounts of virus are produced and excreted by the infant in the presence of circulating antibody. The humoral component appears adequate, and large amounts of antibody are produced, particularly of the IgM variety. An impaired proliferative response of cell-mediated immunity, as measured by lack of responsiveness to phytohemagglutinin, has been demonstrated in these congenital viral infections. Recently, impairment in specific cell-mediated immunity has been demonstrated in the congenital rubella syndrome.

SLOW VIRUS INFECTIONS

Another kind of immunologic imbalance is the type that occurs in certain slow viral infections as described previously. Two types of slow virus infections illustrate certain of the mechanisms of immunity and immune injury involved in these interactions: lymphocytic choriomeningitis of mice and subacute sclerosing panencephalitis (SSPE) of man.

Lymphocytic Choriomeningitis

LCM virus infection of mice serves as a prototype of a slow viral infection in which the host sustains immunologic injury. Mice infected with LCM *in utero* or in the newborn period go on to a carrier state in which they sustain a high level of viremia throughout their lives and excrete large quantities of infective virus in all their secretions. In this steady-state infection, the mouse maintains viral antigens in many tissues. Since conventional serologic methods in the past have failed to detect circulating antibody in these neonatal mice, they were thought to represent the classic example of immunologic tolerance produced by a viral agent. For many years it was thought that these animals were "tolerant"; i.e., no antibody was seen in the presence of large amounts of virus. Recent studies have shown that infant mice infected early do produce small amounts of antibody that, when complexed with a massive amount of antigen, form circulating complexes that are deposited in tissues such as the renal glomeruli and induce renal disease later in the animal's life through a type 3 immune-complex injury. Histologic examination of the brains of neonatally infected carriers has shown little or no evidence of choroidal, meningeal, or parenchymal damage; however, such animals develop a mild and transient choroiditis during the second week of life. Immunofluorescent staining of tissue from the carrier mouse has revealed minimal antigen within cells in the choroid plexus, ependyma, and meninges but widespread infection in several regions of the brain. Other types of viruses that display these characteristics include lactic dehydrogenase virus, Aleutian mink disease virus, and equine infectious anemia virus. This, then, is an example of the effect of an incompletely developed immunologic system on the progress of an immunologically mediated disease in which the host sustains injury not as a result of the virus *per se* but as a result of the effects of the immune response.

Infection of adult animals with LCM, on the other hand, leads to a rapidly fatal disease in which the virus regularly produces a lethal disease within six to eight days. Histologic examination of the brain reveals marked mononuclear cell infiltration in all membranes (meninges, ependyma, and choroid plexus) but litle pathologic change in neurons. In contrast to the neonatally infected mouse, fluorescent antibody staining in tissues of the adult infected with LCM demonstrates a heavy antigen concentration that is localized primarily in the choroid plexus and meninges with little involvement of the brain parenchyma.

More recent studies have shown that treatment of adult mice with cyclophosphamide converts potentially lethal choriomeningitis in the adult mouse into a nonfatal carrier infection similar to that seen in the neonatally infected mouse, with persistence of viral antigen in the carrier. These studies have indicated that the adoptive transfer of immune,

TABLE 16–11. Comparison of Effects of Age or Immunosuppression on Manifestations of LCM in the Mouse

Mouse	Site of Virus Replication		Path-ology	Chorio-menin-gitis	Disease Entity
	Membranes	*Parenchyma*			
Adult	++++	±	−	+	Acute chorio-meningitis
Newborn	±	++++	−	−	Carrier state
Adult and cyclo-phosphamide	±	++++	−	−	Carrier state
Adult and cyclo-phosphamide and adoptive transfer of immune lymphocytes	++++	±	−	+	Acute chorio-meningitis

but not normal, lymphoid cell into the drug-induced carriers results in acutely fatal choriomeningitis, histologically similar to classic LCM. These results are summarized in Table 16–11.

The results suggest that in the adult mouse the manifestations of acute choriomeningitis may be the result of cell-mediated immune injury by sensitized lymphocytes and not the effects of antibody as in the neonatal model. Thus, in LCM the status of the immune response has been shown to affect the manifestations of the disease.

Subacute Sclerosing Panencephalitis

SSPE is a chronic, fatal, inclusion body encephalitis of children and adolescents that usually develops several years after an initial exposure to natural measles virus or possibly live measles vaccine. Recently, the disease has been shown to follow the congenital rubella syndrome. The relationship of these viruses to SSPE is now well established. Fibroblast cultures of brain tissues of SSPE patients have shown the presence of suppressed intracellular measles or rubella virus and viral antigen on the surface of cells. Completely enveloped virus has not been detected in the fluid from these cultures. SSPE therefore represents an abortive type of measles infection occurring in partially permissive cells. (The immune response that is directed to this virus stands in marked contrast to that described for LCM. These differences are illustrated in Table 16–12.)

In newborn hamsters inoculated intracerebrally with human measles virus, neurologic signs of encephalitis developed. When the virus was inoculated into hamsters containing maternally derived measles-neutralizing antibody, the onset of acute encephalitis was blocked, but a chronic silent infection was established. When these chronically infected animals were treated with cyclophosphamide, however, several developed tremors, and infectious virus was isolated from the brains at autopsy. Thus, the effects of cyclophosphamide in this animal model were exactly opposite those seen in LCM. More recent

TABLE 16–12. Comparison of Two Experimental Slow Virus Infections

	LCM	MEASLES
Virus	LCM	Measles virus or SSPE variant
Animal	Mouse	Hamster, man
Age	Fetal or newborn: *chronic infection*	Newborn or weanling: *fatal infection*
	Adult: *acute infection*	Adult: *silent infection*
Effect of maternal antibodies	Form antigen-antibody complexes with resultant disease	Prevent acute encephalitis; lead to latent infection
Effect of cyclophosphamide	Convert acute infection in adult into asymptomatic infection	Convert latent infection into acute infection

studies have indicated that a chronic infection can be established *in vitro*.

There are a number of conflicting reports in the literature regarding the role of immune factors in the pathogenesis of SSPE. Originally, an immunologic imbalance between humoral and cell-mediated immunity was suggested as a pathogenetic mechanism for the progressive disease SSPE. Burnet suggested that an altered state of immunity (tolerance) might exist in which selective inhibition of cell-mediated immunity to measles virus resulted, while measles antibody–forming capacity remained intact. More recently, cell-mediated immunity has been shown to be normal and alterations of immunity may stem from the presence of "blocking factors" that interfere with the expressions of immunity. These blocking factors may be similar to those described in cancer and appear to consist of free antigen or complexes of viral antigen and antibody (Chapter 19).

ABERRATIONS INVOLVING THE SPECIFIC IMMUNITY MECHANISMS

Another type of immunologic imbalance leading to severe clinical sequelae results when one compartment of the specific immunologic apparatus, either humoral or cell-mediated, is selectively stimulated or, alternatively, when one compartment is congenitally absent or deficient.

Abberations of the Antibody Component

In addition to their protective role in viral immunity, it is now well established that antibodies are important in the pathogenesis of viral disease. If serum IgG antibody is stimulated in the absence of local secretory IgA, severe reactions can occur. For example, respiratory syncytial virus (RSV) disease occurs most frequently during the first six months of life, at a time when circulating maternal IgG antibody is present in the infant's serum. Since IgA antibody does not cross the placenta, the infant is susceptible to such localized infections as RSV. When infection occurs, maternal IgG antibody permits the formation of antigen-antibody complexes that damage the lungs. Thus, even the maternal gift of IgG can be deleterious in certain types of viral infection.

Another type of immunologic imbalance is known to occur following the use of inactivated (killed) vaccines and results in the selective stimulation of serum IgG without a concomitant stimulation of secretory IgA antibody. This effect has been seen in children immunized with either killed RSV or measles virus vaccines. Following natural infection with RSV or measles virus, these children develop a severe disease that is more intensified than that seen in unimmunized children. It has been suggested that this type of immunologic imbalance occurs because of an anomalous situation in which the killed vaccine stimulates predominantly serum IgG antibody but not secretory antibody. Because of the secretory antibody deficiency, upon subsequent exposure to natural virus, a viral replication can occur within the respiratory tract. Since only limited IgG antibody is available and the viral antigen is in relative excess, antigen-antibody complexes occur that lead to immunologic injury. This damage may be restricted to the lungs, in the case of RSV infection, or may be generalized, as in the case of measles, with skin and pulmonary manifestations (atypical measles) (Chapters 20A and 23).

Aberrations Involving the Cell-Mediated Component

A deficiency in the host's cell-mediated immunity may render him susceptible to repeated or protracted infections. For example, infants born with defects of the thymic-dependent immune system are prone to viral infections, including vaccinia necrosum following the use of smallpox vaccine and Hecht cell pneumonia following natural measles. The well-known exacerbation of herpes zoster in older individuals with malignant disease may represent a failure of the surveillance mechanism of the host; in any patient with herpes zoster, a very careful search for malignant conditions should be made. These examples illustrate the effect of impaired cell-mediated function on viral susceptibility of the host whose resistance is dependent upon this mechanism of immunity.

ABERRATIONS DUE TO VIRUSES THAT PERSIST: IMMUNE-COMPLEX DISEASE AND VIRUS-INDUCED CELL-MEDIATED IMMUNOPATHOLOGY

In certain chronic virus infections of man and animals the interplay of ongoing viral replication and a continuing host immune response have been shown to lead to an immune-complex (type 3) or cell-mediated immune (type 4) form of immunopathology. These mechanisms, described in greater detail in Chapters 13 and 20, seem to contribute to tissue injury because of the persistence of viral antigen. In addition, virus antibody complement (V-Ab-C) complexes have been shown to act as blocking factors, inhibiting cell-mediated immunity in a fashion analogous to that seen in malignant disease (Chapter 19). Listed in Table 16–13 are some viral infections in which these various mechanisms of injury have been shown to occur.

ABERRATIONS DUE TO HERPES AND HEPATITIS VIRUSES

The herpes and the hepatitis viruses are two groups assuming increasing importance in medicine today because of their frequency and

TABLE 16–13.

| | | EVIDENCE FOR IMMUNE COMPLEXES | | |
Species	Infection	*In Injury*	*Blocking Factors*	CMI
Man	Hepatitis B	+	−	?
	Epstein-Barr (EB)	+	−	±
	Dengue hemorrhagic fever	+	−	?
	Subacute sclerosing panencephalitis (measles rubella)	+	+	+
	Multiple sclerosis	−	+	?
Animal	Lactic dehydrogenase	+	−	
	LCM − infant mouse	+	−	
	− adult mouse	−	−	+
	Oncorna viruses	+	+	+
	Aleutian disease	+	−	
	Equine infectious anemia	+	−	
	Hog cholera	+	−	

After Oldstone, M. B. A., and Dixon, F. J.: Immune complex disease associated with viral infections. In A. L. Notkins (ed.): Viral Immunology and Immunopathology. New York, Academic Press, 1975.

their ability to become latent or persistent in the host with clinically apparent sequelae. The following discussions will briefly highlight some of the recent observations concerning these viruses, together with their immunologic implication and disease processes.

The Herpes Viruses

There are four currently known types of viruses in the herpes group. These are listed in Table 16–14 with their common clinical characteristics.

TABLE 16–14. The Herpes Viruses of Man

Type	Usual Age of Onset (years)	Usual Clinical Manifestations
H. hominis type 1 type 2	0–20	Cold sores (herpes labialis) Genital herpes (herpes genitalis) Neonatal herpes
Cytomegalovirus	0–20	Congenital CNS Infectious mononucleosis (heterophil negative)
Varicella-zoster (V-Z)	0–10	Chickenpox Shingles (herpes zoster)
Epstein-Barr (EB)	0–10	Infectious mononucleosis (heterophile positive)

Herpes (Simplex) Hominis Viruses—Types 1 and 2.   There are two known types of herpes (simplex) hominis viruses: type 1 usually produces an oral infection and type 2 produces a genital infection. In addition, these viruses can sometimes infect a wide variety of other tissues, such as the skin, the cornea, and the central nervous system, and lead to a generalized form of disease in the newborn or the immunosuppressed patient. Maternal genital infection presents a particular risk to the neonate because of its immature immunologic responses. The most significant features of these herpetic viral infections are their ability to become latent in the nervous system (e.g., dorsal root ganglia) and their capacity to cause recrudescent infections at other sites (e.g., skin, eyes, and central nervous system). As stated previously, the mechanisms of immunity involved in these herpetic infections appear to involve mainly the cell-mediated immune responses and the interplay of both macrophages and lymphocytes. Antibody appears to play a relatively minor role, although it may facilitate antibody-dependent cytotoxicity reactions or may directly affect antibody-mediated lysis (Chapters 6 and 9). In addition, the herpes hominis viruses have been implicated in certain forms of malignant disease in the human (Chapter 19). Women with recurrent herpes genitalis show a threefold increase in cervical carcinoma. Conversely, women with cervical carcinoma have significantly elevated titers of antibody to herpes (simplex) hominis virus.

The immunologic implications of herpetic infections stem largely from the fact that these infections are more frequent in the immunologically compromised host, which includes pregnant women, the newborn, and patients receiving tumor chemotherapy or immunosuppressive agents. In each of these clinical situations, a diminution in specific cell-mediated immunity appears to contribute to the enhanced infection rate.

Cytomegalovirus.   Another ubiquitous member of the group of herpes viruses of man is cytomegalovirus. The major interest in this virus was initially stimulated because of its teratogenic role. The virus is now considered to be the major cause of congenital birth defects. An estimated one of 1000 infants sustains some form of functional disability as a result of intrauterine or perinatal infection. In the older child and adult, the virus may produce a wide spectrum of clinical diseases ranging from a mild form of heterophil-negative infectious mononucleosis with atypical lymphocytes to more severe forms of hepatitis and hematologic disorders. Primary or recurrent infection occurs in the vast majority of patients with renal or bone marrow transplantation, as well as in patients with malignant disease, particularly those receiving cancer chemotherapy. As with the herpes (simplex) hominis infections, all of these appear to be related to depressed cell-mediated immunity. Although not proven, the role of CMV in oncogenesis has been suggested by the recent findings of the capacity of the virus to induce *in* *vitro* transformation and by the elevated titers of antibody to CMV seen in patients with cancer of the cervix.

Varicella-Zoster Virus.   The varicella-zoster (V-Z) virus is the causative agent for both varicella (chickenpox) and herpes zoster. Like the other herpes infections, primary infection is usually seen in childhood, after which the virus becomes latent in dorsal ganglia. In this location the virus may be activated and lead to a recrudescent type of infection consisting of localized vesicular lesions restricted to the dermatomes. The V-Z viruses pose a twofold significance with regard to malignant disease. The significance of the V-Z virus is seen in either primary or secondary immune deficiency states in which the virus is a major cause of opportunistic infection.

Epstein-Barr Virus.   The Epstein-Barr (E-B) virus is now recognized as the causative agent of primary E-B infection in man. The manifestations of this infection appear to be age-related. In the infant, the disease is associated with an upper respiratory infection; in the older child and adult, it causes the syndrome of infectious mononucleosis. Originally identified in the lymphocytes of patients with Burkitt's lymphoma, its precise relationship to this malignant disorder is still unknown. The virus appears to have a selective affinity for infection of the B-lymphocyte, which contains specific receptors for this virus. The subsequent reaction of the T-cell to E-B virus–specific antigens on the B-cell appears to be responsible for the atypical lymphocytes seen in the disease.

A wide variety of antibodies of both virus-specific and heterogeneic antibody responses can be detected in individuals with infectious mononucleosis. The virus-specific antibodies include VCA, EA, MA, and EBNA. In addition to the classic heterophil antibodies, cold agglutinins may be generated during the course of the disease, particularly the anti-I antibodies that occasionally may be associated with hemolytic anemia.

The Hepatitis Viruses

Another major group of viruses that produce latent or chronic infections with immunologic sequelae are the hepatitis viruses. At present, there is evidence for several classes of hepatitis viruses. These are shown in Table 16–15 with some of their characteristics.

Type A.   The agents responsible for what was originally known as "infectious" or "short-incubation hepatitis" is now known as hepatitis virus A. The disease is usually transmitted by the fecal-oral route and produces a self-limited illness that is often subclinical in the young and more severe in the elderly. Unlike other forms of hepatitis, chronic hepatitis is rarely seen, if it occurs at all. Several antibody tests are now available for the detection of hepatitis type A, including complement fixation, immune electron microscopy, immune adherence, and ra-

TABLE 16–15. Viral Hepatitis: Characteristics

CHARACTERISTIC	TYPE A	TYPE B	TYPE NON-A, NON-B
Disease			
Incubation period (days)	30 (15–50)*	90 (21–180)	50 (15–160)
Severity (acute)	mild to moderate	moderate to severe	mild to moderate
Chronicity	probably no	yes	yes
Epidemiology			
Mode of spread			
Blood, blood products	rare	yes	yes
Fecal contamination	yes	probably no	probably no
Close personal contact	yes	yes	probably yes
Etiologic agent			
Size (nm)	27	42	?
Nucleic acid	? probably RNA	DNA	?
Classification	? picornavirus	no existing classification	?

*Average and range
(After Dr. Robert H. Purcell)

dioimmunoassay. The control of hepatitis A depends on interrupting the transmission of virus, e.g., improved personal and public hygienic measures. The administration of immune serum globulin (ISG) to exposed individuals before or shortly after exposure is also recommended (Chapter 24).

Type B. The second type of virus, responsible for what was known originally as "serum hepatitis," is hepatitis type B. As with type A, infection is more commonly seen in the lower socioeconomic groups and occurs primarily at an early age. Unlike infection with hepatitis A, the acute illness is more severe and has a greater predilection for producing chronic infection. Up to 10 per cent of clinical cases are associated with a chronic carrier state that is sometimes manifested in apparent chronic carriage of the virus, or more frequently as chronic active or chronic passive hepatitis (Chapter 20).

Although type B hepatitis was originally thought to occur only following the parenteral administration of blood or blood products, e.g., transfusion, recent studies have demonstrated that the virus can be passed vertically from mother to newborn by venereal transmission and by any of a variety of external secretions such as saliva, breast milk, or genital secretions.

The virus consists of two basic components: (1) a core, which contains the hepatitis B core antigen (HB_cAg), and (2) the coat, which contains the hepatitis B surface antigens (HB_sAg). Among the major antigenic specificities are the *d*, *y*, *w*, and *r*. These occur as allelic pairs—*adw*, *ayw*, *adr*, and *ayr*. Other minor antigenic variations, consisting of four subspecificities of *w*, (*w1*, *w2*, *w3*, *w4*), have also been detected. These major and minor specificities have epidemiologic consisting of four subspecificities of *w*, (*w1*, *w2*, *w3*, *w4*), have also been detected. These major and minor specificities have epidemiologic importance since they suggest that several types of hepatitis virus B may exist in a worldwide distribution, in comparison to type A, in which only a single type has been described.

An additional antigen, E (HB$_e$Ag), appears during many hepatitis virus infections. Although not part of the surface of the hepatitis virus B, it may be a virus-specified antigen playing a role in intracellular virus synthesis or an excess viral DNA polymerase not incorporated into the virus core. The detection of HB$_e$Ag and virus-specific DNA polymerase in the serum correlates well and is an important marker of infectivity.

A large number of immunologic tests have been developed for the detection of hepatitis B antigens and antibodies. The most widely used include radioimmunoassays and passive hemagglutination tests. Diagnosis is usually based on the identification of HB$_s$Ag in acute-phase sera. Although several reports have appeared concerning cell-mediated immune responses to hepatitis virus B, they have not been substantiated and their specificity and significance await further clarification.

The control of type B transfusion-associated hepatitis has been effectively achieved by screening for the presence of HB$_s$Ag by very sensitive immunologic techniques. The screening of donor blood for HB$_s$Ag by blood banks has resulted in a decrease in the incidence of transfusion-associated hepatitis from as high as 50 per cent to less than 10 per cent in some studies.

The significance of persistent excretion of hepatitis B antigens is seen in certain forms of chronic hepatitis. This will be described in greater detail in Chapter 20.

Although hepatitis virus B has not been cultured *in vitro*, "subunit" vaccines have been prepared from HB$_s$Ag that has been purified from the plasma of individuals chronically infected with the virus. Such vaccines have proved to be safe, immunogenic, and effective in preventing hepatitis in chimpanzee experiments and in preliminary studies in the human.

Type Non-A, Non-B Hepatitis.   A third type of hepatitis appears to be caused by an agent that is unlike that of type A and type B viruses. This agent has been arbitrarily designated "non-A, non-B" virus or viruses. Serologic tests for this virus are nonexistent, but several epidemiologic studies indicate that the agent more closely resembles the agent for hepatitis type B than type A.

NEOPLASIA AND AUTOIMMUNITY

It appears that neoplasia and autoimmunity occur as frequent sequelae in individuals with deficiencies of cell-mediated immunity. Many have speculated that this increase in incidence of both neoplasia and autoimmunity may reflect an increased susceptibility to infections—more frequently with viral agents—due to defects in immunologic surveillance. The continued persistence of antigen may in turn lead to an "autoimmune" state or the transformation to a malignant state.

PROJECTIONS FOR THE FUTURE

The immunologic mechanisms described make it apparent that the major emphasis for the management of viral infection is on prevention. This has been made possible through the use of vaccines (Chapter 23), the most effective of which are those viral vaccines that most closely mimic natural disease. Experience has shown that some inactivated viral vaccines may have harmful effects, since they selectively lead to an immunologic imbalance that leads to a state of hypersensitivity rather than to protective immunity.

The therapeutic use of interferon has become available for the treatment of viral infections. Certain interferon stimulators, such as polyinosinic acid, may be used to stimulate the nonspecific immunologic apparatus, resulting in the inability of virus to replicate. In our lifetime, the increased knowledge of virus-host relationships may eventually lead to the elucidation of the underlying causes and prevention of malignant disease in man.

SUGGESTIONS FOR FURTHER READING

Alford, C. A., Jr., and Whitley, R. J.: Treatment of infections due to *Herpes virus* in humans: A critical review of the state of the art. J. Infect. Dis., *133* (supplement):A101–A108, 1976.

Bellanti, J. A., and Artenstein, M. S.: Mechanisms of immunity to virus infection. Pediatr. Clin. North Am., *11*:558, 1964.

Bellanti, J. A.: Biologic significance of the secretory IgA globulins. Pediatrics, *48*:715, 1971.

Bellanti, J. A., Catalano, L., and Chambers, R. W.: Herpes simplex encephalitis: Virologic and serologic study of a patient treated with an interferon inducer. J. Pediatr., *78*:136, 1971.

Davis, B. D., Dulbecco, R., Eisen, H. A., Ginsberg, H. S., and Wood, W. B., Jr.: Microbiology. 2nd ed., New York, Harper & Row, Publishers, 1973.

DeClercq, E., and Merigan, T. C.: Current concepts of interferon and interferon induction. Annu. Rev. Med. *21*:17, 1970.

Evans, A. S.: Viral Infections of Humans. Epidemiology and Control. New York, Plenum Medical Book Company, 1976.

Feinstone, S. M., Kapikian, A. Z., Purcell, R. H., Alter, H. J., and Holland, P. V.: Transfusion-associated hepatitis not due to viral hepatitis type A or B. New Engl. J. Med., *292*:767–770, 1975.

Fenner, F.: The Biology of Animal Viruses. Vol. 1. Molecular and Cellular Biology. Vol. 2. The Pathogenesis and Ecology of Viral Infections. New York, Academic Press, Inc., 1968.

Finter, N. B.: Interferons. Philadelphia, W. B. Saunders Company, 1966.

Gajdusek, D. C., Gibbs, C. J., Jr., and Alpers, M.: Slow, Latent and Temperate Virus Infections. United States Department of Health, Education and Welfare, Public Health Service, 1965.

Hilleman, M. R.: Prospects for the use of double stranded ribonucleic acid (poly I:C) inducers in man. J. Infect. Dis., *121*:196, 1970.

Johnson, R. T.: Subacute sclerosing panencephalitis. J. Infect. Dis., *121*:227, 1970.

Krugman, S., and Gershon, A. A.: Progress in Clinical and Biological Research. Vol. 3. Infections of the Fetus and the Newborn Infant. New York, Alan R. Liss, Inc., 1975.

McCollum, R. W.: Infectious mononucleosis and the Epstein-Barr virus. J. Infect. Dis., *121*:347, 1970.

Notkins, A. L.: Viral Immunology and Immunopathology. New York, Academic Press, Inc., 1975.

Peterson, J. M., Dienstag, J. L., and Purcell, R. H.: Immune response to hepatitis viruses. *In* A. L. Notkins (ed.): Viral Immunology and Immunopathology. New York, Academic Press, 1975.

Remington, J. S., and Klein, J. O.: Infectious Diseases of the Fetus and Newborn Infant. Philadelphia, W. B. Saunders Company, 1976.

Tomasi, T. B., Jr., and Bienenstock, J. : Secretory immunoglobulins. Adv. Immunol., *9*:2, 1968.

Youmans, G. P., Paterson, P. Y., and Sommers, H. M.: The Biologic and Clinical Basis of Infectious Diseases. Philadelphia, W. B. Saunders Company, 1975.

Zeman, W., Lennette, E. H., and Brunson, J. G.: Slow Virus Diseases. Baltimore, The Williams & Wilkins Company, 1974.

Chapter 17 ⎯⎯⎯⎯⎯⎯⎯⎯⎯⎯⎯⎯⎯⎯⎯⎯⎯⎯⎯⎯

MECHANISMS OF IMMUNITY
TO PARASITIC DISEASES
Ray H. Cypess, D.V.M., Ph.D.

Parasitic diseases result in large-scale morbidity, mortality, and economic loss for man and his domestic animals in both industrialized and developing countries. Essentially, the immunologic responses of the host to parasitic infection are governed by the same principles that govern responses to other infectious agents, but they involve more complex host-parasite interactions.

Although parasitic organisms were among the first disease agents to be studied, a great deal of the early progress in this field centered on morphologic descriptions, the elucidation of life cycles, studies of mechanisms of transmission, and development of new chemotherapeutic agents. In recent years, there has been increased attention focused on the *in vitro* cultivation and biochemical aspects of these organisms and the response of the host to infection with these parasitic agents. Despite progress in the prevention and control of some parasitic diseases, the advances have not matched those made with other infectious agents. The slow development of the field of immunoparasitology can be attributed largely to several factors. First, because of their complex life cycles and host specificity, it has been difficult to culture these agents *in vitro*, so that the availability of antigenic materials for analysis has been limited. Second, the complexity of their developmental cycles has resulted in not only a multiphasic antigenic stimulation in the host but also a diversified functional (e.g., protective) and nonfunctional set of immune responses. Third, there has been a lack of success in developing attenuated strains suitable for vaccination with methods normally used in other fields of microbiology, e.g., temperature-sensitive mutants and *in vitro* growth of organisms in tissue culture were employed. Finally, the lack of a vinculum between parasitologists and immunologists has impeded progress. Nevertheless, the current renaissance in the fields of immunology and immunopathology has stimulated greater interest in the role of immunologic factors in these host-parasite systems, and these agents have become useful models for the study of immunologic responses, e.g., IgE production.

418

MAJOR GROUPS OF ANIMAL PARASITES

The parasites affecting man are grouped as protozoan (unicellular) or metazoan (multicellular) organisms. In addition to their morphologic differences, there are other characteristics displayed by these two groups that determine the degree and type of pathologic and immunologic responses accompanying infection by these agents.

Infections by protozoa are often *intracellular* in several or all of the tissue-invading stages of the organism. These agents rapidly undergo multiplication within the host, and the disease spectrum produced may proceed as a rapid fulminating syndrome. In contrast, the metazoa are primarily *extracellular*, do not normally multiply in the definitive host, and result in the development of a more chronic localized disease accompanied by nonspecific symptoms.

Much of the information on immunoparasitology is derived from studies in both laboratory and domestic animal populations. These studies have shown that, as with other host-parasite relationships (i.e., involving viruses, bacteria, and fungi), resistance to infection by both multicellular and unicellular parasites is conditioned by innate and naturally acquired factors. These experimental studies have also demonstrated that manifestations of immunity operate in two ways: (1) some affect the parasite directly, i.e., the inhibition of penetration and infection, the retardation of development, the decrease in the duration of patency (i.e., latency), the inhibition of multiplication, resulting in a depression of parasitemia, the reduction of fecundity, the elimination of residual parasitic populations, and the alteration of structural and physiologic components; and (2) some operate indirectly to modify the effects of the parasite within the host and result in a reduction of morbidity and mortality. The extent to which these phenomena occur in man has not been fully established.

IMMUNE RESPONSE TO PARASITIC INFECTIONS

There is ample evidence that man exhibits innate resistance to many of the animal parasites, a resistance that may vary, depending upon host characteristics (race, age, physiologic status, and nutritional status). It has been difficult to document whether or not man develops acquired immunity to many of the metazoa (nematodes, cestodes, trematodes), and much of the information concerning this question has been derived indirectly from epidemiologic studies. Indeed, if acquired immunity does develop in man, its expression may not result in complete removal of the agent, i.e., sterile immunity. It is only in rare instances that one sees sterile immunity against these agents in any host system, and in many parasitic infections the immune state is defined as one in which the parasite numbers are controlled at a low pathogenic level and hyperinfection of the host does not occur, e.g., synergism. One could hypothesize that sterile immunity does not occur with *any* group of agents, but since animal parasites are large, their presence, even in low numbers, is more readily apparent.

Parasites contain a variety of somatic and metabolic antigens, some of which are stage-specific and transitory in nature; others persist and may continually stimulate a diversity of immunologic responses. Host responses to these agents are further complicated by the fact that many parasites share antigenic moieties not only with other infectious agents but also with antigens of the host. For example, extracts of *Trichinella spiralis* have been reported to cross-react with A_2 human blood group substance, *Ancylostoma, Ascaris, Filaria, Onchocerca, Trichuris, Echinococcus, Fasciola, Schistosoma, Salmonella typhi, Treponema, Giardia,* and human serum albumin. It is therefore not surprising that these agents stimulate a multitude of both humoral and cell-mediated immune responses that can be detected by a wide variety of *in vitro* and *in vivo* assays. Moreover, infection with these organisms can have immunopotentiative effects to other antigens (Chapter 10). To date, the role of these responses in the pathogenesis of parasitic disease is not clear, nor is the relationship between these responses and immunity well defined. In spite of an often rapid and exaggerated humoral and cell-mediated immune response to infection, many of these parasites remain viable within the host for extended periods of time (Fig. 17–1). The failure of a host to develop acquired immunity under natural conditions may result from any of the following:

(1) Limited tissue invasion by the agent that results in little or no stimulation of the immune response, e.g., intestinal helminths: *Enterobius vermicularis, Taenia* spp.; *protozoa: Entamoeba histolytica, Giardia lamblia.*

(2) The inaccessibility of the agent to the immune system owing to the intracellular location of the protozoa, e.g., *Toxoplasma gondii* in neurologic tissue, *Trypanosoma cruzi* in the myocardium, *Plasmodium vivax* in exoerythrocytic stages.

(3) The encapsulation of the agent, e.g., tissue protozoa: *T. gondii;* tissue helminths: *Trichinella spiralis, Echinococcus granulosis.* Despite the formation of a cyst, however, stimulation of the host by parasitic antigens may still take place. Encapsulation alone, therefore, may not entirely account for the ability of the parasite to survive.

(4) Infection of the host in subthreshold doses. Since metazoa do not multiply within the host, the amount of antigen available for the stimulation of the immune system may be limited by the size of the infecting dose.

(5) The ability of the agent to alter its antigenic composition during infection, e.g., African trypanosomiasis or the incorporation of host proteins onto the parasite, e.g., *Schistosoma* spp., resulting in a failure of host recognition of the organism.

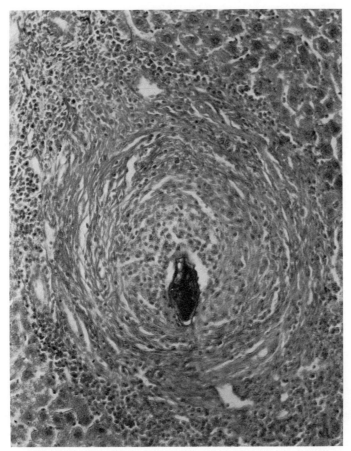

Figure 17-1.   Section of liver from a patient with schistosomiasis. Egg of *Schistosoma mansoni* is seen within the center of a granuloma, containing a heavy infiltration of eosinophilic leukocytes. Hematoxylin and eosin stain, × 100.

(6) The release of large amount of soluble and particulate antigens, which may result in the possible development of tolerance. Alternatively, these antigens alone or complexed with antibody may function as "blocking" factors similar to these described in patients with malignant disease (Chapter 19). Examples of these organisms include blood and tissue protozoa: *Plasmodium* spp., *Leishmania donovani;* blood and tissue metazoa: filaria, *Schistosoma* spp.

(7) The ability of the agent to evade the arsenal of nonspecific and specific immune responses. For example, many of the metazoa, e.g., *Toxocara*, and other migrating larval stages, e.g., schistosomes, have been shown to survive long periods of time within the infected host.

(8) The capacity of the organisms to replicate within phagocytic cells of the host, e.g., *Toxoplasma* in macrophages.

Thus, depending on the specific host-parasite factors involved, e.g., developmental cycle, location, and tissue invasion, any or all of these mechanisms may determine the failure of the host to develop acquired immunity.

IMMUNITY TO PROTOZOA

The type and level of immune responses induced by protozoan infections are influenced by their site of colonization and the extent of tissue involvement, e.g., intracellular *versus* extracellular, localized (intestinal) *versus* systemic (in blood or tissue). In general, humoral responses are elicited in response to stages of the parasite that circulate in the blood, and cell-mediated immune reactions are seen with those agents with intracellular development. In contrast to the metazoa, these protozoan parasites do not usually induce immediate-type hypersensitivity skin responses, and eosinophilia is not a common feature of these infections.

Intestinal Protozoa

In the human alimentary tract, the lumen is the most frequent site of colonization. Tissue invasion occurs only with the ciliate, *Balantidium coli,* and the amoeba, *Entamoeba histolytica.* The third intestinal protozoa of clinical importance to man, the flagellate *Giardia lamblia,* occurs either free in the lumen or attached to the mucosal surface of the villi of the small intestine.

The most frequently studied intestinal amoeba, *E. histolytica,* is the causative agent of both acute and chronic amoebic dysentery in man. The amoeba, ingested with contaminated food or water, encysts and colonizes in the intestinal tract. Occasionally, it may become invasive and penetrate tissues locally (intestinal amebiasis) or systemically (extraintestinal amebiasis). The infection may be asymptomatic or symptomatic. Of the latter, the most frequent manifestation is intestinal amebiasis. Hepatic amebiasis is the most common form of extraintestinal amebiasis (Fig. 17–2). The prevalence of this disease has been difficult to assess because of the lack of a simple direct diagnostic test. Very little is known about acquired immunity in man and the lack of an adequate animal model has limited experimental studies. There is no evidence for the development of resistance to reinfection, which may be related to the inaccessibility of the parasite to the immune mechanisms of the host. The principal success in immunologic studies to date has been in the development of serodiagnostic tests (indirect hemagglutination, precipitin, particle agglutination, fluorescent antibody). Because antibody response follows the invasion of the intestinal mucosa or colonization within the liver, these tests are most useful in establishing

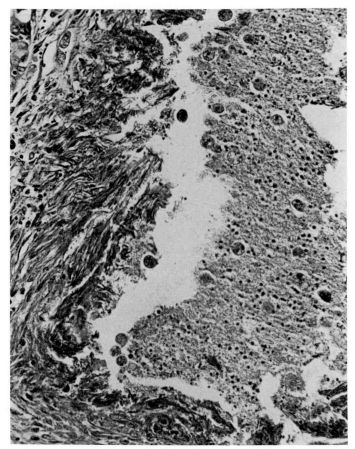

Figure 17–2. Section of liver from a patient with an amoebic liver abscess. Note the massive destruction of liver parenchyma with minimal surrounding cellular reaction. Hematoxylin and eosin stain, × 125.

exposure to the parasite. Negative results with the indirect hemagglutination and precipitin tests are of clinical importance in excluding suspected cases of extraintestinal amebiasis. Nonetheless, the occurrence of cases in which no antibody can be detected limits their diagnostic value.

Although the protective effect of local antibody has been demonstrated in a number of systems, including those involving bacterial, fungal, and viral agents, a similar role for secretory IgA or local cellular immunity against intestinal protozoa has not been established. The functions of IgA in localized immunity to microbial agents have been described previously (Chapter 14) and include its neutralizing or coating effect on epithelial surfaces that prevents attachment or penetration of the organism.

Blood and Tissue Protozoa

Trypanosoma. There are two major groups of trypanosomes containing species that parasitize man. The first group, *Stercoraria,* is characterized by transmission from host to host of infective forms that occur in the feces of insect vectors and multiply intracellularly in the muscle, macrophage, and other cells. An example is *T. cruzi,* the agent of American trypanosomiasis (Chagas' disease). The second group, *Salivaria,* is characterized by transmission from host to host of infective forms that occur in the saliva or mouth of the insect vector and multiply not intracellularly but in the lumen of blood vessels and in tissue spaces (*T. gambiense* and *T. rhodesiense,* the causative agents of African trypanosomiasis). Protective antibodies can be demonstrated in the sera of animals after experimental and natural infections with the *Salivaria,* but to date there is no immunizing procedure that will protect man against natural infection. Patients with African trypanosomiasis may exhibit a rapid and marked increase in IgM globulins in serum and cerebrospinal fluid, but most of this immunoglobulin response is nonspecific. This elevation of CSF IgM globulins is of diagnostic importance. In animal models, infection with *Salivaria* produces selective IgG immunosuppression to nonrelated antigen. Whether this immunosuppression occurs in areas of endemic trypanosomiasis is unknown.

Leishmania. Leishmaniasis, an important protozoan disease, evolves in several clinical forms that appear to depend on the host's immunologic response to the parasite. The two major forms of the disease are a *cutaneous* and a *visceral* type. Cutaneous leishmaniasis is caused by a variety of leishmania species and is expressed clinically as a spectrum of disease. The three major forms are: (1) diffuse cutaneous leishmaniasis (DCL), characterized by an absence of specific delayed hypersensitivity to leishmania, disseminated nodules, and poor response to treatment; (2) lupoid leishmaniasis, characterized by a well-developed specific delayed hypersensitivity, local scar formation with peripheral spread of lesions but no metastasis, and a variable response to treatment; (3) cutaneous leishmaniasis (oriental sore), the most common form, in which delayed hypersensitivity develops after a variable period of time and single lesions may take one to two years to heal. In DCL, the patients handle intercurrent infections normally, respond positively to skin tests with nonrelated antigens, and exhibit no apparent alterations in serum immunoglobulin levels.

Visceral leishmaniasis (kala azar) is caused by infection with *L. donovani.* This form of the disease is characterized by heavy parasitization of systemic macrophages, a lack of specific delayed hypersensitivity, and a massive hyperglobulinemia. After successful treatment of kala azar, the delayed hypersensitivity response returns and the host exhibits an immunity to reinfection. The intradermal test for delayed hypersensitivity reactions in leishmaniasis is termed the leishmanin skin

(Montenegro) test and a positive reaction correlates with *in vitro* lymphocyte transformation to leishmanial antigens.

Plasmodium.   The infectious cycle of malaria is illustrated schematically in Figure 17–3. Following the bite of an infected anopheline mosquito, sporozoites are introduced into the bloodstream and migrate directly to the liver, where they multiply within parenchymal cells. In experimental studies in rodents and primates the administration of irradiated sporozoites has been shown to induce immunity to subsequent challenge infections. In rodents, immunity to the sporozoite has been shown to be T-cell-dependent; however, immunity to the exoerythrocytic stage is both T- and B-cell-dependent. How to apply these findings to man is currently under active investigation and holds greater promise for the development of an effective vaccine for malaria. The major problem has been the production of adequate numbers of sporozoites and the extreme lability of the organisms when stored. The recent development of methods for the *in vitro* cultivation of large numbers of erythrocytic parasite stages represents a major advance toward the development of an effective vaccine.

The exoerythrocytic stages apparently do not stimulate an immune

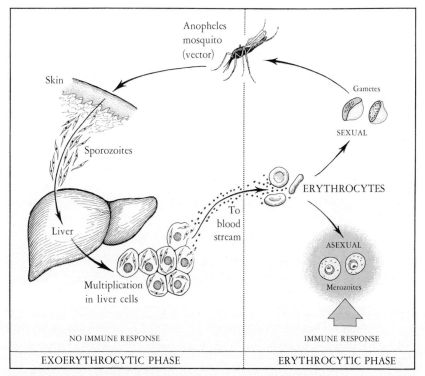

Figure 17–3.   Schematic life cycle of malaria. Note that detectable immune responses are directed against erythrocytic phase.

response, and following exoerythrocytic development, the liver cells burst, releasing merozoites into the peripheral circulation. The rapid multiplication of erythrocytic stages releases an abundance of antigens and results in the induction of specific and nonspecific host responses. This situation is expressed as a rise in specific and nonspecific immunoglobulins, a marked proliferation and hyperactivity of the reticuloendothelial system, and alterations in various lymphoid organs. The precise function these various responses play in the cessation of the parasitic cycle is not clear. Since in endemic populations the newborn is protected from infection by maternally transferred antibody, it is clear that humoral antibody plays some role in the development of acquired immunity.

Field reports in areas where malaria is endemic indicate that children produce low antibody titers in response to vaccination with tetanus toxoid. This association of immunosuppression has also been observed in experimentally induced malaria in rodents. A depression of various components of the complement system is also observed in man and animals, and it is clear that infection with this parasite results in multiple alterations in the immune system. It has been suggested that the predisposition to Burkitt's lymphoma in restricted regions of Africa may stem from these immunologic alterations seen after infection of these populations with malaria (Chapter 19).

Toxoplasma. One of the most important of the intracellular parasitic infections in the United States is toxoplasmosis. *T. gondii* is an obligate intracellular parasite that may circulate briefly in the blood in the trophozoite form. Infection of man is usually acquired by the ingestion of oocysts from cat's excreta or cysts present in inadequately cooked meat. The disease may take several forms ranging from the most common asymptomatic form to an acute syndrome representing infectious mononucleosis to a more acute disseminated infection or congenital infection. Congenital infection, the most serious form, occurs as a result of maternal infection with parasitemia and transmission of the organisms of the fetus (Fig. 17–4).

Recent studies have shown that neonates with congenital toxoplasmosis have an elevation in IgM and IgM *Toxoplasma* antibody. These infants may also exhibit other alterations in immunoglobulin development: retarded development of serum IgA and excessive production of IgM and IgG, the degree of increase of IgM and IgG possibly associated with the severity of infection. A similar elevation in levels of IgM and IgG is seen in congenital rubella, cytomegalic inclusion disease, and syphilis (Chapter 26).

There is substantial evidence that immunocompetent hosts develop immunity to toxoplasmosis and that the basis for this immunity involves both humoral and cellular components. It appears that antibody functions against extracellular organisms free in blood or extracellular fluid. Also, since the organism is killed by macrophages. and defects in

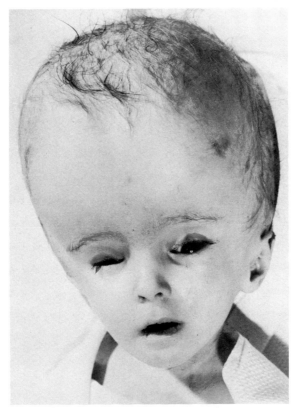

Figure 17-4. Photograph of an infant with congenital toxoplasmosis. Note extreme hydrocephalus. (Courtesy of Dr. Leon Jacobs.)

cellular immunity (as in Hodgkin's disease or following corticosteroid therapy) predispose to fatal dissemination, a role of CMI is implicated in immunity to this organism.

IMMUNITY TO METAZOA

Immediate and delayed hypersensitivity are commonly associated with helminthic parasitic infections in both man and animals. Why this group of agents so frequently stimulates these reactions is unknown. Possible explanation for this association may be related to the nature of their antigens, the chronicity of their infections, permitting persistence of antigens, or their location at mucosal membranes during either developmental or adult stages, thereby allowing the interaction of the proper receptors with the allergens. For example, there are different portals of entry for different organisms. The skin is an important and common portal of entry for some of the helminthic infections, e.g., hookworm. In others, the gastrointestinal tract assumes significance, e.g., ascariasis. The significance of this is that different routes of presentation of antigen may selectively favor the stimulation of one or another type of immune response, e.g., humoral *versus* cellular immunity, and may also influence the sequence of involvement of immunologic responses, e.g., local *versus* systemic antibody.

Intradermal tests for the immediate, delayed, and mixed reactions have been described in man for hookworm, ascariasis, dracontiasis, enterobiasis, filariasis, strongyloidiasis, trichinosis, paragonimiasis, clonorchiasis, schistosomiasis, diphyllobothriasis, echinococcosis, and taeniasis. Many of the data on hypersensitivity reactions related to helminths in humans need to be re-examined and verified, since many of the antigens used for skin testing were often inadequate in regard to their method of preparation, purity, and standardization.

Since many helminths are potent inducers of homocytotropic antibodies (e.g., IgE), and immediate hypersensitivity reactions, it is not surprising that local or systemic eosinophilia is often observed in parasitized hosts. The association of IgE and eosinophilia is well established in parasitic infections, as well as in other allergic conditions. Whether these two events are causally related or coincidental is unknown. The development of eosinophilia is most marked in helminthic infections in which developmental stages invade and migrate to tissues, e.g., ascariasis, dracontiasis, filariasis, strongyloidiasis, and trichinosis (Fig. 17–5), and often persist at high levels in man involving nonhuman helminths, e.g., *Angiostrongylus, Toxocara, Brugia, Strongyloides, Ancylostoma, Gnathostoma.* The precise role that these hypersensitivity reactions play in the acquired immunity in these diseases is not known but parasitized hosts often exhibit a variety of symptoms that may be manifestations of both immediate and delayed hypersensitivities. In the case of immediate hypersensitivity these include the urticaria, pruritus, asthma-like signs, abdominal pain, and acute diarrhea observed in ascariasis; the muscle pain, fever, rashes, and edema in trichinosis; and the urticaria, asthma-like signs, subcutaneous edema, and generalized lymphadenopathy in schistosomiasis. In the case of delayed hypersensitivity the symptoms include the formation of associated granulomas with the egg stage in schistosomiasis and capillariasis; the granulomas associated with the larval stages of *Toxocara, Trichinella,* and *Filaria;* and a component of the intestinal inflammation observed in trichinosis, trichostrongylosis, and other gastrointestinal helminthiases.

Of recent interest has been the observation that under certain experimental conditions, several helminths, i.e., *Nippostrongylus, Fasciola,* and *Trichinella,* potentiate reaginic antibody responses to nonrelated antigens. This potentiating effect by helminths may be of clinical significance in the etiology of urticaria, asthma, and other related phenomena, but further investigations need to be undertaken in human populations before these associations can be substantiated.

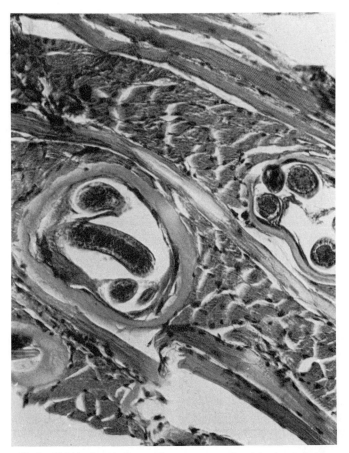

Figure 17–5. *Trichinella spiralis,* rat. Larvae encapsulated in the skeletal muscle of a rat. The intense inflammatory reaction that characterized the early stages of the infection is no longer present and has been replaced by a protective fibrous capsule, within which the larvae may remain quiescent but infective. Hematoxylin and eosin stain, × 100.

THE ROLE OF ANIMAL PARASITES IN THE IMMUNOLOGICALLY COMPROMISED HOST

Like certain fungi, bacteria, and viruses, certain parasitic agents can cause the compromised host to develop a fatal disseminated disease following infection or relapse of a latent infection. Of particular significance in this regard are *Toxoplasma gondii, Pneumocystis carinii,* and *Strongyloides stercoralis.*

Toxoplasma may persist in a latent form in many tissues in the human host. Defects in cellular immunity, in the inflammatory responses, and in antibody formation have been shown to predispose the host to disseminated *toxoplasmosis.* This predisposition has also been induced by corticosteroids in cases of *Toxoplasma* and *Strongyloides* diseases. The development of disseminated toxoplasmosis has been reported as a complication in malignant disease and organ transplantation, and is frequently associated with other opportunistic pathogens.

PNEUMOCYSTIS CARINII

Pneumocystis carinii is an example of a parasite of low-grade virulence that presents a clinical problem only in the immunologically compromised host (Chapters 14 and 22). The organism induces a pneumonitis with characteristic clinical and pathologic findings. Three groups of susceptible hosts have been defined as follows: (1) premature or debilitated infants, (2) individuals with primary immunologic deficiency disorders, and (3) individuals who have malignant disease or are receiving immunosuppressive therapy and demonstrate an immunologic deficit.

The first group is composed of premature or debilitated infants, particularly when maintained in nurseries. In this setting, the organism may be transmitted from one infected infant to other infants within the nursery. The carriers in these cases are presumed to be nursery personnel.

A second group is made up of those individuals with a basic underlying immunologic deficiency, genetic or acquired (Chapter 22). It has been observed that patients with deficient function of the thymic-dependent system, e.g., thymic dysplasia, are particularly vulnerable to this form of pneumonitis. In certain families of individuals with thymic dysplasia, all siblings have died of *Pneumocystis carinii* pneumonitis. Further immunologic imbalance in individuals with primary immunologic deficiency states may have been contributed to by the use of antibiotics.

A third group, those individuals undergoing immunosuppressive therapy or with certain malignant diseases, are also predisposed to *Pneumocystis carinii* pneumonitis. A high proportion of infections have been seen in individuals with lymphoid malignancies, especially Hodgkin's disease. The depression of lymphocyte-mediated immunity in Hodgkin's disease has been well established and points to an association between the thymic-dependent system of lymphocytes and susceptibility to *Pneumocystis carinii* pneumonitis. Of particular diagnostic value in this situation is the lymphopenia that may accompany the lymphoid malignancy.

Pneumocystis carinii pneumonitis has a characteristic clinical course. In infants and in individuals with primary immunologic deficiency diseases, the onset is insidious, with an increasing state of dyspnea and progressive cyanosis and a dry, nonproductive cough. In individuals with secondary immunologic deficiencies, such as those treated with immunosuppressive agents, the onset may be sudden and the pulmonary symptoms progressive within several days. Physical examination usually reveals rales and rhonchi and decreased breath sounds. Most remarkable is the lack of systemic reaction to this infection; many patients are usually dyspneic and cyanotic even in the absence of fever, malaise, or anorexia. The laboratory findings include the demonstration of a ventilation-perfusion deficit with a relatively normal pH and pCO_2 in the face of severe cyanosis. Pulmonary compliance is markedly decreased; low arterial oxygen saturation can be brought to near-normal levels or normal levels by high concentrations of oxygen.

The disease is mainly confined to the lungs. Although infiltration of the spleen and liver with cysts has been reported, little or no dysfunction of these tissues occurs. A severe interstitial fibrosis and a characteristic intra-alveolar exudate are the pathologic lesions induced by *Pneumocystis carinii*. The parasites are difficult to demonstrate in tissue with conventional staining, but may be readily visualized with silver impregnation techniques such as the Gomori methenamine silver stain (Fig. 17–6). The cyst is approximately one fifth the size of an erythrocyte. The double outer membrane of the cyst distinguishes it from other cells within the lung parenchyma (Fig. 17–6). The cyst can sometimes be seen in sputum specimens or tracheal washings. Since there is diffuse involvement of both lungs, an open lung biopsy and frozen section may be necessary to confirm the diagnosis. The x-ray findings parallel the pathologic process. The lung parenchyma reveals a diffuse interstitial infiltration involving the lower lung fields of the hilum (Fig.

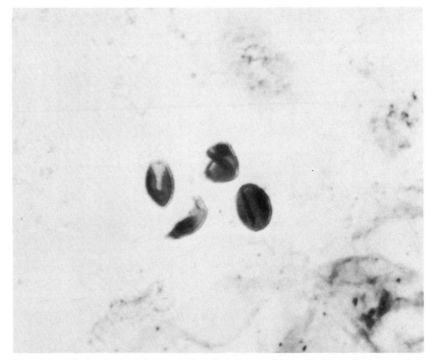

Figure 17–6. Cyst of *Pneumocystis carinii* from a frozen section of an open lung biopsy stained with Gomori's methenamine silver. The double outer membrane of the cyst helps to distinguish this structure from other cell types. Original magnification, × 930. (From Bradshaw, M., Myerowitz, R. L., Schneerson, R., Whisnant, J. K., and Robbins, J. B.: *Pneumocystis carinii* pneumonitis. Ann. Intern. Med., 73:775, 1970.)

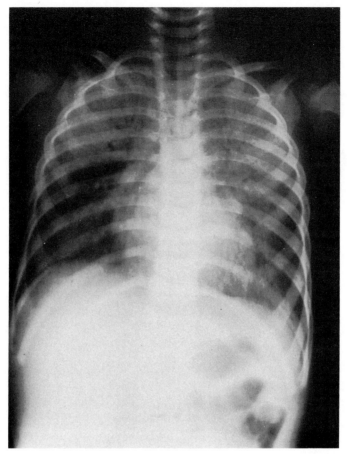

Figure 17–7.   Chest roentgenogram of a five-year-old child with *Pneumocystis carinii* pneumonitis. (From Bradshaw, M., Myerowitz, R. L., Schneerson, R., Whisnant, J. K., and Robbins, J. B.: *Pneumocystis carinii* pneumonitis. Ann. Intern. Med., *73*:775, 1970.)

17–7). Rupture of the lung parenchyma with spontaneous pneumothorax has also been reported.

Successful treatment of affected individuals with pentamidine isethionate has been reported. This drug may produce some toxic effects, particularly a bleeding diathesis secondary to a thrombocytopenia. More recently, the use of trimethoprim-sulfadiazine has been introduced; its toxicity is considerably less.

The nature of the infecting parasite is unknown. Information concerning the pathogenesis of human infection has been hampered by the inability to grow the organism *in vitro*. Very recently, an *in vitro* method has been introduced, but additional studies have not been completed. The disease may be induced in laboratory animals by treating them with immunosuppressive drugs or cytotoxic agents, e.g., cyclophosphamide. Serologic techniques for the diagnosis of the disease are hindered in humans, since most affected individuals have immunologic deficiency states and are therefore incapable of an antibody response. Since the detection of the organism in the environment is not possible, the mode of spread of this parasite in nature is unknown.

ATYPICAL PARASITISM IN MAN

It is becoming increasingly clear that even in the industrialized urban environment man is exposed to a number of zoonotic animal parasites. In 1950, the isolation of a nematode larva from the liver of a two-year-old girl with chronic eosinophilia led to the discovery that nematodes of lower vertebrates have the ability to penetrate and invade the human host. This syndrome has been termed larva migrans — the migration of larval nematodes in unsuitable hosts. Depending on the location of the migrating stages, larva migrans may be separated into three groups: cutaneous, visceral, and subcutaneous-visceral. A number of helminths have since been shown to induce this syndrome (Table 17–1); within this group, visceral infections by dog and cat ascarids of the genus *Toxocara* have received the most attention.

Patients with visceral larva migrans due to *Toxocara* show a variety of symptoms, the most significant of which are as follows: absence of ova of *Ascaris* in the feces; hypergammaglobulinemia, particularly IgM with decrease in serum albumin; increase in isohemagglutinin titer; elevated and persistent eosinophilia; splenomegaly; hepatomegaly; fever; cough; neurologic or ocular lesions, e.g., chronic endophthalmitis with retinal detachment; and granulomatosis. Previously, definitive diagnosis was made only by isolating the larvae from infected host tissue (Fig. 17–8), a procedure that is not reliable. More recently, utilizing a genus- and stage-specific antigen from *Toxocara*, an enzyme-linked immunosorbent assay (ELISA) has been developed that shows high specificity and sensitivity.

TABLE 17–1.   Agents Reported to Cause Visceral Larva Migrans

Ascaris lumbricoides
Ascaris suum
Strongyloides stercoralis
Capillaria hepatica
Gnathostoma sp.
Dirofilaria immitis
Angiostrongylus cantonensis
Toxocara canis
Toxocara cati

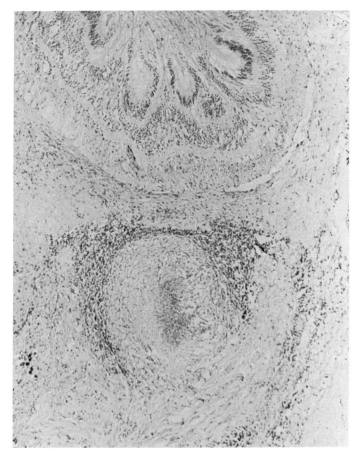

Figure 17–8. *Toxocara canis*, human. *A*, Section of retina from a child diagnosed as having retinoblastoma. Larvae of *Toxocara canis* are seen within a granuloma surrounded by lymphocytic infiltrations. Hematoxylin and eosin stain, × 44.

IMMUNOPATHOLOGIC ELEMENTS IN PARASITIC INFECTIONS

The parasitic infections represent the example *par excellence* for conditions of tissue damage by any of the four mechanisms of immunologic injury (Chapters 13 and 20). This stems, in large part, from the persistence or release of parasites or host-cell antigens during the course of infection and the relative inefficiency of the host in eliminating these antigens or cross-reacting antibodies to the host, e.g., Chagas' disease.

Certain immunologic factors have been observed in conjunction with parasitic infections that have also been associated with the development of immunopathologic phenomena in other infectious diseases. These include (1) the release of large amounts of antigen during the

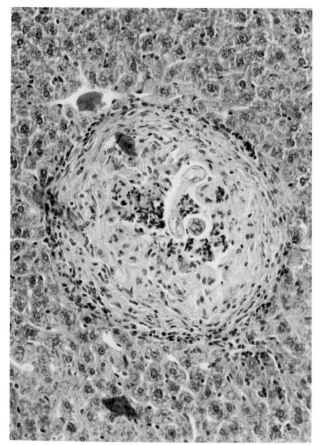

Figure 17–8. *Continued.* *B,* Section of liver from a 23-month-old child whose only clinical findings was a marked eosinophilia. Larvae of *T. canis* are seen within a granuloma surrounded by a fibrous capsule. Minimal cellular reaction surrounds the capsule. Hematoxylin and eosin stain, × 250.

course of infection; (2) the persistence of antigen in many tissues and in the circulation; (3) the alteration and destruction of host tissue; (4) the presence of antigenic components shared by the host and the parasite; and (5) the chronicity of the infections. Nevertheless, direct evidence for immunopathologic complications in many of these infections is limited and as yet not fully understood. Most of the investigations in autoimmunity in parasitic infections have been directed to malaria and trypanosomiasis, in which the presence of cold agglutinins, rheumatoid factor, antinuclear factors, and heterophil antibodies have been observed. In addition, the presence of soluble malaria antigen, the renal deposition of specific immunocomplexes, and the formation of autoantibody has been observed in malaria patients. In the case of schistosomiasis mansoni and japonica, both experimental studies in animals and observations of natural infections in humans support the concept of immune complexes in the pathogeneses of schistosomal renal disease. Other parasitic diseases in which autoimmune factors are suspected are filariasis and ascariasis.

SUGGESTIONS FOR FURTHER READING

Brown, I.N.: Immunological aspects of malaria infection. Adv. Immunol., *11*:267–340, 1969.

Hudson, R. J.: Moderated immunologic responsiveness in parasitic infections. Adv. Vet. Sci. Comp. Med., *17*:87–117, 1973.

Larsh, J. E., Jr., and N. F. Weatherly: Cell-mediated immunity in certain parasitic infections. Curr. Top. Microbiol. Immunol., *67*:113–37, 1974.

Marcial-Rojas, R. A., ed.: Pathology of Protozoal and Helminthic Disease. Baltimore, Williams & Wilkins Co., 1971.

Ogilvie, B. M., and V. E. Jones.: Immunity in the parasitic relationship between helminths and hosts. Progr. Allergy, *17*:93–144, 1973.

Pifer, L. L., Hughes, W. T., and Murphy, M. J.: Propagation of *Pneumocystis carinii in vitro*. Pediatr. Res., *11*:317, 1977.

Smithers, S. R.: Recent advances in the immunology of schistosomiasis. Br. Med. Bull., *28*:49–54, 1972.

Soulsby, E. J. L., ed.: Immunity to Animal Parasites. New York, Academic Press, 1971.

Symposium on toxoplasmosis. Bull. N. Y. Acad. Med., *50*:107–240, 1974.

Turk, J. L., and Bryceson A. D. M.: Immunological phenomena in leprosy and related diseases. Adv. Immunol., *13*:209–261, 1971.

MECHANISMS OF IMMUNITY TO FUNGAL DISEASES

Joseph A. Bellanti, M.D.

Fungi are a class of infectious agents that have classically been regarded as "plantlike" in their organization and structure. One of the outstanding properties of most of the pathogenic fungi, which is not shared by any of the other microorganisms, is the ability to exist in nature as a branching, twiglike structure (vegetative or a mold form) and in the tissues of the host as a unicellular, oval, or spheric form (the yeast phase). This property, termed dimorphism, is one of several properties of fungi that differentiate them from bacteria.

The effects of fungi on man have been both beneficial and harmful. As a class of microorganisms, they have a diverse number of properties that are beneficial to man, including their role in fermentation reactions and their biosynthetic capability in the production of antibiotics and in maintaining the geochemical structure of the earth's soil. Their pathogenic relationship to man, however, often poses serious problems for the physician. In this chapter we shall focus on the host defense mechanisms involved in the immunity to fungus infections.

In contrast to his success with bacteria, parasites, and some viruses, which have been controlled by chemotherapy, immunization, and public health measures, man has shown a notable lack of success in removing fungal pathogens from his environment. In fact, with the advent of chemotherapy for bacterial diseases there has been a change in the flora within the host, resulting in some cases in fungal overgrowth. The fungi present a second problem to the physician because of the limited number of therapeutic measures available for the treatment of fungal diseases. Thus, in spite of the widespread prevalence and occurrence of fungi, the mechanisms of immunity to them have been only recently elucidated, and considerably less is known of fungal immunology than of viral or bacterial immunology.

PATHOGENESIS OF FUNGAL DISEASES

In order to understand the mechanisms of immunity involved in fungal diseases, it is necessary first to describe the various types of interaction that a fungus can have with a host. The eventual outcome of such an interaction will depend upon (1) the properties of the fungus and (2) the status of the host in which the interaction occurs.

LOCALIZED VERSUS GENERALIZED INFECTION

The properties of fungi that are important in pathogenicity include their ability to establish localized infection at the portal of entry and their ability to become invasive and establish generalized infection. Examples of localized infection include those fungal infections restricted to body surfaces, such as those caused by the *Candida* or the dermatophytes. Fungal infections of a more generalized nature include histoplasmosis, coccidioidomycosis, and blastomycosis. Certain fungi have a polysaccharide capsule that may be of importance in resisting phagocytosis in a manner similar to that described for the encapsulated bacteria (Chapter 15).

ACUTE VERSUS CHRONIC INFECTION

A second important consideration in the pathogenesis of fungal infections is whether a disease is *acute* or *chronic*. The chronicity reflects adaptation of the fungus to its host. Those fungal infections that are characterized by the initiation of an acute inflammatory process have been most responsive to disposal by the host's immune mechanisms and also to treatment; those that establish quiet residence with minimal tissue damage are most apt to continue as parasites in man. In general, if the defense mechanisms of the host are adequate to resist the initial attack by fungus, the disease will be acute and self-limiting. If, on the other hand, the nature of the virulence factors of the organism or the size of the initial inoculum can overwhelm the host defense factors, or if the defense mechanisms are incompletely developed or suppressed, then the eventual outcome will be unfavorable for the host and will lead to chronic systemic, and sometimes fatal, infection. With the development of chronic infection, there is development of a prominent delayed hypersensitivity with granuloma formation.

EFFECT OF ENVIRONMENTAL FACTORS

Environmental conditions affect the host fungus relationship. For example, the aridness of the western United States is associated with high incidence of fungal diseases such as coccidioidomycosis (San

Joaquin fever). It seems that the immune system of otherwise normal individuals is ineffective under these conditions. It may be related to either a high concentration of pathogen in these areas or diminished efficiency of the nonspecific immune responses in the host. A pathogen in high enough concentration can overwhelm the defense mechanisms of the normal host. Other types of fungal infections are more commonly seen with different environmental conditions, such as occupations in which the skin is subjected to immersion in water, predisposing the host to superficial fungal infections of the skin. These two examples illustrate the effect of the external environment on the host-parasite relationship involved in fungal infections.

CLASSIFICATION OF FUNGAL DISEASES

The various types of fungal diseases, the mycoses, may be classified according to the following types: (1) opportunistic, (2) cutaneous, (3) subcutaneous, and (4) systemic (Table 18–1).

OPPORTUNISTIC FUNGI

Perhaps the most common of the fungi infecting man are the so-called opportunistic fungi (Table 18–1). These fungi are normally non-pathogenic in healthy humans but may behave as virulent organisms in

TABLE 18–1. Types of Mycotic Diseases of Man Caused by the Pathogenic Fungi

TYPE OF MYCOTIC DISEASE	FUNGUS	PORTAL OF ENTRY	TYPE OF DISEASE
Opportunistic	*Candida albicans, Aspergillus* spp., *Phycomycetes (Mucor, Rhizopus)*	Mucous membranes, skin and respiratory tract	Thrush, vulvovaginitis, pneumonitis
Cutaneous	*Microsporum, Trichophyton, Epidermophyton*	Skin, hair, and nails	Tinea corporis, tinea capitis, onychomycosis
Subcutaneous	*Sporotrichum schenckii*	Break in skin and lymphatics	Ulcerating nodular abscess with lymphangitic spread
Systemic	*Cryptococcus neoformans Coccidioides immitis Histoplasma capsulatum Blastomyces dermatitidis*	Respiratory tract, skin	Pneumonia, skin, CNS, or other systemic involvement

individuals with depressed immune function—the newborn, patients with lymphoreticular malignancy, patients receiving immunosuppressive therapy, or patients in other clinical situations, e.g., diabetes or the use of broad-spectrum antibiotics. The fungi included in this group are the *Candida, Aspergillus,* and *Phycomycetes.* Under circumstances in which either nonspecific or specific factors are depressed, these fungi may establish a variety of localized or generalized, acute or chronic types of infection (Fig. 18–1). Of these, *Candida* is the most common and the

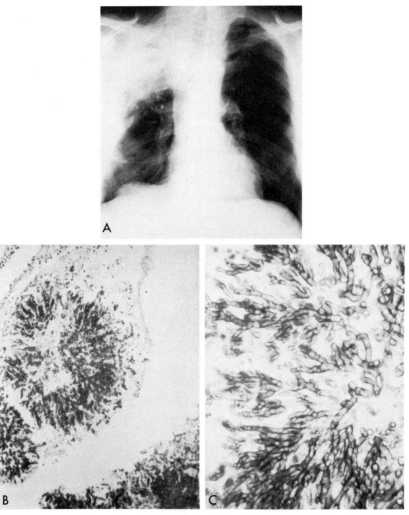

Figure 18–1. Aspergillus infection in a 57-year-old male with bronchogenic carcinoma. *A,* X-ray of chest showing area of increased density in right upper lobe. *B,* Section of lung showing hyphae of *Aspergillus fumigatus* in the wall of a pulmonary abscess. Hematoxylin and eosin stain, ×100. *C,* Same section of lung as shown in *B,* photographed under increased magnification, ×600. (Courtesy of Dr. John Guerrant.).

most important of the opportunistic fungi pathogenic for man. This organism inhabits the normal mucous membranes of the mouth, vagina, and intestinal tract. Thrush and vaginitis are examples of infections of the mucous membranes caused by *Candida*. Thrush, a localized infection of the mucous membranes of the mouth and pharynx consists of discrete whitish patches, is seen during the early newborn period and in young infants, and is presumably acquired by passage through the birth canal. It is also seen in individuals receiving broad-spectrum antibiotics or with depressed specific immunity, such as in patients receiving immunosuppressive therapy. A second type of involvement of the mucous membrane is vulvovaginitis. This infection affects the mucous membranes of the female genital tract, consists of whitish patches, and is usually associated with or occurs during pregnancy or diabetes. It is to be stressed once again that the pattern of disease cannot be described merely as a function of the pathogen but rather must be viewed in total perspective with the host response.

These opportunistic fungal infections may be acute and self-limited or chronic and occasionally disseminated, particularly in very immature infants or individuals with severely depressed immune functions. These opportunistic fungi may become invasive and involve virtually every tissue of the body. A particular form of candidiasis is seen in children with immune deficiency diseases involving the thymic-dependent tissues (Chapter 22). This is associated with a chronic form of mucocutaneous candidiasis, involving the mucous membranes of the mouth, the respiratory and gastrointestinal tracts, and the skin and the nails, that is often serious and life-threatening. This presenting clinical picture is so common that if candidiasis is seen beyond the newborn period in individuals not receiving antibiotics a diligent search should be made for diseases of the lymphoproliferative system or for an immunologic deficiency, particularly of the thymic-dependent limb of immunity.

Another type of involvement with these opportunistic fungi is seen in clinical situations in which prosthetic valves or devices are used in the human, e.g., the use of cardiac valves or ventricular valves in the treatment of hydrocephalus. These prostheses act as foci of infection and, since they are avascular, are not accessible to the normal clearing mechanisms available to the host, i.e., phagocytosis.

CUTANEOUS FUNGI

A second type of infection produced by fungi involves the epidermis and its appendages (hair and nails). These infections are referred to as the *dermatomycoses;* the fungi responsible for these infections are referred to as dermatophytes (Table 18–1). Included within this group are members of the following genera: *Microsporum, Tricophyton,* and *Epidermophyton.* These fungi have a predilection for keratin-rich tissues such as the skin, hair, and nails. They appear to have the capacity to degrade keratin and use its breakdown products as a nutritional source.

These fungi can produce infections of the scalp (tinea capitis), of the skin (tinea corporis), or of the nails (onychomycosis) (Table 18–1). Infection of the scalp due to *Microsporum canis* or *Microsporum audouini* occurs most frequently in childhood. Conversely, infection of the skin (e.g., athlete's foot) very rarely occurs in children and is more commonly seen in adults. The immunity mechanisms controlling these types of infection are poorly understood but appear to involve both nonspecific and specific immunologic events. For example, the resistance of adults to ringworm of the scalp has been attributed mainly to the increase in secretion of saturated fatty acids with antifungal activity at puberty. The increased susceptibility of adults to infection of the skin may be related to factors that promote fungal growth, e.g., excessive sweating (hyperhidrosis).

Immunity cannot always be explained in terms of classic specific immunologic reactions. Although fungistatic factors have been noted in the sera of individuals with and without infection, they are not associated with the immunoglobulins. Cell-mediated immunity appears to be an important immunity mechanism during the course of most fungal infections. Since antibody occurs in individuals with and without an infection, antibody determinations offer little diagnostic or prognostic value. Certain localized manifestations of the skin occur during the course of fungal infections and are referred to as "id" reactions. The mechanism of these reactions is one of delayed hypersensitivity. The role of these reactions in immunity is unclear.

SUBCUTANEOUS FUNGI

A third type of infection caused by fungi is the *subcutaneous* type of infection. An example of these fungi is *Sporotrichum*. They are distributed in soil and on plants and are introduced into the body by penetration of the skin with contaminated splinters, thorns, and soil. Once established, infections tend to be localized in subcutaneous tissues and become associated with chronic draining ulcerated lesions. There may be involvement of the regional lymph nodes and, occasionally, systemic spread. Immunity mechanisms appear to include nonspecific and specific antibody and cell-mediated factors.

SYSTEMIC FUNGI

The systemic mycoses, the fourth type of infection caused by fungi, are the most serious. Fungal infections of this type include cryptococcosis, coccidioidomycosis, histoplasmosis, and blastomycosis (Table 18–1). Specific immune responses are stimulated in these diseases and

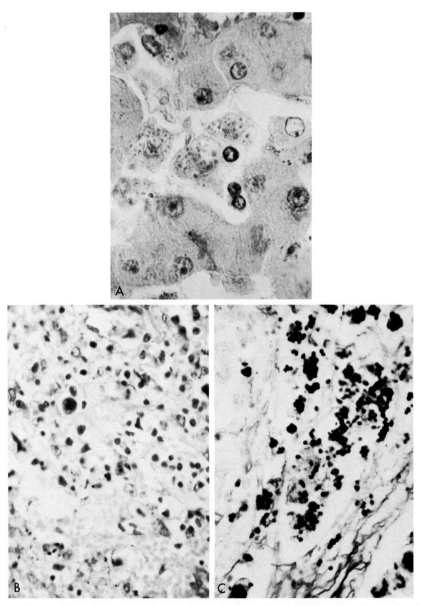

Figure 18–2. Disseminated histoplasmosis in a 60-year-old male who died of myeloid metaplasia. *A*, Section of liver showing the *Histoplasma capsulatum* within Kupffer cells. Hematoxylin and eosin stain, ×600. *B*, Section of spleen showing *Histoplasma capsulatum* within macrophages. Hematoxylin and eosin stain, ×100. *C*, Section of lymph node showing *Histoplasma capsulatum* in tissue. Silver methenamine stain. ×100. (Courtesy of Dr. Daniel Mohler.)

appear to be important mechanisms of resistance. Thus, the development of serum antibody, including precipitins, agglutinins, and complement-fixing antibodies, offers both diagnostic and prognostic value.

The pathogenesis of these infections usually invokes entry of the pathogen by inhalation into the respiratory tract or by introduction through a break in the skin (Fig. 18–2). Following a limited replication at a local site, the organism may be removed by nonspecific factors (macrophages) in which it may persist for long periods of time. Following infection, an inflammatory response characterized by granuloma formation is seen (Chapter 12). In many of the infections, such as histoplasmosis, liquefaction (caseous) necrosis may develop and recovery may be associated with roentgenographic evidence of calcification.

In addition, cell-mediated immunity (delayed hypersensitivity) may develop. Thus, the injection of purified blastomycin, coccidioidin, or histoplasmin is associated with the development of a cutaneous delayed-hypersensitivity reaction. The effector mechanisms by which these cell-mediated events effect recovery have been described (Chapter 9). These cell-mediated responses also offer important diagnostic aid.

WORKING HYPOTHESIS OF THE ROLES OF THE VARIOUS ELEMENTS OF THE IMMUNE RESPONSE DURING FUNGAL INFECTIONS

Starting with a nonimmune susceptible host, a primary encounter with fungus would be countered by the nonspecific barrier presented by the intact skin and mucous membranes. If these are surmounted, the next barriers encountered are the nonspecific humoral factors, such as antifungal properties of sebum. If these are overcome, an infection may be initiated. This might take the form of a *localized* infection, e.g., thrush; or it may be more extensive, as in the case of cutaneous and subcutaneous infections; or it may be even more extensive, with systemic involvement. The pulmonary lesions of systemic infections may be localized within macrophages, e.g., granuloma formation. If these barriers are not effective, however, there may be widespread generalized dissemination of the fungus to deep-seated organs, such as the brain. In all these host-fungus interactions, but particularly in the case of the more extensive infections, there are stimulated specific immunologic factors consisting of antibody and delayed hypersensitivity. The precise role of these specific factors in the recovery of these infections is unclear. Cell-mediated immunity, however, appears to be an important effector mechanism in these deep-seated chronic infections and probably exerts its effect by the same interactions with macrophages as described for bacterial diseases (Chapter 15).

CLINICAL STATES IN WHICH ABERRATION OF THE IMMUNE RESPONSE LEAD TO PREDISPOSITION TO FUNGAL INFECTIONS

TRAUMA

Trauma appears to be a predisposing condition in the successful establishment of many fungal infections, especially those of the chronic granulomatous type. Trauma to either the mucous membranes or the skin provides a portal of entry for fungi.

AGE

The very young and the very old are predisposed to fungal infections, particularly the opportunistic fungi, presumably owing to either immaturity or senescence of the immune system. In the case of infants, infections are usually self-limited and disappear as the child grows. Whereas most adults possess agglutinins and delayed-hypersensitivity reactions to *Candida,* the neonate usually manifests neither. The development of both antibody and delayed hypersensitivity occurs with maturation because of an exposure to these pathogens.

METABOLIC STATES

Many types of metabolic derangements, including diabetes and pregnancy, are associated with overgrowth of fungi. The precise role of the metabolic derangement is incompletely understood but might be related to enhanced growth as a result of increased glucose in extracellular fluids.

TREATMENT WITH ANTIBIOTICS OR IMMUNOSUPPRESSIVE AGENTS

The overgrowth of fungi is widely known to occur during the course of treatment with broad-spectrum antibiotics, wherein the ecologic balance of microbial growth is disturbed. The opportunistic fungi are usually involved in these interactions. As described earlier, the specific defects of the immunologic system, particularly those involving the thymic-dependent system, may present with overwhelming fungal infections, e.g., mucocutaneous candidiasis. Patients receiving immunosuppressive therapy, e.g., metabolites or steroids, or with lymphoproliferative diseases, e.g., leukemia or lymphomas, may also present with these fungal infections. Therefore, with any patient who develops fungal infection, these factors should be taken into consideration and a diligent search made for underlying diseases.

CLINICAL CONDITIONS THAT RESULT FROM HYPERSENSITIVITY TO FUNGI

There are three probable outcomes that result from the interaction between the host immune response and fungus. The degree to which fungal antigen persists or is reintroduced will determine the expression of the host's reaction. If fungal antigen is successfully eliminated by the inflammatory response and phagocytosis, or if a specific immune response is stimulated with the development of delayed hypersensitivity and antibody, then no further host interaction is seen. If the fungus is not successfully eliminated or is reintroduced in either a live or killed form, the persistence of fungal antigen causes further host interaction. For example, if the IgE reagins are stimulated, the patient could express symptoms of asthma (Type I reaction). If precipitating antibody is stimulated and fungal antigen is reintroduced via the respiratory tract, antigen-antibody complexes might result and could be associated with such diseases as farmer's lung (Type III reaction); the persistence of fungal antigen could also result in granuloma formation, with the development of delayed hypersensitivity locally or at distal sites in the skin, e.g., "id" reactions (Type IV reaction).

SUMMARY

The immune mechanisms displayed by the host in antifungal defense are best viewed according to the type of fungal infection that occurs: (1) opportunistic, (2) cutaneous, (3) subcutaneous, and (4) systemic. The fungal pathogens as a group evoke both nonspecific and specific factors of immunity, and the participation of these various factors is directly correlated with the degree of penetration of the fungus into the host. Cell-mediated immunity (delayed hypersensitivity) appears to be a most important defense mechanism in most types of fungal infections. Congenital or iatrogenic depression of the immune function predisposes the host to fungal infections.

SUGGESTIONS FOR FURTHER READING

Burnet, J. H.: Fundamentals of Mycology. London, Edward Arnold (Publishers) Ltd., 1968.

Chandler, J. W., Smith, T. K., Newberry, W. M., Jr., Chin, T. D. Y., and Kirkpatrick, C. H.: Immunology of the mycoses. II. Characterization of the immunoglobulin and antibody responses in histoplasmosis. J. Infect. Dis., *119*:247, 1969.

Conant, N. F., Smith, D. T., Baker, R. D., Callaway, J. L., and Martin, D. S.: Manual of Clinical Mycology. 3rd ed. Philadelphia, W. B. Saunders Company, 1971.

Davis, B. D., Dulbecco, R., Eisen, H. A., Ginsberg, H. S., and Wood, W. B., Jr.: Microbiology. 2nd ed. New York, Harper & Row, Publishers, 1973.

Kirkpatrick, C. H., Chandler, J. W., and Schimke, R. N.: Chronic mucocutaneous moniliasis with impaired delayed hypersensitivity. Clin. Exp. Immunol., *6*:375, 1970.

Kirkpatrick, C. H., Rich, R. R., and Bennett, J. E.: Chronic mucocutaneous candidiasis: Model building in cellular immunity. Ann. Intern. Med., *74*:955, 1971.

Newberry, W. M., Jr., Chandler, J. W., Chin, T. D. Y., and Kirkpatrick, C. H.: Immunology of the mycoses. I. Depressed lymphocyte transformation in chronic histoplasmosis. J. Immunol., *100*:436, 1968.

Pepys, J.: Hypersensitivity Diseases of the Lungs Due to Fungi and Organic Dusts. Monographs in Allergy. Vol. 4. Basel and New York, S. Karger, 1969.

Sawaki, Y., Huppert, M., Bailey, J. W., and Yagi, Y.: Patterns of human antibody reactions in coccidiodomycosis. J. Bacteriol., *91*:422, 1966.

IMMUNE DEFENSE MECHANISMS IN TUMOR IMMUNITY

W. T. Kniker, M.D.,
and Joseph A. Bellanti, M.D.

An aberration or imbalance in the surveillance mechanisms of the host immune system is now believed to be involved in the development of neoplasms. Such an association has been investigated in animals for many decades and may be applicable to man. A tumor cell, either transplanted or induced, represents a foreign configuration to the host in which it arises. The immune mechanisms operable against tumor cells are the same as those marshaled in response to any other foreign configuration.

Most of the responses in tumor antigenicity and in specific tumor immunity closely resemble those that apply to allograft rejection phenomena involving relatively weak transplantation antigen systems. Antigens arise in many tumors as a consequence of the neoplastic change and are specific for each tumor or group of tumors. These antigens are referred to as tumor-specific transplantation antigens (TSTA) or tumor-specific antigens (TSA). They are cell-surface antigens and evoke a specific immune response when injected into an appropriate host. The implication of these findings is that the origins of these newly acquired antigens are influenced by the oncogenic agent. The antigens are under genetic control and are transmitted to the descendants of these altered tumor cells. A knowledge of them may allow for their ultimate utilization in the diagnosis and treatment of certain human neoplasms.

The recent widespread use of immunosuppressive agents in graft recipients has been associated with an increased incidence in malignant disorders after organ transplantation. In addition, accumulated data have shown that children with immunologic deficiency diseases have an increased risk of neoplasia (Chapter 22). This increased incidence is shown in Table 19–1.

448

TABLE 19–1.   Evidence of Malignancy in Primary Immunodeficiency Syndromes*

Disease	Incidence	Estimated Risk
Congenital X-linked immunodeficiency	6/approx. 100	6%
Severe combined system immunodeficiency	9/approx. 400	2%
IgM deficiency	6/approx. 70	8%
Wiskott-Aldrich syndrome	24/approx. 300	8%
Ataxia-telangiectasia	52/approx. 500	10%
Common variable immunodeficiency	41/approx. 500	8%
Total	138/approx. 1870	7%

*From Kersey, J. H., Spector, B. D., and Good, R. A.: Primary immunodeficiency diseases and cancer: the immunodeficiency-cancer registry. Int. J. Cancer, *12*:333–47, 1973.

THE CONCEPT OF TUMOR ANTIGENICITY

During the early part of this century, many attempts were made to develop a "cancer vaccine." These efforts, using outbred strains of animals, met with almost uniform failure because of the histocompatibility differences, which were unknown at that time. By using a genetic approach with inbred animal strains that are histocompatible, the activity of tumor-specific antigens (TSA) could be studied. Such techniques have made it possible to identify the host reaction to tumor-specific antigens.

RESPONSES TO ALLOGENEIC TUMOR TRANSPLANTATION

In two dissimilar individuals, the transplantation of tumor tissue can have one of three outcomes: (1) *rejection* due to incompatibility, (2) *acceptance* and growth (*enhancement*) of the tumor transplant or (3) inhibition due to a nonspecific tumor cytolytic effect (*allogeneic inhibition*). These are shown schematically in Figure 19–1.

With the first outcome, if a normal tissue, such as skin, were transplanted between two genetically dissimilar animals, A and B, the graft would be rejected as a result of the dissimilarity of the normal transplantation antigens (Chapter 3). If tumor cells were transplanted from A to B, the graft would be rejected owing to two types of incom-

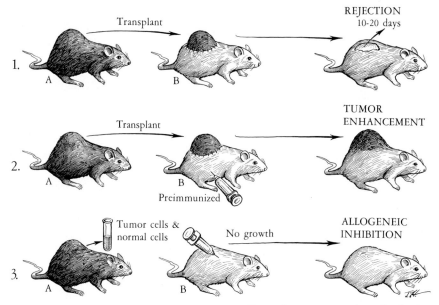

Figure 19–1. Types of responses seen after allogeneic tumor transplantation in the mouse.

patibility: (1) that due to the dissimilarity of natural histocompatibility antigens and (2) that due to the tumor graft itself, which contains unique tumor-specific antigens (TSA) foreign to the recipient host. In both cases, the graft would be promptly rejected because of tissue incompatibility.

A paradoxical effect is seen in the second outcome, in which animal B is *preimmunized* to the tumor antigens either actively or passively (Fig. 19–1). The net effect is one of increased tumor growth, or enhancement. Two mechanisms have been proposed to explain this anomalous effect: (1) the antibody may combine with the tumor antigens before reaching a lymph node, thereby preventing an immune response (afferent blockade), or (2) the antigen-combining sites on the tumor may be masked by being coated with antibody (efferent blockade) (Chapter 24). Preimmunization does not always cause tumor enhancement, however; in some cases, tumor growth is delayed and animals are protected. Apparently the quality of immunity in the sensitized animals and the relative dose of transplanted tumor cells determine the outcome.

A completely nonspecific consequence of tumor transplantation between two dissimilar hosts is seen in the third outcome (Fig. 19–1). Mixing of tumor cells with normal cells prior to tumor implantation results in tumor cell destruction or inhibition. This phenomenon, referred to as allogeneic inhibition, is believed to represent a reaction between dissimilar cell surfaces.

RESPONSES TO SYNGENEIC TUMOR TRANSPLANTATION

In contrast to the responses seen between allogeneic hosts, syngeneic hosts provide genetic similarity so that the effects of the tumor-specific antigens are their major differences. These models have provided useful information concerning tumor antigens. Despite the fact that such genetic models provide information concerning TSA, the physician should be aware that in patients the allogeneic effects are the rule.

Although spontaneous tumors with no known etiology may arise in man and in animals, there are two experimentally induced groups that may serve as models for malignant tumors in man (Table 19–2).

Methylcholanthrene (MCA) produces tumors that are representative of those induced by chemical and physical agents. These agents induce unique tumor-specific antigens. Regardless of morphologic similarity, each new tumor induced by the same agent possesses a TSA specificity unique for each tumor (Fig. 19–2). Thus, resistance to one chemically induced tumor does not prevent growth of a second tumor induced by a different chemical, even though the two tumors may be morphologically identical. The strength of the tumor-specific antigens on the cell surface is thought to be directly related to the length of the latent period between the application of the oncogen and the development of the tumor—the shorter the latent period, the greater, in general, the strength of the antigen. The mechanism for emergence of the unique TSA is unknown but has been postulated to be related to derepression of DNA (Fig. 19–3). Supporting this hypothesis are the cross-reactions seen between certain tumors and embryonic tissues. Such cross-reaction with fetal tissues has been observed in patients with carcinoma of the colon (carcinoembryonic antigen) or of the liver (α-fetoprotein).

In contrast, these characteristics differ from those seen in tumors induced by viruses (Fig. 19–4). The virus-induced tumors have antigens that cross-react even though morphologic appearance differs. Such cross-reactivity, shared by both DNA and RNA viruses, is presumably due to the ability of viral nucleic acid to be incorporated into the genetic material of the host. In spite of the cross-reactivity, there are fundamental differences in the ability of viruses to induce tumors (Fig. 19–5). The DNA viruses produce an *integrated infection* through which the host cell's properties are transformed; however, cell growth persists in the absence of fully infectious virus (Chapter 16). From within the cell, the virus specifies the production of unique transplantation antigens on the cell surface, as well as the production of other virus-specific antigens (Fig. 19–5).

The integrated type of infection is not seen in hosts normally infected with the virus; it is seen only in an unnatural host (e.g., newborn) to which it is artificially transmitted. For example, the SV-40

TABLE 19–2.   Types and Antigenic Characteristics of Tumor Formation

Group	Example of Agent	Type of Tumor Induced	Antigenic Specificity (TSTA)	Result of Primary Infection or Exposure		
				In Newborn	*In Adult*	*In Adult Thymectomized as Newborn*
Chemical or physical agents	Methylcholanthrene (MCA)	Sarcoma Leukemia Carcinoma	Individual for each tumor	Tumors after maturity; no tolerance	Solid immunity	Increased tumor incidence
Viruses DNA viruses	Polyoma SV-40 Adenoviruses	Heterogeneous Sarcoma Undifferentiated sarcomas	Cross-react within group	Tumors after maturity; no tolerance	Solid immunity	
RNA viruses	Rous sarcoma virus (RSV) and avian leukosis viruses	Avian leukemia and sarcoma	Cross-react within group, generally	Tumors after maturity; no primary response; animals can be immunized	Not susceptible to infection	
	Murine-leukemia-sarcoma complex (Friend, Maloney, Rauscher [FMR], and Gross*)	Murine leukemia, sarcoma	Cross-react within group but also TSA specificity	Tumors after maturity;* tolerance	Solid immunity	Leukemia prevented when infected in newborn
	Mammary agents	Mammary carcinoma	Cross-react within group but also TSA specificity	Tumors after maturity; tolerance	Solid immunity	
Spontaneous	Unknown	Many types	Individual for each tumor	Unknown	Unknown	Unknown

*Gross virus capable of inducing tumors in newborn; virus contains type-specific antigens.

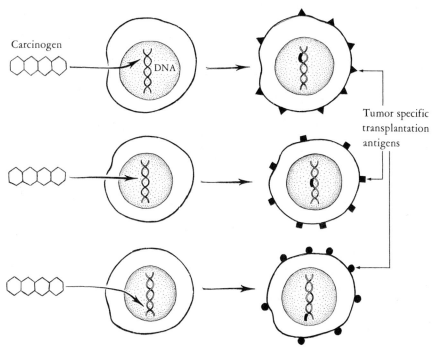

Figure 19-2. Schematic representation of development of tumor antigens by a chemical carcinogen. Note that when cells of identical genetic identity are transformed by the same chemical carcinogen, each new tumor has its own unique antigenic specificity regardless of morphologic appearance.

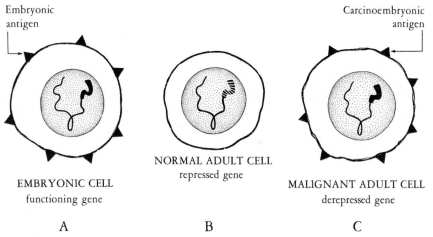

Figure 19-3. Postulated mechanism of emergence of carcinoembryonic antigens. *A*, A normal embryonic antigen produced by a functioning gene within an embryonic cell. *B*, Repression of the gene (*dotted line*) with no further elaboration of the embryonic antigen in the adult cell. *C*, Derepression of the gene in the malignant cell with reappearance of the embryonic antigen (carcinoembryonic antigen) on the surface of the cell.

virus normally infects monkeys and results in an inapparent or respiratory infection. When this virus is transferred to the newborn hamster, however, sarcoma develops in the absence of its usual disease expression. Since the virus seems to be restricted to the nucleus, there is no shedding of infectious virus and consequently no development of a state of tolerance (Chapter 10). As the newborn develops, there is an increased incidence of tumor with little demonstrable evidence of antibody formation. In adult animals, however, the DNA-virus infections lead to a state of immunity, with elimination of virus and no evidence of tumor formation. Adults previously thymectomized during the neonatal period show an increased tumor incidence when infected during adult life. The implication of this model for the physician is the possibility that other species could transmit viruses to man, particularly *in utero* or during the neonatal period, with such aberrant effects of viral infection as malignant tumors. Such a relationship of "horizontal transmission" has been suggested between the feline viruses and human leukemia.

The pathogenesis of malignant disorders in the case of the RNA viruses appears to be quite different. With the notable exception of RSV, RNA viruses produce steady-state infections (Chapter 16). The maturation of these lipid-rich viruses occurs at cell surfaces, where they are extruded by "budding" (Fig. 19–5). These viruses are fully infectious and are acquired congenitally by "vertical transmission"; they freely circulate and produce a state of tolerance (Chapter 10). In con-

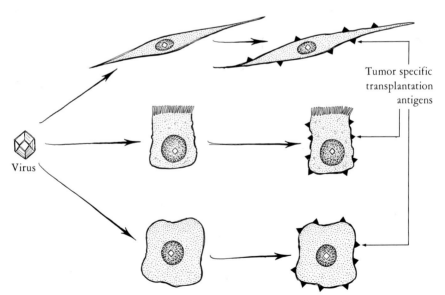

Figure 19–4. Schematic representation of the development of tumor-specific antigens (TSA) by a tumor virus. Note that although the morphologic appearance may vary, each tumor induced by a single virus contains the same TSA on the cell surface.

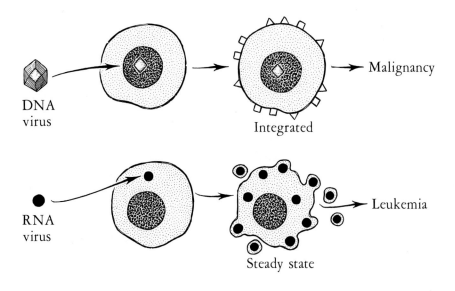

DNA
virus

Integrated

Malignancy

RNA
virus

Steady state

Leukemia

Fully infectious DNA virus

Portion of DNA virus incorporated
in nucleic acid of cell

Virus specific antigen

Tumor specific transplantation antigen (TSTA)

RNA virus prior to release

Fully infectious RNA virus with
incorporated cell membrane

Figure 19–5.   Schematic representation of the types of tumors seen in response to oncogenic viruses.

trast to the DNA viruses, they produce in their natural hosts a high level of viremia that is sustained. Thus, the steady-state viruses show the criteria for the induction of tolerance as follows: (1) a high-dose inoculum of viral antigen, (2) the persistence of virus-specific antigen, and (3) the development and persistence of tumor-specific antigens. Infection of adults who have a fully developed immunologic system results in active immunity, elimination of virus, and a reduced incidence of tumor formation. In contrast to the response to DNA viruses, adults previously thymectomized in neonatal life show a decreased tumor incidence when infected with RNA viruses during adult life.

Huebner has suggested an hypothesis by which RNA viruses can be carried in the genetic material of the host. In this model, an RNA virus ("oncogene") infects the cell and becomes integrated into the host's DNA. Either spontaneously or after activation by a variety of environmental stimuli (e.g., radiation and carcinogenic chemicals), the virus expresses itself, and tumor formation may ensue. Animal RNA tumor viruses are able to reverse the normal flow of transmission of genetic information from DNA to RNA to protein by using an enzyme to produce DNA from RNA messenger molecules. The enzyme is an

RNA-dependent DNA polymerase and is also called reverse transcriptase. The fact that high levels of reverse transcriptase activity have been found in human leukemia cells and other neoplastic cells suggests associated RNA viruses. This finding is not unique to neoplasia; elevated enzyme activity can also be found in embryonic tissues, normal cells, and cells injected with nononcogenic tumor viruses.

EVIDENCE FOR VIRUS INVOLVEMENT IN HUMAN ONCOGENESIS

No virus has as yet been proved to be the etiologic agent causing any human cancer, although several viruses from human and animal sources have oncogenic abilities in laboratory animals. Recent demonstration of C-type particles in human and nonhuman primate placentas suggests the presence of vertically transmitted potentially oncogenic RNA viruses. A viral etiology in sarcomas is strongly suggested by the finding of common antigens in a wide variety of sarcomas. Antibodies to the common antigens are found in 80 per cent of patients with sarcoma and 25 per cent of their close relatives, an incidence far greater than that in normal individuals or patients with other forms of cancer. Although elevated levels of antibody to herpesvirus hominis type 2 in women with cervical cancer suggest an etiologic association, the evidence remains circumstantial.

BURKITT'S LYMPHOMA

Burkitt's lymphoma provides the most suggestive evidence for a human malignancy of viral etiology. The disease was first described by Burkitt in 1958 as a multiple visceral and jaw tumor in children who lived in restricted areas of Africa (Fig. 19–6). Since then, Burkitt's lymphoma has been reported in other parts of the world, including North America.

Evidence has been obtained for a viral etiology of the tumor by the demonstration of membrane-bound virus particles (Epstein-Barr or EB particles) in tissue culture cells derived from tumor biopsy material (Fig. 19–7). The evidence suggests that it is a DNA virus of the herpes group (Chapter 16). In many ways, this virus–host cell interaction resembles an integrated infection.

Serologic studies have revealed a high incidence of EB antibody in the sera of normal American children (35 per cent) and adults (85 per cent), as demonstrated by immunofluorescence. These data suggest that either the same virus or a similar one is occurring with a high frequency in the United States. Of African patients with Burkitt's lymphoma, close to 100 per cent have high serum titers of antibody to the EB virus. In the United States, a similar frequency of EB antibody has been detected among patients with nasopharyngeal carcinoma.

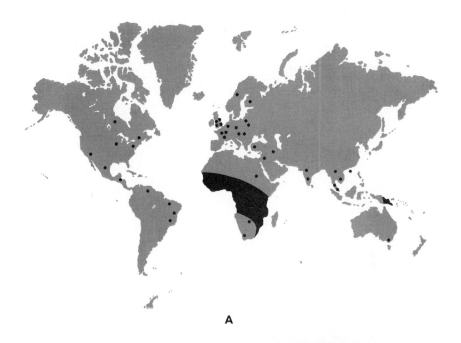

A

Figure 19-6. *A*, Map of world showing worldwide distribution of Burkitt's lymphoma. *B*, Photograph of a seven year old boy with Burkitt's lymphoma of the mandible. (Courtesy of National Institutes of Health.)

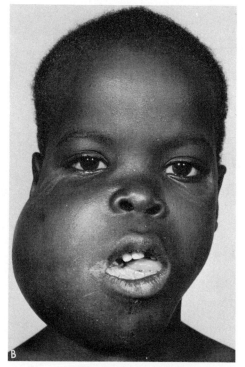

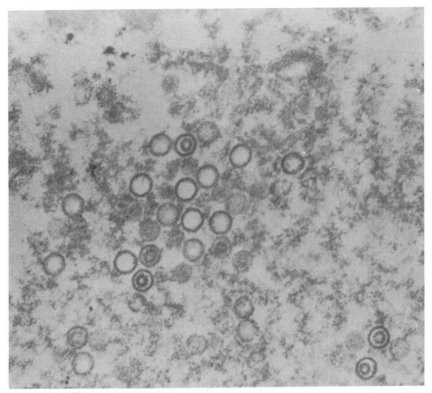

Figure 19–7. Electron micrograph of EB virus from a patient with Burkitt's lymphoma. ×32,000. (Courtesy of Dr. Paul H. Levine.)

Study of individual EB virus–induced antigens on Burkitt lymphoma cells differentiates immune responses in patients. Antibodies to membrane antigens correlate with the clinical course and are highest in tumor regression and lowest in tumor progression. Antibodies to (cytoplasmic) *capsid* antigens have no clinical relevance and are found in humans with a wide variety of disorders. Antibodies to *early* antigens (EA) and *precipitating* antigens are found during active phases of Burkitt's lymphoma only (Chapter 16).

On the basis of serologic findings, EB virus has subsequently been shown to be related to infectious mononucleosis. Lymphocytes from patients with infectious mononucleosis behave in many respects like the lymphoma cells from patients with Burkitt's disease. Both appear as transformed cells and acquire the propensity for increased growth potential *in vitro*. Recently, a receptor for the EB virus was demonstrated on the surface of the B-cell. The atypical lymphocyte of infectious mononucleosis has recently been identified as a transformed T-cell. Thus, the evidence suggests an etiologic role for EB virus in Burkitt's lymphoma, nasopharyngeal carcinoma, and infectious mononucleosis.

CHARACTERISTICS OF THE IMMUNE RESPONSE IN HOST RESISTANCE TO TUMORS

The host possesses both nonspecific and specific mechanisms of response to tumor formation. In tumor rejection, as in protection from infecting agents, the host immune response is directed toward the maintenance of homeostasis (Chapter 2). The homeostasis can be altered toward establishment of the tumor or in favor of the host.

NONSPECIFIC FACTORS

There is evidence that nonspecific, nonimmunologic factors may be of paramount importance in determining the fate of neoplastic cells in a host. Presumably, mutations induced by viruses, chemicals, physical factors, and radiation occur frequently. Why, then, are occasional clones able to evade recognition long enough to establish themselves as cancerous disease? The cancer cell appears to have a metabolic edge: it has lost contact inhibition and no longer responds to controlling influences that regulate the activity of other cells. It manufactures a variety of unique products: some are transplantation-type antigens (TSTA), some reflect an expressed virus, and some are fetal, indicative of a derepressed state. Other products of the tumor cell may be of crucial importance to the survival of the cancer cell since they seem to evade many facets of host defense, such as chemotaxis, phagocytosis, and killing by macrophages, killing by lymphocytes, and lymphocyte transformation with release of mediators necessary for expression of cell-mediated immunity (Chapter 9). Moreover, several suppressive products of cancer cells have been found (e.g., inhibition of chemotaxis); some are dialyzable and thermolabile, and others are heat-stable proteins. Their significance in the establishment and maintenance of the cancer state *in vivo* remains speculative.

SPECIFIC FACTORS

The Case for Immunologic Surveillance

The concept of "immunologic surveillance" states that malignant disorders occur when there is failure of the immune system to recognize and destroy neoplastic cells before they become established in the body. This concept is supported by the observed higher incidence of malignancy in patients with immunologic deficiency syndromes or immune suppression secondary to drugs.

Immunologic Deficiency States

The immunologic deficiency states comprise a heterogeneous group of inborn and acquired defects of the lymphoreticular tissues that may involve defects of the humoral (B) or the thymic (T) system, or both (Chapter 22). These diseases are characterized by an increased susceptibility to infection as a common clinical sign that reflects their defective defense function. The same defects that lead to this aberration in defense from infectious disease also give rise to defects in surveillance and result in an increased risk of neoplastic change. Children with immunologic defects have a high incidence of tumors, which constitute one of the major causes of death. These tumors usually involve malignant disorders of the lymphoreticular tissues, especially the thymus. Although the group as a whole is at risk, the apparent increase in malignancy appears to affect primarily those subjects with defects of the thymic-dependent tissues. These tumors have been described in patients with ataxia-telangiectasia, Wiskott-Aldrich syndrome, and acquired hypogammaglobulinemia (see Table 19–1). This increased susceptibility to neoplastic change provides clinical support for a relationship between resistance mechanisms and tumor formation.

Immunosuppression

Patients whose immune systems have been suppressed are vulnerable to viral and bacterial infections and are also susceptible to neoplasia. In the several thousand organ transplants that have been performed throughout the world, an increased incidence of subsequent neoplasia has been reported. The possibility exists that unsuspected neoplastic tissue may have been transplanted or that immunosuppression has led to the genesis of a primary tumor.

It has been suggested that, in humans, Burkitt's lymphoma might represent an inadequate immunologic defense against EB virus infection, most normal infected individuals limiting the viral expression to the clinical disease infectious mononucleosis. The EB virus appears to infect B-lymphocytes, and normally, the T-lymphocytes make an appropriate immunologic response, perhaps including antimitotic suppressor cells. Plasma from convalescent infectious mononucleosis patients contains factors that inhibit incorporation of tritiated thymidine in normal resting lymphocytes *in vitro;* such activity is not present in plasma from normal patients or those in the acute phase of infectious mononucleosis. It may be that the lymphoma occurs only in those patients who are relatively immunologically deficient, either innately or as a result of malarial infection, malnutrition, or other factors.

The Case Against Immunologic Surveillance

Because many cancer patients appear to be immunologically intact and do make an appropriate, vigorous immune response to their cancer, many workers have begun to question the validity of the concept of immunologic surveillance. They note that bona fide immune deficiency chiefly is associated with lymphoreticular malignancy and not with solid tumors of other organ systems. It is not yet understood how a clone of transformed cells is able to "sneak through" the host's multiple recognition mechanisms to become established. In individuals with essentially normal immune function, it may be that the neoplastic cells possess protective advantages. In some instances, tumor-specific antigens may be weak and of low density on the cell membrane (Table 19–3); in such cases, the host's immune response could not be vigorous.

Immunoselection. A possible antibody-mediated effect that may be applicable to man is *immunoselection*. Antigenic specificity does not appear to be altered during serial passage. It has been postulated that immunologic factors suppress those cells with the most surface antigenicity and "select" those cells with the least surface antigenicity. For example, if a tumor is passed repeatedly through animals immune to TSTA, a tumor is obtained that has lessened antigenicity and lessened susceptibility to the effects of antibody-mediated cytotoxicity. In a manner consistent with the phenomenon of immunoselection, tumors with the highest concentration of surface antigen, such as the RNA-induced tumors, are most likely to lose antigenicity, as contrasted with DNA tumors with weak antigens, which lose little or no antigenicity through passage. This phenomenon has been used in the laboratory in selecting clones of tumor cells with varying concentrations of surface antigen. The importance of immunoselection in the growth of human tumors has yet to be demonstrated but it may represent a mechanism by which a neoplastic cell with low antigenicity may "sneak through" the antibody-mediated surveillance mechanisms of the host.

In other cases, the tumor may induce an inappropriate immune response. In multiple myeloma, macrophages are induced to make a material that suppresses antibody formation by normal B-lymphocytes (a feedback inhibition?) (Chapter 21). In other cases, the tumor appears to stimulate T-suppressor lymphocytes more than it does killer lymphocytes and helper T-lymphocytes. In conclusion, it is obvious that most human patients with cancer of any sort possess specific cell-mediated immunity and specific antibodies against tumor-associated

TABLE 19–3. The Relationship Between Relative Concentration of Tumor-Specific Antigens and Biologic Effects

Relative Surface Concentration	Types of Tumors	Susceptibility to Complement-Mediated Cytotoxicity *in vivo*	Enhancement
High	RNA viruses	++++	+
Low	DNA viruses, chemical, spontaneous	±	++++

antigens (TAA) of their autochthonous tumors. It is not clear why, in those individuals with progressing or disseminating cancer, such demonstrable immune responses are not adequate to control the tumor; some of the probable explanations are described in later sections.

Cell-Mediated Immunity in Cancer

In many animal tumor systems and in most studied cancer patients, specific lymphocyte killing of autochthonous or allogeneic tumor cells (Chapter 9) can be demonstrated. Newer radioisotope cytotoxic assay procedures have replaced the more cumbersome colony-inhibition method in many laboratories. Tumor immunity has also been demonstrated against membrane-bound or solubilized antigens by lymphocyte transformation or release of mediators such as MIF and LIF from sensitized lymphocytes. Moreover, it is likely that other mediators, such as blastogenic factor, transfer factor, immune RNA, and interferon, participate in the *in vivo* cell-mediated response against tumor antigens (Chapter 9). It should be emphasized that since these cell-mediated immune responses to tumor antigens can be demonstrated in appropriate tests *in vitro* during all stages of disease, central or afferent tolerance to TAA does not exist (Chapter 10).

In cell-mediated immunity, the attraction, immobilization, and activation of macrophages is an important element that augments the already existing nonspecific macrophage attack on a tumor cell. Thus, the importance of the macrophage in cellular defense against tumors cannot be overemphasized. Among leukocytes, activated macrophages have the unique ability to recognize malignant cells and to selectively kill them, leaving normal cells or benign tumor (transformed) cells unharmed.

Antibody-Mediated Immunity in Cancer

In many tumor-bearing individuals, specific antibodies can be demonstrated. Some evidence suggests that tumor-specific antibody can be detrimental to the host. In experimental situations, tumor-specific antibody administered before transplantation of tumor or infection by oncogenic virus leads to tumor enhancement (afferent limb—suppression of response). Other studies suggest that antibodies attach to the surface of tumor cells, thereby blocking or masking attachment sites for cytotoxic lymphocytes and cytolytic antibodies (efferent limb).

Plasma from individuals with progressing tumor may inhibit lymphocyte- and complement-mediated killing of tumor cells *in vitro*; such effect has been ascribed to the presence of "blocking antibody." More recent studies, however, have shown that plasma blocking activity is due to tumor antigen-antibody complexes or free tumor antigen, rather than antibody per se. In autochthonous tumors, neoplastic cells, cell fragments, soluble antigens, and tumor antigen-antibody complexes circulate. Indeed, tumor antigen-antibody complexes have been found deposited in glomerular capillaries in various tumor systems in the human. Therefore, it seems most likely that the observed blocking of tumor immunity reflects the large antigen mass associated with the host's tumor burden, leading to high-dose tolerance (efferent and central limbs). A similar situation exists in certain of the slow virus infections, e.g., SSPE (Chapter 16). Passively administered antibody to TAA reduces blocking activity of plasma *in vitro* and has been shown to halt tumor progression *in vivo*. Such activity has been termed "unblocking antibody."

Antibodies specific for tumor antigens have been shown to kill tumor target cells in two ways; both appear to operate *in vivo*. The first way is complement-dependent; IgG and IgM antibodies fix to antigenic sites on target cells and activate the complement cascade. Terminal C8 and C9 components bring about lysis by the classic pathway. The second cytocidal pathway is independent of complement and is known as antibody-dependent, cellular cytotoxic (ADCC) reaction (Chapter 9). Once tumor-specific IgG antibody fixes to target cell membrane, there is an alteration of the Fc portion of the heavy chain. Mononuclear cells, referred to as killer cells, need not be sensitized, are attracted, and kill the target cell in direct contact. Although the precise identity of killer cells is not known, lymphocytes and macrophages have been suggested (Chapter 9).

IMMUNOLOGIC PHENOMENA ASSOCIATED WITH STATE OF DISEASE

At any stage of cancer, including early localized disease, factors that inhibit phagocyte chemotaxis, phagocytosis, and target cell killing can be found in the plasma of a significant number of patients. These factors are produced either by tumor cells or by immune regulatory cells.

During active progression or dissemination of some tumors, certain other phenomena have been noted that probably occur generally (Table 19–4). There is seeding of interstitial fluid and blood with cancer cells, cell fragments, and membrane-associated soluble antigens. These neutralize lymphocytes and combine with specific antibody, blocking an effective immune response at the site of tumor cells. Plasma levels of antibody to TAA are low or not measurable. With advanced or disseminated cancer, specific or general immune suppression may occur, possibly manifested by diminished numbers of circulating T-lymphocytes, disappearance of delayed hypersensitivity in the skin

TABLE 19–4. The Relationship Between Various Immunologic Parameters and the Clinical State in Cancer Patients

Immunologic Parameter	Material Tested	Tumor Progression or Dissemination	Tumor Remission
Delayed hypersensitivity to multiple antigens	*In vivo* (skin)	Often decreased	Normal
Number of T-lymphocytes	Blood	May be decreased	Normal
Tumor-associated antigens (TAA)*	Plasma or serum	Present	Absent
Cytotoxic antibodies to TAA	Plasma or serum	Absent or low titer	Present
Effect of Plasma or Serum on:			
Host lymphocyte killing of target cell		Blocking activity (TAA-antibody complexes)	Unblocking activity (free antibody to TAA)
Lymphocyte transformation by antigens and mitogens		May inhibit	No effect
Release of lymphokines		May inhibit	No effect
Phagocyte function: chemotaxis, phagocytosis, target cell killing		May inhibit (even in early, localized cancer)	No effect

*TAA = Tumor-associated antigens, dispersed on cell membranes or solubilized from cell membranes.

(anergy), and decrease in lymphocyte transformation and release of mediators after mitogen or antigen stimulation *in vitro*. These phenomena persist as long as the tumor progresses; their presence at the time of diagnosis portends a poor prognosis.

During remission of tumor, findings are the opposite. In the plasma, there are no TAA and no blocking factors; the level of specific antibodies for tumor-associated membrane antigens are found to be high. Levels of antibodies to membrane antigens appear to be more relevant than do those nuclear or cytoplasmic antigens measured by other techniques such as complement fixation. Tumor-specific immunity and general immune function are intact; there is no anergy *in vivo* or *in vitro*. Subsequent appearance of TAA or blocking factors in the plasma and decline in titer of tumor-specific antibody is indicative of tumor exacerbation. These changes in immunologic parameters may precede clinical manifestations of tumor recurrence by weeks or months.

IMPLICATIONS FOR THERAPY

For a variety of cancers, cure rates and incidence of remission have been steadily improving. This is due in part to the cooperation of surgeons, radiologists, oncologists, and immunologists who jointly manage cancer patients, applying multiple modalities at appropriate times. Surgical removal and radiation therapy probably serve to reduce the bulk of tumor mass; chemotherapy eliminates the majority of persisting tumor cells (Table 19–5). The expectation is that the host's innate and acquired defenses will be able to control surviving cancers cells or eliminate them entirely.

The aim of immunotherapy is to augment such antitumor defenses (Chapter 10). Many approaches are under study, and thus far there have been varying degrees of questionable or limited success (Table 19–5). One approach is the augmentation of nonspecific phagocytosis and killing of tumor cells by macrophages. Application of infectious BCG mycobacteria has been the most widely used approach; administration of nonliving *Corynebacterium parvum* is increasingly being employed. Glucan, a pyran copolymer derived from microorganisms, is also being evaluated. Levamisole is an antihelminthic drug that appears to be efficacious in stimulating CMI and macrophage function. In leukemia and some solid tumors, beneficial results have been demonstrated with such prolonged adjuvant treatments.

A related approach has been carried out successfully in such

TABLE 19–5.   Therapeutic Goals in Treatment of Cancer

A. Primary: Reduction of tumor mass (antigen load)
    1. Surgical extirpation
    2. Radiation
    3. Chemotherapy
B. Secondary: Augment body defenses (immunotherapy)
    1. Nonspecific
        a) Adjuvants of CMI and macrophage function
            −BCG
            −*C. parvum*
            −glucan
            −levamisole
        b) Topical delayed hypersensitivity to unrelated antigen (DNCB)
    2. Specific
        a) Passive−unblocking serum
        b) Active−immunization with autologous or homologous processed tumor cell antigens, with or without adjuvant
        c) Adoptive
            −thymus soluble products
            −transfer factor or immune RNA
            −transplantation of fetal thymus or immunocompetent cells, e.g., bone marrow

---

localized tumors of the skin as keratoses, basal cell carcinoma, squamous carcinoma, and melanoma. Dinitrochlorobenzene (DNCB) is a contactant that induces cell-mediated immunity readily. When applied topically to skin tumor sites, the ensuing DNCB-specific delayed-hypersensitivity reaction brings about the "nonspecific" regression of tumor by local accumulations of killer lymphocytes and activated macrophages.

Augmentation of tumor-specific immunity can be passive, active, or adoptive. As indicated previously, passively administered "unblocking" serum containing a high titer of tumor-specific antibody has been associated with clinical remission; others have reported no particular benefit or even tumor enhancement. Since a cancer patient is already immunized to autochthonous tumor antigens, danger of tolerogenesis or of tumor enhancement by antibody seems more theoretical than real.

Much effort has been extended toward increasing active immunity to tumor antigens. At surgery, tumor sites have been cauterized, frozen, chemically burned, and enzymatically treated to alter endogenous TAA *in situ*. *In vitro*, tumor cells have been irradiated, freeze-thawed, and treated with neuraminidase to expose more antigen sites or to denature tumor antigens. Upon injection of treated cells or solubilized TAA into the same or a homologous host, with or without adjuvant, the expectation is that the host can make a more vigorous and varied immune response to the tumor.

Adoptive measures remain the most alluring, with the hope of transferring to the host missing ingredients of defense from a healthy immune donor. Thymosin, a hormone extracted from bovine or human thymus (Chapter 2), has been shown to enhance T-lymphocyte immunity in individuals with primary or secondary immune deficiency. Transfer factor, a dialyzable, nonimmunogenic message material from T-lymphocytes, seems to transfer specific reactivity to new antigens *de novo* as well as to boost pre-existing immunity in the manner of an adjuvant (Chapters 9 and 22). Both agents are under study in patients with cancer. Immune RNA in animals protects against otherwise fatal infectious disease in susceptible hosts; its applicability to the human is currently under study. Transfer of immunocompetent lymphoid tissue in the form of bone marrow transplants has been used in the treatment of leukemia. This approach is not yet practical and is still considered experimental. There are serious problems: the tumor-bearing recipients will reject a bone marrow graft unless the recipient is immunosuppressed. There is always the risk of serious overwhelming infection, and if the bone marrow takes, a graft-versus-host reaction is possible. Transplants of fetal thymus theoretically might augment CMI that is depressed and avoid problems of graft rejection.

At this time, it is fair to say that the efficacy of immunotherapy in the treatment of tumors is not yet proved. Indeed, the vital role of specific immunity in control of most tumors in most individuals is not defined. It is possible that nonimmunologic, nonspecific defense mechanisms or even tumor cell characteristics per se will prove to be more critical in determining the success of host defense against neoplasms.

SUGGESTIONS FOR FURTHER READING

Alexander, P.: The nature of the immunological interaction between the host and the tumor. Can. J. of Otolaryngol., *4*:1, 36–38, 1975.

Alexander, P., Eccles, S. A., and Gauci, C. L. L.: The significance of macrophages in human and experimental tumors. *In* H. Friedman, and C. Southam (eds.): International Conference on Immunobiology of Cancer. Vol. 276. New York, New York Academy of Sciences, 1976, pp. 124–133.

Anderson, V., Kuer, M., and Bendixen, G.: In vitro demonstration of cellular hypersensitivity to tumour antigens in man. Ser. Haematol., *5*:3–21, 1972.

Baldwin, R. W., Embleton, M. J., Jones, J. S. P., and Langman, M. J. S.: Cell-mediated and humoral reactions to human tumors. Int. J. Cancer, *12*:73–83, 1973.

Chang, R. S., and Spiva, C. A.: Suppression of spontaneous in vitro transformation of autologous leukocytes by plasma from convalescent and post-convalescent injection mononucleosis patients. J. Natl. Cancer Inst., *55*:803, 1975.

Currie, G.: Immunological aspects of host resistance to the development and growth of cancer. Biochim. Biophys. Acta, *458*:135–165, 1976.

Harris, J., and Copeland, D.: Impaired immunoresponsiveness in tumor patients. Ann. N.Y. Acad. Sci., *230*:56–85, 1974.

Hellström, I., Hellström, K. E., Sjögren, H. O., and Warner, G. A.: Serum factors in tumor-free patients. Cancelling the blocking of cell-mediated tumor immunity. Int. J. Cancer, *8*:185–191, 1971a.

Hellström, I., Sjögren, H. O., Warner, G. A., and Hellström, K. E.: Blocking of cell-mediated tumor immunity by sera from patients with growing neoplasms. Int. J. Cancer, *7*:226–237, 1971b.

Irie, K., Irie, R. F., and Morton, D. L.: Evidence for in vivo reaction of antibody and complement to surface antigens of human cancer cells. Science, *186*:454–456, 1974.

Kerbel, R. S.: Mechanisms of tumor-induced immunological deficiencies and their possible significance in relation to the use of immunopotentiators in tumor-bearing hosts. Biomedicine, *20*:253–261, 1974.

Khoo, S. K., Warner, N. L., Lie, J. T., and Mackay, I. R.: Carcinoembryonic antigenic activity of tissue extracts: A quantitative study of malignant and benign neoplasms, cirrhotic liver, normal adult and fetal organs. Int. J. Cancer, *11*:681–687, 1973.

Kniker, W. T., Ganaway, R. L., and Smith, K. O.: Suppression of lymphocyte transformation by fetal and tumor factors. Fed. Proc., *33*:749, 1974.

Lewis, M. G., Hartman, D., and Jerry, L. M.: Antibodies and anti-antibodies in human malignancy: an expression of deranged immune regulation. *In* H. Friedman, and C. Southam (eds.): International Conference on Immunobiology of Cancer. Vol. 276. New York, New York Academy of Sciences, 1976, pp. 316–327.

Morton, D. L., Homes, E. C., Eilber, F. R., and Wood, W. C.: Immunological aspects of neoplasia; a rational basis for immunotherapy. Ann. Intern. Med., *74*:587–604, 1971.

Nelson, D. S.: Immunity to infection, allograft immunity and tumor immunity: Parallels and contrasts. Transplant. Rev., *19*:226–254, 1974.

Perlmann, P., Perlmann, H., and Wigzell, H.: Lymphocyte-mediated cytotoxicity in vitro. Induction and inhibition by humoral antibody and nature of effector cells. Transplant. Rev., *13*:91–114, 1972.

Perlmann, P., O'Toole, C., and Unsgaard, B.: Cell-mediated immune mechanisms of tumor cell destruction. Fed. Proc., *32*:153–155, 1973.

Pilch, Y. H., and Golub, S. H.: Lymphocyte-mediated immune responses in neoplasia. Am. J. Clin. Pathol., 62:184–211, 1974.

Smith, R. T.: Tumor specific immune mechanisms. N. Engl. J. Med., 287:439, 1972.

Snyderman, R., and Pike, M. C.: Defective macrophage migration produced by neoplasms. In M. A. Fink (ed.): The Macrophage in Neoplasia. New York, Academic Press, 1976.

Snyderman, R., and Pike, M. C.: An inhibitor of macrophage chemotaxis produced by neoplasms. Science, 192:370, 1976.

Ting, C. C., and Herberman, R. B.: Humoral host defense mechanisms against tumors. Int. Rev. Exp. Pathol., 15:93–152, 1976.

Vanky, F., Stjensward, J., Klein, G., Steiner, L., and Lindberg, L.: Tumor-associated specificity of serum-mediated inhibition of lymphocyte stimulation by autochthonous human tumors. J. Natl. Cancer Inst., 51:25–32, 1973.

Waldmann, T. A., Strober, W., and Blaese, R. M.: Immunodeficiency disease and malignancy. Various immunologic deficiencies of man and the role of immune processes in the control of malignant disease. Ann. Intern. Med., 77:605–628, 1972.

Wilson, R. E., Alexander, P., Rosenberg, S. A., and Simmons, R. L.: Horizons in tumor immunology. A seminar. Arch. Surg., 109:17–29, 1974.

Winters, W. D.: Immunovirology. In D. Shottenfield (ed.): Cancer Epidemiology and Prevention. Springfield, Illinois, Charles C Thomas, 1975, pp. 207–230.

Wybran, J., Hellström, L., Hellström, K. E., and Fudenberg, H. H.: Cytotoxicity of human rosette-forming blood lymphocytes on cultivated human tumor cells. Int. J. Cancer, 13:515–521, 1974.

Section Three

CLINICAL APPLICATIONS OF IMMUNOLOGY

Chapter 20

IMMUNOLOGICALLY MEDIATED DISEASES

Joseph A. Bellanti, M.D.

Introduction: The Concept of Immunologically Mediated Disease

The basic function of the immunologic system is to detect and eliminate from the body any substance recognized as *foreign.* In performing this function, the host employs a wide variety of cells and cell products, each interacting with one another in the removal of this material (Chapter 11). Usually, such interactions are efficient and successful without detriment to the host. Occasionally, however, when the type of antigen presented to the system or the reactivity of the host is inappropriate, perturbations occur that lead to harmful sequelae – the *immunologically mediated diseases.*

The summation of the total immunologic capability of the host to all foreign matter is shown schematically in Figure 20–1.

There are three types of responses through which all foreign substances can proceed, the progression of which depends upon two factors: (1) the nature of the substance (Chapter 4) and (2) the genetic constitution of the host (Fig. 20–1) (Chapter 3).

The *nonspecific (primary)* response, the most primitive type, consists of those ancient responses to the first encounter with a foreign configuration – *phagocytosis* and *inflammation.* If the substance (e.g., carbon particles) is completely eliminated at this stage, the host's response terminates. Some substances, however, are not completely eliminated at this stage and reflect antigen persistence.

If the primary encounter leads to a processed product (antigen), the *specific (secondary)* or more sophisticated responses are stimulated (Fig. 20–1). These consist of two possible effector mechanisms: (1) B-lymphocyte-mediated humoral immunity with the elaboration of antibody (IgE, IgM, IgG, IgA, and IgD) and (2) T-lymphocyte-mediated antigen elimination. A sophisticated addition to these mechanisms is the capacity to enhance the immunologic responses through the actions of complement, the coagulation sequence, and a bank of "memory cells" if antigen is re-encountered. If antigen is successfully eliminated, the immunologic response terminates. Normally, most antigens are successfully eliminated at this stage without detriment to the host.

If antigen still persists, the *tissue-damaging (tertiary)* responses are called into play. Antigen persistence may result from the nature of the antigen itself or from some genetic defect in antigen processing. If antigen persists, four types of immunologic interactions can be elicited: Types I, II, III, and IV (Chapter 13). These responses are no longer beneficial to the host and are manifested as disease phenomena, the *immunologically mediated diseases* (IMD). These may be either temporary or permanent, depending upon the efficiency of antigen elimination (Fig. 20–1). If antigen can be removed or eliminated, the tertiary response is terminated with minimal discomfort to the patient (e.g., penicillin hypersensitivity). However, if the tertiary response is ineffective and antigen still persists, the more harmful sequelae of the immune response emerge, e.g., "autoimmune disease." This represents a maximal deleterious, self-perpetuating attack of an aberrant immune response in which the host sustains injury. It has

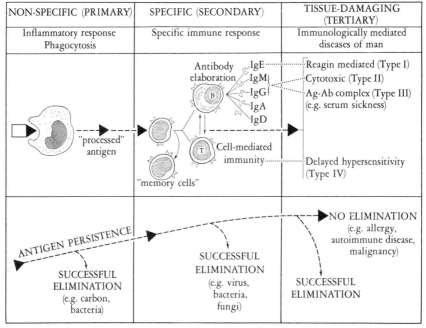

Figure 20–1. Schematic representation of the total immunologic capability of the host based upon efficiency of elimination of foreign matter.

been postulated that a failure in surveillance with persistence of antigen could also be involved in malignant disorders (Chapter 19).

TYPES OF IMMUNOLOGICALLY MEDIATED DISEASES

It should be recalled that the immune response does not occur as an isolated event *(in vacuo)*; every foreign configuration may stimulate several immunologic systems. Certain compartments of the immunologic system, however, may be selectively stimulated, depending upon the nature of the antigen, its configuration, the degree of macrophage processing, and the route by which antigen is introduced into the host (Chapter 7).

Immunologically mediated diseases may be viewed as three general types, depending upon the nature of the antigen — those involving *exogenous, allogeneic,* or *autologous* antigens. Examples of each are listed in Table 20–1.

Thus, antigens that make contact topically may favor the stimulation of the secretory immunoglobulin system (IgA or IgE). These responses serve useful functions normally. In some individuals, the local production of IgE may lead to undesirable allergic symptoms characteristic of atopic diseases, e.g., hayfever reaction to pollen. Also, the genetic controls of the immunologic system are expressed as variations in immunologic responsiveness between individuals (Chapter 3). These variations depend not only on the nature of the antigen but also on a number of modifying factors, including age and the emotional and nutritional status of the host. Recently, the association of the HLA system and immune responsiveness, as well as the recent knowledge of the cellular interactions of T-helper and T-suppressor cells, has been implicated in the expression of allergic disease (Chapters 3 and 7). Regardless of the precipitating factors, whether involving host or

TABLE 20–1. The Immunologically Mediated Diseases of Man

TYPE OF ANTIGEN	EXAMPLE OF DISEASE RESPONSE
Exogenous	Atopic diseases and reactions to environmental allergens, e.g., tree and grass pollens
Allogeneic	Alloantigens (including transplantation, blood transfusions, and erythroblastosis fetalis)
Autologous	Autoimmune diseases, e.g., systemic lupus erythematosus (SLE)

antigen, if aberrations are established, *immunologic imbalance* is created, with resultant IMD (Chapter 2).

EFFECTOR MECHANISMS OF IMMUNOLOGIC INJURY

Basically, the mechanisms responsible for immunologically mediated diseases comprise four categories that were presented in Chapter 13 and are summarized in Table 20–2.

The first of these, the anaphylactic (cytotropic), or Type I, reaction, is mediated primarily by the IgE reaginic antibodies. These immunoglobulins are cytotropic and have a characteristic property of binding to mediator cells, e.g., mast cells or their circulating counterpart, the basophils. Following reaction with antigen, subsequent release of pharmacologically vasoactive amines accounts for the clinical symptoms of these diseases (Chapter 13). The target organs most commonly involved are the *gastrointestinal tract*, the *skin*, and the *respiratory tract*. This reaginic response is seen in the normal individual but, when aberrant, is responsible for most of the atopic allergic diseases of man (atopy).

The cytolytic (cytotoxic), or Type II, reaction is usually mediated through complement-fixing properties of antibody. Also included in this type are the antibody-mediated reactions that require the participation of cellular elements. This may occur by any of three mechanisms, each of which involves the cytotoxic effect of antibody with antigen on a cell surface. In one type, the reaction of antibody with antigens on the surface of a particle enhances the phagocytosis of the particle (opsonization) with its subsequent intracellular destruction. A second cytotoxic effect of antibody is its direct reaction with surface antigens that together with complement lead to the destruction of the cell through antibody-mediated cytolysis (Chapter 6). The third type of cytotoxic reaction is that in which antibody, through its participation with killer cells, can function in antibody-dependent cellular cytotoxicity (ADCC) reactions (Chapter 9). The best studied of these cytotoxic reactions are the antibody-mediated, complement-directed cytotoxic reactions. The effector mechanisms in these cases are mediated primarily by IgG or IgM antibody directed toward target cells, e.g., circulating blood cells (Table 20–2). The clinical manifestations of these diseases may present as hemolytic anemia, leukopenia, or thrombocytopenia.

A third category of immunologically mediated diseases is the immune complex, or Type III (Arthus), type. These reactions have assumed increased clinical significance and have been implicated in several immunopathologic states, including a variety of vasculitides, systemic lupus erythematosus and glomerulonephritis. The mechanism

TABLE 20–2. Mechanisms of Immunologically Mediated Diseases According to Gell and Coombs

Type	Target Organs	Clinical Manifestations	Mechanisms
I. Anaphylactic (Cytotropic)	Gastrointestinal tract Skin Lungs	Gastrointestinal allergy, urticaria, atopic dermatitis, rhinitis, and asthma	IgE and other immunoglobulins
II. Cytolytic (Cytotoxic)	Circulating blood elements (red cells, white cells, and platelets)	Hemolytic anemia, leukopenia, thrombocytopenia, hemolytic disease of newborn, and Goodpasture's disease	IgG, IgM, and phagocytes (opsonization) and mononuclear cells (ADCC) reactions, or antibody-mediated complement cytolysis
III. Arthus: Immune complex (Serum sickness)	Blood vessels of: Skin, joints, kidneys, and lungs	Serum sickness, systemic lupus erythematosus, nephrosis of quartan malaria, and chronic glomerulonephritis	Antigen-antibody complexes (IgG)
IV. Cell-mediated (Delayed hypersensitivity)	Skin Lungs CNS Thyroid Other organs	Contact dermatitis Tuberculosis Allergic encephalitis Thyroiditis Primary homograft rejection	Sensitized T-lymphocytes
V. Mixed types: I and III		Allergic bronchopulmonary aspergillosis	IgE and precipitating IgG antibodies
III and IV		Extrinsic allergic alveolitis	Antigen-antibody complexes and cell-mediated immunity

of injury is mediated by antigen-antibody complexes that form in moderate antigen excess (Chapter 8). In this form, the soluble aggregates fix complement, circulate in the vascular system, and then may deposit in vascular endothelium, where they initiate a sequence of destructive inflammatory reactions in tissues, e.g., blood vessels, skin, joints, kidneys, and lungs, or may participate in the destruction of circulating cellular elements. The resultant clinical entities are exemplified by acute glomerulonephritis, serum sickness, and certain drug reactions.

The fourth mechanism of immunologic injury is the cell-mediated (delayed hypersensitivity), or Type IV, reaction. Unlike the previous three mechanisms, this response does not involve humoral antibody but is mediated by the action of sensitized T-lymphocytes. As described in Chapters 9 and 11, the action of T-cells may involve direct cytotoxic effects or the elaboration of lymphokines and the recruitment of other cells, e.g., macrophages.

A.   Immunologically Mediated Disease Involving Exogenous Antigens (Allergy)

Robert T. Scanlon, M.D., and
Joseph A. Bellanti, M.D.

Classically, the term "allergy," coined by von Pirquet, referred to a state of altered reactivity (Chapter 13). Subsequent modifications of the term's meaning have equated allergy with hypersensitivity. Since the concept of immunity presented throughout this book has been one of a reaction to foreignness, allergy is best viewed as a specialized case of immunity in which the reaction to foreign material terminates in a deleterious outcome. Allergy may be considered as one of several types of immunologically mediated disease of man directed at exogenous antigens.

There are four general types of allergic diseases seen in man. These include the *atopic reactions,* the *drug sensitivities, serum sickness,* and *contact dermatitis.*

Allergic diseases manifest imbalance primarily through three target organs—the *gastrointestinal tract,* the *skin,* and the *respiratory tract.* A

TABLE 20-3.   Routes and Types of Antigens That Give Rise to Allergic Manifestations

Route	Example of Antigen	Immunologic Mechanism	Disease Manifestation
1. Ingestants	Foods	Type I	Gastrointestinal allergy
	Drugs	Types I, II, III	Urticaria, atopic manifestations
			Immediate drug reaction
			Hemolytic anemia
			Serum sickness
2. Inhalants	Pollens	Type I	Allergic rhinitis
	Dusts		Bronchial asthma
	Molds		
	Aspergillus fumigatus	Types I, III	Allergic bronchopulmonary aspergillosis
	Thermophilic actinomycetes	Types III, IV	Extrinsic allergic alveolitis
3. Injectants	Drugs	Types I, II, III	Immediate drug reaction
			Hemolytic anemia
			Serum sickness
	Bee stings	Type I	Anaphylaxis
	Vaccines	Type III	Localized Arthus reaction
	Serum	Type I	Anaphylaxis
4. Contactants	Poison ivy	Type IV	Contact dermatitis

common feature to all three is their exposure to the external environment, which provides a common route of entry for exogenous agents.

The most common routes and types of antigens that give rise to allergic manifestations are shown in Table 20–3, together with their suspected immunologic mechanisms and disease manifestations.

CLINICAL MANIFESTATIONS OF GASTROINTESTINAL ALLERGY

Gastrointestinal (GI) allergy may be defined as hypersensitivity to certain exogenous substances, usually foods, that gain access to the body via the gastrointestinal tract, are manifested primarily through vomiting, diarrhea, or abdominal pain, and at times may be of such severity as to result in malabsorption or protein-losing enteropathy. These may also be accompanied by skin manifestations (e.g., atopic eczema and urticaria) and respiratory tract manifestations (e.g., rhinitis and asthma) (Fig. 20–2). This symptom complex of diarrhea and vomiting after the ingestion of certain foods encompasses a syndrome of varying etiology of which GI allergy may be a component. Conditions other than allergy to food that can produce this same clinical picture include the following entities: disaccharidase deficiency, gluten-sensitive enteropathy (celiac disease), cystic fibrosis, and galactosemia. Foods most frequently implicated in gastrointestinal allergy are milk, chocolate, citrus fruits, eggs, wheat, nuts, peanut butter, and fish.

Gastrointestinal allergy is manifested clinically by the rejection of the foreign antigen through vomiting and diarrhea. The small infant may present with restlessness, spasmodic pain, and crying characteristic of colic. Although some of these symptoms are thought to be mediated through the IgE reaginic response via the liberation of vasoactive substances (Chapter 13), other non-IgE-mediated mechanisms may also be operative in some cases. In addition, the clinical syndrome of growth retardation, gastrointestinal symptoms (e.g., bleeding), iron deficiency anemia, and recurrent pulmonary disease with hemosiderosis has been reported in association with the finding of milk precipitins in sera of small infants (Heiner's syndrome). Although a Type III antigen-antibody complex response has been suggested as a possible mechanism of injury in this syndrome, the evidence is indirect and inconclusive.

Several difficulties exist in attributing this symptom complex to gastrointestinal allergy. When food is the offending agent, the active immunogen may be the degradative product of the food, whose identity may escape detection. Further, antigens may be added to foods in the form of drugs, additives, or preservatives. For example, cows with

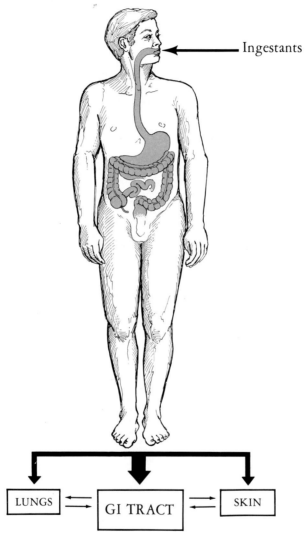

Figure 20-2. Schematic representation of the clinical manifestations of gastrointestinal allergy.

mastitis are treated with penicillin and yield milk containing trace amounts of this antibiotic. Thus, a penicillin hypersensitivity unrelated to milk protein may be masked by the ingestion of trace amounts of the drug. Also, current nutritional practices including food additives such as preservatives, sweeteners, and coloring agents, e.g., tartrazine (red dye 2), may further complicate the identification of the etiologic agent. Recently, these agents have been implicated in the pathogenesis of certain hyperkinetic learning disabilities of childhood. A second difficulty in establishing the diagnosis of gastrointestinal allergy is a lack of incontrovertible immunologic evidence. Although precipitating antibody has been found in the sera and stools of infants suspected of being sensitive to milk, evidence suggests that similar antibodies are also present in otherwise normal infants and in individuals recovering from gastroenteritis. Nonetheless, there is suggestive evidence that hypersensitivity to food substances may play a role in the pathogenesis. For example, isolated segments of guinea pig ileum sensitized by exposure to serum antibody manifest smooth muscle contracture after exposure to antigen (Shultz-Dale reaction) (Chapter 13). More recently, RAST has been employed to measure IgE-associated antibodies to a variety of allergens, including foods. The significance of these observations awaits further elucidation.

As described in Chapter 5, the secretory IgA immunoglobulins are found in abundance at mucosal surfaces such as the gastrointestinal tract where they appear to function primarily in local immunity to infectious agents. The attachment of these immunoglobulins to mucosal cells may also protect the intestinal cell from penetration by other antigens, e.g., allergens. For example, a decrease in IgA content in the infant may occur in severe diarrheal diseases and in marasmus, as well as in isolated IgA deficiency, conditions that may favor the development of allergic sensitization. The precise relationship of the secretory IgA system and the IgE system is unknown, but it has been suggested that the deficiency of IgA could allow the absorption of potentially allergenic substances that could result in IgE production with subsequent local or systemic reactions.

Although gastrointestinal allergy is primarily a reaction to dietary antigen, it should be emphasized that dietary antigen need not manifest itself solely by gastrointestinal symptoms but can also lead to involvement of other shock organs, such as the *skin* and *lungs.*

CLINICAL MANIFESTATIONS OF ALLERGIC DISEASE OF THE SKIN

The skin is another frequently involved shock tissue. The manifestations of allergic reactions in skin may be classified under two broad categories: (1) the *immediate,* e.g., urticaria, and (2) the *delayed,* e.g., contact dermatitis. These disorders may be induced by ingested food, drugs, or contactants. Although the main shock organ is the skin, secondary involvement may also include the respiratory tract and the gastrointestinal tract (Fig. 20–3).

The mechanisms underlying the immediate reaction involve the release of vasoactive amines primarily through the IgE reagin Type I response; the "delayed" reactions may involve other types, including

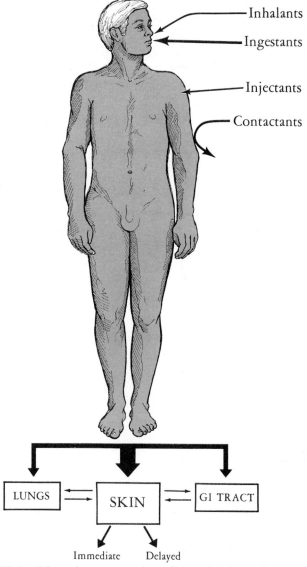

Figure 20–3. Schematic representation of the clinical manifestations of allergy affecting the skin.

Type IV (delayed hypersensitivity), independent of circulating antibody. The immediate reactions are triggered primarily by ingestants and injectants and, at times, inhalants; the delayed reactions are caused primarily by contactants (Table 20–3).

Atopic Eczema and Contact Dermatitis

The clinical appearance and the histologic features of the lesions of atopic and contact dermatitis are similar; the two differ in their mechanisms of production and their distribution. Atopic dermatitis is commonly grouped with the immediate-type hypersensitivities, and elevated levels of IgE are commonly seen. The basic defects of atopic dermatitis are unknown but may be due to sebum deficiency allowing free skin water to absorb edema fluid, transepidermal water loss by evaporation due to deficiency of water-binding agents (e.g., urea), and a very low pruritic threshold perhaps resulting from a genetic difference in pain fiber associated with pruritus (cyclic nucleotide imbalance). The immunologic basis for atopic dermatitis, however, is even less well understood. Although elevated levels of IgE are commonly seen, the histopathologic features in no way represent those of a Type I reaction. The lesions of atopic dermatitis may be generalized and are characterized by erythematous, papular, vesicular lesions that may weep and ooze, particularly in the small infant. In this age group, the lesions are usually distributed on the cheeks, forehead, wrists, extensor surfaces of the forearms, and lower extremities (Fig. 20–4). After the age of two years, the skin tends to be thickened, scaly, and lichenified, and the distribution becomes confined predominantly to the flexor surfaces of the antecubital and popliteal areas (Fig. 20–5).

The lesions of contact dermatitis may also show erythema, papules, vesicles, and bullae in the acute stage and, when chronic, become thickened, scaly, and lichenified. Histopathologically, both atopic and contact dermatitis demonstrate vasodilatation of blood vessels of the corium, resulting in intracellular edema in the malpighian layer of the epidermis. This is followed by an inflammatory reaction in the underlying dermis and subsequent parakeratosis, scaling, and acanthosis (Fig. 20–6). An important differentiating point is the distribution of the two lesions; the multiple area involvement of atopic dermatitis stands in marked contrast to the localization of lesions generally found in contact dermatitis. This restriction and localization is the key differentiating point between the two entities (Fig. 20–7).

The immunologic mechanisms for the two conditions are known to differ. Contact dermatitis expresses itself through the Type IV mechanism of delayed hypersensitivity mediated by sensitized lymphocytes. The etiologic agent is a simple chemical or other compound of low molecular weight, e.g., hapten, including the many substances that characterize our complex environment. These include plants (poison ivy), cosmetics,

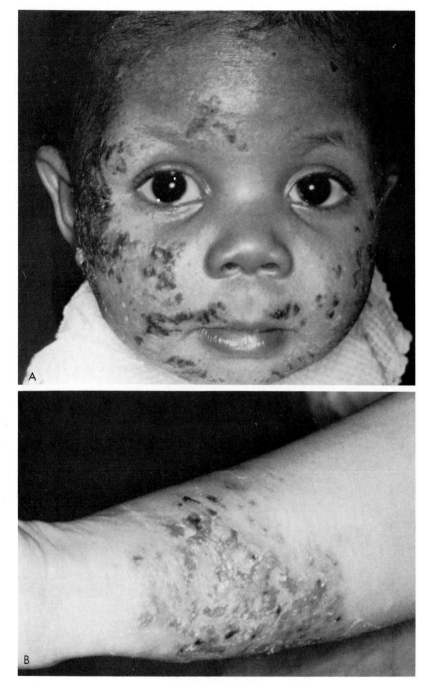

Figure 20–4. Photographs of the lesions of atopic eczema in the infant. Note the distribution on the face (*A*), on the surfaces of the lower forearms (*B*), and on the back (*C*). (Courtesy of Dr. James P. Rotchford.)

Illustration continued on the opposite page

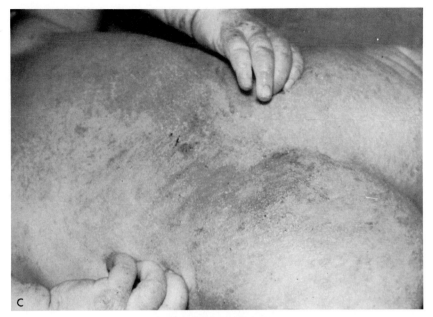

Figure 20–4 Continued.

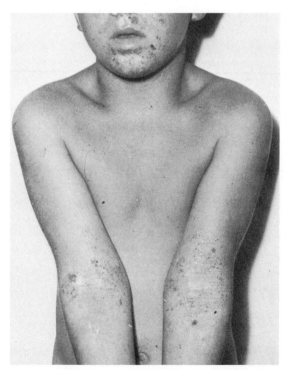

Figure 20–5. Photograph of the lesions of atopic eczema in an older child showing the distribution on the face and flexor surfaces of the antecubital areas. (Courtesy of Dr. James P. Rotchford.)

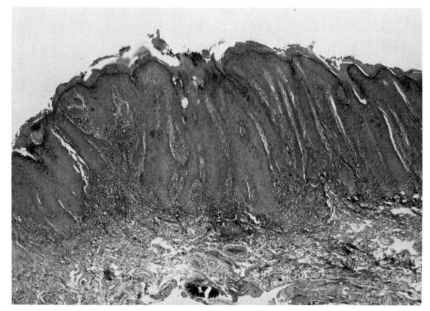

Figure 20-6. Photomicrograph of the skin lesion of atopic dermatitis showing the characteristic inflammatory reaction in the dermis with parakeratosis and acanthosis. Hematoxylin and eosin stain. ×120. (Courtesy of Dr. George H. Green.)

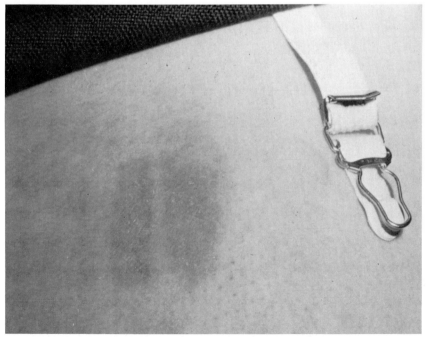

Figure 20-7. Photograph of the thigh of a patient with contact dermatitis due to nickel sensitivity (garter). Note the localization of the lesion to the area in contact with the metallic surface. (Courtesy of Dr. James P. Rotchford.)

industrial products, detergents, topical medications, clothing, food, and metals. These agents act as haptens and combine firmly and irreversibly with tissue protein to form a complete antigen (immunogen).

The immunologic mechanism underlying atopic eczema is thought to be associated with the immediate Type I hypersensitivity (Chapter 13). It appears that the reaction of the offending antigen with cell-bound reagin might lead to the release of vasoactive substances with a resultant increased vascular permeability. However, there are a number of other abnormal skin findings seen in patients with atopic eczema whose relationship with the primary disorder is unclear. These include blanching of the skin on stroking (white dermatographism), delayed blanching after injection of acetylcholine, in contrast to the normal erythema, and an exaggerated response in the cold pressor test. Although cellular cyclic AMP has been found to be reduced in the skin of atopic individuals, levels of adenyl cyclase are normal.

URTICARIA

Urticaria, or hives, is a skin manifestation that has an immediate onset and is characterized by erythema and wheal formation (Fig. 20–8).

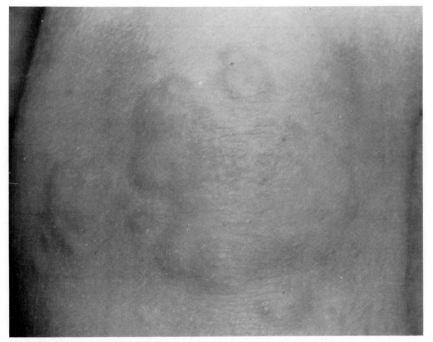

Figure 20–8.   Photograph of the knee of a patient with urticarial lesions of the skin. (Courtesy of Dr. James P. Rotchford.)

The lesions are characteristically evanescent, vary in size and shape, and are pruritic.

From a clinical standpoint, the urticarias are classified as (1) immunologic and (2) nonimmunologic, e.g., physical (cold urticaria), cholinergic, emotional, or produced by histamine-releasing drugs or systemic diseases, such as lymphomas, hyperthyroidism, and malignant disorders. The basic mechanism underlying all of the urticarias involves the localized increase in vascular permeability that occurs through the release of vasoactive amines, e.g., histamine, via any of a number of mechanisms.

The urticarial lesion is explained by the triple response of Lewis: (1) localized vasodilatation (erythema), (2) transudation of fluid (wheal), and (3) flaring due to local axon reflex.

In the immunologic type of urticaria, the release of vasoactive substances from mast cells occurs by any of a number of immunologic reactions, e.g., IgE response, antigen-antibody complexes, or cytophilic mechanisms (Chapter 13). Thus, urticaria can be seen after a penicillin reaction (IgE), during a serum sickness-like reaction (IgE or antigen-antibody complex), or during an incompatible blood transfusion (cytotoxic antibodies). However, the most common causes of urticaria are immunologically related and appear to be associated with infection (acute, e.g., streptococcus and parasitic, or chronic, e.g., dental and genitourinary), foods, and drugs (Table 20–4).

There are two other entities that enter into the differential diagnosis of chronic urticaria: urticaria pigmentosa and hereditary angioedema. Urticaria pigmentosa is characterized by discrete pink papules that are infiltrated by mast cells. When the lesions are stroked, the presence of these cells causes visible wheal and flare formation. This rare and self-limited disease is mediated by mediator release (Fig. 20–9).

TABLE 20–4.   Common Causes of Urticaria

Type	Examples
Infection	Bacteria
	Viruses
	Parasites
	Fungi
Foods	Berries
	Shellfish
	Chocolate
	Nuts
Drugs	Penicillin
	Laxatives
	Tranquilizers
	Aspirin

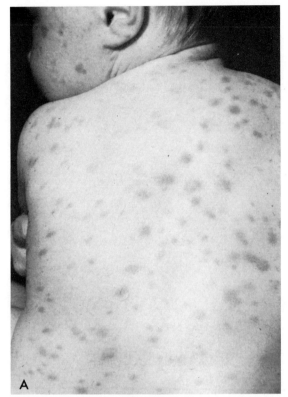

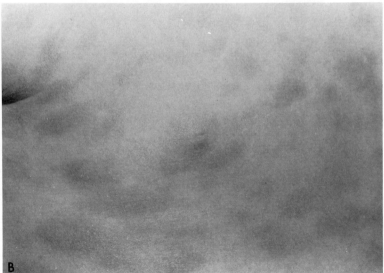

Figure 20-9. Photograph of a patient with urticaria pigmentosa. Note the wide distribution of the lesions (*A*) and the development of visible wheal and flare formation after stroking the affected areas (*B*). (Courtesy of Dr. James P. Rotchford.)

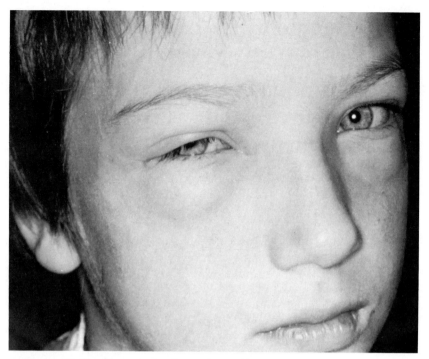

Figure 20–10. Photograph of a patient with angioedema showing the affected eyelids. (Courtesy of Dr. James P. Rotchford.)

Hereditary angioedema (HAE) is a familial disease transmitted as an autosomal dominant trait (Chapter 22). The basic defect is a deficiency of the inhibitor or a nonfunctional inhibitor of C1 esterase that expresses itself as a marked increase in vascular permeability. It presents as a sudden onset of painless urticarial edema, which at times can be life-threatening. It should be pointed out that patients with this disease do not have the classic circumscribed lesions of urticaria (Fig. 20–10) but rather have massive collections of fluid in the subcutaneous tissues (angioedema) (see Fig. 22–13). The diagnosis can be established by demonstration of C1q inhibition or decrease in C4 with normal C3 activities. Treatment of this disorder has traditionally rested with the use of epsilon-aminocaproic acid. Most recently, the use of danazol has shown quite promising results.

ALLERGIC DISEASE OF THE RESPIRATORY TRACT

Further hostility of the environment is manifested through exposure of the host to a variety of noxious agents that assault the respiratory tract. The majority of these insults occur by inhalation of organic and inorganic substances, including dust, pollen, molds, animal

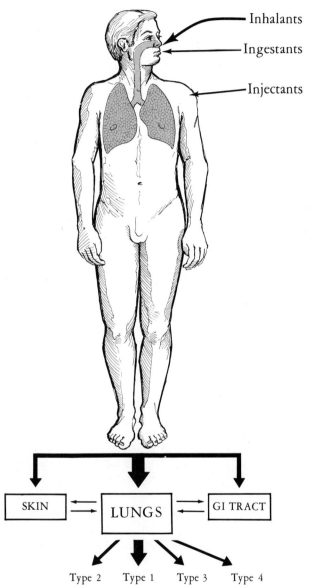

Figure 20–11. Schematic representation of the clinical manifestations of allergic diseases of the respiratory tract.

TABLE 20–5.   Allergic Diseases of the Respiratory Tract

Type	Example of Disease	Example of Antigen	Mechanism
Type I	Allergic rhinitis Bronchial asthma	Pollen	IgE antibody
Type II	Goodpasture's syndrome	Glomerular basement membrane (GBM) antigen	Anti-GBM
Type III	Farmer's lung	Dust of molding hay	Antigen-antibody complexes (together with Type IV)
Type IV	Tuberculosis	Tuberculoprotein	Sensitized lymphocytes

dander, silica, organic dusts, and living organisms (Fig. 20–11). These allergic diseases of the lung may also be triggered by *ingestants* (foods and drugs) or by *injectants* (drugs and vaccines). Examples of allergic diseases of the respiratory tract and their mechanisms of injury are given in Table 20–5.

Allergic diseases of the respiratory tract include several of the mechanisms of immunologic injury. The majority of clinical entities are produced by Type I reactions. Delayed hypersensitivity is a prominent feature of many infectious diseases of the respiratory tract, e.g., tuberculosis. Although such reactivity is not the primary cause of the disease, it contributes to the excessive tissue destruction commonly seen in these infections. In other forms of allergic disease of the lung, mixed forms of immunologic injury are operative.

TYPE I RESPONSE

The major localized anaphylactic categories of disease that affect the respiratory tract include conjunctivitis, rhinitis, and asthma. These respiratory insults are resented by the host, who expresses symptoms of the disease through the harmful action of cytotropic antibodies found at local sites. Although these reactions are primarily IgE-mediated, there is some recent evidence to suggest a pathogenetic role of IgG reagins, e.g., IgG4. After the interaction of antigen with cell-bound reagin, there is the release of vasoactive amines, e.g., histamine, SRS-A, ECF-A, and PAF (Chapter 13), which cause vasodilatation, hypersecretion, edema, and swelling of the (respiratory) mucosa or contribute to the inflammatory reaction. Since there is a continuity of the mucous lining membranes of all components of the respiratory tract (accessory sinuses, nasopharynx, and upper and lower respiratory tract), all components are adversely affected in this allergic attack. The degree to which each is affected will determine the clinical manifestation of the disease. Thus, in the young infant, obstruction with nasal blockage and eustachian tube impedance frequently is accompanied by otitis media, e.g., secretory otitis media.

Asthma

Asthma may be defined as acute intermittent reversible obstructive airway disease. The entity has been classically divided into *extrinsic* asthma, in which an exogenous allergen can be identified, and *intrinsic* asthma, in which no identifiable causative agent can be demonstrated. It should be pointed out, however, that this classification is inadequate, since intrinsic defects may be demonstrated in extrinsic asthma, and extrinsic factors, e.g., microorganisms, have been suggested in intrinsic asthma. Indeed, both show a β-adrenergic blockade, as will be described below.

The central defect in allergic diseases of the lung of atopic individuals is caused by obstruction of the lumen of the lower respiratory tract by bronchospasm, edema, thick secretions, and hyperplasia of smooth muscle and mucus-secreting glands. This leads to ventilatory insufficiency due to obstruction, with wheezing and dyspnea (Fig. 20–12). This inability presents with hyperinflation, expiratory

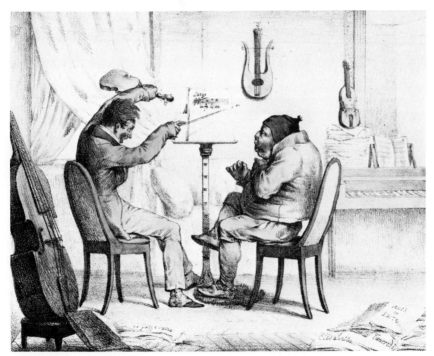

Figure 20–12.   A cartoon caricaturing the respiratory insufficiency of the asthmatic. (Courtesy of the National Library of Medicine.)

wheezes, and musical rales characteristic of lower tract involvement. Radiographic changes may show hyperinflation (Fig. 20–13). There is a striking similarity between these responses of the host and the bronchiolitis seen after infection with respiratory viruses, e.g., respiratory syncytial virus. Indeed, in clinical onset they may be so similar as to create diagnostic confusion until a subsequent course of the disease clarifies the issue. These viral agents have been associated with exacerbation of pulmonary symptoms in the atopic host, e.g., wheezing in asthmatic children.

TYPE II RESPONSE

The classic example of a Type II hypersensitivity reaction involving the lung is Goodpasture's syndrome. The disorder is characterized by diffuse proliferative glomerulonephritis, pulmonary hemorrhage, anemia, and a rapidly progressive course that usually ends in death within a few weeks to months. The pulmonary manifestations are clinically indistinguishable from those seen in idiopathic pulmonary hemosiderosis, and both are associated with pulmonary hemorrhages, hemoptysis, iron deficiency anemia, and hemosiderin-laden macrophages, which are usually demonstrable in smears of the sputum or gastric washings. The characteristic immunologic feature of Goodpasture's syndrome is the finding of antibodies in the serum that are reactive with glomerular basement membrane of the lung and the kidney. These anti-GBM antibodies have been shown to deposit in the

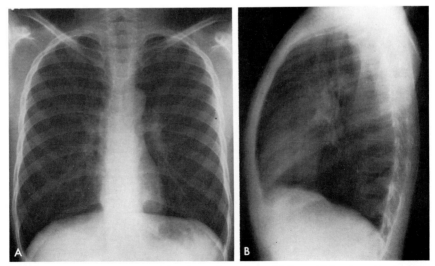

Figure 20–13.   An x-ray of the chest of a patient with bronchial asthma showing the hyperinflation (*A*) and depressed diaphragm (*B*) characteristic of the disease.

kidneys and in the lungs with a characteristic linear pattern of deposition (Chapter 20C).

The course of Goodpasture's syndrome is nearly always fatal. Treatment with corticosteroids may induce temporary remission, but it does not alter the ultimate outcome. A variety of other approaches, including immunosuppressive cytotoxic agents, e.g., azathioprine, exchange transfusion and plasmapheresis have been used but with limited success.

TYPE III RESPONSE

Several hypersensitivity reactions of the lung involve a Type III immune complex–type injury (Table 20–5). They occur in concert with other types of immunologic mechanisms and are described below with allergic diseases of the lung involving injury due to mixed immunologic responses.

TYPE IV RESPONSE

The classic example of the Type IV hypersensitivity reaction in the lung is that seen after infection with tuberculosis. The basic histopathologic feature of this condition is the formation of tubercles containing collections of epithelioid cells, fibrous tissue, and lymphocytes. In this reaction, the sensitized lymphocytes play the major role, independent of circulating antibody. There are other exogenous agents that elicit similar responses. These include silica, coal dust, and beryllium, as well as drugs, e.g., nitrofurantoin (Furadantin). The response to these materials may represent a simple inflammatory episode, although evidence for participation of specific immunologic events is suggested by the similarity in histopathologic appearance of the lesion.

There are a number of other poorly defined pulmonary diseases seen in other clinical conditions, such as rheumatoid arthritis. The association with exogenous agents in these diseases has not been clearly established. The physician should be constantly alert to the possibility of new pollutants and industrial by-products that may produce new immunologically mediated diseases.

MIXED IMMUNOLOGIC RESPONSES: EXTRINSIC ALLERGIC ALVEOLITIS, TYPES III AND IV, AND ALLERGIC BRONCHOPULMONARY ASPERGILLOSIS, TYPES I AND III

Another set of responses of the host to exogenous antigens is that caused by the extensive inhalation of proteinaceous material, as seen in extrinsic allergic alveolitis, or that resulting from the effects of aspergillus, as seen in allergic bronchopulmonary aspergillosis. These diseases appear to involve mixed immunologic responses that allow a basis for classification of their clinical presentations (Tables 20–2 and 20–6).

Extrinsic Allergic Alveolitis (Pulmonary Hypersensitivity Disease)

This form of hypersensitivity disease results from special circumstances of occupation or environmental exposure. A wide variety of thermophylic actinomycetes, molds, and proteinaceous materials have been implicated in this disorder. Examples of the antigens that give rise to these clinical entities are shown in Table 20–7. Unlike the Type I responses, which affect only about 15 to 20 per cent of genetically predisposed individuals under conditions of everyday exposure, these reactions are seen predominantly in the nonatopic individual under conditions of intensive exposure. Moreover, there appears to be a direct

TABLE 20–6. Comparison of the Clinical and Laboratory Findings in Extrinsic Allergic Alveolitis and Allergic Bronchopulmonary Aspergillosis*

	EXTRINSIC ALLERGIC ALVEOLITIS	ALLERGIC BRONCHOPULMONARY ASPERGILLOSIS
Basic nature	nonatopic	atopic
Immunologic basis	Types III and IV	Types I and III
Physical exam	±	wheezing
Skin test	±†	dual positivity (immediate Type I and Type III Arthus in 4–6 hours)
X-ray	pulmonary infiltrates – interstitial	pulmonary infiltrates – lobar
Complications	pulmonary fibrosis	atelectasis, bronchiectasis
Blood	normal	eosinophilia
Sputum	normal	eosinophilia, mycelia
IgE	normal	elevated
Pulmonary function	restrictive	obstructive
Bronchial provocation	delayed (5–6 hours)	immediate and late
Antibody	precipitating (IgG)	precipitating (IgG), non-precipitating (IgE)

*Adapted from Slavin, R. G.: *In* E. Middleton, C. Reed, and E. Ellis (eds.): Allergy: Principles and Practice. St. Louis, C. V. Mosby, 1978 (in press).
†Positive immediate and late in some cases of pigeon breeder's lung.

TABLE 20–7.   Causes of Hypersensitivity Pneumonitis*

Disease	Source of Antigen	Probable Antigens
Vegetable products		
Farmer's lung	moldy hay	thermophilic actinomycetes
		Micropolyspora faeni
		Thermoactinomyces vulgaris
Bagassosis	moldy pressed sugarcane	thermophilic actinomycetes
	(bagasse)	*Thermoactinomyces sacchari*
Mushroom worker's disease	moldy compost	thermophilic actinomycetes
		Micropolyspora faeni
		Thermoactinomyces vulgaris
Suberosis	moldy cork	unknown
Malt worker's lung	contaminated barley	fungi
		Aspergillus clavatus
Maple bark disease	contaminated maple logs	fungi
		Cryptostroma corticale
Sequoiosis	contaminated wood dust	fungi
		Graphium sp.
		Pullularia sp.
		other fungi
Wood pulp worker's disease	contaminated wood pulp	fungi
		Alternaria sp.
Humidifier lung	contaminated home humidifier	thermophilic actinomycetes
	and air conditioning ducts	*Thermoactinomyces vulgaris*
		Thermoactinomyces candidus
Paprika slicer's lung	moldy paprika pods	fungi
		Mucor stolonifer
Grain measurer's lung	cereal grains	unknown
Thatched roof disease	dried grass and leaves	unknown
Tobacco grower's disease	tobacco plants	unknown
Tea grower's disease	tea plants	unknown
Coffee worker's lung	green coffee bean	unknown
Hypersensitivity pneumonitis	sawdust	unknown
Coptic disease	cloth wrappings of mummies	unknown
Animal products		
Pigeon breeder's disease	pigeon droppings	pigeon serum protein
		(albumin, gamma globulin,
		and others)
Duck fever	bird feathers	chicken proteins
Turkey handler's disease	turkey products	turkey proteins
Insect products		
Miller's lung	wheat weavils	*Sitophilus granarius*
Bacterial or viral products		
Hypersensitivity pneumonitis	*B. subtilis* enzymes[a]	*Bacillus subtilis*
Smallpox handler's lung	smallpox scabs	unknown

[a] Probably induces IgE mediated obstructive airways disease in the great majority of cases.

*From Lopez, M., and Salvaggio, J.: Hypersensitivity pneumonitis: Current concepts of etiology and pathogenesis. Ann. Rev. Med., 27:453, 1976.

relationship between the intensity of the clinical symptoms and the circumstances of exposure. For example, a more acute form of the disease is seen after intensive exposure, whereas a low-grade exposure leads to a more chronic presentation. The effect of such agents in extrinsic allergic alveolitis is to stimulate IgG precipitating antibody in the serum, which then forms complexes with antigen and complement in the interstitial tissues of the lung, mediating injury in a Type III reaction (Table 20–6). Recent evidence suggests that a Type IV-mediated reaction may also be involved. The primary effect of these

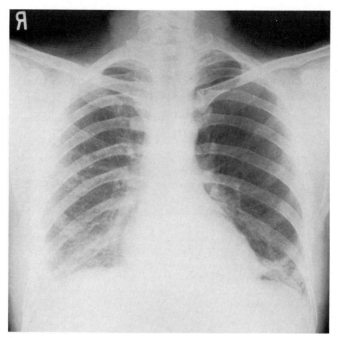

Figure 20–14. An x-ray of the chest of a patient with farmer's lung, showing the "honeycomb" changes in the lungs. (Courtesy of Dr. Sol Katz.)

immunologic reactions is to induce an inflammatory reaction in the lungs with primary involvement of bronchioles and alveoli leading to an interstitial pneumonitis. In contrast to the Type I reaction, this type of allergic disease of the lung is characterized by a restrictive ventilatory defect rather than an obstructive defect. These abnormalities consist of decreased carbon monoxide diffusion, decreased lung compliance, and increased residual volume. Clinically, the condition is characterized by cough, dyspnea, and cyanosis. Wheezing is usually absent, but systemic findings of fever and chills, malaise, and loss of weight are common. Radiographic changes include micronodular infiltrations followed by diffuse fibrosis and "honeycomb" changes affecting particularly the upper lobes (Fig. 20–14). The diagnosis should be suspected on the basis of history, pulmonary function tests, and the finding of precipitins in the serum. Skin tests are of limited value since most antigens lead to nonspecific dermal responses, e.g., thermophylic actinomycetes. A delayed response to bronchial challenge is usually obtained after five to six hours. This procedure should be used with great caution, however, because of the dangers of systemic and pulmonary reactions. Although these responses are mediated primarily by antigen-antibody complexes, as described above, more recent evidence suggests that the late-acting effects of IgE may also be involved.

Allergic Bronchopulmonary Aspergillosis (ABA)

A second type of allergic lung disease whose pathogenesis involves a mixed immunologic response is allergic bronchopulmonary aspergillosis (ABA) (Table 20–6). This is one of several conditions that compose the so-called Loeffler's syndrome or pulmonary infiltration with eosinophilia (PIE) syndrome. Shown in Table 20–8 are the three manifestations of infestation of the host with aspergillus. Aspergilloma, or fungus ball, is an accumulation of the organisms in a pulmonary cavity that can result from a variety of causes, e.g., congenital or bronchiectatic cysts. The disseminated form of aspergillosis occurs as a complication seen primarily in immunosuppressed hosts or in chronic debilitating conditions. Allergic bronchopulmonary aspergillosis is a form of hypersensitivity reaction involving primarily the lung. In contrast to extrinsic allergic alveolitis, ABA occurs primarily in the atopic individual who usually has a long-standing history of bronchial asthma (Table 20–6). The disease occurs as a result of normal exposure to various species of aspergillus, e.g., *A. niger* or *A. fumigatus.* The net effect of such exposure is the production of both IgE nonprecipitating and IgG precipitating antibodies that then participate in immunologic reactions contributing to the tissue injury characteristic of the clinical entity. The most characteristic symptoms of the disease are mediated by Type I IgE-mediated responses, which give rise to the obstructive pulmonary component of the disease. IgG precipitating antibody may also participate in a Type III reaction. A dual skin response is commonly seen, including an immediate Type I (IgE) response and a Type III (Arthus) response seen in four to six hours. The clinical presentation is characterized by low-grade fever, episodic wheezing and dyspnea, and a typical expectoration of golden brown plugs that consist primarily of eosinophils and mycelia. Hyperimmunoglobulinemia E and blood eosinophilia, as well as the finding of a positive precipitating antibody to aspergillus by Ouchterlony double diffusion in agar, are helpful diagnostic aids. The chest roentgenogram classically

TABLE 20–8. Manifestations of the Host After Infestation or Exposure to Aspergillus

Manifestation	Predisposing Condition
Aspergilloma	Cysts, e.g., congenital or bronchiectatic
Disseminated aspergillosis	Immunosuppressed host, e.g., patient receiving azathioprine or chronic debilitating condition (e.g., malignant disorder)
Allergic bronchopulmonary aspergillosis (ABA)	Exposure of the atopic host to aspergillus

reveals transient lobar pulmonary infiltrates that affect different lung areas at different times. Bronchial provocation, when performed, reveals a dual response (immediate and late), as will be described below.

The management of both extrinsic allergic alveolitis and allergic bronchopulmonary aspergillosis rests with the identification of the offending antigen, its removal from the environment where possible or its avoidance, and the use of anti-inflammatory agents, e.g., steroids.

A specialized form of allergic disease of the lung involving mixed immunologic responses is believed to be the basis for the atypical reaction seen after the injection of killed viral vaccines in children (Chapter 23). The two major offenders observed are measles virus and respiratory syncytial virus. After immunization with killed viral vaccines, natural infection resulted in a typical and more devastating disease than occurs in previously nonimmunized children. One hypothesis for these reactions is that selective stimulation of serum IgG antibody had occurred in the absence of local secretory IgA antibody in the respiratory tract. This immunologic imbalance leads to an atypical disease that may have a basis similar to that described for extrinsic allergic alveolitis. Following subsequent exposure to natural measles, an anomalous situation is believed to occur in which viral antigen within the respiratory tract

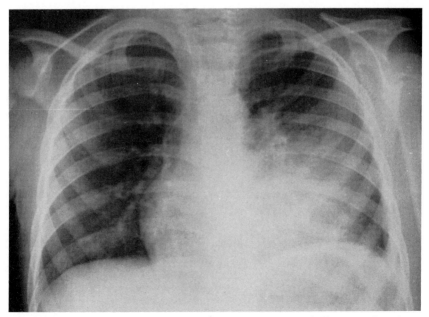

Figure 20-15. An x-ray of the chest showing a pulmonary infiltrate attributed to a Type III reaction occurring in a child with atypical measles who had been previously immunized with killed measles vaccine.

could complex with serum IgG antibody. Such complexes would initiate a Type III reaction in the lung (Fig. 20–15). Children previously immunized with killed measles vaccine who subsequently received live measles vaccine show a localized Arthus reaction at the site of injection (Chapter 23). Immunopathologic staining of biopsy material from these children has revealed the presence of C3, measles and IgG globulin, all present simultaneously within blood vessel walls. Although these histopathologic findings provide direct evidence for the participation of these immune complexes in the pathogenesis of this type of disease, other mechanisms of immunologic injury, e.g., Type I or Type IV, may also be operative in the pathogenesis.

IMMUNOLOGICALLY MEDIATED DISEASES OF UNKNOWN ETIOLOGY ASSOCIATED WITH INFECTION

In many infections caused by various organisms (bacteria, viruses, fungi, and parasites), there are a number of hypersensitivity reactions that occur (Chapters 15, 16, 17, and 18). Some of these are transitory and occur during the course of the disease; others are more protracted and lead to more severe sequelae, e.g., rheumatic fever or acute glomerulonephritis after group A beta hemolytic streptococcal infection. Some acute expressions of acute viral infection might also result in hypersensitivity reactions, e.g., RSV infections that mimic attacks of acute asthma. Indeed, it is still uncertain whether the virus may be infecting selective populations, e.g., atopic individuals, in the expressions of bronchiolitis. These immunologically mediated diseases that are triggered by exogenous agents but affect autologous tissues will be described under the section on autologous antigens.

In summary, the gastrointestinal tract, the skin, and the respiratory tract constitute the primary target organs of the common allergies of man. Although the composition of the initiating agent varies, they are all exogenous in nature. It should be noted that they are all mediated by any of the four mechanisms of immunologic injury. There frequently occurs a transition from one target organ to another. In the most severe case of this nature, the dermal respiratory syndrome, severe eczema progresses to intractable asthma. Indeed, the more elevated levels of IgE immunoglobulins, for example, are seen in those patients with eczema who also have respiratory tract disease. Factors that foster the progression from one target organ to another may be an expression of the genetic constitution of the host, may be related to the quantitative load of antigen, or may represent an insult that overwhelms the immunologic capacity of the individual. It is clear that exogenous antigens evoking these responses should be identified and eliminated from the environment if immunologic balance is to be maintained.

NONIMMUNOLOGIC MECHANISMS INVOLVED IN ALLERGY

Although the immunologic basis of allergic disease has been highlighted in this section, it should be emphasized that another type of imbalance may exist in the allergic individual, i.e., an imbalance of the autonomic nervous system upon which the immunologic imbalance may be superimposed.

The autonomic nervous system is composed of the parasympathetic (cholinergic) and the sympathetic (adrenergic) systems. These two systems generally exert opposing effect on various organs. Between these two systems there appears to exist a balance that maintains a homeostatic control over *mediator cells* and *target cells*. In mediator cells such as the mast cell, for example, the release of vasoactive amines (mediators) can be modulated by both adrenergic and cholinergic agonists; similarly, smooth muscle tone in target cells such as in the bronchial tree can be determined by the balance between sympathetic and parasympathetic activity.

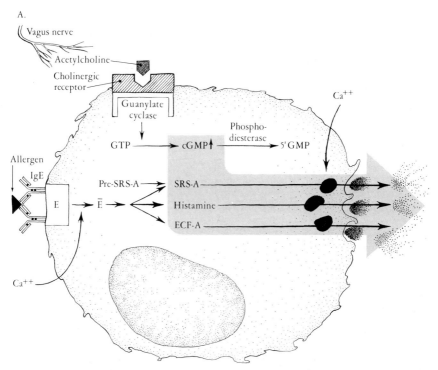

Figure 20–16. Schematic representation of the effects of the sympathetic and parasympathetic responses in allergic mediator release that are mediated through the cyclic nucleotide system. *A*, Effects of elevated cGMP on increased mediator release. *B*, Effects of elevated cAMP on decreased mediator release. *C*, Effects of pharmacologic agonists and antagonists on mediator release. *D*, Role of microtubules in mediator release and inhibition. (*A*, *B*, and *C* adapted from Dr. T. Hubscher.)

Illustration continued on the opposite page

According to current concepts, sympathetic and parasympathetic responses exert their effects through the second messenger system, the cyclic nucleotide system (Fig. 20–16). Stimulation of the parasympathetic system, e.g., vagus, leads to the production of acetylcholine, which converts an inactive form of guanylate cyclase to its active form. This enzyme in turn converts guanosine triphosphate (GTP) into cyclic guanine monophosphate (cGMP). This effect of parasympathetic stimulation can be blocked by the muscarinic antagonist atropine.

In a manner similar to that in which the parasympathetic system affects the levels of cGMP, sympathetic stimulation affects the quantities of cyclic AMP (cAMP). Stimulation of the sympathetic nervous system leads to two types of effects: (1) stimulation of the α receptors leads to decreased intracellular levels of cAMP, and (2) stimulation of the β receptors leads to an elevation of cAMP that occurs through the conversion of the inactive form of adenyl cyclase to its active form, which in turn catalyzes the conversion of ATP to cyclic AMP. The breakdown of both cGMP and cAMP occurs through the actions of the enzyme phosphodiesterase.

The α and β receptors of the sympathetic nervous system are stimulated differentially by various endogenous effector molecules (agonists). Norepinephrine, for example, secreted at the noradrenergic

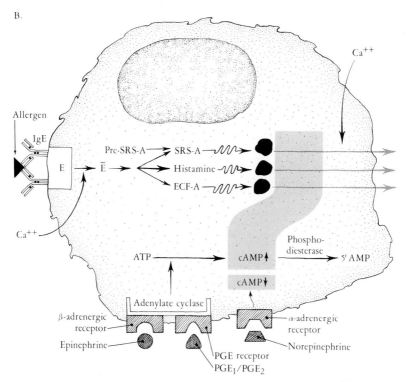

B.

Figure 20–16B *Continued.*
Illustration continued on the following page

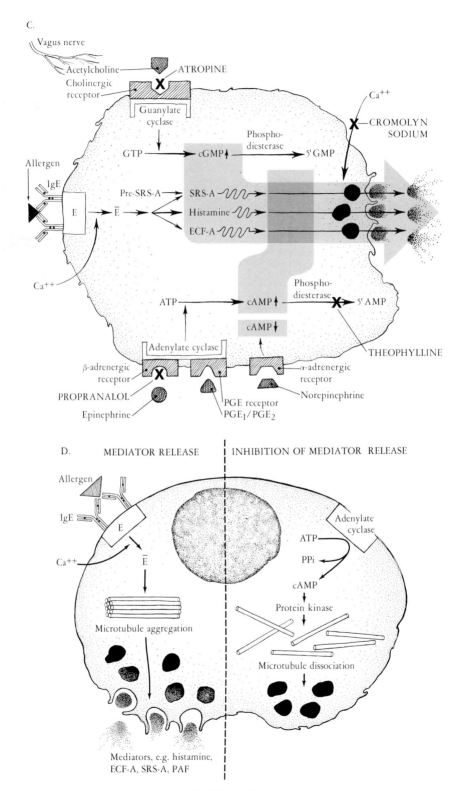

Figure 20–16C and D Continued.

nerve terminals, acts at both α and β receptors, with the α effect predominating. Epinephrine, released by the adrenal medulla, likewise acts on both α and β receptors, but the β effects predominate. There are, in addition, exogenous adrenergic agonists that are specific for the β receptor, e.g., isoproterenol. More recently, it has been demonstrated that there are two types of β receptors, β_1 and β_2, whose distribution in tissues varies. For example, the β_2 receptor is found predominantly in lung tissue, and, as we shall see, the recent development of specific β_2 agonists, e.g., salbutamol, has had particular therapeutic significance in the treatment of bronchial asthma.

PROPOSED MECHANISMS OF RELEASE OF MEDIATORS AND THEIR EFFECTS ON TARGET CELLS

Normally, a balance appears to exist between intracellular levels of cAMP and those of cGMP, the effects of cAMP predominating (Fig. 20–17). As just described, this balance is influenced by both parasympathetic and sympathetic activity, as well as by a variety of other reactants, including inflammatory mediators, e.g., histamine, prostaglandins, and the actual levels of cAMP and cGMP (Fig. 20–17). The relative amounts of these reactants appear to maintain a homeostatic control over both *mediator cells*, e.g., basophils and mast cells, and *target cells*, e.g., smooth muscle cells and mucosal cells. The arbitrary use of these latter terms throughout this book has been defined in Chapters 2, 11, and 13.

Following the interaction of at least two membrane-associated IgE molecules with antigen, a sequence of biochemical events occurs that

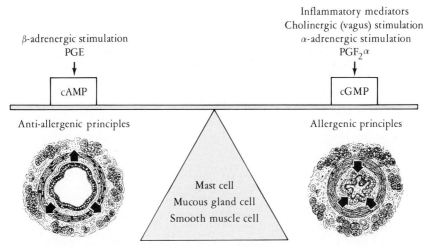

Figure 20–17. Schematic representation of the balance of intracellular cAMP and cGMP and various factors that affect this balance.

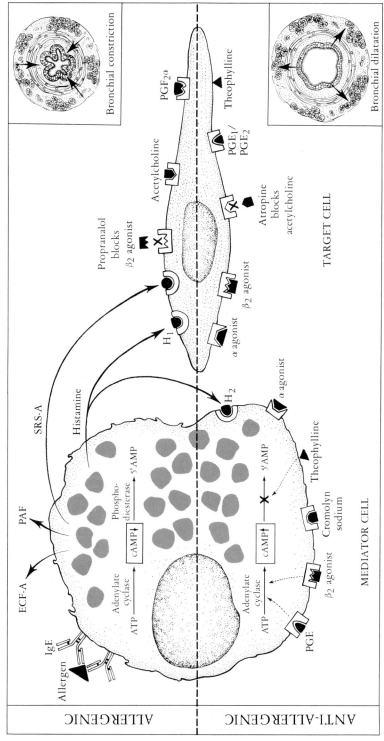

Figure 20–18. Schematic representation of the pharmacologic control of allergic responses by various agents that affect mediator release from mediator cells or the effects of mediators on target cells. (Adapted from Dr. T. Hubscher.)

ultimately leads to the secretion of mediators (Fig. 20–16). This occurs in several steps that include the activation of a proesterase (E) to an active esterase ($\overline{E}$), microtubular aggregation, and finally, the movement of granule-containing mediators to the surface of these cells with the subsequent release of mediators (Fig. 20–16D). Concomitant with these events is a decrease in cellular levels of cAMP. The release of mediators is an energy-requiring step for which ions, e.g., Ca^{++}, must be present. Some mediators (e.g., histamine and ECF-A) are found preformed in the cell; others (e.g., SRS-A) are synthesized from precursors (Fig. 20–16) (Chapter 13). It is now established that agents capable of stimulating adenyl cyclase, e.g., the β-adrenergic agonists, increase the intracellular levels of cAMP and inhibit mediator generation or release, or both (Fig. 20–18). Phosphodiesterase inhibitors such as aminophylline also block mediator release; this occurs because of the elevated levels of cAMP that result from the failure of cAMP catabolism by the inhibition of phosphodiesterase (Fig. 20–16). The net effect of this intracellular buildup of cAMP is microtubular dissociation and an inhibition of mediator release (Fig. 20–16). It should be pointed out that the release of histamine itself can have a negative feedback on this process, since histamine, through its action on the H_2 receptors (Chapter 13), leads to a decreased secretion of mediators (Fig. 20–18).

The relative balance of the cyclic nucleotides also exerts its effect on

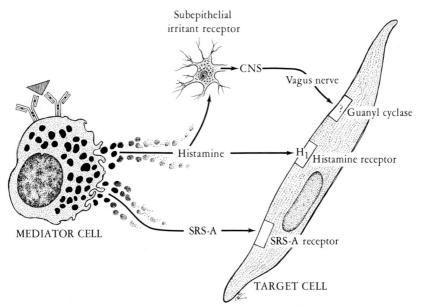

Figure 20–19. Schematic representation of the effects of released mediators on target cells and the indirect mediators in irritant receptors.

target cells by modulating the physiologic state of the cell, e.g., bronchial smooth muscle tone (Fig. 20–18). The effects of raised levels of cAMP lead to a relaxation of smooth muscle, vasoconstriction of blood vessels, or decreased secretion of mucus from target cells; decreased levels of cAMP have the opposite effect. In addition, the release of mediators also has an effect on the target cell, acting presumably through receptors on the surface of the target cells (Fig. 20–19). The mediators can also exert their effects secondarily by affecting subepithelial irritant receptors that can exert a cholinergic effect, e.g., through the vagus, on the target cell (Fig. 20–19).

Thus, the effects of the autonomic balance are twofold: (1) they effect the release of mediators, e.g., histamine, and (2) they lead to effects on target cells, e.g., relaxation of smooth muscle, vasoconstriction of blood vessels, or decreased secretion of mucus. Although less well studied, the effects of cGMP appear to be opposite those of cAMP.

THE NATURE OF THE AUTONOMIC IMBALANCE IN THE ALLERGIC (ATOPIC) INDIVIDUAL

It has been proposed that owing either to a partial β-adrenergic blockade, as originally suggested by Szentivany, or to an inefficiency of the β receptor, an imbalance between intracellular levels of cAMP and cGMP exists in the atopic individual. Such an imbalance would lead to an aberration in the homeostatic regulation of both mediator and target cells in the atopic individual having a tendency toward hyperactive release of mediators and a hyper-responsiveness of target cells. It is known, for example, that the airways and the skin of the atopic individual are more responsive to a wide variety of both specific and nonspecific stimuli than the airways and skin of the normal individual. In the patient with bronchial asthma, one can see the results of this dual effect. The exaggerated response of the airways of the allergic individual that is known to occur after the inhalation of such nonspecific exogenous irritants as smoke, sulfur dioxide, and drugs (e.g., methacholine), as well as endogenous products, e.g., $PGF_2\alpha$, could be accounted for by the hypothesized autonomic imbalance. This response, which appears to be mediated by the irritant receptors (Fig. 20–19), traces its origin from the afferent vagus to the medulla, with completion of the cycle through the efferent vagal nerve endings.

The autonomic imbalance of the allergic individual would also explain the responses of mediator cells. The release of mediators from the mast cells of the allergic individual, for example, would be enhanced by the β blockade owing to decreased intracellular levels of cAMP. This would lead to a further assault on the target cell by the augmentation of target cell responsiveness through these released mediators.

MODIFYING FACTORS

GENETIC PREDISPOSITION

It is well established that there is a genetic predisposition for the development of the atopic diseases of man. These diseases are grouped together, since they are all mediated by a prominent IgE reaginic antibody response. It should be noted, however, that what appears to be heritable is not the specific allergic disease but the capacity to become sensitized to an allergen with which the patient has repeated contact. For example, a mother with asthma whose attacks are precipitated by ragweed may give birth to a child who subsequently suffers from allergic rhinitis, with house dust being the prime offending agent. Furthermore, there is no correlation of an allergen with a specific shock organ. For example, ragweed may trigger allergic rhinitis in one individual and bronchial asthma in another. Recently, there have been associations of allergic disease made with certain histocompatibility types (Chapter 3). Although not definitively proved, a relationship has been suggested between HLA 7 and ragweed hypersensitivity. More recent studies suggest subtle defects in T-lymphocytes (e.g., suppressor cells) that may account for heightened IgE production.

AGE

In achieving immunologic balance, the age of the individual is of critical importance. This is particularly true of the small child in whom the allergic insult may occur prior to complete maturation of the immunologic system. With maturation, the child will develop increasing resistance to many of the infectious agents that at a younger age may be important in initiating his allergic disease. The importance of maturation is also illustrated by the manner in which various diseases present. Tuberculosis in the young infant very often presents in a disseminated miliary form with extrapulmonic involvement; in the older child it is largely restricted to the lungs. These differences are thought to reflect expressions of immunologic maturity. Of particular importance to allergy is the age-related maturation of the IgE system. Age differences have implications in diagnosis, therapy, and predictive value of future disease (Chapter 26).

ROLE OF INFECTION

The role of infection in complicating and triggering allergic disease (asthma) is clear and must be considered in management. Severe bronchospasm and wheezing may initially be triggered by a variety of microorganisms, particularly the respiratory viruses, e.g., RS virus. In other situations, after stimulation by the primary exogenous antigen, these infectious agents may be superimposed upon a primary allergic reaction. Although the mechanism of the precipitation of asthma by infection is not completely understood, it may reflect the stimulation of the irritant receptors of the vagus nerve, as described above.

EMOTIONAL FACTORS

An important concept in the management of the allergic individual lies in appropriate consideration of the role of the emotional factors as both triggering and exacerbating events. It is well known that an attack of asthma may be evoked by an emotional upset. Similarly, the allergic disease may have profound effects on the psychologic development of the individual. As described above, these emotional factors too may exert their effects by way of the autonomic nervous system.

PHYSICAL FACTORS

In addition to the above factors, a variety of physical factors, including heat, cold, exercise, and changes in barometric pressure, may also trigger allergic attacks. Although the precise mechanism of these factors is not completely understood, they are believed to be mediated primarily through the parasympathetic nervous system and initiated by irritation of the afferent receptors in various shock organs.

MANAGEMENT

More than in any other immunologically mediated disease, the causal relationship of persistent antigen is best demonstrated in allergic disease. Symptoms persist precisely as long as the antigen persists. Upon removal of the antigen or blockage of its effect there is a disappearance of the harmful expressions of the immune response. When undertaking the management of the allergic diseases, therefore, there are four points to consider: (1) prevention of the immunologic imbalance, (2) recognition of the immunologic manifestation, (3) identification and removal of the offending agent, and (4) therapy.

PREVENTION OF IMMUNOLOGIC IMBALANCE

Elimination of potential antigens, e.g., foods, animals, and other offending substances, even before the clinical evidence of disease occurs is an important preventive measure. Prior experience, either within a family or derived from prior therapeutic practices, can indicate the preferential avoidance of potential substances known to be allergenic. For example, in other family members in which atopic disease occurs, the use of breast feeding or milk substitutes may prevent the subsequent development of allergy to milk protein. Moreover, since immunologic maturity of the gastrointestinal tract occurs at approximately five months of age, it would seem reasonable to delay, when possible, the introduction of solid foods or at least the most frequently allergenic foods until this time. Furthermore, it has been postulated that the absorption of food proteins or other macromolecules from the gastrointestinal tract may lead to sensitization and subsequent immunization of the older patient manifesting a variety of hypersensitivity diseases, particularly in the IgA-deficient individual. The use of active immunization or the use of human hyperimmune sera rather than foreign sera, e.g., horse serum, in immunotherapy will prevent the development of a serum sickness reaction. Finally, the avoidance of undue exposure to environmental allergens in some of the environmentally induced allergies, e.g., dermatitis and extrinsic allergic alveolitis, may be an important preventive measure in the management of these diseases.

RECOGNITION OF THE IMMUNOLOGIC MANIFESTATION

In order to recognize the immunologic manifestations of immunologically mediated disease, a thorough *history* and *physical examination* must be performed and appropriate *laboratory tests* must be made.

A family history is helpful in identifying patterns of allergic disease in parents or grandparents. Thus, in about 40 per cent of children with severe atopic allergy, a history can be elicited of one parent's having manifest allergy; if both parents have atopic disease, the incidence is raised to approximately 80 per cent in the offspring. In addition to genetic expression, a history of environmental exposure should be obtained. Agents to be looked for include a panorama of foods, inhalants, contactants, or infecting organisms that may be responsible for immunologic imbalance. The history of repeated respiratory–middle ear infections may provide the first clue to the diagnosis of allergic disease, particularly in small children.

Physical examination will reveal signs that vary with the age of the individual and with the length of exposure to the offending exogenous agent. In general, the type and degree of tissue involvement will determine the variety of physical signs. Similarly, appropriate laboratory tests, including nasal smears for eosinophilia, eosinophil counts, sedimentation rates, and appropriate radiographs, may help substantiate the diagnosis of allergic disease (Chapter 26).

IDENTIFICATION OF THE OFFENDING ANTIGEN

Tests of Immediate Hypersensitivity

***In Vivo* Tests.** The most commonly applied technique for the determination of sensitivity to a number of offending agents employs the demonstration of a reaginic effect when small amounts of antigen are introduced either into (*intradermal*) or onto (epicutaneous or prick test) the skin (Chapters 13 and 26). The principle underlying the procedure is based on the immediate-type hypersensitivity reaction that is mediated primarily by cell-bound IgE reaginic antibody. Following the encounter with specific antigen, there is a release of vasoactive substances from the tissue mast cells that results in erythema, induration, and wheal and flare reaction at the site of injection. This response is immediate (within minutes) and its timing assumes diagnostic importance. Occasionally, one encounters late cutaneous allergic reactions (LCAR) that occur four to six hours after the application of the test antigen and appear to be associated with the immediate IgE cutaneous responses. This LCAR may also contribute to the late bronchial provocation reaction as described below.

The P-K, or Prausnitz-Küstner, test represents the passive counterpart of this test and is performed by injecting serum from a positive individual into the skin of a normal recipient. After a latent period of 24 hours, the skin site is injected with specific antigen. If the serum contains reagin, an immediate hypersensitivity reaction is seen. The test is not as commonly used because of the risk of transmitting hepatitis B virus and the development of newer techniques of *in vitro* testing, e.g., RAST. The importance of an immediate skin test reaction is that it is diagnostic in ascertaining the atopic hypersensitivity. This has been particularly useful in the inhalatory antigens but is of limited value in the immunologic imbalance caused by food substances and drugs. The commonly used skin test allergens in allergy include extracts of dusts, molds, pollens, and animal dander.

Immediate-type skin reactivity is not to be confused with other skin tests, such as the Dick and Schick tests, that measure circulating antitoxin (toxin-neutralization) to erythrogenic toxin and diphtheria toxin, respectively, and not mediator release (Chapter 8). These are not mediated by IgE antibody but by classic IgG antibody.

Provocation Tests. Provocation challenge is another method of *in vivo* diagnosis that is sometimes used to further document immediate hypersensitivity states. These procedures include conjunctival, nasal, and bronchial challenge, as well as oral challenge in the case of ingestants. In addition to the use of specific antigens, pharmacologic agents, e.g., methacholine, have also been employed to demonstrate the autonomic imbalance.

There are basically three types of reactions commonly seen after bronchial challenge (Table 20–9, Fig. 20–20). These include the immediate, late, and dual responses. The immediate responses are characterized by a fall in FEV_1 within minutes of challenge, are triggered by the IgE Type I mechanism, and are classically seen in bronchial asthma. Late responses are characterized by a fall in FEV_1 within four to six hours after challenge, are mediated classically by antigen-antibody complexes (Type III) or the late effects of IgE antibody, and are

TABLE 20–9. Types of Responses Seen After Bronchial Provocation in Various Allergic Diseases of the Lung

Type	Functional Response	Mechanism	Example of Disease
Immediate	Fall in FEV, within minutes	IgE (Type I)	Bronchial asthma
Late	Fall in FEV, within 4–6 hours	Type III or late IgE	Pulmonary hyper-sensitivity
Dual	Both immediate and late	Type I Type III or IgE	Allergic bronchopulmo-nary aspergillosis

classically seen in extrinsic allergic alveolitis. The dual responses involve both immediate and late reactions, are triggered by the immediate Type I responses of IgE, the late responses of IgE, or the responses of antigen-antibody complexes (Type III), and are classically seen in acute allergic bronchopulmonary aspergillosis.

In Vitro **Tests.**   There are a variety of *in vitro* tests for the detection of IgE globulin and IgE-associated antibody (Chapter 26). The most commonly employed test for the determination of serum IgE concentrations is the radioimmunosorbent test (RIST). More recently, the PRIST test has been used for the detection of IgE. This assay, which is based on a radioimmunoassay rather than competitive inhibition, has the additional advantages of increased sensitivity and specificity. The principles underlying these procedures have been described in Chapter 8 and are shown schematically in Figure 20–21. Elevated concentrations of IgE are seen in atopic individuals, particularly in older children and adults. In addition, a wide variety of other nonatopic conditions have been associated with elevated IgE concentrations (Table 20–10). The most widely employed test for the detection of IgE-associated antibody is the radioallergosorbent test (RAST), which is represented schematically in Figure 20–21.

Tests of Arthus Hypersensitivity (Type III)

At times, it may be diagnostically helpful to examine for the presence of Type III (Arthus) reactions after the introduction of antigen into the skin. These responses are seen particularly in the mixed forms of hypersensitivity diseases of the lung, e.g., extrinsic allergic alveolitis or allergic bronchopulmonary aspergillosis. The principle underlying this response is based on the formation and subsequent deposition of antigen-antibody complement complexes that initiate an inflammatory dermal reaction within four to eight hours.

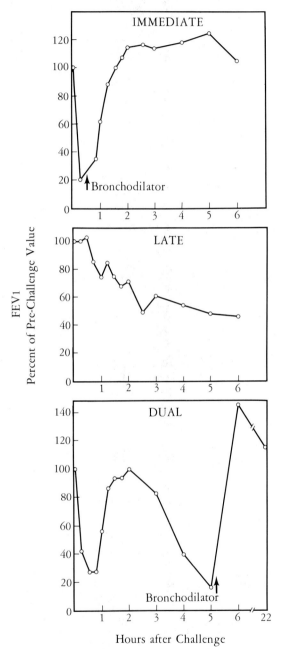

Figure 20–20. Schematic representation of various bronchial provocation responses (immediate, late, and dual) seen in allergic diseases of lung.

Tests of Delayed Hypersensitivity (Type IV)

***In Vivo* Tests.** Other skin tests of the delayed type are used for the assessment of accompanying infectious disease (Chapter 26). These include delayed-hypersensitivity reactions to histoplasmosis, blastomycosis, coccidioidomycosis, cat scratch disease, tuberculosis, and atypical mycobacteria.

Patch Tests. Patch test techniques evoke a skin response in sensitized individuals to surface contactants and represent a form of delayed-type hypersensitivity (Type IV). After application of 24 to 48 hours, an erythematous reaction can be elicited at the site of contact with the offending material. This test is of value in determining contact hypersensitivity. In this situation, the offending agent acts as a hapten conjugated to tissue protein. The offending agents include a variety of dyes, metals, plastics, and organic materials.

***In Vitro* Tests.** *In vitro* tests of delayed hypersensitivity may also be performed. These tests are described in greater detail in Chapter 26 and rely upon the detection of surface markers or morphologic and biochemical responses of T-lymphocytes.

THERAPY

Management of immunologically mediated disease in response to exogenous antigens rests on efforts to adequately identify the causative agent by history, physical examination, and laboratory procedures. If this is to be accomplished, the first role of the physician is to remove the offending agent from the patient. In some cases this is possible, e.g., the removal of household pets, an offending food, or the offending contactant. In other cases, such as with household dust or pollen, total elimination is a physical impossibility. In these cases, a regimen of allergic hyposensitization is often recommended. When the agent is identified as a susceptible bacterium, the offending agent can be eliminated by appropriate antibiotic or chemotherapeutic agents. The use of gamma globulin as a nonspecific adjunct in the treatment of allergic diseases rests on tenuous ground and must be condemned.

Hyposensitization (Immunotherapy)

After identification of the offending exogenous antigen, immunotherapy is frequently employed. This procedure has been shown to be of greater benefit in allergic rhinitis than in bronchial asthma. The procedure involves the injection into the host of gradually increasing doses of antigen, usually to maximal tolerated doses, at varying intervals in an attempt to develop blocking (IgG) antibody protection against these agents. The mechanism of this therapy is thought to be primarily due to the blocking effects of this antibody against reaginic IgE antibody. Re-

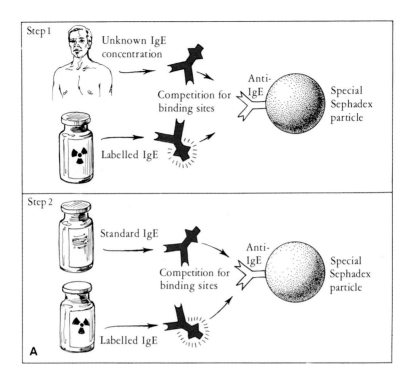

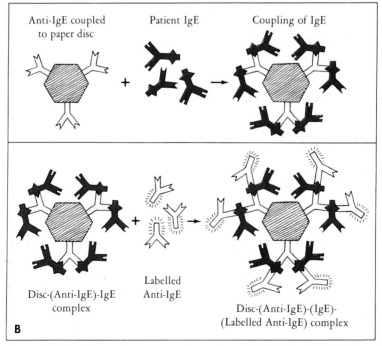

Figure 20–21. Schematic representation of the RIST (A), the PRIST (B), and the RAST (C).

Illustration continued on the opposite page

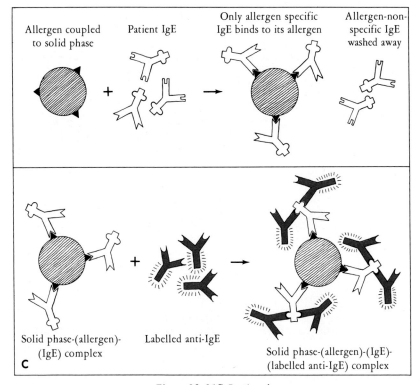

Allergen coupled to solid phase   Patient IgE   Only allergen specific IgE binds to its allergen   Allergen-non-specific IgE washed away

Solid phase-(allergen)-(IgE) complex   Labelled anti-IgE   Solid phase-(allergen)-(IgE)-(labelled anti-IgE) complex

C

Figure 20–21C Continued.

TABLE 20–10.   Clinical Conditions Associated with Elevations of IgE

ATOPIC
Eczema
Allergic rhinitis
Bronchial asthma
Food allergy (?)

NONATOPIC
Parasitic infections
IgE myeloma
Immune deficiency:
    Hypergammaglobulinemia E with recurrent infections
    Wiskott–Aldrich
    Thymic dysplasia
Pulmonary infiltrates with eosinophilia (PIE)
    Loeffler's syndrome
    Bronchopulmonary aspergillosis

cently, the demonstration of IgA blocking antibody in the nasal secretions of individuals undergoing immunotherapy has suggested another possible mechanism for immunotherapy. During the course of immunotherapy, elevated levels of IgE are seen initially; with continued therapy, however, there is a gradual decrease in IgE antibody that generally accompanies the elevation of IgG blocking antibody in the serum. In addition, recent evidence suggests that the development of IgA and IgG blocking antibody in nasal secretions occurs during immunotherapy, and its presence may correlate with improvement. These events are represented schematically in Figures 20–22 and 20–23. It is obvious that such therapy may be ineffective unless accompanied by elimination of other agents to which the patient is sensitive.

Pharmacologic Therapy

With the increased knowledge of the pathophysiologic mechanisms underlying allergic disease, it is possible to provide a more rational approach to the pharmacologic treatment of these diseases.

Antihistamines are frequently used to prevent the symptoms of IgE-mediated atopic allergies. They appear to modify the response and to interrupt the chemical mediation of a number of symptoms of allergic disorders, such as coryza, edema, and itching, characteristic of these entities. They act by antagonizing the effects of histamine. Their use in

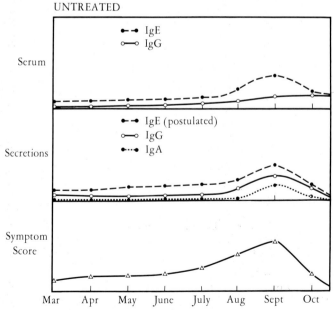

Figure 20–22. Schematic representation of the changes in serum and secretory immunoglobulins and symptom score in untreated allergic individuals.

TREATED

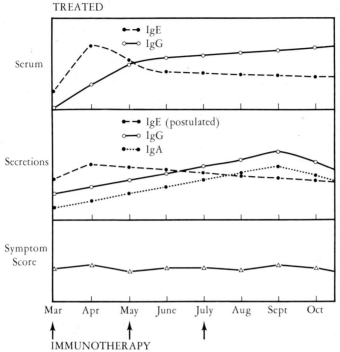

Figure 20–23. Schematic representation of the changes in serum and secretory immunoglobulins and symptom score in treated allergic individuals.

asthma may further enhance the degree of viscosity of mucus owing to their atropine-like effect and may further complicate the obstructive phenomenon characteristic of the asthmatic state. Their use alone in the treatment of this entity, therefore, is not indicated. In addition, other drugs, such as the hydroxyzines, are of benefit in the treatment of urticaria and serum sickness. These drugs have a diverse action that includes an antihistaminic, anticholinergic, and antiserotonin activity.

Another group of drugs is the β agonists that act by stimulating the β receptors (Fig. 20–16). The most efficacious drug for the treatment of immediate hypersensitivity reactions, particularly the anaphylactic, is epinephrine. This drug acts on both β_1 and β_2 adrenergic receptors: (1) β_1 stimulation affects such organs as the heart and skeletal muscle, and (2) β_2 stimulation affects the smooth musculature, blood vessels, and mucus-secreting glands of the lung, for example. The β_1 stimulatory effects of epinephrine are a disadvantage, and various sympathomimetic drugs have been developed by alterations in the basic structure of the epinephrine moiety. These drugs have resulted in agents that contain more β_2 and less β_1 activity and are available both for aerosolization and for systemic use, e.g., isoetharine, metaproterenol, terbutaline, and salbutamol (albuterol).

Another group of drugs that act on the cyclic nucleotide system are the xanthine drugs. Theophylline is one of the most useful drugs in the treatment of asthma. It acts primarily by inhibiting the effects of phosphodiesterase, leading to enhanced levels of cAMP. The drug is best utilized orally or parenterally (5 to 7 mg per kilogram per six hours); however, owing to pharmacokinetic differences in drug metabolism, particularly in children, it is important that blood levels be obtained in order to prevent toxicity; optimal blood levels are usually achieved within the range of 10 to 20 μg per milliliter.

.Disodium cromoglycate (cromolyn) is used in the prevention of bronchial asthma (Fig. 20–16). It is particularly effective in extrinsic asthma and exercise-induced asthma. Its mode of action is to prevent the release of mediators from mediator cells, presumably by preventing calcium influx after the allergen-IgE reaction. Recent reports have suggested toxic reactions to the drug consisting of hypersensitivity pneumonitis, which is reversible upon cessation of the drug.

The corticosteroids have also been useful in preventing or modifying many of the hypersensitivity manifestations of several allergic states, primarily through their anti-inflammatory effect (Chapter 25). They may be applied locally in atopic and contact dermatitis but also have been used systemically in all allergic diseases. Because of side-effects, however, the systemic use of the medication has been reserved for cases refractory to other modes of therapy. The recent development of steroid drugs that can be administered by aerosolization, e.g., beclomethosone and triamcinolone, has provided new approaches to the use of these agents, which have the advantage of producing few or no systemic side-effects when used by the aerosol route. Although local candidiasis and mucosal cell atrophy have been reported after use of these local steroidal preparations, these do not appear to be serious side-effects.

Although systemic use of atropine-like drugs for the treatment of asthma has been avoided in the past because of their drying effects, recent studies have indicated that atropine administered via the aerosol route may be a valuable adjunct in the treatment of bronchial asthma. This approach provides relief of the cholinergic stimulation through its parasympatholytic effect.

INSECT ALLERGY

A specialized group of allergic reactions are those caused by insects. These include those that result from stinging insects (e.g., bees, wasps, yellow jackets, and hornets), from biting insects (e.g., deerfly, blackfly, and the fire ant), or from insect emanations (e.g., caddis fly and cockroach). The mechanisms of these reactions vary with each and may result from the venom (stinging insects), from the salivary secretions (the biting insects), or from inhalation of the allergen (insect emanations). These reactions are for the most part IgE-mediated and may be localized or systemic. The stinging insects produce most serious reactions, which may be life-threatening anaphylactic reactions. The management of these reactions requires a careful history or direct examination of the site (some produce a distinctive lesion, e.g., the fire ant). Preventive measures include avoidance, when possible; however, for those in certain occupations, e.g., agricultural workers and bee keepers, this may not be possible. At the present time, the subject of diagnosis and treatment of allergic reactions to stinging insects with whole-body extracts is controversial. Recent studies indicate that purified specific venom is more effective than whole-body extracts for testing and treatment. Several enzymes have been found in the venom that appear to be potent allergens, e.g., phospholipase A. The continuing development of RAST and histamine-release procedures that can measure the specific antibodies to these allergens may be useful in the future in diagnosis and evaluation of treatment regimen.

ALLERGIC DRUG REACTIONS

Adverse drug reactions have become increasingly common as the number and variety of therapeutic agents have multiplied. It is estimated that between 5 and 10 per cent of hospital inpatients have drug reactions during their stay and that in the general population there is an incidence of appproximately 0.1 to 1 per cent of allergic reactions to any given drug. Moreover, as many as 15 per cent of individuals in the general population believe themselves to be allergic to one or more drugs and therefore may be unnecessarily deprived of an effective drug in a subsequent therapeutic situation. Clearly, it is important to recognize such adverse reactions and to understand their immunologic basis in order to prevent their occurrence and to ameliorate their disease expressions.

CLASSIFICATION OF DRUG REACTIONS

A drug may be defined as any agent used in the diagnosis, treatment, or prevention of disease. In addition to the wide range of drugs currently available to the physician for the treatment of disease, e.g., antibiotics (penicillin), anti-inflammatory drugs (aspirin), anticonvulsant drugs (phenytoin), and local anesthetics (lidocaine), all of which may be associated with adverse reactions, other agents used in the diagnosis of disease, e.g., contrast media (diatrizoate), can also give rise to adverse reactions. The subject of adverse reactions to biologicals used in the prevention of disease, e.g., sera and vaccines, will be taken up in Chapters 23 and 24. Thus, adverse drug reactions can arise during the course of normal therapeutic or diagnostic procedures and can be superimposed upon already existing clinical conditions to create two clinical problems instead of one.

For ease of discussion, the adverse drug reactions are commonly divided into the following groups: (1) *overdosage,* (2) *intolerance,* (3) *idiosyncrasy,* (4) *side-effects,* (5) *secondary effects,* (6) *drug interactions,* and (7) *allergy (hypersensitivity).* Overdosage refers to the symptoms that occur after excessive intake or failure of normal metabolism or excretion of a drug. When the symptoms of overdosage occur at normal pharmacologic doses of the drug, the adverse reaction is referred to as *intolerance. Idiosyncrasy* refers to a qualitatively abnormal response after drug administration that differs from its pharmacologic effect but is not immunologically determined. Idiosyncratic effects generally result from a biochemical variation in drug metabolism. For example, in individuals with G-6-PD deficiency, the ingestion of primaquine results in enchanced red cell hemolysis. A *side-effect* is defined as a therapeutically undesirable but often unavoidable action of a drug, e.g., drowsiness associated with antihistamine therapy. In addition to the primary action of a drug *secondary effects* occasionally are seen, e.g., candidiasis, in patients receiving tetracycline. Another category of adverse drug reactions that is assuming increased clinical importance is that of *drug interaction.* This is defined as the action of one drug upon the effectiveness or toxicity of another. Drug interactions may occur *in vitro* owing to incompatibility of drugs when mixed, or *in vivo* when one drug affects the absorption, protein binding, metabolism, excretion, or interactions at the binding site of another drug. Finally, *allergic (hypersensitivity)* reactions are similar to the idiosyncratic reactions in that both are qualitatively abnormal reactions occurring in small numbers of patients. However, unlike idiosyncracy, the allergic reactions are immunologically mediated. This section will focus primarily on these allergic drug reactions.

Factors Influencing the Development of Drug Allergies

Basically, two groups of factors appear to influence the development of drug hypersensitivity: (1) *drug factors* and (2) *host factors.*

Drug Factors

The immunogenicity of the drug will be affected by its basic nature. For example, some inert drugs, such as the antacids that are composed of simple inorganic chemicals, rarely produce adverse reactions. The capacity to induce an immune response depends upon the capacity of the drug or one of its reactive metabolites to bind to tissue proteins and to then function as a complete immunogen.

Drugs initiating allergic manifestations are usually chemicals of low molecular weight (< 1000 MW) and therefore are not immunogenic in themselves. They act as haptens and must form a firm covalent bond with a tissue protein before an immunologic response can be generated. In some cases, the drug administered is not directly immunogenic, but its degradation products are. The prime example of this is penicillin (Fig. 20–24).

The most frequently used penicillin, benzylpenicillin, produces several distinct breakdown products (Fig. 20–24). When benzylpenicillin is allowed to interact with protein, the major proportion (approximately 95 per cent) forms the benzylpenicilloyl (BPO) haptenic group, the "major" haptenic group. A small proportion of the benzylpenicillin degrades further to produce a number of metabolites, including benzylpenicilloic acid, benzylpenaldic acid, and penicillamine. These may all act as haptens, combining with protein to form antigenic determinants collectively known as the "minor" determinants. These

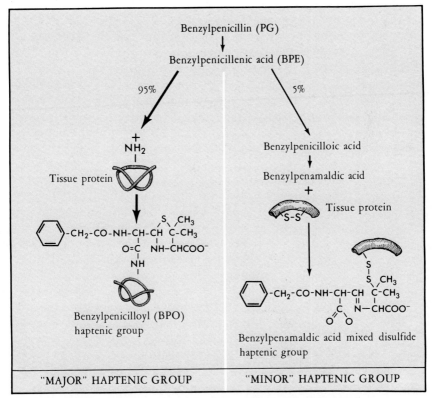

Figure 20–24. Schematic representation of the breakdown products of penicillin thought to be important in penicillin hypersensitivity. (After Levine, B.: Genetic factors in hypersensitivity reactions to drugs. Ann. N.Y. Acad. Sci., *151*:988, 1968.)

"minor" haptenic groups have major clinical importance, however. Although IgE antibodies are directed against both major and minor antigenic determinants, most of the IgE reaginic antibody responsible for severe immediate hypersensitivity drug reactions are directed against the minor determinants.

Other clinical reactions related to these metabolic degradation products of drugs are seen. Drugs may cross-react because their basic structures are similar or the degradation products are antigenically related. For example, multiple semisynthetic penicillins have been produced by the modification of the side chain attached to the beta-lactam ring of the penicillin nucleus. Since most of the immunologic reactivity of the penicillin nucleus is directed to the 6-aminopenicillanic acid nucleus common to all, variations of the side chain have little effect in decreasing cross allergenicity between penicillin and other homologues. Thus, oxacillin, nafcillin, ampicillin, and carbenicillin produce the same types of allergic reactions in penicillin-allergic individuals as does benzylpenicillin.

Although a wide variety of drugs have been implicated in allergic drug reactions, the more common drug allergens include: *antibiotics* (e.g., penicillin), *anti-inflammatory agents* (e.g., aspirin), and *chemotherapeutic agents* (e.g., sulfonamides). Collectively, these drugs account for 80 to 90 per cent of allergic drug reactions encountered in the human.

Another factor influencing drug allergy is the route by which the drug is administered. Topical application of a drug has the greatest capacity for inducing sensitivity, e.g., contact sensitivity; oral administration has the least. The likelihood of reactions following parenteral administration is considered intermediate. Thus, commonly used effective antibiotics that have a potential systemic use should not be used topically, and, except in serious life-threatening infections, the oral route is preferred.

The degree of exposure to a drug may also affect the likelihood of sensitization. The induction period, the time between drug administration and onset of symptoms, varies from one individual to another. In general, the immediacy of onset of the allergic drug reaction is proportional to the degree of prior exposure. Reactions of later onset may reflect the results of an ongoing sensitization. Although prolonged administration of drugs at higher doses would suggest a greater likelihood of sensitization, clinically this does not appear to be the case. The more a drug is used, however, the more likely a drug reaction will develop in any susceptible individual. Furthermore, it should be noted that a drug reaction can be seen in individuals without known prior administration of the drug. For example, penicillin reactions have been observed in individuals who have received the drug for the first time. This presumably represents sensitization by trace amounts of penicillin in food, milk, or nature.

Host Factors

Age. Drug allergy, although appearing in all ages, is seen less frequently in the young. This may reflect the developmental immunologic deficiency of the younger patient or simply the lower degree of exposure to drugs required for sensitization at this age.

Genetic Makeup of the Individual. The fact that only a small proportion of the population is affected indicates a genetic predisposition to drug hypersensitivity rather than a drug effect per se. Information concerning genetic controls operative in drug allergies is limited. However, many clinical and experimental observations have been made recently that suggest the relationship between drug hypersensitivity and genetic regulation. Although allergic drug reactions, particularly to penicillin, have been thought to occur with greater frequency in atopic individuals, more recent evidence has not confirmed this impression. Furthermore, the atopic state does not predispose to the development of contact sensitivity or the immune-complex type of drug allergy.

Conceptually, genetic controls may be operative in any of the following types of mechanisms (Fig. 20–25): (1) metabolic degradation of a drug, (2) the capacity to elaborate components of the immunologic array, (3) structural integrity of the receptor site on tissue cells, and (4) the elaboration of pharmacologically active mediators.

Metabolic Degradation of a Drug. As described above, the allergic drug reaction is often directed against metabolic degradation products of the drug. Thus, it is apparent that in the allergic individual, the development of drug hypersensitivity may be a function of genetically determined differences in drug metabolism.

Elaboration of the Immunologic Array. The varieties of reactions to a drug are as different as the genetic constitutions of the individuals who receive it. Again, penicillin serves to illustrate this variation of immunologic response (Fig. 20–25*B*). Some individuals produce IgE antibodies that result in various urticarial reactions. Others produce IgM antibodies complexed with penicillin that have been associated with exanthematous skin reactions. In still others destruction of hematopoietic cells is produced, resulting in hemolytic anemia, granulocytopenia, or thrombocytopenia. The nature of the control of these mechanisms is still unclear.

The mechanisms by which a drug produces blood dyscrasias are unknown. Four mechanisms have been proposed (Fig. 20–25*C*). The first mechanism is that of IgE-mediated injury. Anaphylactic reactions are those reactions that involve the release of vasoactive amines from mediator cells and can involve Type I (homocytotropic), Type II (cytotoxic), or Type III (anaphylotoxin) responses, as described in Chapter 13. The most frequent and most serious are the IgE responses. Mimicking the anaphylactic reactions are those in which the release of vasoactive substances from mediator cells occurs by nonimmunologic mechanisms, e.g., bee venom, anesthesia, or drugs. These reactions are sometimes termed *anaphylactoid.*

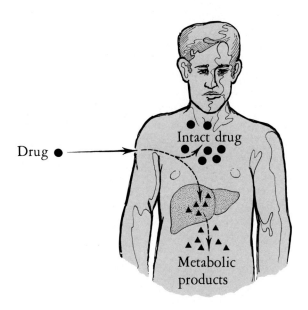

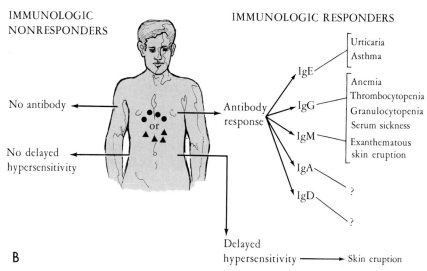

Figure 20-25. Schematic representation of the points at which genetic mechanisms may be operative in drug hypersensitivity: (1) metabolic degradation of a drug (*A*), (2) the capacity to respond with the elaboration of components of the immunologic array (*B*), (3) the structural integrity of the receptor sites on tissue cells (*C*), and (4) the elaboration of pharmacologically active mediators (*C*) as shown in the four types of mechanisms of immunologic injury.

Illustration continued on the opposite page

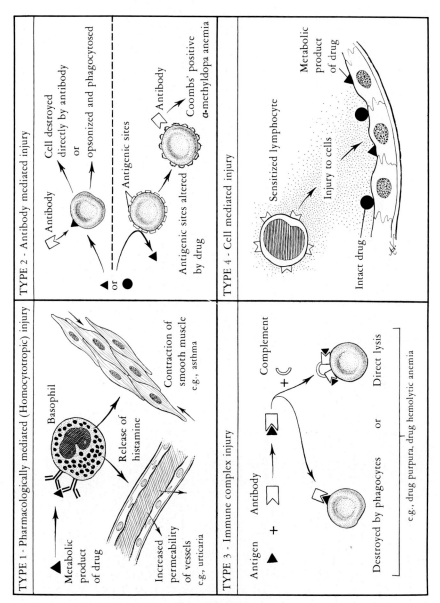

Figure 20–25 *Continued.*

The second mechanism was postulated by Ackroyd, who demonstrated the presence of platelet-lysing antibodies in the sera of patients who had received the drug apronalide (Sedormid). When platelets, drug, and complement were added *in vitro*, the platelets were lysed. The platelet cell was assumed to contain the carrier protein that complexed with the drug (hapten), and then antibodies were developed against the platelets (Fig. 20–25*C*, Type II); antibodies to the drug were not demonstrated, however. The nature of this reaction is unexplained on the basis of classic hapten immunology, in which antibodies are usually formed to the hapten, and, therefore, the nature of this reaction is still unclear.

The third mechanism is one of antigen-antibody complexes in which antibodies to the drug and the hapten form soluble complexes (Fig. 20–25*C*, Type III). Subsequent injury of the target cell occurs through the direct cytotoxic effect of these complexes. This phenomenon is reminiscent of the leukopenia and thrombocytopenia seen in serum sickness, in which it has been shown that immune complexes with complement lead to the rapid elimination of these cells from the circulation.

Another mechanism is the type of hemolytic anemia seen in penicillin hypersensitivity, in which the major haptenic antigen (BPO) attaches firmly to the red cell surface and antibodies are directed to the hapten. This antibody then coats cells, which produce a positive Coombs test, after which the red cells are removed. This phenomenon has been referred to as "passive" hemagglutination of "passive" hemolysis (Fig. 20–25*C*, Type II).

A fourth mechanism involves alteration of cell surface antigens by drugs such as alpha-methyldopa (Fig. 20–25*C*, Type II). This mechanism leads to autoantibody formation, and this will be described later.

The complexes of drug with antibody can also result in a more generalized serum sickness reaction with involvement of skin, joints, and kidney. Finally, contact hypersensitivity to penicillin has resulted from the repeated handling of the drug by medical personnel. While the capacity to become allergically sensitive to all drugs probably is under complex genetic control, it has been postulated that a genetic polymorphism exists to respond to certain immunogens with the production of reaginic antibody, the atopic condition. Atopic individuals appear to be more susceptible to reactions mediated by reaginic antibody than nonatopic individuals. Recent studies in humans and animals suggest the existence of genes that control the capacity to respond to specific allergens and others that regulate the amounts of IgE synthesized under the influence of suppressor T-cells (Chapter 3). Moreover, in the case of contact hypersensitivity, recent work suggests that the expression of these hypersensitivity states can be regulated by suppressor T-cells (Chapter 10). This knowledge concerning the genetic controls of immunologic reactivity should provide new approaches to the prevention and therapy of allergic drug reactions in the future.

Receptor Sites. Several explanations have been proposed to explain drug allergies on the basis of variability of tissue receptor sites or differences in binding of the drug with products of the immune response (Fig. 20–25*C*). For example, alpha-methyldopa administration has been associated with the appearance of a positive Coombs test in certain individuals. The autoantibody has been shown to be of the IgG warm active type and has shown specificity for the Rh locus. Presumably, tissue receptors at the Rh locus are modified by the drug or its products. These observations suggest that a genetic control may exist at the tissue receptor sites, accounting for drug hypersensitivity in some individuals.

Elaboration of Pharmacologically Active Mediators. The elaboration of pharmacologically active mediators may also be a controlling factor in the development of drug allergy. Inbred strains of animals show striking variations in histamine release. Variations in response to a single drug also occur within a strain. These observations have not been substantiated in man, but the great variability in urticarial lesions, for example, from individual to individual suggests that the elaboration of these mediators may be under genetic control and may account for the variability of drug reactions in man (Fig. 20–25C). As described above, the anaphylactic reaction may be an example of this phenomenon.

CLINICAL VARIETIES OF DRUG REACTIONS

The clinical manifestations of drug reactions are varied and can affect virtually every tissue of the body. For ease of discussion, the clinical varieties of drug reactions can be divided into: (1) *systemic* and (2) *cutaneous* The common manifestations of both are shown in Table 20–11 and Table 20–12, together with examples of drugs known to cause these various manifestations.

TABLE 20–11. Clinical Patterns of Adverse Drug Reactions: Systemic

MANIFESTATION	EXAMPLE OF DRUG
Drug fever	Para-aminosalicylic acid
Anaphylaxis	Penicillin
Serum sickness syndrome	Penicillin, serum
Pulmonary manifestations	
Bronchial asthma	Aspirin
	Nitrofurantoin
Hypersensitivity lung disease	Cromolyn
Loeffler's type syndrome (pulmonary infiltrate with eosinophilia (PIE))	Para-aminosalicylic acid
Interstitial fibrosis	
Vasculitis	Sulfonamide
Hematologic-lymphoreticular manifestations	
Eosinophilia	Phenytoin (Dilantin)
Thrombocytopenia	Chlorothiazides
Hemolytic anemia	Alpha-Methyldopa (Aldomet)
Lymphadenopathy	Phenytoin (Dilantin)
Hepatic manifestations	
Cholestasis	Phenothiazines
Hepatocellular damage	Iproniazid
Collagen-vascular manifestations	
Vasculitis	Penicillin
Polyarteritis	Sulfonamides
SLE-like	Hydralazine

TABLE 20–12.   Clinical Patterns of Adverse Drug Reactions: Cutaneous

Manifestation	Example of Drug
Contact dermatitis	Penicillin, paraben esters
Urticaria and angioedema	Salicylates
Exanthematous eruptions	Barbiturates
Erythema multiforme–like eruptions (Stevens-Johnson syndrome)	Phenytoin (Dilantin)
Erythema nodosum	Iodides and bromides
Purpuric eruptions	Sulfonamides
Exfoliative dermatitis	Barbiturates
Fixed drug eruptions	Phenolphthalein
Photosensitivity	
Phototoxicity	Chlorpromazine
Photoallergy	Sulfonamides

Systemic Varieties of Drug Reactions

Drug Fever.   One aspect of drug reactions is drug fever. This condition is characterized by a temperature elevation seen during the course of drug administration. The diagnosis of this condition may be at times perplexing, since the drug is usually an antibiotic, e.g., penicillin, that is being used in the treatment of an ongoing infection in which fever may also be seen. Drug fever should always be suspected if a prolonged febrile response occurs in the patient after adequate antibiotic therapy. Drug fever may be associated with a vasculitis characterized by multiple small vessel inflammation. If allowed to continue, the drug can lead to severe organ damage. Early recognition of the condition is therefore mandatory.

Anaphylactic, Accelerated, and Late Reactions.   Classification of allergic drug reactions can be based on the time of onset of symptoms after administration of the drug (Table 20–13). The most serious drug reactions occur within minutes of drug administration and are characterized by urticaria, hypotension, and shock. When the reaction is life-threatening, it is termed *anaphylactic* or *anaphylactoid*. These reactions are *immediate* and are mediated primarily by the IgE reaginic antibodies, which in the case of penicillin hypersensitivity are directed toward the minor haptenic groups of the molecule. *Accelerated* reactions begin from 1 to 72 hours after drug administration and are almost always manifested by urticaria. They occasionally take the form of morbilliform eruptions and laryngeal edema, which are associated with antibodies directed toward the major antigen. The *late* reactions begin three days after therapy and are seen as various forms of skin eruptions, serum

TABLE 20–13.   Clinical Types of Allergic Drug Reactions*

IMMEDIATE	ACCELERATED	LATE	USUALLY LATE
Urticaria	Urticaria	Urticaria	Hemolytic anemia
Hypotension	Morbilliform eruptions	Exanthematic	Thrombocytopenia
Asthma	Laryngeal edema	skin reactions	Granulocytopenia
Laryngeal edema		Serum sickness–	Stevens-Johnson
		like reactions	syndrome
		Drug fever	Acute renal insufficiency
			Lupus-like syndrome
			Cholestatic jaundice

*After Levine, B. B.: Genetic factors in hypersensitivity reactions to drugs. Ann. N.Y. Acad. Sci., *151*:988, 1968.

sickness, and drug fever (Fig. 20–26). More rarely, the unusually late reactions, which are listed in Table 20–13, are seen. Although it is not known with certainty, the accelerated drug allergies are thought to be mediated by IgE, and the late allergic reactions are thought to be mediated by soluble antigen-antibody complexes in which the antibodies are primarily of the IgG and IgM varieties. The unusually late reactions are triggered by a variety of immunologic mechanisms and are less readily classified. For example, some are associated with IgG cytolytic (Type II) reactions, e.g., hemolytic anemia; others with antigen-antibody complexes (Type III), e.g., thrombocytopenia; and still others with unknown mechanisms, e.g., the Stevens-Johnson syndrome.

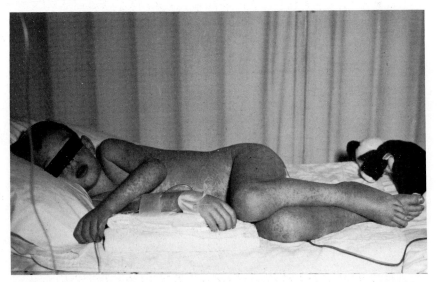

Figure 20–26.   Photograph of a child with a late drug reaction due to ampicillin. Note the generalized exanthem, edema of the extremities, and involvement of the joints characteristic of a serum sickness–like reaction.

Serum Sickness Syndrome. The syndrome of serum sickness was originally described after the use of foreign serum in passive immunization. The reaction resulted from the vehicle of the heterologous serum (Chapter 24). This response is no longer commonly seen after the use of heterologous serum, since whenever possible, human sources of antibody are now used in immunotherapy. It has since been observed that some drugs may also induce a serum sickness–like syndrome. Clinically, the syndrome is characterized by low-grade fever, urticaria, facial edema, pain and swelling of the joints, and lymphadenopathy. Occasionally, other complications occur, such as periarteritis nodosa, Guillain-Barré syndrome, brachial plexus neuritis, optic neuritis, and nephritis.

Pulmonary Manifestations. The lung is occasionally the primary target organ of injury during the course of many adverse drug reactions (Table 20–11). Bronchial asthma, which is the most common pulmonary manifestation of a drug reaction, can occur following the systemic use of drugs such as aspirin. Other forms of hypersensitivity lung disease have been seen following the administration of drugs used in therapy, e.g., nitrofurantoin. Some pulmonary drug reactions are accompanied by the pulmonary infiltration with eosinophilia (PIE) syndrome, e.g., para-aminosalicylic acid. Other drugs can lead to chronic forms of pulmonary injury with fibrosis, e.g., busulfan. Although the precise mechanisms of immunologic injury involved in lung injury are unknown, it has been suggested that with some drugs, e.g., nitrofurantoin, Types II and III injury may be involved in the acute form of the disease and Type IV mechanisms may be operative in the chronic forms. The lung may also be involved in allergic vasculitis, which is usually one of the systemic manifestations of the collagen-vascular diseases.

Hematologic-Lymphoreticular Manifestations. Each of the circulating blood elements can be adversely affected in allergic drug reactions by any of the mechanisms described previously (Table 20–11). Eosinophilia may accompany other adverse drug reactions or may be the sole manifestation of drug hypersensitivity. Its presence, therefore, should alert the clinician to the possibility of an adverse drug reaction. Thrombocytopenia is also a well-known complication; it presents clinically with petechiae or, rarely, with hemorrhage. A wide variety of drugs can produce this clinical syndrome, e.g., chlorothiazides. Hemolytic anemia due to immunologically mediated injury of red cells, e.g., alpha-methyldopa (Aldomet), must be differentiated from the idiosyncratic form that stems from a deficiency of the enzyme glucose-6-phosphate dehydrogenase, e.g., primaquine. Lymphadenopathy is also a common feature of many allergic drug reactions, particularly as part of the serum sickness syndrome. However, it may be present as an isolated event ("pseudolymphoma"), particularly with the anticonvulsant drugs, e.g., phenytoin.

Hepatic Manifestations. The liver can be involved in two types of adverse drug reactions: (1) *cholestasis* and (2) *hepatocellular damage.* Intrahepatic cholestasis is associated primarily with the phenothiazines, which give rise to a clinical picture of biliary obstruction that is usually reversible upon cessation of the drug. The second type of hepatic reaction is that of hepatocellular damage resembling the clinical picture of viral hepatitis. This is a more serious sequela and may not be reversible; it is seen with drugs such as the monoamine oxidase inhibitors, e.g., iproniazide.

Collagen-Vascular Manifestations. Drug allergy should be suspected in the differential diagnosis of all collagen-vascular diseases, since the two diseases can mimic each other. A clinical picture of vasculitis including polyarteritis nodosa with involvement of the skin, musculoskeletal system, kidneys, lungs, and peripheral nerves has been seen after the use of penicillin and the sulfonamides, as well as with a wide variety of other drugs. Other vascular involvements, e.g., Wegener's granulomatosis, allergic granulomatosis, and temporal arteritis, also occur and are less commonly associated with drug administration.

The drug-induced systemic lupus erythematosus–like picture is a well-recognized syndrome following the administration of several drugs, e.g., hydralazine and procainamide (Chapter 20C). This presents with manifestations indistinguishable from those of systemic lupus erythematosus (SLE), e.g., fever, rash, arthritis, and the presence of antinuclear antibodies. It is uncertain whether the mechanism of this reaction is a drug effect per se or whether the drug is selecting the individual genetically predisposed to the natural disease.

Nephropathy. The kidney may be affected in adverse drug reactions either as a glomerulonephritis or as an interstitial nephritis. Several of the anticonvulsants, e.g., trimethadione (Tridione), have been associated with the development of the clinical picture of the nephrotic syndrome indistinguishable from that of the minimal disease type. An interstitial nephritis with tubular damage has been observed after the administration of the penicillins, particularly methicillin. Although a Type III mechanism of injury has been implicated, antitubular membrane antibodies (ATM) have also been demonstrated in this entity.

Neurologic Manifestations. The nervous system has also been involved as the adventitious target of injury in adverse drug reactions. Several drugs have been known to produce a postvaccinal encephalomyelitis–like picture, as well as a peripheral neuritis, either alone or as part of the serum sickness–like syndrome (Table 20–11).

Cutaneous Varieties of Drug Reactions

Contact Dermatitis. An allergic eczematous contact dermatitis may be produced by drugs that are applied topically to the skin or mucous membranes and can be exacerbated after the systemic administration of drugs (Table 20–12). Physicians, nurses, and pharmacists are particularly likely to develop such reactions during the course of handling such drugs, e.g., penicillin; dentists are susceptible to similar problems from handling local anesthetics. A particular problem of increasing importance associated with contact sensitization is that of the paraben esters, which are used as preservatives in creams and lotions.

Urticaria and Angioedema.   Urticaria and angioedema can occur as isolated events but may be part of the serum sickness–like reaction. In either case, a diligent search for a drug etiology should be made in every patient. A long list of drugs is associated with this clinical picture; the most common are penicillin and the salicylates.

Exanthematous Eruptions.   A wide variety of exanthems may accompany adverse drug reactions. These range from erythematous macular, papular lesions to petechial purpuric lesions and very often may be confused with the common viral exanthems (Fig. 20–26). A wide variety of drugs may produce these lesions; the most common offenders are the barbiturates, penicillin (particularly ampicillin), and the anticonvulsants, e.g., phenytoin.

Of special interest are the two major types of drug eruptions due to ampicillin: (1) a toxic reaction, and (2) an immunologic reaction. After the administration of ampicillin, a florid erythematous eruption may be seen within the first week of therapy. This may be exaggerated in patients with infectious mononucleosis or other viral infections. These toxic reactions associated with ampicillin are not immunologically mediated, and the eruptions subside promptly after the drug is stopped. These reactions may be triggered by toxic impurities in the preparations. With recent improvements in the preparation of ampicillin, however, more purified preparations of the drug are available that have fewer of these toxic reactions. In addition to these toxic reactions, the truly immunologically mediated reactions to ampicillin may occur because of the cross-reacting 6-aminopenicillenic acid nucleus. These reactions may present clinically with urticaria or with more life-threatening sequelae characteristic of true penicillin hypersensitivity.

A particularly important variant of cutaneous drug eruptions is that of the erythema multiforme eruption due to drug allergy and its malignant variant that affects the mucous membranes, the Stevens-Johnson syndrome. Erythema multiforme should be suspected whenever the classic features of erythema with typical bull's eye, sharply circumscribed lesions with central clearing (iris lesions) are present. The Stevens-Johnson syndrome should be suspected whenever the mucous membranes are involved, e.g., mouth, anus, vulva, and conjunctivae. A wide variety of drugs have been implicated in the pathogenesis of these diseases, e.g., phenytoin.

Exfoliative Dermatitis.   Extensive erythema and scaling with shedding of the superficial skin characterize the severe adverse drug reaction exfoliative dermatitis. Death is frequent, particularly in the debilitated or the elderly. Commonly involved drugs include the heavy metals, the barbiturates, and the sulfonamides.

Fixed Drug Eruptions.   Fixed drug eruptions consist of isolated lesions recurring in the same site each time the specific drug is given. This finding is virtually pathognomonic of this type of drug hypersensitivity. Common causes include phenolphthalein, barbiturates, and sulfonamides.

Photosensitivity Reactions After being exposed to sunlight, patients receiving drugs may exhibit adverse reactions. These reactions presumably involve the interaction of a drug and light energy at a restricted wave length (2800–4300 Å). This may occur with direct sunlight or filtered or artificial light. There are two types of photosensitivity reactions: (1) phototoxicity and (2) photoallergic. The phototoxic reactions are nonimmunologic and occur in a significant number of individuals after the first exposure to a drug when adequate light and drug concentrations are present. Clinically, the reaction resembles an exaggerated sunburn, occasionally with vesiculation. Demethylchlortetracycline (Declomycin) and chlorpromazine (Thorazine) have been associated with these reactions. The photoallergic reactions, on the other hand, generally present with an eczematous phase and can also mimic allergic contact dermatitis. These reactions appear to have an immunologic basis and can be differentiated from phototoxic reactions by the fact that only a small fraction of patients exposed to the drug and light will exhibit them. They usually do not occur immediately but may require incubation periods of days or months. Further, the concentration of drug required to elicit these reactions is usually lower than with phototoxic reactions, and there appears to be a significant cross-reactivity with other drugs of similar structure.

Local Anesthetics

Another important aspect of drug reactions is that of adverse reactions to local anesthetics. The three major types of adverse reactions to these agents, in the order of decreasing frequency, are: (1) toxic, (2) vasovagal, and (3) allergic. The toxic reactions arise primarily from overdosage, e.g., rapid absorption after accidental intravascular injection. The manifestations of toxic reactions include central nervous system stimulation, excitement, nausea, vomiting, and occasionally, convulsions with coma and respiratory and cardiac failure. Other undesirable side-effects are the manifestations arising from the sympathomimetic effects of epinephrine, which is often mixed with the local anesthesia to delay absorption. The symptoms consist of anxiety, tremor, tachycardia, and occasionally hypertension; syncope may accompany a vasovagal reaction following dental anesthesia. The allergic reactions, which are relatively infrequent, are immunologically mediated and range from the immediate Type I reaction, e.g., urticaria, to contact hypersensitivity (Type IV).

The local anesthetics are commonly divided into two groups, based upon the presence or absence of the para-aminophenyl nucleus. Group I, the "procaine group," contains the para-aminophenyl nucleus and includes such drugs as procaine (Novocain), benzocaine, and tetracaine (Pontocaine); group II drugs lack the para-aminophenyl nucleus and include lidocaine (Xylocaine), mepivacaine (Carbocaine), and dibucaine (Nupercaine). The clinical importance of this division is that patients allergic to drugs in one group can safely receive drugs in the other.

Contrast Media

Reactions to contrast media, although mimicking allergic reactions, do not appear to have an immunologic basis. They occur within the first few hours after administration of the contrast medium and range from vasomotor reactions, e.g., light-headedness, syncope, pruritus, and urticaria, to the more serious sequelae of coma and death. Although the precise mechanism is unknown, these agents are believed to initiate their effects through mediator release in susceptible individuals. Although these reactions occur three to five times more frequently in atopic individuals, this does not prove that they have an allergic origin. It appears that there are fewer reactions occurring after intra-arterial injection than after intravenous administration. The reactions are not more commonly seen in allergic individuals, and the use of intradermal, ocular, and oral tests is not reliable. Recent studies have suggested that prior administration of antihistamines or steroids to individuals with previous reactions may lessen the severity of these adverse reactions.

Response to Protein Hormones

A variety of reactions to protein hormones have been described. Of particular importance are the reactions to insulin. These may take two forms: (1) insulin allergy and (2) insulin resistance. Although both may involve antibody to insulin, insulin allergy involves an IgE-mediated reaction, and insulin resistance involves circulating IgG, IgA, and IgM antibodies.

Insulin allergy may be characterized by immediate hypersensitivity, e.g., urticaria or anaphylaxis. The management of insulin allergy includes the change of insulin from one species to another or the use of recrystallized insulin. If these procedures are ineffective, the judicious use of desensitization has been suggested. Recently, the use of highly purified forms of insulin, e.g., monocomponent or single-peak insulin, has been shown to be associated with a significantly lower incidence of insulin allergy; this suggests that these reactions may be more related to contaminating proteins than to the insulin itself.

The presenting features of insulin resistance are the appearance of excessive requirements for insulin, i.e., greater than 200 units daily, in the absence of other complications, e.g., diabetic acidosis. The management of insulin resistance usually involves the use of steroids.

It has recently been shown that protein hormones, e.g., insulin, ACTH, and growth hormone, require binding to a membrane receptor for their action. Conditions of hormone resistance have been shown to be related to impairment in hormone-receptor interaction. In the case of insulin resistance, a cause of this interference relates to two effects of antibody: (1) antibody directed to the insulin molecule, preventing the interaction of insulin with its receptor; and (2) antibody directed to the receptor itself, which blocks the hormone receptor from interacting with the insulin. Recently, in myasthenia gravis, antibody to the acetylcholine receptor has been demonstrated to be associated with interference of neurotransmission characteristic of this disease. Paradoxically, in certain patients with thyrotoxicosis, antibody to TSH receptors may actually be responsible for the disease state. For example, in certain patients with Graves' disease, thyroid-stimulating immunoglobulins (TSI), which may represent autoantibodies to the thyroid thyrotropin receptors, are present and lead to a stimulation of thyroxine production (Chapter 20C).

DIAGNOSIS AND TREATMENT

The diagnosis of drug hypersensitivity rests primarily on a high index of suspicion and on disappearance of symptoms upon discontinuance of the drug. Except in the case of penicillin hypersensitivity and hypersensitivity of protein hormones, skin tests are usually unreliable. This lack of reliability is related to the lack of knowledge of the precise nature of the haptenic determinants responsible for these reactions.

In the case of penicillin hypersensitivity, skin tests employing both major and minor antigenic haptenic groups may be used in a predictive way. Only the major haptenic groups are available commercially. Recently, it has been suggested that as an alternative to the use of the minor haptenic determinants, which are not available commercially, skin testing may be performed with freshly prepared solutions of benzyl-penicillin, which conjugates with skin proteins to form the appropriate minor antigenic determinants. Skin tests are limited to IgE reactions. There are no assays that can predict risk with the other immunopathologic states associated with drug hypersensitivity. On the basis of retrospective analysis of the results of skin testing with these preparations, it has been estimated that approximately 95 per cent or more of the potential anaphylactic reactors can be identified. Scratch tests are usually performed prior to intradermal testing. Negative skin tests, however, do not rule out the possibility of late drug reactions, e.g., morbilliform or exanthematic skin reactions, or serum sickness–like reactions, since these are mediated by non-IgE mechanisms, e.g., IgG or IgM.

Other tests of drug hypersensitivity include *in vitro* tests of histamine release and lymphoproliferative responses to the drug. These tests also suffer from a general lack of availability and a lack of reliability. The recently introduced radioallergosorbent test (RAST) for penicillin and the major BPO antigen allows the detection of some IgE antibodies. Although this provides some additional information, it cannot be used solely for the exclusion of IgE responses.

Treatment

The treatment of drug hypersensitivity, as in other cases of immunologically mediated disease, rests upon removal of the offending agent (drugs). In life-threatening situations, epinephrine is the drug of choice, along with other supportive measures. In the other types of drug hypersensitivity, symptomatic treatment using antihistaminics and corticosteroids may be employed.

B. Immunologically Mediated Disease Involving Homologous Antigens

Chester M. Zmijewski, M.D.

The homologous antigens, or alloantigens, constitute tissue identity and differentiate one member of the species from another (Chapter 3). They are sometimes referred to as isoantigens. When alloantigens are involved in immunologically mediated disease, the process is referred to as alloimmunization. In contrast to the immunologic expressions of immunologically mediated disease due to exogenous antigens (Types I, II, III, and IV), the predominant effector mechanism seen in alloimmunization is an antibody-mediated (cytolytic) reaction (Type II).

The homologous antigens are of importance to clinical medicine, and immunologically mediated disease related to these antigens forms three broad categories: (1) disorders due to donor incompatibility resulting from transfusions or pregnancy, (2) disorders due to homologous tissue transplantation, and (3) disorders due to postulated tumor-specific transplantation antigens (TSTA) that may develop during the course of malignant disease (Chapter 19). The immunologically mediated diseases associated with homologous antigens are listed in Table 20–14 with examples.

In describing alloimmunization, a clear distinction should be made between the response of the host to alloantigens from another member of the same species and the response to alloantigens that have been altered within the host by exogenous agents. For example, multitransfused patients may develop antibodies to red cell, white cell, and platelet

TABLE 20–14. Immunologically Mediated Diseases Associated With Homologous Antigens

CATEGORY	EXAMPLE OF ANTIGEN	EXAMPLE OF DISEASES
Transfusion or pregnancy	Red blood cell (ABO, Rh_0 incompatibility)	Hemolytic transfusion reactions, hemolytic disease of newborn
	White blood cell	Nonhemolytic transfusion reactions, neonatal granulocytopenia
	Platelets	Thrombocytopenic purpura, neonatal thrombocytopenia
	Gamma globulin	Hypersensitivity reactions to gamma globulin, prolonged physiologic hypogammaglobulinemia, nonhemolytic transfusion reactions
Organ transplantation	Histocompatibility antigens (HLA)	Graft rejection; graft-versus-host reaction (GVH)
Tumor antigens	Tumor-specific transplantation antigens (TSTA)	Malignant disorders

alloantigens that can lead to systemic reactions; viral infections, such as measles, may alter platelet alloantigens so as to induce an immunologically mediated attack on platelets (thrombocytopenic purpura) within the host. The development of antibody to homologous platelet alloantigens from other individuals is clearly different from the development of antibody to altered platelet alloantigens within the same individual.

The most frequent and clinically important alloimmunizations are the Rh_0 and ABO incompatibilities. These result from allosensitization to red blood cell antigens not present in the host. They present as hemolytic disease of the newborn (erythroblastosis fetalis) or as transfusion reactions. The genetic principles that underlie these incompatibilities were presented in Chapter 3.

In the case of Rh_0 and ABO alloimmunization, IgG and IgM antibodies seem to be of primary clinical importance. The naturally occurring anti-A and anti-B antibodies are IgM and are postulated to be the result of exposure to antigens of similar structure (natural antibodies). Blood group antibodies acquired as the consequence of alloimmunization are "immune," or IgG in type. On a molecular basis, the IgM antibodies have twice the hemolytic activity of IgG antibodies. Only the IgG antibodies, however, can cross the placenta and give rise to hemolytic disease of the newborn. In contrast, both IgM and IgG antibodies have been associated with transfusion reactions.

TRANSFUSION REACTIONS

The generic term *transfusion reaction* refers to a variety of immune and nonimmune complications occurring during or after the transfusion of whole blood or blood products (Fig. 20–27). Examples of nonimmune complications include infection secondary to transfusion of contaminated blood (hepatitis) and cardiac failure due to the rapid transfusion of blood. The immune complications result from the passive transfer or active formation of antibodies to foreign alloantigens of red cells, white cells, platelets, or gamma globulin; less commonly, immune complications may also result from the passive transfusion of allergic antibodies that can initiate hypersensitivity phenomena in the recipient (e.g., reagin-mediated urticaria).

IMMUNOLOGIC ASPECTS

From a practical standpoint, the most commonly occurring and clinically important types of transfusion reactions are those that result in the destruction of red blood cells—the hemolytic transfusion reactions (Table 20–15). The signs and symptoms of these reactions are due to the hemolysis of red blood cells and consist of chills, fever, pain in the lower back, and hemoglobinuria. The hemolytic reactions may be either *immediate* or *delayed* in onset (Table 20–15).

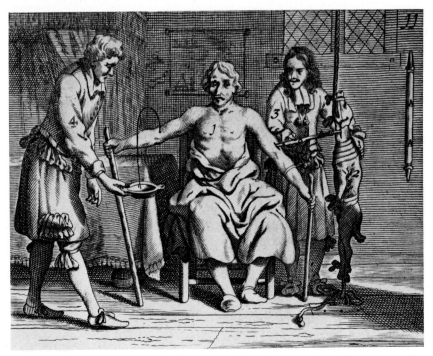

Figure 20–27.   Engraving of a blood transfusion from an animal donor to man by Johann Scultetus, Leyden, 1693. (Courtesy of National Library of Medicine.)

TABLE 20–15. Types of Hemolytic Transfusion Reactions

	TYPE	SYMPTOMS
Immediate		
Major incompatibility	Antibody in recipient's plasma; antigen on donor's cells	Chills, fever, pain, and shock
Minor incompatibility	Antibody in donor's plasma; antigen on recipient's cells	Mild transient hemolytic anemia, self-limiting
Delayed	Delayed onset of antibody production	Late onset of hemolytic anemia

The immediate reactions are due to the presence of preformed antibody and may be of two types: *major* and *minor* incompatibilities. The distinguishing feature between these two types of reactions is the origin of the antibody. The more severe transfusion reactions are seen when antibody is present in the recipient's plasma (major incompatibility). If the antibody is in the donor's plasma, it is diluted upon entering the recipient's circulation and is less likely to produce a severe reaction (minor incompatibility). In contrast, in the delayed type, the transfusion reaction is late in onset and occurs only after antibody is induced through active immunization.

The prevention of a hemolytic transfusion reaction begins with proper compatibility testing (cross-matching). These tests reveal the presence of antibodies directed against either donor or recipient red blood cell antigens. Since blood group antibodies have a wide spectrum of serologic activity dependent upon their immunochemical properties, these tests are usually carried out under a variety of conditions (Chapter 8). The tests conducted at room temperature in saline detect primarily IgM antibodies with low thermal amplitude ("complete" or "saline-active" antibodies). Certain IgG antibodies are detected by performing the test at 37° C in albumin ("incomplete" or "albumin-active" antibodies). Still other IgG antibodies directed against deeply situated receptors in the erythrocytes are detected only by the antiglobulin (Coombs) technique. In addition, the recent findings implicating anti-IgA antibodies in the pathogenesis of transfusion reactions might suggest the desirability of testing the sera for the presence of these antibodies (Chapter 8).

CLINICAL MANAGEMENT

The immediate management of a transfusion reaction requires the prompt cessation of the transfusion at the earliest signs suggesting a reaction while maintaining a continuous intravenous infusion for the direct administration of medications, if necessary (Table 20–16). After

TABLE 20–16. Immediate Treatment of Hemolytic Transfusion Reactions

1. Stop blood
2. Give 1000 ml. of 10 per cent mannitol solution or
3. Give 1000 ml. of normal saline
4. If diuresis continues, repeat 2 and 3 until hemoglobinuria occurs
5. If diuresis does not occur, suspect renal tubular necrosis and anticipate hemodialysis with concurrent exchange transfusion
6. Do not use vasopressor drugs

the blood has been stopped, plasma hemoglobin, which is potentially toxic to the kidney, is removed by osmotic diuretics (10 per cent mannitol) and liberal fluids. This is continued until hemoglobinuria has ceased. If a diuresis does not occur, the possibility of acute renal failure secondary to renal tubular necrosis should be entertained and a program of appropriate fluid restriction instituted. Vasopressor drugs, which may reduce renal perfusion and clearance of hemoglobin, should be avoided.

If it is anticipated that a patient will receive multiple transfusion, e.g., for aplastic anemia, the use of buffy coat–poor red cells without platelets and white cells will reduce the probability of alloimmunization to non–red cell antigens. This will, in turn, reduce the incidence of nonhemolytic transfusion reactions caused by this type of alloimmunization, which will be described later.

HEMOLYTIC DISEASE OF THE NEWBORN

Hemolytic disease of the newborn (HDN) is a condition character-ized by enhanced fetal red cell destruction due to the hemolytic action of maternal antibody transferred across the placenta (see Fig. 4–1). The clinical signs of HDN are explicable on the basis of the hemolytic process (anemia and jaundice) or the sequelae of increased red cell regeneration (erythroblastosis and hepatosplenomegaly). The consequences of ane-mia are the major causes of intrauterine death and include heart failure and, in severe cases, generalized edema (hydrops fetalis).

MECHANISMS OF SENSITIZATION

Although the most frequent fetomaternal incompatibility is that of the ABO system (fetal A and maternal O), the symptoms of the disease are usually relatively mild. Severe hemolytic disease of the newborn is more commonly caused by Rh incompatibility. The antibody most frequently responsible for the disease is the anti-Rh_0 (D); as previously described, only the IgG antibody can cross the placenta and express this disorder.

Antibody formation in the mother can occur through prior transfusion of incompatible cells or more commonly as a consequence of previous pregnancies (Fig. 20–28). It has been shown that fetal red cells can be detected in the blood of randomly selected postpartum women in approximately 71 per cent of cases. There is a variability, however, in maternal production of antibody to these cells that appears to be dependent upon genetic constitution, the number of immunizing cells, and the type of red cell antigen transferred. In general, in the case of Rh_0 incompatibility, the severity of the disease is directly proportional to the number of affected pregnancies. The risk of Rh_0 immunization is diminished if a concurrent ABO incompatibility coexists between the mother and fetus. Any Rh_0-positive cells that enter the Rh_0-negative mother's circulation are destroyed immediately, preventing maternal anti-Rh_0 antibody formation. This observation has formed the basis for

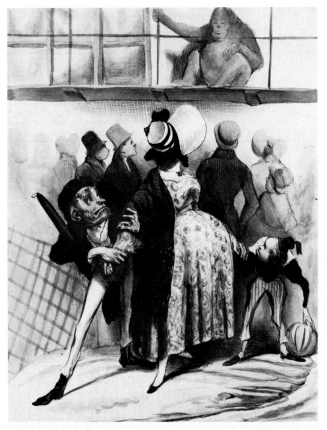

Figure 20–28. Caricature illustrating superstitious fears of prenatal influences on the fetus. A hunchbacked husband and son urge the pregnant mother not to look at an orangutan to avoid malformation in the unborn infant. (Courtesy of National Library of Medicine.)

the most effective method of prevention of Rh_0 sensitization by immuno-suppression through the use of specific anti-Rh_0 antibody. This will be described more fully later.

Regardless of the blood group incompatibility responsible for HDN, an anemia develops that is characterized by a fall in hemoglobin concentration and an increase in the number of nucleated red cells (erythroblasts) in the peripheral circulation; this latter finding gives rise to the term erythroblastosis fetalis. The anemia is more severe in the case of Rh_0 incompatibility.

In addition to anemia, the hemolysis of erythrocytes causes increased amounts of bilirubin pigments to appear in the infant's circulation. In intrauterine life, potentially toxic quantities of indirect bilirubin are excreted through the placenta and are conjugated to direct water-soluble bilirubin in the maternal liver. Postnatally, however, the excess indirect bilirubin cannot be conjugated by the immature neonatal liver, and toxic quantities of indirect bilirubin may accumulate. If they attain sufficiently high concentrations in plasma, the lipid-soluble indirect bilirubin pigment may deposit in brain tissue, resulting in kernicterus with permanent cerebral damage.

DIAGNOSIS

Immunologic Tests

Routinely, the red blood cells of expectant mothers are typed for ABO and Rh_0 blood types. Their plasmas are screened for the presence of "irregular" antibodies other than the normally expected anti-A or anti-B that may have been induced by a previous pregnancy or transfusion. If the mother is Rh_0-negative, the father should be tested to determine his Rh_0 status. If he is found to be Rh_0-negative, no possible incompatibility exists; if he is Rh_0-positive, the possibility exists that the child may also be Rh_0-positive. Although the probability of HDN in the first newborn child is quite low, it is possible that this pregnancy could induce alloimmunization of the mother. In subsequent pregnancies the possibility of the child being Rh_0-positive remains the same but the disease probability increases. The risk depends upon whether the father is homozygous or heterozygous for Rh_0 (D) antigen. After delivery and after every subsequent delivery of an Rh_0-positive baby, the mother should be given anti-Rh_0 globulin within 72 hours of delivery in order to prevent sensitization (Chapter 24).

In addition, during the pregnancy of an Rh_0-negative woman who has a chance of carrying an Rh_0-positive fetus, Rh_0 serum titers should be measured to determine whether active immunization has occurred. Once stimulation has occurred, significant antibody titers persist for many years. Therefore, in such a situation, a single specimen would be uninformative. However, a rise in anti-Rh_0 antibody titer during the course of an individual pregnancy would indicate that an active allo-immunization is in progress. Thus, the possibility of HDN can be assessed from antenatal antibody titers, although the definitive diagnosis can only be made by other techniques.

In patients with a high probability of HDN, prenatal diagnosis can also be established by amniocentesis and spectrophotometric examination of the amniotic fluid for the presence of hemoglobin breakdown pigments. If the diagnosis is established, the risk of fatal HDN can be reduced by the use of intrauterine transfusion of compatible red blood cells. Care should be taken to use blood that has been treated to remove lymphocytes. Transfusion of lymphocyte-contaminated blood has given rise to graft-versus-host reactions during the course of intrauterine transfusions.

After birth, the diagnosis of HDN is established on the basis of clinical and laboratory findings. Jaundice within the first 24 hours of life accompanied by an anemia almost invariably indicates HDN. Evidence to substantiate the diagnosis rests on immunohematologic and chemical laboratory tests. The immunohematologic techniques may be employed for the detection of antibody sensitization of red blood cells. Fetal erythrocytes may be tested directly for antibody coating using the direct Coombs test. Indirect evidence for antibody sensitization may be obtained by screening the maternal plasma against a panel of red blood cells with known antigenic specificity to identify antibodies in her serum that would be potentially harmful to the fetus.

In addition, through the combined use of the direct antiglobulin test and the adult serum-albumin slide sensitization test (Witebsky test), it may be possible to further differentiate ABO sensitization from Rh_0 sensitization. Both tests can be performed on cord blood in every suspected case. Both tests are usually positive in the case of HDN owing to Rh_0 sensitization; usually only the Witebsky test, however, is strongly positive in ABO sensitization (Table 20–17). A positive direct anti-globulin test in the absence of obvious Rh_0 incompatibility may be indicative of sensitization with one of the other less frequently harmful blood group systems, e.g., Duffy or Kell. Since the mother is the source of antibody, a specimen of her blood should be obtained in every case for cross-matching with prospective donors for exchange transfusions and also for further characterization of the injurious alloantibodies.

TABLE 20–17. Immunologic Tests for Detection of Red Cell Sensitization in Hemolytic Disease of Newborn

Type of HDN	Coombs'	Witebsky
Rh_0	+	+
ABO	0 or weakly positive	+

Chemical Tests

Since the intensity of a positive antiglobulin test does not indicate the severity of the disease, hemoglobin and bilirubin determinations are often performed as indicators of red cell destruction. These tests should always be performed in conjunction with the preceding serologic tests. Cord hemoglobin values below 14 gm per 100 ml are considered abnormal. Bilirubin levels require an accelerated rate of rise as an index for exchange transfusion. Althought a level in excess of 20 mg per 100 ml has been used as a guide for exchange transfusion, the decision is more complex since several other critical factors will influence the therapy, e.g., anoxia, prematurity, low birth weight, and serum albumin concentration.

TREATMENT

Exchange transfusion has literally saved the lives of thousands of children and prevented untold numbers of infirmites, such as mental retardation, deafness and cerebral palsy. The purpose of exchange transfusion is to (1) correct the anemia and restore cardiac function, (2) remove sensitized red cells and therefore the source of additional bilirubin, and (3) remove the accumulated bilirubin.

PREVENTION

The use of specific antibody in suppressing the immune response is a well-established technique. It has been used successfully in the prevention of Rh_0 alloimmunization in the human. The principles and mechanisms of this form of immunosuppression were presented in Chapter 10, and the clinical use of the material is described in Chapter 24.

Rh_0 immune globulin is indicated in Rh_0-negative mothers whose newborns are shown to be Rh_0-positive. The preparation is administered within 72 hours of delivery, since this is the time that the greatest number of fetal cells are in the maternal circulation. The material can also be used to prevent immunization due to the transfusion of Rh_0-positive blood to Rh_0-negative women of childbearing age. This has been done successfully in many cases with Rh_0-negative women. Once sensitization has occurred, however, this form of therapy is ineffective.

IMMUNOLOGICALLY MEDIATED DISEASE INVOLVING WHITE CELL AND PLATELET ALLOANTIGENS

Alloimmunizations to white cell and to platelet antigens are analogous in their clinical expressions. Both are seen in multitransfused patients and may occur in multiparous women. They account for nonhemolytic transfusion reactions after blood transfusions. These reactions consist of chills, fever, dyspnea, cardiac abnormalities, and pulmonary edema. These antibodies, when present in the sera of pregnant women, have been shown, on occasion, to cause neonatal granulocytopenia and neonatal thrombocytopenia.

IMMUNOLOGICALLY MEDIATED DISEASE INVOLVING GAMMA GLOBULIN

Alloimmunization to gamma globulin has been observed in individuals receiving gamma globulin injections and also in multiparous females. These antibodies have been associated with hypersensitivity reactions, such as localized reactions consisting of swelling and tenderness, and with generalized anaphylactic reactions. In addition, they have been implicated in the prolonged physiological hypogammaglobulinemia of infancy owing presumably to the passive transfer of antibody directed to paternal gamma globulin types (Chapter 22). These data indicate that gamma globulin therapy should not be used indiscriminately, since it may have undesirable effects. Furthermore, the development of antibodies to IgA globulins has been reported to account for approximately 80 per cent of nonhemolytic transfusion reactions. These antibodies can be of two types: (1) one type that reacts with all forms of IgA (panreactive) and usually occurs in individuals lacking IgA, and (2) another type that is directed against a single genetic form of IgA and can arise in anyone who has been sensitized by transfusion or some other means (Chapter 5).

ORGAN TRANSPLANTATION

Michael C. Gelfand, M.D.

The science of organ transplantation originated more than a thousand years ago with the grafting of skin to repair congenital defects. Today, organ transplantation from one individual to another or within the same individual from one location to another is an accepted therapeutic measure of modern medicine. Virtually every organ except the central nervous system has been transplanted (Table 20–18). In the treatment of end-stage kidney disease alone, over 50,000 renal transplants have been performed, and each year more than 10,000 new kidney transplants will be done throughout the world. Additional productive years have been added to the lives of patients seriously debilitated with severe heart disease, liver failure, or chronic obstructive pulmonary disease through transplantation. Essentially normal lives have been restored to patients with end-stage kidney disease or a variety of forms of bone marrow failure by transplantation of kidneys or bone

TABLE 20–18.   Organ Transplants

Type of Transplant	Example of a Clinical Indication	Complications
Skin	Burns	Rejection, infection
Bone marrow, thymus	Thymic dysplasia, DiGeorge syndrome	Rejection, graft-versus-host reaction
Kidney	End-stage kidney disease	Destruction of graft due to underlying disease process, rejection, infection due to overzealous immunosuppression
Heart	Arteriosclerotic heart disease, congenital heart disease	Rejection
Liver	Congenital biliary atresia	Rejection
Lungs	Chronic obstructive pulmonary disease	Rejection
Pancreas	Pancreatic insufficiency, diabetes, chronic pancreatitis	Rejection
Cornea	Cornea destruction	Opacification

marrow cells. Sight may be re-established by the grafting of cornea, one of the most exciting organ transplants of all since the cornea may be preserved for extended periods of time in organ banks, may be freely transplanted between individuals, and is not readily rejected. Moreover, the privileged condition of the corneal transplant has not only provided evidence for the importance of lymphatic drainage in inducing sensitization of the host but also, more important, represents the desired ideal situation for future transplantation in which organs might someday be preservable and used interchangeably among patients.

In spite of increasingly expanding experience, organ transplantation remains, at best, an imprecise science. This is partly because our knowledge of the various technical, biochemical, and immunologic aspects of transplantation remains incomplete and partly because the clinical aspects of every transplant are different. In experimental organ transplantation in animals, many of these variabilities are controlled by the use of highly inbred animals as recipients or donors, or both. Factors such as age, sex, environmental exposure, tissue antigens, diet, and so forth may be standardized. Since this is not readily accomplished in human organ transplantation, each transplant situation must be approached with considerable individualization.

Nevertheless, the careful analysis of data from experimental and clinical organ transplantation has provided a number of useful general principles of organ transplantation. This section will present the guiding principles that are largely applicable to all organ transplants, highlighting problems of special clinical interest concerning the transplantation of specific organs.

TERMINOLOGY

Living and Cadaveric Donor Grafts

The term by which a graft is known depends on the origin of the graft and its relationship to the recipient. Thus, in human organ transplantation, a graft may be obtained from a living donor (in the case of duplicated organs such as the kidney) or from a recently deceased individual (as necessary in the case of an essential organ such as the heart or liver). Grafts from the former category are called living donor grafts and those from the latter are called cadaveric donor grafts.

Auto-, Iso-, Allo-, and Xenografts

Four types of grafts may be identified, depending on the relationship of the donor to the recipient (Chapter 3). An autograft is a graft taken from and transplanted to the same individual, for example, skin transplanted from the thigh to the chest in a patient with a severe burn. Autografts are not rejected since they are derived from the recipient himself. A graft from an identical twin is called an isograft. This type of graft is also not rejected, since it is antigenically identical to the recipient and is similar to transplantation between inbred littermate animals.

The vast majority of grafts are allografts, exchanged between individuals of the same species but having different tissue antigens. With the exception of the identical twin transplant, all human-to-human organ grafts are allogenic grafts.

The xenograft is not often used in clinical organ transplantation. In this situation, the graft is transplanted between individuals of different species, for example, a baboon liver transplanted into a human with liver failure. Xenografts are generally rapidly rejected since we are not yet successful in transplanting across species lines.

Histocompatibility Antigens

The cell surface proteins that give an organ its recognizable antigenicity and evoke the rejection phenomenon are referred to as histocompatibility antigens (Chapter 3). In all animal species studied sufficiently, similar antigens have been identified on the surface of the nucleated cells of the transplanted tissue. These glycoprotein molecules are responsible for the induction of rejection and appear to be inherited in a systematic fashion, in all cases bearing a relationship to parental antigens.

Histocompatibility Complex

The strip of chromosome that codes for the histocompatibility antigens of man is known as the histocompatibility or HLA complex (Chapter 3). Mice and rats have analogous systems known as H-2 and AGB, respectively, that have been carefully studied and have provided much of our understanding of the HLA complex of man. In these systems, there are genes capable of coding for the production of cell surface antigens, which can be recognized by the recipient as self or foreign. On each of two chromosomes there are at least four known loci, each containing a series of codominant allelic forms. At present, in man, 51 antigens have been recognized in the HLA system; 20 on locus A, 20 on locus B, 5 on locus C, and 6 on locus D (see Table 3–3). Each individual inherits one chromosome from each parent and thus one allele from

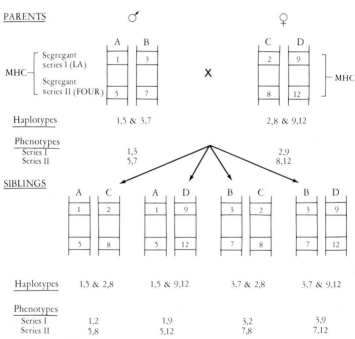

Figure 20–29. One antigen determined by genes at each of the two segregant series (I and II) defines the haplotype. The genotype is composed of both haplotypes present in the diploid cell. The phenotype describes the presence of antigens of the segregant series without reference to their position on the chromosome. In the absence of recombination, only four possible genotypes can result from the mating as shown. Note that genetic material closely associated with the two segregant series will also be transmitted in a similar fashion. (Modified from Glasork, R. J.: Transplantation, immunology, and the dialysis patient. *In* S. G. Massry, and A. L. Sellers (eds.): Clinical Aspects of Uremia and Dialysis. Springfield, Illinois, Charles C Thomas, 1976.)

each of these four loci from each parent. A parent will share exactly half of the antigens with an offspring, and siblings may share all, some, or none of these antigens (Fig. 20–29).

One of the very important distinctions among the antigens of the various loci within the histocompatibility complex is that the gene product antigens of the various loci are capable of stimulating recognition by different limbs of the immune response. The A and B loci antigens stimulate recognition by the humoral immune system, i.e., the serologically determined (SD) antigens, whereas the D locus appears to stimulate recognition by thymus-derived (T-) lymphocytes, i.e., the lymphocytically determined (LD) antigens. Thus, sensitization against antigens of the A or B locus induces circulating antibodies against the specific antigens of these loci. Indeed, this is the basis of the technique that was first used to identify the alleles of the A and B loci. In contrast, individuals sensitized against the antigens of the D locus will have enhanced mixed lymphocyte culture reactivity.

DONOR-RECIPIENT MATCHING

The closer the match between the donor and the recipient, the more likely it is that the transplant will be successful. This is clearly apparent when graft survival in identical twin donor-recipient pairs is compared to that in unrelated pairs. Indeed, bone marrow transplantation almost invariably met with dismal failure until the development of methods of typing and matching donor bone marrow.

The general principles of donor-recipient matching are illustrated in Table 20–19. The first two principles are inviolable, whereas the remainder are relative requisites. Transplantation will not be successful in the presence of ABO incompatibility. It can, however, be performed in the presence of incompatibilities of minor blood group, including Rh.

TABLE 20–19.   Principles of Donor-Recipient Matching

Principle	Method Used for Testing
1. No transplantation across ABO incompatibility	Hemagglutination
2. No transplantation in presence of positive cross-match	Lymphocytotoxicity, leukagglutination
3. Attempt to obtain best HLA match from ABO-compatible potential donors	Lymphocytotoxicity
4. Attempt to obtain transplant from donor inducing least mixed lymphocyte response from ABO-compatible, satisfactorily matched, potential donors	Mixed lymphocyte culture reactivity

A positive cross-match, i.e., when the recipient has demonstrable circulating antibodies against the tissue antigens of the donor, is also a contraindication to transplantation. Such circulating cytotoxic antibodies are routinely tested for by incubating donor lymphoid cells in recipient serum in the presence of a source of complement. After a period of incubation, a marker of cell death (such as trypan blue) is added to the cell suspension and the proportion of dead cells is counted. The presence of significant numbers of dead cells indicates a positive cross-match.

The lack of histocompatibility between recipient and donor is not a contraindication to transplantation; however, in most cases, every effort is made to obtain the closest possible antigenic match for the recipient. This is done by tissue typing, i.e., identifying the antigens of loci A, B, and C on the cells of the recipient by means of monospecific antisera obtained from sensitized individuals and performing a series of individual cross-match tests with the recipient's lymphoid cells. The same is done with the cells of all potential donors, and in the absence of other critical factors, the closest match is selected to be the donor. Critical factors that might eliminate a potential donor include ABO incompatibility, antibodies in the recipient against the donor's cells, medical disability of the donor, and unwillingness to donate an organ.

Living related donors may be further matched to recipients by evaluating D locus compatibility. Compatibility for this locus is evaluated by mixed lymphocyte culture reactivity (MLC), i.e., the degree to which recipient lymphocytes undergo blast transformation on exposure to donor lymphocytes (Chapter 9). To date, the mixed lymphocyte response of the recipient is only evaluated prospectively in living donor transplantation situations. The MLC test requires a number of days to perform and therefore requires too much time to evaluate the recipient's response to cells of a cadaveric donor. In studies done retrospectively, low response of recipient lymphocytes to cadaveric donor cells is associated with better allograft survival.

IMMUNOBIOLOGY OF REJECTION

Rejection may be defined as the process by which the immune system of the host recognizes, becomes sensitized against, and attempts to eliminate the antigenic differences of the donor organ. With the exception of autografts and isografts, some degree of rejection occurs with every transplant. For the present, until clinically applicable methods of inducing unresponsiveness are developed (Chapter 10), the function of immunosuppression is to control the host's natural response and to prevent rejection of the graft.

The prototype of the immunobiology of rejection is primary (first-set) rejection (Chapter 10). In this form of rejection, the host encounters the histocompatibility antigens on the surface of the cells of

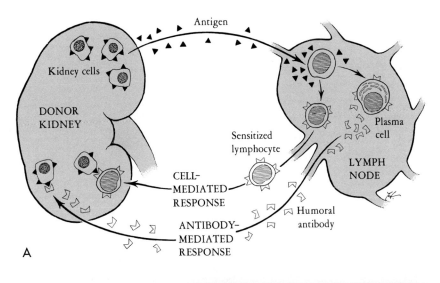

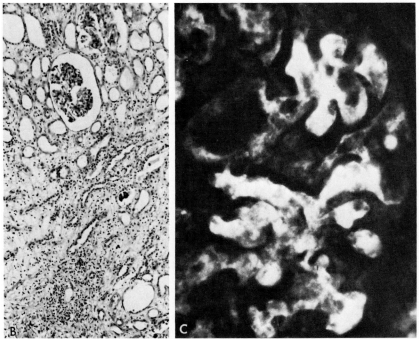

Figure 20–30. Pictorial representation of a kidney undergoing rejection. *A*, Schematic representation of the mechanism of the sensitization process that results in the ultimate acute rejection of a donor tissue. *B*, Photomicrograph of a kidney undergoing acute rejection, showing infiltration of lymphocytes and plasma cells in the interstitial tissues with tubular atrophy also apparent. Hematoxylin and eosin stain, ×120. *C*, Photomicrograph showing the fluorescent antibody staining of a kidney undergoing acute rejection. Note the localization seen along glomerular basement membranes. Original magnification ×800. (*B*, Courtesy of Dr. Abner Golden; *C*, courtesy of Dr. Heinz Bauer.)

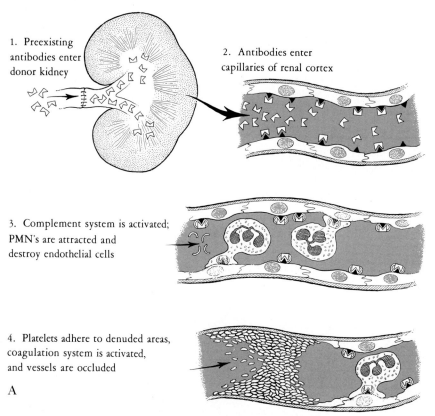

1. Preexisting antibodies enter donor kidney

2. Antibodies enter capillaries of renal cortex

3. Complement system is activated; PMN's are attracted and destroy endothelial cells

4. Platelets adhere to denuded areas, coagulation system is activated, and vessels are occluded

A

Figure 20–31. Pictorial representation of a kidney undergoing *hyperacute* rejection within minutes of transplantation. *A,* Schematic representation of the mechanism of blood vessel occlusion.

Illustration continued on the opposite page

the transplant for the first time. In some as yet poorly described manner locally or within regional lymph nodes, macrophages process antigenic material and present it to B- and T-lymphocytes for sensitization (Fig. 20–30). Sensitized lymphocytes may then enter the peripheral circulation directly or may proceed via lymphatics to the thoracic duct and then enter the peripheral circulation. Upon arriving in the grafted organ and encountering the specific antigens of the graft, sensitized lymphoid cells initiate immune injury. The immune injury may be mediated by either the humoral or cellular limb of the immune response in a variety of ways: (1) directly, by cytotoxic T-cells (K-cells); (2) indirectly, by soluble T-cell mediators of immune injury (lymphokines); (3) by B-cell–mediated (humoral) antibody; or (4) by antibody-dependent cellular cytotoxicity (ADCC) attack on the target organ. This process of primary rejection is the classic model and can become clinically evident after the first week post transplantation.

In contrast to primary rejection is hyperacute rejection. In this type

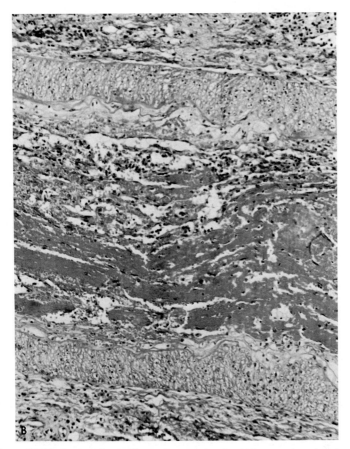

Figure 20–31 *Continued.* B, Photomicrograph of a kidney undergoing hyperacute rejection and showing thrombosis of a major interlobar renal artery. Hematoxylin and eosin stain, ×120. (Courtesy of Dr. Abner Golden.)

of rejection, the recipient has been sensitized to the histocompatibility antigens of the graft by previous transfusions, pregnancy, or transplantation. Circulating cytotoxic antibodies to the HLA antigens of the graft may be found in the serum of recipients hyperacutely rejecting their grafts. Upon completion of the vascular anastomosis, there is prompt deposition of antibody along the vascular endothelium with activation of the complement and the coagulation systems, resulting in fibrin deposition, polymorphonuclear leukocyte infiltration, platelet thrombosis, and prompt coagulative necrosis with invariable loss of the graft (Fig. 20–31).

Acute rejection describes the clinical situation associated with the abrupt onset of signs and symptoms of rejection. The graft is tender, and it is heavily infiltrated with mononuclear and inflammatory cells.

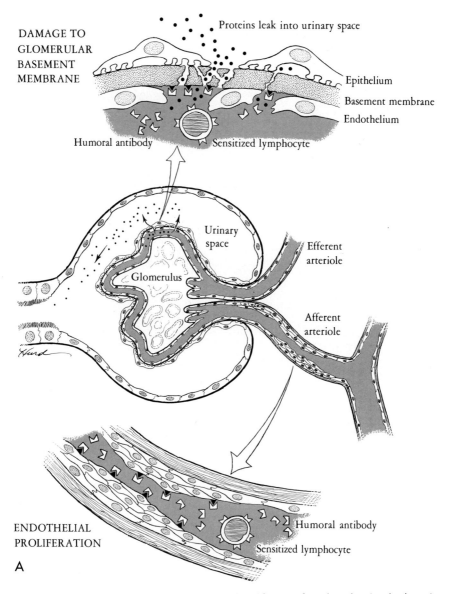

DAMAGE TO
GLOMERULAR
BASEMENT
MEMBRANE

Proteins leak into urinary space

Epithelium

Basement membrane

Endothelium

Humoral antibody   Sensitized lymphocyte

Urinary
space

Efferent
arteriole

Glomerulus

Afferent
arteriole

ENDOTHELIAL
PROLIFERATION

Humoral antibody

Sensitized lymphocyte

A

Figure 20–32. Pictorial representation of a kidney undergoing *chronic* rejection. *A,*
Schematic representation of the tissue destruction seen in the chronic rejection of a kidney.
Illustration continued on the opposite page

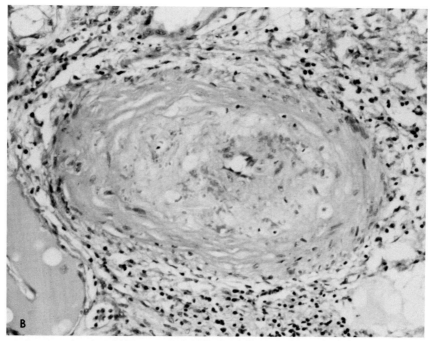

Figure 20–32 *Continued.* *B,* Photomicrograph of a kidney undergoing chronic rejection and showing marked intimal thickening with constriction of the lumen of a renal artery. Note the mucinous appearance of the intima. Hematoxylin and eosin stain, ×360. (Courtesy of Dr. Abner Golden.)

Nevertheless, this type of rejection may respond to immunosuppressive therapy with resolution.

Chronic rejection occurs after an extended period of time and is characterized by gradual loss of function of the graft. On histopathologic examination, the chronically rejected organ appears infiltrated with large numbers of mononuclear cells predominantly of the T-cell line, although B-cells may also be involved. This type of rejection is indolent and is often unresponsive to immunosuppressive therapy (Fig. 20–32).

DIAGNOSIS AND TREATMENT OF REJECTION

The clinical diagnosis and treatment of allograft rejection are extremely challenging for the transplantation immunologist, since there is neither a precise method to make the diagnosis nor any universally accepted or "correct" treatment. This is, in part, related to the fact that no two recipients, donors, or recipient-donor pairs are identical. For example, the underlying state of health of one recipient will differ from that of another, or the type of organ being transplanted might differ. Some of these variables are listed in Table 20–20. Nevertheless, a

TABLE 20–20. Some Factors Affecting Organ Transplantation Between Individual Donor-Recipient Pairs

Recipients
1. Immunologic integrity
2. Previous sensitization
3. Presence of other diseases affecting immune response (e.g., uremia)
4. Presence of disease that might affect metabolism of immunosuppressive drug (e.g., liver disease)
5. Presence of systemic condition that might be exacerbated (e.g., diabetes or hypertension)
6. Need for other medication (e.g., allopurinol)
7. Nutritional status
8. Patient compliance

Donors
1. Type of organ being transplanted
2. Relationship to recipient
3. Degree of match with recipient
4. If cadaver donor, cause of death

number of clinically helpful symptoms and signs of rejection have been identified and are listed in Table 20–21. Fever, myalgias, and localized graft tenderness are frequently observed symptoms; hypertension, leukocytosis, and hypocomplementemia are useful biochemical signs in the diagnosis of graft rejection. In addition, depending on the type of organ being transplanted, there are more specific signs and symptoms to be observed. In renal transplantation, for example, oliguria, lymphocy-

TABLE 20–21. Symptoms and Signs of Rejection

Symptoms
    Fever
    Malaise
    Graft tenderness

Signs
    General
        Hypertension
        Leukocytosis
        Hypocomplementemia
        Elevated sedimentation rate
    Organ-Specific Signs
        Renal: Rising BUN
                Rising creatinine
                Lymphocyturia
                Hematuria
                Proteinuria
                Oliguria
        Heart: Arrhythmias
                Rising cardiac enzymes
        Liver: Rising alkaline phosphatase
                Rising bilirubin
                Rising liver enzymes

TABLE 20–22.   Principles of Immunosuppression

1. Use highest dose of treatment during early post-transplantation period to prevent sensitization
2. Combination drug regimens are often more effective than a single-drug regimen
3. Taper immunosuppression when possible
4. If effective, low-dose or alternate-day regimens are associated with reduced side-effects
5. Treat rejection promptly and aggressively
6. In severe infection or leukopenia, immunosuppression may have to be greatly reduced or stopped to prevent patient death
7. Do not overtreat. There is no successful transplant in a dead patient

turia, hematuria, proteinuria, and rising serum urea nitrogen and creatinine may be seen. In heart transplantation, the development of cardiac arrhythmias may signal incipient rejection.

The treatment of rejection varies considerably depending on the type of transplant and the institution; however, there are a number of generally applicable principles of immunosuppression, which are described in Chapter 25 and shown in Table 20–22. The goal of immunosuppression is to prevent or minimize sensitization, because once sensitization has occurred, the suppression of the immune response becomes considerably more difficult. For this purpose, the recipient receives the largest dose of immunosuppression just prior to or during the first week after transplantation, the period during which primary sensitization occurs. In the unfortunate instance in which the recipient has been presensitized, prompt graft rejection (hyperacute or accelerated) will ensue, defying in most cases the most strenuous attempts at immunosuppression. If no early rejection occurs, the drugs used for immunosuppression are tapered over succeeding days to weeks until a stable maintenance dose is achieved.

In the event of the development of an acute rejection episode, the dose of immunosuppressive agents being used may be increased or different drugs may be added to the regimen until the rejection is brought under control or the graft is lost.

Immunosuppressive Agents

The drugs used for immunosuppression fall into three general categories: anti-inflammatory agents, antimetabolites, and cytotoxic agents (Chapter 25). Table 20–23 lists the commonly used immunosuppressive agents and their mechanisms of action.

Anti-Inflammatory Agents.   The major anti-inflammatory and perhaps the major agents used for immunosuppression are the adrenocortical steroids, e.g., prednisone, prednisolone, and methyl-prednisolone. These agents provide broad, nonspecific, anti-inflamma-

TABLE 20–23.   Immunosuppressive Agents Used in Organ Transplantation

Type of Agent	Mechanism
I. Anti-inflammatory Adrenocortical steroids: Prednisone, prednisolone, methylprednisolone	Stabilizes lysozomes, impairs antigen recognition and processing Lymphocytolysis, impairs antibody synthesis
II. Antimetabolites Azathioprine, 6-mercaptopurine	Impairs nucleic acid synthesis and pyrimidine ribonucleotide
III. Cytotoxic Alkylating agents: Cyclophosphamide, chlorambucil	Causes inter- and intrastrand DNA cross-linkage with alteration of DNA helix
X-irradiation	Karyorrexis, destruction of DNA helix
Antilymphocyte globulin	Immune cytolysis

tory action by stabilizing lysosome membranes. In addition, steroids have a variety of other functions in suppressing the immune response, including prevention of antigen recognition and the effector limb of lymphocyte function (Chapter 25).

Antimetabolites.   A number of agents with antimetabolic properties have been used in immunosuppression. The purine antagonist azathioprine and its active metabolite 6-mercaptopurine competitively inhibit effective purine nucleotide synthesis, thereby resulting in faulty RNA synthesis. The alkylating agents cyclophosphamide and chlorambucil also have antimetabolic effects, since these agents include breaks in the cross-linkage of the DNA helix with faulty relinkage and subsequent cell death.

Cytotoxic Agents.   This large category includes a variety of agents. X-irradiation, whether total-body, local to the graft, or delivered extracorporeally to cells of the bloodstream, has cytolytic properties especially on rapidly reproducing cellular elements such as lymphoid cells undergoing sensitization. In addition, antilymphocyte serum or globulin, an antibody produced in animals (usually the horse) against human lymphocytes, is of help in suppressing the immune response by destroying or inactivating circulating lymphocytes (Chapter 24). Steroids, azathioprine, the alkylating agents, and certain antibiotics such as actinomycin-D also have cytotoxic capabilities. The steroids are predominantly effective in ablating recirculating lymphocytes, the alkylating agent cyclophosphamide is effective against both T- and B-lymphocytes, azathioprine predominantly affects T-lymphocytes, and actinomycin-D is cytotoxic for a variety of dividing cells.

Immunosuppressive Treatment Regimens

Most treatment regimens are designed to combine the effects of various immunosuppressive agents so as to provide a multifocal attack on the immune response. For example, many regimens include a corticosteroid to prevent sensitization, ablate lymphocytes, impair antibody synthesis, and suppress inflammation plus an antimetabolite to inhibit the transmission of the message of antigen sensitization and to provide additional lymphocytolysis. An alkylating agent such as cyclophosphamide may be added for its additional cytotoxic properties, especially against B-lymphocytes. X-irradiation or antilymphocyte serum may be added to enhance cytotoxicity. In the treatment of rejection episodes, boluses of intravenous corticosteroids are frequently added to the standard regimen, with tapering upon successful reversal of rejection.

Consequences of Suppression of Immune Response

Immunosuppressive therapy provides one of the rare opportunities in clinical medicine to be *too* successful. Since most immunosuppressive regimens are nonspecific assaults on immune responsiveness, successful efforts to prevent normal graft rejection must invariably be accompanied by depression of host immune defenses. Fortunately, in most instances, alterations in immunocompetence do not result in major complications. For example, delayed hypersensitivity to an intradermal antigen such as PPD may disappear during immunosuppressive therapy. This is a rather trivial consequence; however, the reactivation or new acquisition of tuberculosis during therapy is an example of a more significant complication.

There are three major complications of immunosuppression: (1) increased susceptibility to infection; (2) development of neoplasms; and (3) graft-versus-host disease (Table 20–24). Infection represents the most important category and includes common and uncommon infectious agents. When approaching the diagnosis of infection in the immunosuppressed host, it is appropriate to consider first the more common organisms. Pneumonia is still more likely to be caused by pneumococcus, and urinary tract infection is more likely to be caused by *Escherichia coli*. Nevertheless, the immunosuppressed individual has a considerably increased risk of having pneumonia caused by *Pneumonocystis carinii* or cytomegalovirus and having urinary tract infection caused by Candida.

In most instances, infections in the transplant recipient can be successfully treated with routine antimicrobial therapy. In the event of overwhelming infection or infection caused by an uncommon organism for which treatment may be ineffective (such as disseminated herpes), it may be of utmost importance to restrict or even stop immunosuppres-

TABLE 20–24. Consequences of Immunosuppression

1. Infections
Common organisms
Pneumococcus
Escherichia coli
Uncommon organisms
Pneumocystis carinii
Cytomegalovirus
Candida
2. Neoplasms
Lymphomas
Reticulum cell sarcoma
Skin and lip carcinomas
3. Graft-versus-host disease
Dermatitis
Diarrhea
Fever
Failure to thrive
Death (if severe)

sive treatment to allow recruitment of host immune defenses or to employ antiviral chemotherapy, e.g., ARA-a. In some cases, such infections result in loss of the graft; however, the ultimate survival of the host must be the primary objective. Frequently, the goals of host survival and graft survival are not easily separated. In renal transplantation, the host may be kept alive by returning to hemodialysis in the event of graft failure; however, in cardiac transplantation, it is virtually impossible to save the patient who loses his graft.

The second category of undesired consequences of immunosuppression is neoplastic transformation. Since the normal immune response provides surveillance against the development of neoplasms, it is not unexpected that the immunosuppressed host is at higher risk to develop neoplasms (Chapter 19). The risk of lymphoma developing in the immunosuppressed transplant recipient appears to be increased 35-fold, with reticulum cell sarcoma occurring at 300 times the expected frequency. Of less serious clinical consequence, but also occurring with considerably increased frequency in the transplant recipient, are cancers of the skin and lip.

Perhaps the clearest example of excessive immunosuppression of the host is the development of graft-versus-host (GVH) disease. This entity lies at the far end of the spectrum of host-graft symbiosis and results when the host is so totally immunosuppressed that the donor lymphoid cells transplanted along with the graft are able to become sensitized and mount an unchallenged immune response against the host. The GVH phenomenon is well described in experimental transplantation where immunoincompetent neonatal F_1 hybrid mice are injected with parental immunocompetent spleen cells. The parental cells recognize and mount an immune response against the F_1 host cells, but the neonatal host cells fail to recognize the parental cells as foreign. In the ensuing reaction, recipient mice develop a clinical syndrome characterized by failure to thrive, runting, diarrhea, dermatitis, and eventually death. In effect, in GVH disease, the host is "rejected" by the uninhibited immune assault of donor lymphoid cells. GVH occurs infrequently (or only subclinically) in most instances; however, in bone marrow transplantation, because the recipient is often spontaneously or intentionally severely depleted of immunocompetent cells, GVH disease is not an uncommon complication.

Specific Organ Transplantation

In this section, the problems relating to specific organ grafts will be presented. In most cases, general principles of organ transplantation are appropriate; however, each organ transplanted provides specialized challenges to the transplantation surgeon and immunologist.

Renal Transplantation.   The successful renal transplant provides the most effective rehabilitative therapy for patients with end-stage renal disease. This is because the kidney provides not only excretory function but also a number of metabolic functions such as vitamin D metabolism and erythropoietin production. Hemodialysis or peritoneal dialysis may provide satisfactory substitution for excretory function, but metabolic functions are not adequately replaced. A dramatic example of this is transplantation of a normal kidney into a patient with Fabry's disease, in which renal failure results from the deposition of glycolipid in the kidney due to absence of α-galactosidase. After renal transplantation, levels of the enzyme as high as 10 per cent or more have been observed, suggesting that renal transplantation has resulted not only in restoration of renal function but also in partial reversal of the underlying enzyme deficiency.

Over 50,000 renal transplants have now been performed, providing the majority of current clinical experience in organ transplantation. This experience has emphasized the importance of careful management of the transplant recipient with avoidance of excessive immunosuppressive therapy. With good matching, the current success rate at two years is about 75 per cent for living related donor transplants and 50 per cent for the cadaveric donor transplants (Fig. 20–33). Moreover, living related donor transplantation is generally associated with fewer and more easily reversible complications, allowing for a smoother post-transplantation course. For these reasons, many transplant centers prefer to do living related donor transplantation whenever possible. Graft survival statistics in renal transplantation actually have not changed significantly in a number of years; however, patient survival rates have increased, suggesting progress in medical management of the transplant recipient.

The general principles of organ transplantation described above are applicable in renal post-transplantation follow-up; however, two types of

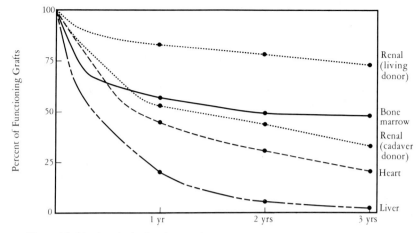

Figure 20–33 Survival of various cadaver and living related donor transplants.

complications are of special importance in renal transplantation. In a small number of patients, technical or surgical problems such as leakage of urine from the newly implanted ureter, stenosis of the newly anastomosed renal artery, or the collection of lymph around the kidney may occur. These technical problems may result in graft loss; however, prompt corrective surgical intervention is usually successful.

A second complication specific for renal transplantation is graft loss secondary to return of the original disease. This was first noted in identical twins in whom no rejection should occur, yet a large proportion of recipients of twin renal grafts had loss of function. Analysis revealed that the loss of function in the transplant resulted from return of glomerulonephritis, the original disease. More recently, the list of diseases that recur after renal transplantation has been expanded to include such diseases as anti–glomerular basement membrane disease, diabetes, and oxalosis (Table 20–25).

Bone Marrow Transplantation. As of 1977, over 500 bone marrow transplants had been performed throughout the world for a variety of conditions of bone marrow failure but primarily for severe combined immunodeficiency disease (SCID) and aplastic anemia.

SCID is a rare congenital disorder in which the functional capacities

TABLE 20–25. Diseases Found to Recur After Renal Transplantation

Glomerulonephritis
    1. Focal sclerosing glomerulonephritis
    2. Membranoproliferative glomerulonephritis
    3. Rapidly progressive glomerulonephritis
       (Anti-GBM-type)
Henoch-Schönlein purpura
Polyarteritis
Oxalosis
Diabetes

of both T- and B-cell lines are absent or severely depressed (Chapter 22). Prior to 1968, the disease was incurable and invariably fatal, usually within the first year of life. Over the last decade, more than 70 children with this disorder have been treated by bone marrow transplantation. Of those treated in this way, nearly 30 per cent remain alive as long as eight years after transplantation. Almost two thirds of children who receive HLA-A and B identical and mixed lymphocyte culture unreactive bone marrow cells survive for at least six months. Children receiving HLA-A or B nonidentical but MLC unreactive marrow have a 38 per cent chance of six months' survival; however, of those receiving MLC-incompatible marrow, only 5 per cent survive six months. These results emphasize the critical importance of MLR matching and the less critical but additional importance of HLA matching.

Of those children who did not survive, nearly all died of infection within the first four months after transplantation. A second major problem in bone marrow transplantation for SCID is GVH disease. GVH is more severe in males, in males receiving bone marrow from females, and in older children (over six months of age) than it is in females and younger children.

Bone marrow transplantation in the treatment of aplastic anemia is associated with approximately a 50 per cent one-year survival. In those patients surviving a year there is virtually no increased mortality at two or three years, showing that a full "take" has occurred by one year. Younger patients (21 years) have better survival rates than older patients. Again, sepsis and GVH disease are the most common causes of death.

Cardiac Transplantation. The era of cardiac transplantation was ushered in with fantastic excitement, perhaps because of the mystique attributed to that organ; however, the overall results of cardiac transplantation have been somewhat disappointing. Approximately 500 heart transplants have been performed and although there are many long-term survivors, sudden death from myocardial infarction or complete atrioventricular conduction block in patients apparently doing well has prevented the proliferation of centers performing this procedure. Nevertheless, groups actively pursuing cardiac transplantation report 50 per cent one-year survival and 30 to 40 per cent two-year survival.

The same general principles hold true with heart transplants as with other organ transplants; however, there are some special problems. The recipient cannot lose his graft and still survive, as he can in kidney transplantation. Except in rare circumstances, there can be no living donor heart transplantation. In cardiac transplantation, the recipient is, in most instances, otherwise uncompromised. This is different from the recipient in kidney or bone marrow transplantation, in which the recipient is immunosuppressed by uremia in the former instance or by the absence of immunocompetent cells in SCID or aplastic anemia.

It is probably too early to draw any significant conclusions regarding the future of cardiac transplantation. Certainly, heart disease is a major public health problem, and when successful, cardiac transplantation has provided from months to many years of added functional life. The vital nature of the heart, and thus the lack of available time in which to reverse the effects of rejection, makes successful cardiac transplantion exceedingly difficult.

Transplantation of Other Organs.   More than 300 liver transplants have been performed with some success but a very high failure rate. It has been suggested that this high failure rate is in part related to the special difficulty encountered in liver transplantation. Of special note are the surgical difficulties encountered in the successful reconstruction of the biliary duct. Nevertheless, survivals as long as five years have been reported, and hepatic transplantation has been life-saving in the presence of irreversible hepatic failure without major secondary systemic decompensation.

Other organs that have been transplanted include the lung and the pancreas. Experience with transplantation of these organs is still too small to provide significant conclusions as to their success rates.

FUTURE PROSPECTS

A major breakthrough in the field of organ transplantation has now been eagerly awaited for a number of years. The hoped-for major increase in graft survival of more closely tissue-matched transplants has not been forthcoming. More potent methods to suppress the immune response, although quite possible in the near future, will likely remain nonspecific, more powerful general attacks on the immune system and will thus result in a higher likelihood of immunosuppressive complications.

From the present viewpoint, any future advances in organ graft survival will out of necessity be derived from some form of specific or selective alteration of immune responsiveness of the recipient-graft pair. One way this might occur is through immunologic tolerance — the induction of a state of immunologic unresponsiveness to a specific antigen but not to others. Such states have been achieved experimentally by the induction of blocking antibodies, by a noncytotoxic form of specific antibody, and by the establishment of tolerance in the recipient through high- or low-dose antigen administration or the creation of chimerism in the recipient. All these methods are very exciting experimentally and applicable in theory but have not been successfully applied to clinical organ transplantation.

Another area that may be ultimately more difficult is the alteration or removal of the antigens of the donor organ with replacement of these antigens by those of the recipient. This would in effect result in an autograft or isograft situation and, if maintained, indefinite graft survival.

Whatever method is achieved, it is clear that the future of organ transplantation requires some form of more specific control of the immune response. If more specific immunoregulation is not forthcoming in the near future, allograft organ transplantation might well be replaced by functional artificial organ implantation, if or when technologic advances provide safe, reliable artificial hearts, kidneys, livers, or lungs.

SUMMARY

Immunologically mediated diseases involving homologous antigens include disorders resulting from immunization to those antigens that differentiate one member of the species from another, the alloantigens. The process by which this occurs is called alloimmunization. These disorders may arise as a consequence of a maternal-fetal relationship surrounding pregnancy, transfusions, or transplantation.

Since all these entities are expressions of the host's response to genetically controlled antigenic specifications, a knowledge of these genetic factors is essential for the prevention and management of these disorders.

C. Immunologically Mediated Disease Involving Autologous Antigens

Joseph A. Bellanti, M.D., John J. Calabro, M.D., and Michael C. Gelfand, M.D.

In a minority of the population there occur disorders known as autoimmune diseases. In these, the cardinal feature is tissue injury caused by an apparent immunologic reaction of the host with its own tissues. In most individuals, there exist within the host "self-recognition" and tolerance of all body components; however, in autoimmune disease, there exists the anomalous condition that Ehrlich referred to as "horror autotoxicus," in which a self-destructive process occurs directed by one's own immune system.

A clear distinction must be made between *autoimmune response* and *autoimmune disease*. The term autoimmune response refers to the demonstration of an autoantibody directed to a "self" antigen or reactivity of lymphocytes sensitized to a "self" antigen. The autoimmune response may or may not be associated with autoimmune disease. Although it is thought that autoimmune diseases result from tissue damage by autoimmune responses, it is not known whether the autoimmune phenomena are a cause, a result, or a concomitant finding in autoimmune disease. In spite of extensive animal experimentation, the autoimmune responses as a cause of human disease remain a hypothesis.

It is common to see autoimmune phenomena in association with infectious diseases. Cold hemagglutinins are commonly seen after infection with *Mycoplasma pneumoniae* and are sometimes associated with hemolysis. Yet there exists no evidence that this autoimmune response results in a self-perpetuating protracted autoimmune disease.

The unfortunate use of the term autoimmune disease, implying a primary attack of the host against itself, arose prior to current knowledge of immunologic mechanisms of tissue injury (Chapter 13). The terms "collagen," "collagen-vascular," and "connective tissue" diseases have likewise imposed additional semantic problems. These terms focus undue attention on the connective tissue, which is only one of several tissues involved. The immunopathology of autoimmune disease may manifest itself by any of the mechanisms of tissue injury described in Chapter 13. Autoimmunity may be considered a tertiary manifestation of the immune response directed at antigen whose inappropriate processing leads to destruction of host tissues. This view differs from the classic concept of a primary attack of the host against its own tissues.

THEORIES OF PATHOGENESIS OF THE AUTOIMMUNE DISEASES

Three hypotheses have been proposed to explain the mechanism and manifestations of autoimmune disease (Fig. 20–34).

The first hypothesis, the *forbidden-clone theory*, postulates a clone of mutant lymphocytes arising through somatic mutation (Fig. 20–34*A*). Mutant cells that carry a surface antigen recognized as foreign (antigenically positive mutant) would be normally destroyed. However, according to this theory, mutant cells that lack surface antigen (antigenically negative mutants) would not be destroyed. With the proliferation of these antigen-deficient mutants (forbidden clones), these cells would be capable of reacting with target tissues because of genetic dissimilarity. The phenomenon is analogous to a genetically incompatible lymphocyte graft-versus-host reaction (Chapter 3).

The second hypothesis, the *sequestered-antigen theory*, is based on the phenomenon of tolerance induction in the fetus (Chapter 3) (Fig. 20–34*B*). According to this theory, during embryonic development,

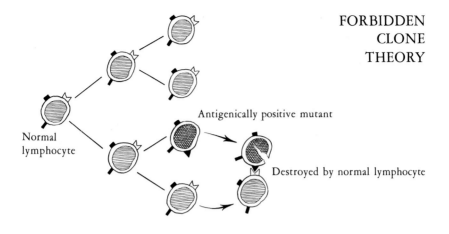

FORBIDDEN
CLONE
THEORY

Antigenically positive mutant

Normal
lymphocyte

Destroyed by normal lymphocyte

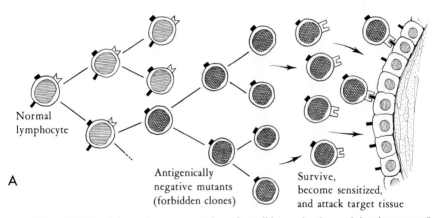

Normal
lymphocyte

A

Antigenically
negative mutants
(forbidden clones)

Survive,
become sensitized,
and attack target tissue

Figure 20–34. Schematic representation of possible mechanisms of development of autoimmunity. *A*, Forbidden-clone theory. *B*, Sequestered-antigen theory. *C*, Immunologic deficiency theory. Note that immunologic deficiency can lead to emergence of deleterious clones or to immunologic injury secondary to persistence of microbes.

Illustration continued on the following page

tissues that are exposed to the lymphoreticular system are recognized as "self." Those that are anatomically separated or sequestered from the lymphoreticular system are not identified as "self." These antigens occur in tissues such as the lens of the eye, the central nervous system, the thyroid, and the testes. In later life, exposure, through trauma or infection, of the sequestered tissue antigens to the lymphoreticular system results in autoimmune disease.

Both these concepts are based on the premise of *hyperactivity* of the immune response, which through autoantibody formation or sensitized lymphocytes (delayed hypersensitivity) would lead to the production of an autoimmune disease.

SEQUESTERED ANTIGEN THEORY

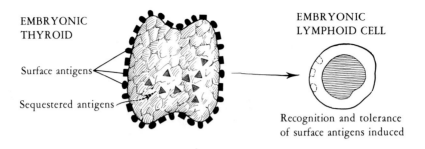

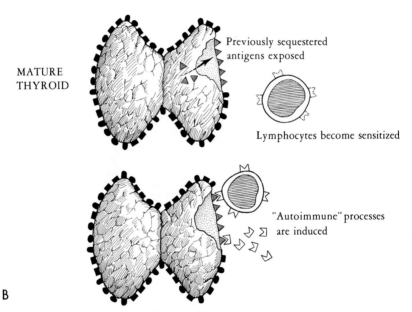

Figure 20–34 *Continued.*

Illustration continued on the opposite page

A third hypothesis, the concept of *immunologic deficiency*, is based on a hypoactive or a deficient immunologic system (Fig. 20–34C). It derives its support from the clinically observed relationships between immunologic deficiency syndromes and the increased incidence of autoimmune abnormalities (Chapter 22). These relationships have been extrapolated largely from data obtained in experimental animals. Injury would occur through the emergence of mutant lymphocytes or as a consequence of persistence of microbial antigen (Fig. 20–25C). From these observations, it has been postulated that otherwise normal individuals who develop autoimmune disease may, in fact, have a more subtle form of underlying immune deficiency predisposing them to the autoimmune states.

IMMUNOLOGIC DEFICIENCY THEORY

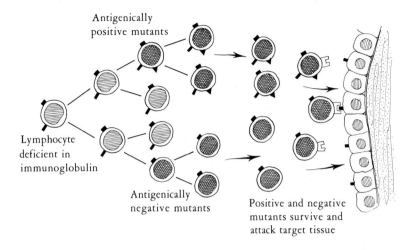

Antigenically
positive mutants

Lymphocyte
deficient in
immunoglobulin

Antigenically
negative mutants

Positive and negative
mutants survive and
attack target tissue

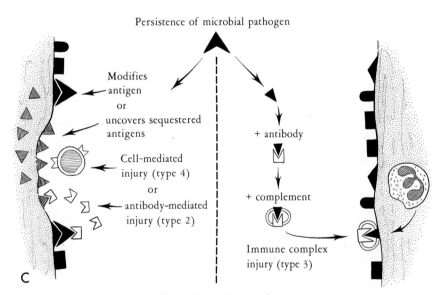

Persistence of microbial pathogen

Modifies
antigen
or
uncovers sequestered
antigens

Cell-mediated
injury (type 4)
or
antibody-mediated
injury (type 2)

+ antibody

+ complement

Immune complex
injury (type 3)

C

Figure 20–34 Continued.

Finally, any concept that seeks to explain the development of the autoimmune state must take into account the genetic control of the immune system (Chapter 3). Familial patterns and sex distributions (for example, showing a female predominance) characterize most of the autoimmune disorders. More recently, the discovery of the association of certain histocompatibility antigens with a variety of diseases suggests that the immune response (Ir) gene in humans may be closely linked to

TABLE 20–26. HLA Antigens and Human Disease

DISEASE	ANTIGEN	DISEASE	ANTIGEN
Ankylosing spondylitis	B27	Psoriasis	B13, B17
Reiter's syndrome	B27	Pemphigus	B13
Reactive arthritis (Yersinia, Salmonella, and Shigella infections)	B27	Multiple sclerosis	A3, B7, B18, D2
		Myasthenia gravis	B8
Rheumatoid arthritis	D_w4	Acute anterior uveitis	B27
Systemic lupus erythematosus	B8, B15	Chronic glomerulonephritis	A2
Diabetes mellitus (insulin-dependent)	B8, B15, D_w3	Hodgkin's disease	B5
Graves' disease	B8	Chronic myelogenous leukemia	A3
Addison's disease	B8, D_w3	Acute lymphocytic leukemia	A2, B12
Celiac disease	D_w3, B8		
Chronic active hepatitis	B8	Lymphosarcoma	B12
Pernicious anemia	B7	Primary Sjögren's syndrome	D_w3

the HLA loci on the sixth chromosome (Chapter 3). The most notable association is the relatively high risk of the development of ankylosing spondylitis or Reiter's syndrome in HLA-B27–positive individuals, who have an inherited susceptibility to develop spondylitis or Reiter's syndrome from a variety of antigenic stimuli. Other associations between human diseases and HLA antigens are shown in Table 20–26.

CLASSIFICATION

The autoimmune diseases are grouped into the *systemic* and *organ-specific* diseases (Table 20–27). Systemic disorders are those in which major involvement is seen in more than one organ, and the organ-specific diseases are those in which the major effect involves a single organ.

SYSTEMIC AUTOIMMUNE DISEASES

SYSTEMIC LUPUS ERYTHEMATOSUS (SLE)

Seen mainly in females, SLE is a generalized disorder that expresses itself as a vasculitis involving many organ systems. The primary target

TABLE 20–27. Autoimmune Diseases

I. Systemic
Systemic lupus erythematosus (SLE)
Rheumatoid arthritis, ankylosing spondylitis
Sjögren's syndrome
Polyarteritis nodosa
Polymyositis and dermatomyositis
Progressive systemic sclerosis (Scleroderma)
Mixed connective tissue disease

II. Organ-Specific

Organ	Disease Manifestation
Blood	Anemia, leukopenia, thrombocytopenia
Central nervous system (CNS)	Allergic encephalitis, demyelinating diseases
Endocrine	Thyroiditis, Addison's disease, hypoparathyroidism
Gastrointestinal	Pernicious anemia, ulcerative colitis, regional ileitis, gluten-sensitive enteropathy
Liver	Chronic liver disease
Kidney	Goodpasture's syndrome, acute post-streptococcal nephritis
Muscle	Myasthenia gravis
Heart	Rheumatic fever
Eye	Uveitis, sympathetic ophthalmia
Skin	Dermatitis herpetiformis, lupus erythematosus, bullous pemphigoid, pemphigus vulgaris

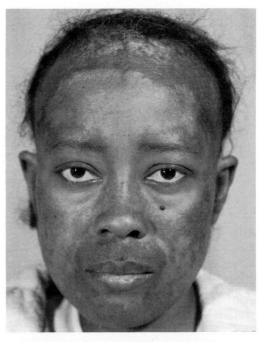

Figure 20–35. Photograph of a patient with systemic lupus erythematosus (SLE) showing the skin lesions and alopecia. (Courtesy of Dr. F. Paul Alepa.)

cells are the hematopoietic system, skin, joints, and kidney (Fig. 20–35). These are involved in a variety of ways by a vast array of antibodies (Table 20–28). Antibodies to red cells, white cells, and platelets account for the hemolytic anemia, leukopenia, and thrombocytopenia, respectively. A prolonged clotting time is occasionally seen in association with antibody to clotting factors. Antibody to nuclear material may complex with antigen and lead to injury of vascular tissues, glomerular membrane of the kidney, or synovial lining of the joints (Fig. 20–36). The extensive antibody formation is reflected by the hypergammaglobulinemia characteristic of many of the autoimmune diseases. Except for damage to blood cells, the autoantibody alone does not seem to initiate tissue damage directly. Damage is thought to occur primarily through the deposition of these antigen-antibody complexes (Type III reaction). As in many of the complex-induced vascular disorders, certain tissues are more vulnerable to injury than others. These tissues include the small blood vessels, glomeruli, joints, spleen, and heart valves.

Pathogenesis. A genetic predisposition, termed "lupus diathesis," has been implicated on the basis of increased incidence in twins and the existence of autoimmune disease in the families of patients with lupus erythematosus. Transient lupus-like syndromes have occurred after prolonged use of drugs such as hydralazine and procainamide (Chapter 20A). In the genetically susceptible individual, certain exogenous factors such as ultraviolet light, certain drugs, and a variety of infectious agents may serve as antigens or produce antigens that trigger self-destructive immunologic responses.

Evidence obtained from the experimental animal also suggests a genetic etiology. In inbred New Zealand black (NZB) strains of mice, a lupus-like syndrome occurs consisting of LE cells and glomerular lesions. In addition to a genetic predisposition, the finding of virus-like particles in these mice raises the possibility of an infectious etiology leading to the autoimmune state. There is recent evidence that suppressor T-cells or a soluble immune response suppressor (SIRS) substance may be deficient in NZB mice (Chapter 10). Although the precise function of suppressor T-cells in the human is unknown, they seem to play an important role in immunologic regulation and in the

TABLE 20–28. Common Manifestations of SLE

MECHANISM	MANIFESTATION
Antibody to RBC	Coombs' + hemolytic anemia
Antibody to WBC	Leukopenia
Antibody to platelets	Thrombocytopenia
Antibody to clotting factors	Prolonged clotting time
Extensive antibody formation	Hypergammaglobulinemia
Antigen-antibody complex: blood vessels	Vasculitis
Antigen-antibody complex: glomeruli	Nephritis
Antigen-antibody complex: synovial membrane	Arthritis

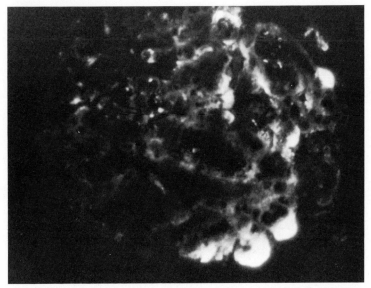

Figure 20–36. Photomicrograph of a kidney of a patient with SLE showing the characteristic irregular immunofluorescent deposition of IgG globulins along the glomerular basement membrane. Original magnification ×100. (Courtesy of Dr. Heinz Bauer.)

prevention of autoantibody production. It might follow, then, that a deficiency of suppressor cell function might allow B-cells to escape from this normal regulatory mechanism and proceed to produce autoantibodies. The descriptions of myxovirus subparticles in renal biopsy material from human cases of systemic lupus erythematosus accentuate this possibility in man (Fig. 20–37). The significance of these findings is as yet unknown.

Immunologic Tests. The lupus erythematosus (LE) cell is a polymorphonuclear leukocyte that has ingested nuclear material complexed with antinuclear antibody (Fig. 20–38).

Tests for the presence of these cells are used to verify the diagnosis of SLE. Peripheral blood or bone marrow is incubated at 37° C, and LE cells are then sought. Antibodies may also be directed against protein or other nuclear materials. Some antibodies are detected by fluorescence (fluorescent antinuclear antibody); others are detected by ammonium sulfate precipitation techniques. (Chapter 8).

Antinuclear antibodies (ANA) have the capacity of complexing with antigen and fixing complement. When the disease is most active, particularly with renal involvement, there is diminished circulating complement in the sera of these individuals, which assumes both diagnostic and therapeutic significance since levels become normal with successful therapy.

Tests for ANA are currently being used to screen for SLE. Since ANA and LE cells also occur in patients receiving drugs, a careful

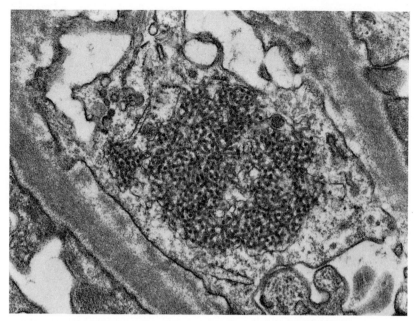

Figure 20-37. Microtubular structures seen in a kidney biopsy of a patient with SLE. ×32,000. (Courtesy of Dr. Theodore Pincus; from Pincus, T., Blacklow, N. R., Grimley, P. M., et al.: Glomerular microtubules of systemic lupus erythematosus. Lancet, 2:1058–61, 1970.)

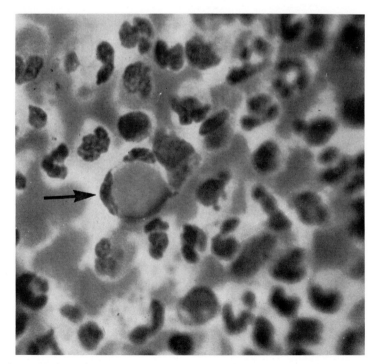

Figure 20-38. Photomicrograph of a lupus erythematosus (LE) cell. Note the amorphous intracytoplasmic inclusion within the polymorphonuclear leukocyte. ×1200. (Courtesy of Dr. S. Gerald Sandler.)

history of drug ingestion should be obtained. Complement levels may provide a useful guide in both the diagnosis and management of the disease, particularly with renal involvement. Rare SLE patients with deficiency of the second or fourth component of complement should also be identified (Chapters 6 and 22). Anti-DNA antibody and DNA binding are newer tests that have a high specificity for SLE and are used serially to assess disease activity. These tests are negative in drug-induced and discoid lupus. Of interest is the recent disclosure that immunofluorescent microscopy of skin reveals immunoglobulin deposition at the dermoepidermal junction in over 90 per cent of specimens from involved skin and in over 50 per cent from uninvolved skin in patients with SLE. In contrast, in discoid lupus, the deposits are noted only in involved skin.

The treatment of SLE rests primarily on the use of immunosuppressive drugs (cytotoxic drugs and steroids) that are employed in an attempt to inhibit antibody formation. Steroids also exert an anti-inflammatory action that is probably more important than their immunosuppressant activity (Chapter 25).

RHEUMATOID ARTHRITIS (RA)

Rheumatoid arthritis is another disease that may involve many organ systems by producing vasculitis (Fig. 20–39). The most frequent site of injury in adults is the synovial lining of joints (Fig. 20–40). More widespread lesions may occur, particularly in children.

Pathogenesis and Etiology. The etiology of RA is unknown. Several etiologies have been postulated, including metabolic derangements and infectious agents (bacteria and mycoplasma). Recently, indirect evidence has been presented for viruses in synovial membranes of patients with RA. A mild arthritis is known to accompany some viral infections. For example, following natural rubella or rubella immunization, approximately one third of adults develop transient rheumatoid arthritis–like effects.

Genetics. Families of probands affected with RA show an increased incidence of connective tissue disorders (e.g., SLE). Furthermore, children with immune deficiency (e.g., agammaglobulinemia) have an increased incidence of connective tissue diseases (e.g., rheumatoid arthritis). Hence, there may exist underlying genetic factors determining the susceptibility of patients to RA, but they are complex and, at present, ill understood.

Immunologic Findings. Rheumatoid factor (RF) is an IgM globulin that has the capacity to react with IgG globulins *in vitro*. There are other antiglobulins of the IgG and IgA variety. The stimulus for the production of RF is not known. This factor is found in the sera and synovial fluid of adult patients with established rheumatoid arthritis but is seldom seen in juvenile RA. From recent investigations, it now appears that children with RA, unlike adults, are more apt to have IgG rather than IgM RF, which is not detectable by the usual agglutination tests such as latex fixation. Although RF is diagnostically useful, it is not specific for the disease and is found in a host of other diseases, including the connective tissue disorders. The test for RF is carried out using various carrier substances as a vehicle for the gamma globulin (latex, bentonite, and erythrocytes).

Because the rheumatoid factor–gamma globulin–complement complex has been found in synovial fluids, RF has been implicated as a causative factor of the chronic inflammatory joint disease of RA. Unlike the case of SLE, a lowered serum complement level is rarely seen in the sera of patients with RA. Since the complexes are localized primarily within the joints, lowered complement levels have been found in the

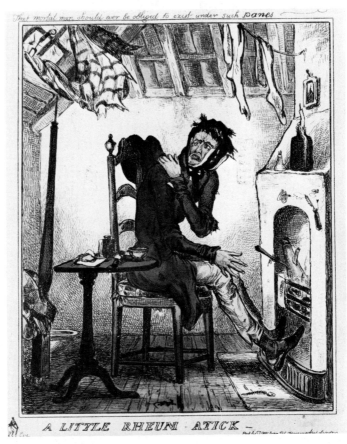

Figure 20–39. Caricature of a patient with "rheum-atick"; "that mortal man should ever be obliged to exist under such panes." (Courtesy of National Library of Medicine.)

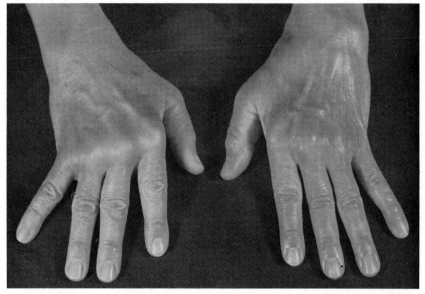

Figure 20–40. Photograph of the hands of a patient with moderately advanced rheumatoid arthritis. Note the deformities of the metacarpal-phalangeal joints with atrophy of the hypothenar muscles and ulnar deviation. (Courtesy of Dr. F. Paul Alepa.)

joint fluids of patients with RA. Synthesis of RF has also been demonstrated within the synovia of affected joints.

Immunologic Tests. In adults, the major differentiating test for RA is the serum RF test. In the systemic or acute febrile form of juvenile RA, the onset of illness often resembles that of an acute infectious process with high fever, rash, leukocytosis, and a rapid sedimentation rate. In children, the definitive diagnosis of RA may have to await the development of joint manifestations.

Treatment of RA is directed primarily at relieving joint pain and inflammation. Commonly used drugs include the salicylates, other nonsteroid agents, steroids, gold, and the antimalarials. Most patients are benefited by these agents and physiotherapy. Since the steroids carry several undesirable side-effects, they should be used with caution and at the lowest dose possible. The benefits of azathioprine, cyclophosphamide, and d-penicillamine are also currently being investigated.

ANKYLOSING SPONDYLITIS (AS)

Ankylosing spondylitis (AS) is a systemic rheumatic disorder characterized by inflammation of the sacroiliac and spinal apophyseal (synovial) joints. Consequently, back pain is a frequent presenting complaint, although the disease can begin in peripheral joints and, rarely, even with acute iridocyclitis. AS affects 10 times more men than women and begins most often between the ages of 20 and 40.

Although the precise etiology of AS remains uncertain, evidence for the influence of genetic factors appears to be mounting. AS has long been suspected of having a genetic background, first because of the striking familial clustering observed among patients and second because of a high concordance rate found in monozygotic twins. More recently, the disclosure of an unusually high frequency of the inherited antigen HLA-B27 in up to 96 per cent of patients and 50 per cent of first-degree relatives provides overwhelming evidence of a genetic linkage in this disorder.

The frequent associations between AS and such seemingly unrelated disorders as ulcerative colitis, regional enteritis, Reiter's syndrome, and psoriasis have, until recently, been unexplained. It now appears that among these underlying disorders, patients with the B27 antigen are those who are primarily destined to develop AS. In fact, it has been estimated that the risk of developing AS is 40 times greater in patients with ulcerative colitis carrying the B27 than in those without the antigen.

Precisely how this genetic relationship links the susceptible individual to the eventual development of AS is unknown. However, recent reports provide evidence of antibody formation and immune complex deposition in AS. Consequently, the pathogenesis of AS may evolve in the following manner. Variable inciting factors, such as ulcerative colitis, might precipitate the evolution of spondylitis in a genetically predisposed individual having the B27 marker. The disease may then be perpetuated by a self-destructive attack of the immune response against "altered self."

Key drugs in management include indomethacin and phenylbutazone, each of which promptly suppresses joint inflammation and discomfort, thereby allowing patients to undertake lifelong supportive measures such as postural training and therapeutic exercise. For rare patients with advanced kyphoscoliosis, vertebral wedge osteotomy may prove beneficial.

Sjögren's Syndrome (SS)

Sjögren's syndrome (SS), in its primary form, consists of keratoconjunctivitis sicca (dry eyes) and xerostomia (dry mouth). However, SS more often occurs secondary to RA or one of the connective tissue disorders such as SLE, scleroderma, or polymyositis. One of the most characteristic features of SS is the remarkable immunolgic reactivity detected in serum. LE cells, ANA, RF, and hypergammaglobulinemia are frequently present; antibodies against RNA, salivary duct, lacrimal gland, smooth muscle, mitochondria, and thyroid gland may also be found. There is an increased frequency of renal tubular acidosis in SS.

Lymphoma may also develop in these patients, particularly in those with the primary form of SS.

Anti–salivary duct antibodies, demonstrated by indirect immuno-fluorescence of human salivary and lacrimal glands, occur more frequently in patients with SS and RA than in those with primary SS. These antibodies appear to block (react with and cover) determinants on ductal lining cells that might otherwise be attacked by sensitized lymphocytes. Recently, an association of HLA-D_w3 has been made with the primary Sjögren's syndrome.

Diagnosis is confirmed by salivary technetium pertechnetate scinti-scanning, which is more sensitive than sialography, and labial biopsy. Treatment includes supportive measures such as the use of artificial tears and steroids or immunosuppressive drugs for serious systemic manifestations such as vasculitis.

NECROTIZING ANGIITIS

Necrotizing angiitis encompasses a group of entities characterized by segmental inflammation of arteries. Polyarteritis nodosa (PN) has a predilection for males and involves both median and small arteries whereas hypersensitivity angiitis involves only small arteries. Clinically, it is often difficult to distinguish PN from hypersensitivity angiitis except that marked cutaneous involvement suggests hypersensitivity angiitis, which is often caused by drugs, notably sulfonamides and penicillin. The toxic appearance of patients with either disorder reflects the variable and widespread organ involvement that results from diffuse vascular occlusion. Treatment includes high doses of steroids and occasionally the addition of other immunosuppressive drugs. The prognosis is better for hypersensitivity angiitis; surviving patients should avoid implicated drugs.

Henoch-Schönlein's purpura affects small arteries of the skin, joints, and gastrointestinal tract (Fig. 20–41). Purpura, gastrointestinal bleeding, and focal glomerulonephritis frequently accompany the angiitis. Recently, biopsies of purpuric lesions have revealed bright granular deposits of IgA, C3, and fibrin-fibrinogen in capillaries and connective tissue of the dermis, findings that may be useful diagnostically, particularly in atypical cases. In Wegener's granulomatosis, vasculitis occurs in the upper respiratory tract, lung, and kidney; in Takayasu's (pulseless) disease, it occurs in the aorta and its major branches; and in giant cell arteritis, it occurs in the temporal and other cranial arteries.

Pathogenesis and Etiology. The presence of immune complexes of the hepatitis B antigen (HB_sAg) in affected tissues, including the kidney, has recently been demonstrated in 30 to 40 per cent of patients with PN. Otherwise, the etiology of these conditions remains unknown. The immunopathologic hallmark of these entities, however, is a vasculitis similar to an immune complex–type injury. Laboratory

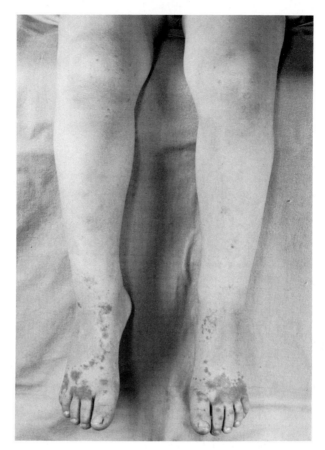

Figure 20–41. Photograph of the lower extremities and feet of a child with Henoch-Schönlein's purpura. Note the purpuric lesions characteristically localized to the skin of the lower extremities.

findings include a leukocytosis and occasionally eosinophilia. With kidney involvement, there may be a heterogeneity of cellular elements found within the urinary sediment ("telescoped urine"). Biopsy is the sole means of confirming a diagnosis and should be obtained from an affected area.

POLYMYOSITIS (DERMATOMYOSITIS)

Polymyositis is another systemic autoimmune disorder characterized pathologically by degeneration and inflammation of skeletal muscle. Clinically, the disease is manifested by weakness of the shoulder and pelvic girdle muscles. Dermatomyositis is a form of polymyositis in which there is also involvement of the skin (Fig. 20–42).

Pathogenesis and Etiology. The etiology of these conditions is obscure, although evidence for a cell-mediated mode of immune injury of muscle continues to mount. Of interest is an overall incidence of a malignant disorder seen in up to 20 per cent of cases. This incidence is related to the age of the host, being highest in the aged. Therefore, in any older adult with these diseases, a diligent search for neoplasm should be undertaken, particularly when the onset is acute. Laboratory findings include elevated serum muscle enzymes (transaminase, aldolase, and creatine phosphokinase) and abnormal electromyographic tracings. The diagnosis can be substantiated by muscle biopsy. Treatment includes the use of immunosuppressants, e.g., steroids.

PROGRESSIVE SYSTEMIC SCLEROSIS (PSS; SCLERODERMA)

PSS is a chronic illness of unknown etiology characterized by a fibrous thickening of the skin (scleroderma) and several internal organs (gastrointestinal tract, heart, kidney, and lungs). Two thirds of the patients are female.

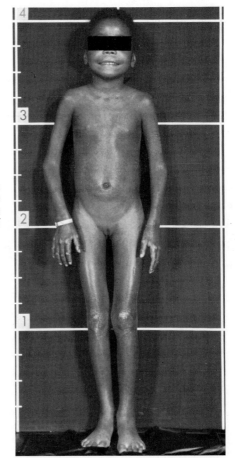

Figure 20-42. Photograph of a patient with dermatomyositis. Note the atropy of the skin and the wasting of the proximal musculature. (Courtesy of Dr. F. Paul Alepa.)

Increased levels of immunoglobulins, ANA (particularly of the speckled and nucleolar patterns), and DNA binding in children with PSS and localized scleroderma (morphea and hemiatrophy) are evidence for an antigen-mediated pathogenesis. *In vitro* examination of scleroderma skin fibroblasts demonstrates an increase in collagen synthesis, suggesting that the basic defect in PSS is one of disordered regulation or activation of the fibroblast. Currently, there is no effective therapy, although d-penicillamine holds some promise, particularly for the localized forms of PSS.

Mixed Connective Tissue Disease (MCTD)

This designation is reserved for patients with combined clinical features of RA, SLE, PSS, and polymyositis. Patients exhibit polyarthritis, diffusely swollen hands, Raynaud's phenomenon, disturbed esophageal motility, myositis, lymphadenopathy, and hypergammaglobulinemia. Typically, patients have positive ANA of the speckled pattern. Diagnosis is confirmed by the demonstration of high titers of antibody to extractable nuclear antigen (ENA). MCTD serum antibody does not react with the antigen when it is pretreated with ribonuclease, unlike the case in SLE. In MCTD, renal involvement is rare and serum complement levels are normal. Most patients respond readily to corticosteroids. Prognosis seems favorable but long-term follow-up of patients has not yet been possible.

Summary

In these systemic diseases, it is apparent that the etiology has remained obscure. With the exception of polyarteritis nodosa, they are often manifested as a group of diseases in which a preponderance of females is seen. In cases in which immunopathologic data are available, there also exists a vasculitis that seems to be the hallmark of these diseases. This is reminiscent of damage seen in the experimental form of immune complex–type injury (Chapter 13). The diagnosis is established by the clinical pattern and, in some, by appropriate laboratory tests. Treatment in most of these is accomplished by the use of immunosuppressive agents. An autoimmune etiology is suggested by the multiplicity of immune phenomena that often accompany these disorders and account for their protean manifestations.

SPECIFIC ORGAN DISEASES

Autoimmune Hemolytic Anemias (AHA)

The AHA are a heterogeneous group of anemias characterized by a hemolytic process associated with red cell–specific antibodies in the serum. Some of the antibodies agglutinate red cells (agglutinins); others lyse them (hemolysins) in the presence of complement. Since these antibodies are directed against the patient's own red cells, they are called autoantibodies. The AHA are classified according to physical characteristics of the antibodies (Table 20–29).

The most common of the AHA are the warm agglutinin group, consisting of idiopathic and secondary types. In these patients, the antibodies are of the IgG class and show limited complement-fixing ability. In the *idiopathic* type, which accounts for more than half of all cases of AHA, the etiology remains obscure. On long-term follow-up, however, some of these patients develop lymphoma. In the secondary type, anemia occurs in association with one of many diseases or after the use of drugs.

In the cold agglutinin group, antibodies of the IgM class have the ability to fix complement and react in the cold ($4° C$), primarily against the I blood group. These anti-I autoantibodies are found in such diseases as atypical pneumonia *(Mycoplasma pneumoniae)*, infectious mononucleosis, and cold agglutinin disease (Chapter 21).

The cold autohemolysins (Donath-Landsteiner type) are found in a third group of AHA associated with paroxysmal cold hemoglobinuria and variable infections, including viral. This disease was first described in patients with tertiary syphilis. The antibodies are IgG and uniformly fix complement. Owing to avid complement fixation, most red cells are lysed before they reach phagocytic cells, producing rapid intravascular hemolysis with the hemoglobinemia and hemoglobinuria characteristic of the disease.

Etiology.   The etiology of AHA is unknown. It has been postulated that exogenous agents (drugs and viruses) may alter antigenic structure of the red cell membrane, resulting in susceptibility of the erythrocyte to hemolysis. In patients who develop AHA there may be a genetically determined susceptibility to develop autoantibodies that in some cases

TABLE 20–29.   Characteristics of Red Cell Autoantibody

Type	Antibody Type	Ability to Fix C′	Type of Disease
Warm agglutinins ($37° C$)	IgG	Rare	Idiopathic: > 50 per cent; secondary: lymphoproliferative diseases, tumors, viral diseases, sarcoidosis and drugs, SLE
Cold agglutinins ($4° C$)	IgM	Frequent	Infectious mononucleosis (anti-i), *M. pneumoniae* (anti-I), cold agglutinin disease (kappa chain)
Cold hemolysins ($4° C$)	IgG	Usually	Donath-Landsteiner antibody (variable infections)

may be associated with immunologic abnormalities, e.g., an inherited or acquired partial failure to form immunoglobulins.

Diagnosis. The major diagnostic criteria used in differentiating the AHA from other forms of anemia are the presence of spherocytes in the peripheral smear and a positive antiglobulin reaction (Coombs' test) for autoantibody. Temperature-dependent agglutination reactions will help identify the specific type of autoantibody (Table 20–29).

Therapy. In the warm agglutinin types, steroids are useful drugs, but other immunosuppressive agents, such as azathioprine, may be employed if the patient fails to respond. Splenectomy may also benefit some patients unresponsive to steroids. In the cold agglutinin group, no specific treatment is required for the postinfectious type; cytotoxic agents are useful in the idiopathic variety. In paroxysmal cold hemoglobinuria, drug therapy has been unsuccessful, although transfusions with blood previously warmed to 37° C are often beneficial.

ENDOCRINE

Autoimmune antibodies have been found in disorders of the thyroid, adrenal, pancreas, and parathyroid glands. The most extensively studied and most frequently occurring are diseases involving the thyroid gland.

Thyroid Gland

The diseases of the thyroid gland in which autoimmune factors have been found are *thyroiditis* and *Graves' disease.*

Thyroiditis is a condition in which varying degrees of destruction of the gland with inflammatory infiltration occur. The patient may present with either *acute, subacute,* or *chronic* manifestations of the disease, which are defined by the degree of inflammation and its duration. The immunologic nature of thyroiditis was clarified by studies in which the disease was produced in rabbits by injecting thyroid tissue emulsified in complete Freund's adjuvant. Although originally thought to be mediated by antibody, it is now felt that the primary mechanism of immunologic injury may involve other mechanisms, e.g., cell-mediated injury.

Acute thyroiditis may be either suppurative or nonsuppurative. There is evidence that the nonsuppurative form may have an immunologic basis. It presents with fever, sore throat, and an enlarged, tender thyroid gland. Symptoms of hyperthyroidism may be present, and the serum thyroxine concentration may be elevated. Symptoms may resemble those of infection, and there may be an elevated white count and a rapid sedimentation rate. The possibility of thyroiditis should be seriously considered in any patient who presents with hyperthyroidism. The female to male ratio is 6:1.

A less fulminating clinical picture occurs in *subacute thyroiditis.* This may or may not be preceded by acute thyroiditis. In this condition, there occurs a tender nodular thyroid gland or a localized goiter that may be confused with carcinoma. Although at one time considered a rare entity, subacute thyroiditis is now being recognized more commonly. Characteristically, patients are euthyroid and no abnormalities in thyroid function are detected.

In chronic lymphocytic thyroiditis (Hashimoto's thyroiditis), the patient has progressed through acute and subacute phases (Fig. 20–43). He may remain euthyroid or may develop varying degrees of hypothyroidism. Depletion of the gland may be total, resulting in myxedema. In the classic form, a diffusely enlarged, nontender gland is found. In cases with myxedema, physical examination may reveal either a goiter or a small, firm thyroid gland with the findings of depressed thyroid function.

As a result of newer immunologic discoveries, Graves' disease is now considered to be a multisystem disorder in which three clinically distinct entities exist: (1) hyperthyroidism due to a diffuse goiter, (2) infiltrative ophthalmopathy (exophthalmos), and (3) infiltrative dermopathy ("localized pretibial myxedema"). These three components may present individually or in combination with each other. The manifestations of

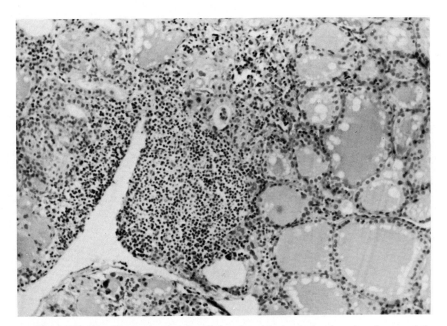

Figure 20-43. Photomicrograph of the thyroid gland showing the characteristic changes of chronic thyroiditis (Hashimoto's thyroiditis). Note the destruction of the normal architecture of the gland with heavy infiltration of mononuclear cells. Hematoxylin and eosin stain, ×100. (Courtesy of Dr. Byungkyu Chun.)

infiltrative ophthalmopathy and infiltrative dermopathy are more commonly seen in the adult patient in whom a higher incidence of antibodies is encountered.

The association between Graves' disease and Hashimoto's disease is becoming more frequently recognized. The two entities frequently coexist and indeed may represent different manifestations of a common spectrum. Circulating antibodies as well as *in vitro* lymphoproliferative responses to various constituents of thyroid are commonly found in both. Moreover, pathologic changes of Hashimoto's disease are frequently seen in the thyroid gland of patients with Graves' disease. In addition to circulating antibodies, which may respresent autoimmune phenomena, antibodies have been described in these two diseases that appear to regulate cellular activity and may actually contribute to the hyperthyroidism. These include a long-acting thyroid stimulator (LATS), a LATS protector activity (LPA), and thyroid-stimulating immunoglobulins (TSI). It is unclear at present whether these activities represent three distinct antibodies or whether they may all be different manifestations of the same antibody specificity, differing only in the methods employed for their detection. These antibodies are detected by means of bioassay–LATS by its *in vivo* ability to enhance the release of thyroid hormone and LPA by its ability to prevent the neutralization of LATS by an inactivator normally present in human thyroid extract. TSI appear to represent autoantibodies directed to thyrotropin receptors, capable of binding to the receptor and stimulating the production of cyclic AMP and the excessive production of thyroid hormone.

Pathogenesis.   The points at which aberrations might occur in immunologic disease of the thyroid are depicted schematically in Figure 20–44. Thyroglobulin is normally transported from the colloidal space into acinar cells by means of a process of pinocytosis. Within the acinar cells, a protease releases thyroxine from a macromolecular protein complex. Normally, thyroglobulin does not enter the circulation in significant amounts. The released thyroxine enters capillary structures surrounding the acinar cells and is transported to peripheral tissues. If the macromolecular complex is not cleared by the protease or is released intact, it may pass into the circulation and induce an immune response with resultant "autoimmune" damage to the thyroid (Fig. 20–44). This may be seen after trauma or infection. More recently, genetic factors have been implicated in the pathogenesis of chronic thyroiditis both in the human and in the experimental animal. With the recent descriptions of LATS, LPA, and TSI, it is thought that these additional antibodies may play a role in the pathogenesis of both Graves' disease and chronic lymphocytic thyroiditis.

Immunologic Tests.   There are several immunologic tests useful for the detection of antibodies to thyroid tissues. Antithyroglobulin antibodies can be detected by precipitation techniques, latex agglutination, the tanned red cell (TRC) test, and radioimmunoassay. Microsomal

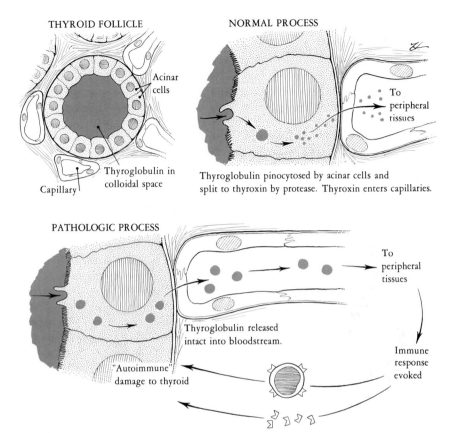

THYROID FOLLICLE

Acinar cells

Thyroglobulin in colloidal space

Capillary

NORMAL PROCESS

To peripheral tissues

Thyroglobulin pinocytosed by acinar cells and split to thyroxin by protease. Thyroxin enters capillaries.

PATHOLOGIC PROCESS

To peripheral tissues

Thyroglobulin released intact into bloodstream.

"Autoimmune" damage to thyroid

Immune response evoked

Figure 20–44. Schematic representation of points at which aberrations might occur in immunologic disease of the thyroid gland.

antibodies are detected by complement fixation, cytotoxicity tests, immunofluorescence of unfixed thyroid epithelial cells, radioimmun-oassay, and hemagglutination tests. The microsomal antigen is intimately associated with lipoproteins of thyroid extracts and is attached to the membranous portion of smooth endoplasmic reticulum. The second antigen of acinar colloid, a protein distinct from thyroglobulin, is also detected by immunofluorescence (Fig. 20–45). The staining for this antibody is brightest in Hashimoto's thyroiditis, although it is not specific for this disorder and can be seen frequently in the sera of patients with thyrotoxicosis and cancer of the thyroid. Thyroid-specific cell surface antibodies have been detected by immunofluorescence on living suspensions of human thyroid cells. The significance of these antibodies is unknown.

Long-acting thyroid stimulator (LATS) has been detected in approximately 50 per cent of patients with Graves' disease. Circulating thyroid-stimulating immunoglobulins (TSI) have been detected in 90

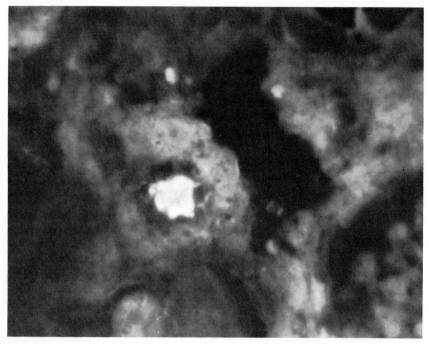

Figure 20–45. Presence of antibody to thyroid colloid in the serum of a patient with chronic thyroiditis as revealed by indirect immunofluorescence. (Courtesy of Dr. Heinz Bauer.)

per cent of patients with Graves' disease and in 15 per cent of cases with Hashimoto's. Although hyperthyroidism may characterize certain phases of thyroiditis, the overall thrust of the self-destructive process of Hashimoto's disease appears to be directed toward the relentless production of chronic inflammation with lymphocytic infiltration and glandular destruction and the eventual attrition of thyroid function and hypothyroidism. The cause of the exophthalmos of Graves' disease is unknown. However, recent studies demonstrating the presence of thyroglobulin in the orbital muscle of patients with this disease may provide a basis for cell-mediated immune injury in the pathogenesis of this entity.

The various forms of thyroiditis can be distinguished by means of a variety of thyroid function and antibody studies (Table 20–30). In the acute form, the most common pattern is that of an increased PBI along with a diminished iodine-131 uptake. Antithyroid antibodies are usually not detected in acute thyroiditis. In subacute thyroiditis, thyroxine levels are frequently normal, but an increase in circulating nonthyroxine iodinated compounds may be detected. Iodine-131 uptake is frequently normal. Antithyroid antibodies are not usually present in subacute thyroiditis. In the chronic form, thyroid function may be normal or decreased, depending upon the degree of thyroid involvement. Antithyroid antibodies are usually detected. In Graves' disease, the PBI is elevated, the radioactive uptake of ^{131}I is increased and antithyroid antibodies, particularly LATS and TSI, are present.

Pancreas

Circulating antibodies to insulin have been found in the sera of diabetic patients, which may contribute to insulin allergy (IgE) or insulin resistance (IgG, IgA, or IgM) (Chapter 20A). However, antibodies have not been regularly encountered in untreated patients. More recently, insulin resistance has been described in untreated patients and appears to be related to two types of antibody: (1) antibody directed to the insulin molecule, and (2) antibodies directed to the insulin receptor. In both situations, the interaction of insulin with its receptor appears to be blocked. Insulin antibodies produced in animals have also provided the basis for a useful test for the radioimmunoassay of insulin concentrations.

Recently, thyroid and gastric autoantibodies have been found in the sera of diabetic patients without clinical thyroid disease or pernicious anemia. These autoantibodies were more commonly detected in the insulin-dependent (juvenile-onset) type and more frequently detected in females. These findings may be one aspect of the heterogeneity of this endocrine disorder.

Adrenals

The finding of antibody to adrenal tissues in patients with Addison's disease has been reported. These antibodies have been detected by immunofluorescence or complement fixation. The significance of these findings is at present obscure.

Parathyroids

Idiopathic hypoparathyroidism occurs with greater frequency in children than in adults and is more common in females than in males.

TABLE 20–30.   Thyroid Function and Antibody Studies in Various Thyroid Diseases

	PBI/T4*	RAI**	THYROID ANTIBODIES
Thyroiditis			
Acute	N or ↑	N or ↓	0
Subacute	N	N	0
Chronic	N or ↓	N or ↓	+
Graves' disease	↑	↑	±

*PBI/T4—serum thyroxine determination: protein-bound iodine (PBI) or radioactive displacement method (T4).

**RAI—radioactive ^{131}I uptake.

Associated disorders may accompany hypoparathyroidism, including idiopathic Addison's disease, alopecia totalis, pernicious anemia, and moniliasis. Antibodies to thyroid, adrenal, and gastric tissues have been detected. Reasonably conclusive evidence has been obtained for an autosomal recessive mode of transmission of a defect underlying these variably associated disorders when clusters of two or more are present. It should be noted that there is also an association of hypoparathyroidism with developmental failure of the thymus-dependent immune system in the DiGeorge syndrome (Chapter 22).

Central Nervous System

Autoimmune diseases of the central nervous system may occur spontaneously or may follow immunization or infectious diseases. Autoimmune encephalitis in the human was first described after the use of Pasteur rabies vaccine grown in rabbit spinal cord. These early observations led to experimental studies in rabbits showing that experimental autoimmune encephalitis (EAE) could be produced by the injection of neurologic tissue homogenates incorporated in Freund's complete adjuvant. It was subsequently demonstrated that this experimental disease could be transferred by the adoptive transfer of lymphocytes but not by serum, suggesting that EAE is a disease of delayed-type hypersensitivity. While the role of circulating antibrain antibodies is not understood, it is possible that antibodies may also be operative in immunologic injury.

The demyelinating diseases of man are of three major types, including (1) acute hemorrhagic encephalopathy, (2) acute disseminated encephalomyelitis, and (3) a chronic form, e.g., multiple sclerosis. These disease entities are shown in Table 20–31, together with their histopathologic features.

Acute hemorrhagic encephalopathy is the most fulminating form and closely resembles EAE. It is primarily a disease of adults and is seen usually in association with an upper respiratory tract infection. There is an explosive onset followed by a relatively short course of illness that is almost uniformly fatal. Histopathologic features include perivascular infiltrates of polymorphonuclear leukocytes in brain tissues.

The second clinical form is the acute disseminated encephalomyelitis seen after inoculation of rabies vaccine and is also a sequela of a variety of infectious diseases (postinfectious type). One distinguishing feature is the relatively long latent period between infection or immunization and appearance of the disease. This period of time may range from a few days to two weeks. Unlike the case in the acute hemorrhagic variety, the onset of encephalitis is not explosive, and the clinical course is characterized mainly by signs of increasing intracranial pressure. Histopathologic features include a perivascular infiltration of mononuclear cells in brain tissues with fewer polymorphonuclear

TABLE 20–31.   Demyelinating Diseases of Man*

	ACUTE *Acute Hemorrhagic Encephalopathy*	SUBACUTE *Acute Disseminated Encephalomyelitis, Rabies, Postinfectious*	CHRONIC *Multiple Sclerosis*
Type of illness:	Explosive	Acute	Chronic
Duration:	Hours or days	Days or weeks	Weeks or years
Histopathologic features:	Focal disseminated perivascular	Focal disseminated perivascular	Focal disseminated perivascular
Cell type:	RBC; PMN	Mononuclear, histiocytes	Very few mono- cytes and histiocytes
Myelin destruction:	± to +	+ to ++	++
Axon and nerve cell damage:	±	±	±
Astrocyte proliferation:	±	+	++
Outcome:	Death	Recovery	Chronic relapsing progressive disease

*From Paterson, P. Y.: The Demyelinating Diseases. *In* M. Samter and H. L. Alexander (eds.): Immunological Diseases. Boston, Little, Brown and Company, 1965.

leukocytes than in the acute hemorrhagic form. Mortality rates vary from 20 per cent in the case of measles to as high as 50 per cent in the case of postvaccinal encephalitis. Survival is the rule, although most patients are left with residual changes or have relapses over a number of months.

Multiple sclerosis is characterized by a chronic course with many relapses. A number of infectious disease pathogens have been implicated but none have been confirmed. The finding of an elevated spinal fluid gamma globulin in 80 per cent of patients is a distinguishing feature. Histopathologic features include degeneration of myelin with considerably less perivascular infiltration than that seen in the other forms. The Guillain-Barré syndrome is another form of neurologic disease with immunologic features. It is a polyneuritis of unknown etiology characterized by peripheral nerve involvement. This entity may follow a variety of infectious diseases or may occur as a sequela of immunization, e.g., swine influenza immunization (Chapter 23).

Working Hypothesis.   Immunologically mediated diseases affecting the central nervous system include a consideration of "slow virus" infections (Chapter 16). In virus infections of the central nervous system, the physician is confronted with a spectrum of diseases that may be either a manifestation of the viral infection itself or an expression of the immunity mechanisms directed against it. These events are shown schematically in Figure 20–46. At one end of the spectrum, the pathologic events of encephalitis resulting from herpes simplex infection represent a direct invasion of the central nervous system by virus. Mumps virus also invades the central nervous system before or after parotitis appears. Varicella and measles encephalitis usually follow

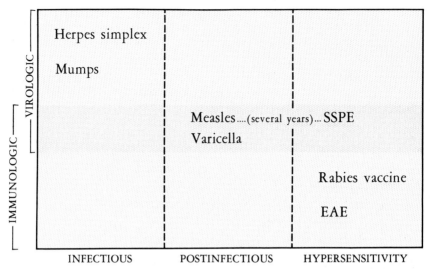

Figure 20–46. Schematic representation of etiologic factors in viral encephalitis.

a viremia, and clinical findings are referred to as postinfectious types. In the postinfectious encephalitides, it has been difficult to culture virus directly from central nervous system tissue, although inclusion bodies have been observed in brain tissue of children with encephalitis (Fig. 20–47). At the other end of the spectrum, the encephalitis that follows

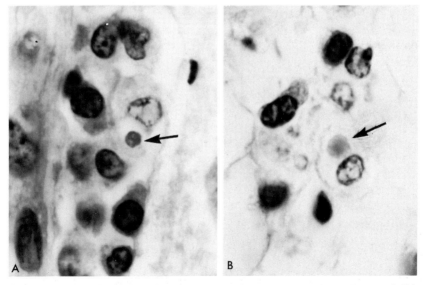

Figure 20–47. Photomicrograph of brain of child who died of measles encephalitis, showing measles inclusion bodies after natural measles (*A*) and after immunization with live measles vaccine (*B*). Hematoxylin and eosin stain, ×2100. (Courtesy of Dr. John Adams.)

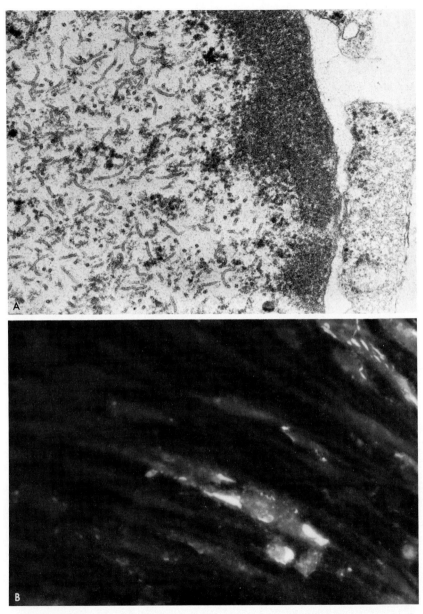

Figure 20–48. Demonstration of measles antigen in brain biopsy of patient with subacute sclerosing panencephalitis (SSPE). *A*, Demonstration of measles virus nucleocapsids (microtubules) in the cytoplasm of glial cells by electron microscopy ×74,250. *B*, Demonstration of measles antigen within glial cells by direct immunofluorescence. (Courtesy of Dr. Luiz Horta-Barbosa.)

administration of rabies vaccine represents an example of a pathologic process resulting from hypersensitivity. The isolation of measles virus from brain biopsy specimens of children with subacute sclerosing panencephalitis (SSPE) suggests that measles virus may be present in an incomplete or masked form (Fig. 20–48). These recent observations concerning incomplete (slow) viral infections offer interesting explanations for what were previously considered autoimmune diseases of the nervous system.

GASTROINTESTINAL

Many lines of evidence suggest that both the stomach and the intestines may be involved in autoimmune processes. Diseases that are triggered by immunologic processes are listed in Table 20–32 and include pernicious anemia, regional ileitis, ulcerative colitis, and gluten-sensitive enteropathy.

Pernicious Anemia (PA)

Pernicious anemia is a disorder characterized by inflammation and subsequent atrophy of the gastric mucosa with inability to secrete hydrochloric acid, intrinsic factor, and pepsin. This is followed by the development of a macrocytic anemia. Up to 95 per cent of patients with this disorder have serum antibody directed against parietal cells or intrinsic factor. Recently, antibody has been found in the gastric juice, and lymphoid cells have been found to infiltrate gastric mucosa. The sera of patients with pernicious anemia contain antibody that, when mixed with intrinsic factor, interferes with the absorption of vitamin B_{12}. It is not known whether these antibodies are the result or the cause of the disease. The fact that some patients improve after treatment with steroids reinforces the possibility of an autoimmune basis for PA. This effect, however, may merely be a consequence of anti-inflammatory action of steroids.

Family studies in first-degree relatives of patients with PA indicate a threefold increase in the incidence of gastric parietal antibody, gastritis, and achlorhydria. In addition, there are thyroid antibodies in about 50 per cent of patients with PA and their relatives. About one third of

TABLE 20–32. Autoimmune Diseases Affecting the Gastrointestinal Tract

REGION	DISEASE
Stomach	Pernicious anemia
Intestine	Regional ileitis Ulcerative colitis Gluten-sensitive enteropathy (Celiac disease)

TABLE 20–33. Types of Serum Antibody Found in Patients with Pernicious Anemia

Autoantigen	Antibody Test
Gastric parietal cell antigen	Complement-fixation (CF)
	Immunofluorescence (FA)
Intrinsic factor	Blocking antibody
	Binding antibody

patients with Hashimoto's disease have antibodies to gastric parietal cytoplasm with no clinical manifestations of PA.

Immunologic Tests. Antibodies in the sera of individuals with PA are of two types: (1) those directed against the microsomal fraction of gastric mucosal cells (these are detected by complement-fixation test or by immunofluorescence) and (2) those directed against intrinsic factor. These antibodies bind with preformed intrinsic factor B_{12} complex (binding antibody) or those that block the combination of intrinsic factor with antibody (blocking antibody) (Table 20–33). The application of these tests in clinical medicine is important in differentiating PA from other causes of megaloblastic anemia.

Ulcerative Colitis

Ulcerative colitis is a chronic disease affecting primarily the large bowel and is characterized by bloody diarrhea, abdominal pain, weight loss, and anemia. The pathogenesis is unknown but thought to be autoimmune on the basis of circulating antibody to colonic tissue. Enteric infection may be the triggering event. There is evidence for a genetic predisposition in this disorder with a slightly increased female to male ratio among those affected.

Immunologic Tests. Three types of antibodies have been demonstrated against colonic tissue: (1) an IgM hemagglutinin, (2) a precipitating antibody, and (3) an immunofluorescent antibody. Their importance in the pathogenesis of ulcerative colitis is uncertain. Antibody-containing serum does not cause cytotoxicity to cells in culture, whereas lymphocytes from affected patients do. This suggests that cell-mediated immune mechanisms may be more important than humoral antibody in the pathogenesis of ulcerative colitis.

Regional Ileitis (Crohn's Disease)

Regional ileitis is a chronic disease of unknown etiology characterized by granulomatous inflammatory changes of the ileum that sometimes involve other parts of the gastrointestinal tract as well. Antibodies to heterologous colon have been demonstrated in regional ileitis. Although suspected, an autoimmune basis has never been substantiated.

Gluten-sensitive Enteropathy (GSE; Celiac Disease)

This syndrome is characterized by malabsorption of fats and carbohydrates. Diarrhea appears to be triggered by ingestion of the gliadin fraction of gluten, a protein found in grains. It is not known precisely how this effect is mediated. There may also occur a hypersensitivity reaction to the gliadin fraction itself. Recently, HLA-D$_w$3 and B8 have been associated with GSE. High antibody titers to gliadin have also been detected in affected patients. The antibodies that mediate these reactions are of the IgA and IgM type, which are also the principal immunoglobulins at mucosal sites. Moreover, IgA deficiency occurs more frequently in celiac patients than in the general population. This is probably related to common factors underlying both IgA deficiency and GSE.

Immunologic Mechanisms of the Gastrointestinal Tract

The gastrointestinal tract is endowed with specific defense mechanisms in addition to nonspecific defense mechanisms provided by the intact mucosa, pH unfavorable for the growth of most pathogens, proteolytic enzymes, and competitive inhibition of commensal bacteria. These specific defense mechanisms include humoral IgG antibodies and secretory IgA antibodies (coproantibody), which are synthesized locally (Chapter 5). Recent evidence indicates that lymphocytes that can mediate immunologic reactions alone (T-cell-mediated immunity) or in conjunction with antibody (ADCC reactions) are known to exist in the lamina propria of the gastrointestinal tract.

AUTOIMMUNE DISEASE OF THE LIVER

Immunologic disorders have been implicated as a cause of a number of different acute and chronic diseases of the liver (Table 20–34).

TABLE 20–34.   Liver Diseases with Immunologic Features

1. Viral hepatitis
a. acute
b. chronic
2. Drug-induced liver disease
3. Biliary cirrhosis
4. Portal cirrhosis

Infectious Hepatitis (Type A) and Serum Hepatitis (Type B)

At least two viruses have been found to cause hepatitis: hepatitis virus A (infectious hepatitis) and hepatitis virus B (serum hepatitis). Other cases of hepatitis, although not well-characterized, appear to be caused by non-A, non-B viruses (Chapter 16). Type A virus is commonly associated with fecal-oral spread and a disease of short duration; type B virus is transmitted via the parenteral route and is associated with a disease of considerably longer incubation. However, recent evidence suggests a considerable overlap between these two entities.

Immunologic phenomena have long been thought to play a role in the pathogenesis of diseases caused by these viruses. Antibody to extracts of liver have been detected in the sera of patients with both forms of hepatitis. In more chronic forms of the disease, elevated levels of serum gamma globulin are found, and there is a lymphocytic infiltration of the liver, suggesting an immunologic component.

An antigen originally termed the Australia antigen, Au/SH, and now known as hepatitis B surface antigen (HB_sAg) (Chapter 16) has also been detected in the sera of patients with hepatitis. Recent findings have suggested that the HB_sAg represents a subunit of the surface protein of hepatitis B virion, and a variety of techniques are available for its detection, including precipitation, counter-immune electrophoresis, and radioimmunoassay. There is evidence to suggest a genetic predisposition controlling the prevalence and persistence of this antigen in certain individuals, e.g., those with Down's syndrome. The original description of Australia antigen among inbred Australian aborigines itself suggested a genetic expression.

It has been reported that the severity of hepatitis may vary according to the amount and persistence of HB_sAg antigen in the host. In one study in which the presence of virus alone was detected, it was not associated with active disease. When smaller amounts of antibody were produced, viral antibody complexes and free excess antigen were found, indicating antigen excess. In this case, chronic active disease resulted, resembling in many respects a serum sickness–type of immunologic injury (Chapter 13). In a fatal case, viral antibody complexes were detected in the serum, indicating relative antibody excess. These data offer interesting possibilities for a basis of immunologic injury of the liver mediated by antigen-antibody complexes. Several recent reports also suggest, but do not prove, the participation of cell-mediated injury. HB_sAg has also been detected in affected tissues of patients with periarteritis nodosa.

Chronic Liver Disease

Hepatitis virus B infection can serve as a model of an infection in which immunologic factors may play a role in the pathogenesis of chronic liver disease.

Liver involvement after hepatitis B infection can be divided into the following categories: (1) acute fulminating hepatitis (acute liver necrosis and acute yellow atrophy), (2) acute hepatitis (classic hepatitis B, serum hepatitis, and acute subclinical hepatitis), (3) chronic active hepatitis, (4) chronic persistent subclinical hepatitis with exacerbations, (5) asymptomatic chronic carrier state of HB$_S$Ag, and (6) neonatal hepatitis. At one end of the spectrum is acute fulminant infection with massive hepatocellular destruction and rapid death. The vast majority of cases of hepatitis B follow a second pattern characterized by a variable incubation period, a short episode of clinical symptoms, HB$_S$Ag antigenemia, and fairly rapid clinical and biochemical recovery within four to six weeks, followed by a rapid reversion to an HB$_S$Ag-negative state. In some cases, particularly in children, the acute infection may be entirely subclinical. A third category is chronic active hepatitis, characterized by a variable symptomatology with a protracted debilitating course with biochemical evidence of disease, HB$_S$Ag antigenemia, and progressive liver destruction and cirrhosis. Chronic persistent hepatitis is associated with intermittent symptomatology with exacerbations, abnormal biochemical findings, but chronic liver disease that is usually progressive. In young women, a variant of chronic hepatitis has been described in which clinical and laboratory manifestations were suggestive of SLE (lupoid hepatitis or plasma cell hepatitis) (Fig. 20–49). Originally thought to be a variant of SLE, the entity is now considered to be a form of chronic persistent hepatitis. Another category is the asymptomatic chronic carrier state in which the patient is free of symptoms and normal biochemical findings in the face of persistent HB$_S$Ag in the blood and secretions. The chronic carrier state constitutes a risk for transmission via blood, saliva, and genital secretions and poses a significant risk in certain professions, e.g., dentists. The next category is neonatal hepatitis (which can take two forms depending on the time of maternal infection). This can present as an acute fulminant infection or a more protracted disease with a subclinical course and persistent antigenemia. The expression of the disease appears to be dependent upon the timing of maternal infection. Neonatal infection can be acquired in one of three ways: (1) transplacental infection from a chronic carrier mother during the last trimester, (2) perinatal transmission of the virus from a mother with acute hepatitis, or (3) perinatal infection from a mother through breast milk or genital secretions.

Drug-induced Liver Disease

A number of drugs induce liver disease on the basis of hypersensitivity. There are basically two forms of drug-induced liver damage: a toxic and a true hypersensitivity reaction (Chapter 20A). No circulating antibodies have been detected in the hypersensitivity type. Treatment is limited to discontinuing the drug.

KIDNEY

Immunologically mediated renal diseases result from the triggering of an inflammatory reaction within the kidney. Inflammation, in most instances, proceeds via immune activation of the complement, coagulation, and kinin systems. Since renal parenchymal tissue is capable of responding to immune inflammatory injury in only a limited number of ways, such as hyperplasia, reduplication, necrosis, and fibrosis (Table 20–35), the nature of the resultant immune injury depends basically

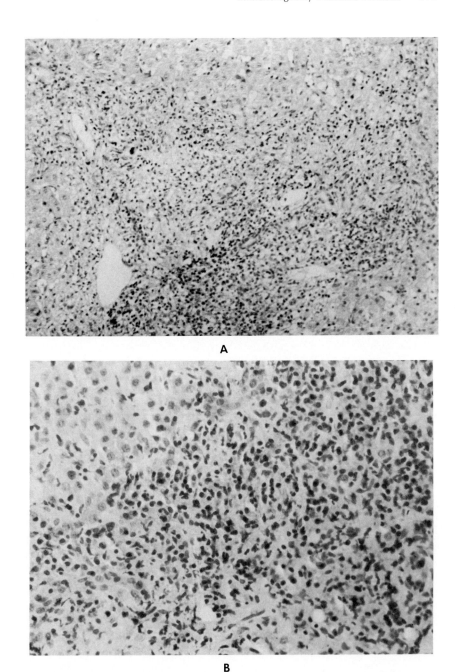

A

B

Figure 20–49. *A,* Photomicrograph of a liver biopsy from a patient with chronic active hepatitis showing liver cell destruction, beginning fibrosis, and prominent infiltration with round cells. Hematoxylin and eosin, ×100. (Courtesy of Dr. Byungkyu Chun.) *B,* Higher magnification of a periportal area of a liver biopsy from a patient with chronic active hepatitis showing infiltration of lymphocytes and plasma cells. Hematoxylin and eosin, ×400. (Courtesy of Dr. Kornel L. Terplan.)

TABLE 20–35.   Renal Parenchymal Tissues and Their Responses to Immune Injury

RENAL PARENCHYMAL TISSUE	RESPONSE
Glomerulus	PMN, mononuclear cell infiltration; sclerosis
Glomerular capillary endothelial cell	Hyperplasia
Glomerular basement membrane	Thickening
Mesangial cell	Hyperplasia
Glomerular visceral epithelial cell	Hyperplasia
Epithelial cell of Bowman's capsule	Hyperplasia (crescent formation)
Interstitium	Cellular infiltration; fibrosis
Tubular epithelial cells	Swelling, necrosis
Interstitial macrophages	Hyperplasia

upon two factors: (1) the type of immune response and (2) its location within the kidney.

Hypersensitivity reactions occurring within the kidney of Types II (cytotoxic), III (immune-complex), and IV (cell-mediated) are associated with development of a variety of specific renal diseases. These types of hypersensitivity reactions may occur in glomerular or tubulointerstitial locations, or both, thus defining the pattern of the disease. Type I (anaphylactic) hypersensitivity has not, as yet, been definitively demonstrated to be associated with specific renal injury (Table 20–36).

Type I (Anaphylactic) Immune Renal Disease

Although no specific renal disease has been definitively ascribed to Type I hypersensitivity, IgE-mediated release of vasoactive amines from mast cells may be of importance in the propagation of a variety of immune inflammatory reactions in the kidney. This concept has been supported by the therapeutic effectiveness of antihistamines in suppressing experimental immune renal injury in animals (Chapter 13).

Type I hypersensitivity has, however, been preliminarily implicated in mediating a form of renal disease associated with Henoch-Schönlein purpura. One report described IgE deposition in the glomeruli of patients with this disease; however, more extensive confirmation is required before IgE is accepted as a definitive pathogenetic factor.

Type II (Cytotoxic) Immune Renal Disease

In this form of hypersensitivity, injury to the kidney results from the combination of antibody with tissue antigens for which it has specificity, with subsequent local activation of the complement and other systems of inflammation. If, for example, antibody is produced with specificity for glomerular basement membrane (GBM), the result is anti-GBM disease.

TABLE 20–36. Patterns of Immunologically Mediated Renal Diseases

Type of Immune Response	Associated Renal Disease	Antigen	Pattern of Deposition of Immune Components		
			Ig	Complement	Fibrin
Type I (Anaphylactic)	1. Henoch-Schönlein purpura (?) 2. Propagation of injury	(?)	Focal mesangial IgE (?)	—	—
Type II (Cytotoxic)	1. Anti-GBM disease	GBM	Linear along GBM	Linear along GBM (sometimes absent)	Extracapillary
	2. Anti-TBM disease 3. Hyperacute rejection	TBM HLA	Linear along TBM Diffuse vascular	Linear along TBM —	— Diffuse cortical vascular
Type III (Immune-complex)	1. Immune-complex GN, e.g., poststreptococcal, serum sickness, hepatitis B, SLE, etc.	Variety of exogenous and endogenous	Lumpy-bumpy in capillary wall	Lumpy-bumpy in capillary wall	Minimal
Type IV (Cell-mediated)	1. Chronic renal allograft rejection 2. Chronic GN	HLA Renal	Diffuse granular Variable	Diffuse granular Variable	Vascular Vascular
Miscellaneous	1. Membranoproliferative GN	None	Often none, occasional IgG in mesangium	C3, subendothelial or intramembranous	Rare
	2. IgG-IgA nephropathy	(?)	IgG and IgA in mesangium	Mesangial, scattered	—

This form of immune renal injury is characterized by the deposition of antibody and complement in a linear fashion along the GBM, as can be shown by direct immunofluorescence (Fig. 20–50 and Chapter 13). Occasionally, the anti-GBM antibody also reacts with other basement membranes, such as lung, producing injury to the pulmonary capillary bed. The syndrome of anti-GBM antibody–mediated immune renal failure and pulmonary hemorrhage is known as Goodpasture's syndrome.

If the anti–basement membrane antibody is directed against tubular basement membrane, the resulting renal disease is predominantly tubulointerstitial. As in anti-GBM disease, the antibody is deposited in a linear fashion along the antigenic tissue for which it is specific (in this case tubular basement membrane). Anti-TBM antibodies are associated with diseases such as anti-GBM disease, systemic lupus erythematosus (SLE), and renal transplant rejection.

One of the most interesting forms of anti-TBM disease is the interstitial nephritis associated with methicillin and other penicillin-like antibiotics. These hypersensitivity renal diseases are characterized by acute oliguria, hematuria, and eosinophilia. On renal biopsy, antibody (IgG) is deposited along the tubular basement membrane. It has been hypothesized that the antibody is directed at the penicillin hapten

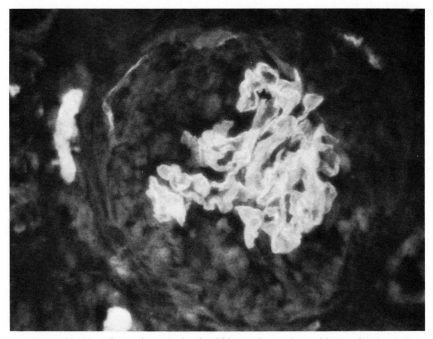

Figure 20-50. Photomicrograph of a kidney of a patient with Goodpasture's syndrome, demonstrated by direct fluorescence microscopy. Note the linear distribution of IgG globulin along the basement membrane and the absence of immunoglobulin in a surrounding crescent. (Courtesy of Dr. Heinz Bauer.)

(Chapter 20A). Since this hapten is concentrated by the renal tubule, antibody localizes along the tubular epithelial cell. An alternative explanation suggests that the penicillin hapten may combine with carrier proteins within the renal tubular cells, resulting in a antigenic hapten-carrier protein complex that elicits specific antibody and becomes the target of Type II attack.

A form of Type II–mediated renal disease that affects the entire kidney is hyperacute renal allograft rejection (Chapter 20B). This form of immune renal injury is associated with high levels of pre-existing antibodies to the histocompatibility antigens (HLA) of the transplant. Upon completion of the vascular anastomosis, there is prompt thrombotic occlusion to the vessels throughout the kidney. It is likely that this diffuse injury results from Type II attack by anti-HLA antibodies against the widely distributed HLA antigens of the renal transplant.

Type III (Immune-Complex) Immune Renal Disease

Immune renal diseases associated with Type III hypersensitivity reactions constitute by far the majority of immunologically mediated renal diseases. In this form of hypersensitivity, inflammation and complement activation result from activation by antigen-antibody complexes. In Type III immune renal disease, these antigen-antibody complexes deposit in the glomerular capillary wall (immune-complex glomerular disease) or in the tubulointerstitium (immune-complex tubulointerstitial renal disease). The antigens that induce the immune-complex glomerulonephritis may be any of a variety of exogenous or endogenous antigens (Table 20–37). In the prototypic disease, post-streptococcal acute glomerulonephritis, the antigen resides in the wall of the streptococcus. Infection with a nephritogenic strain of streptococcus induces production of antibody that combines with the streptococcal

TABLE 20–37. Antigens Associated with Type III Immune Renal Injury

ANTIGEN	EXAMPLES
Exogenous	
Bacterial	Poststreptococcal GN
	Staphylococcal
Viral	Chickenpox
	Hepatitis B
Parasitic	Malaria
	Toxoplasmosis
Foreign serum	Serum sickness
Drugs	Heroin nephropathy (?)
Endogenous	
Nuclear antigens	SLE
Tumor antigens	CEA

antigens to form an immune complex. When these complexes deposit in the glomerular capillary wall, an acute glomerular inflammatory response results with activation of complement, generation of chemotactic components of complement, e.g., $C\overline{567}$, release of lysozymes from polymorphonuclear cells, and subsequent tissue injury. Since the immune complexes probably deposit in a more sporadic fashion in Type III injury than in Type II antibody–mediated anti-GBM disease, it is reasonable that, on immunofluorescence, antibody and complement components appear as lumpy-bumpy structures in the capillary wall (Fig. 20–51).

Endogenous antigens may also result in immune complex–type renal disease, as in the prototypic immune-complex nephritis of SLE. Except for the more diffuse distribution of immune-complex deposition in some forms of lupus nephritis, poststreptococcal and lupus glomerulonephritis look very much alike. In lupus and other immune-complex diseases, the complexes may deposit additionally or preferentially in interstitial structures, resulting in immune injury in tubulointerstitial areas of the kidney.

In contrast to anti-GBM–mediated or anti-TBM–mediated renal diseases, in which antibody fixes directly to antigenic sites, the cause of immune-complex deposition in the glomerular capillary wall is less easily understood. Renal blood flow may explain the delivery of immune complexes to sites of deposition, and the influence of factors such as vasoactive amines to increase permeability of the capillary wall for the movement of antigen-antibody complexes out of the vascular space may help explain how immune complexes arrive at subepithelial sites, where deposition characteristically occurs (Fig. 20–52). Recently, receptors for activated complement have been demonstrated on the visceral epithelial cells of the renal glomerular capillary. These glomerular complement receptors (GCR) may provide the pathogenetic mechanism to explain the fixation of antigen-antibody-complement complexes in these subepithelial sites. The demonstration of specific glomerular receptors for C3 suggests that immune complexes are transported to the glomerulus via the bloodstream, traverse the capillary wall because of the effect of vasoactive amines, and become fixed to subepithelial sites by means of the attraction of C3 within the complex to GCR (Fig. 20–53). This hypothesis is supported by studies of renal biopsies from patients with immune renal diseases. In those biopsies in which *in vivo* deposition of immune complexes in subepithelial sites is demonstrated, the GCR are blocked, suggesting occupation of available binding sites by the complexes.

Type IV (Cell-Mediated) Immune Renal Disease

Type IV immune reactions are characterized by cell-mediated attacks on the target organ. This type of immune renal injury is best

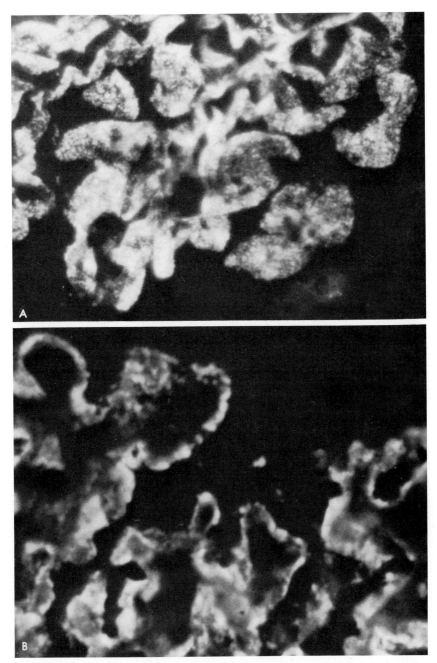

Figure 20–51. Photomicrograph of a kidney of a patient with membranous glomeru-lonephritis demonstrated by direct fluorescence microscopy. *A,* When capillaries are viewed from above, note the diffuse deposition of the complexes. Original magnification, ×400. *B,* Note the subepithelial localization and lumpy character of the immune-complex deposition. Original magnification, ×400. (Courtesy of Dr. Heinz Bauer.)

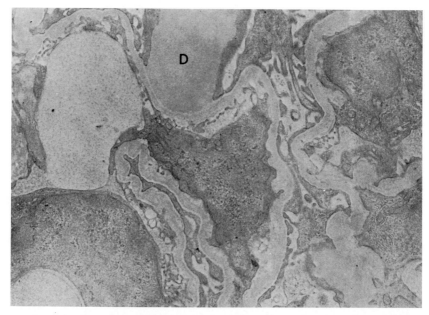

Figure 20–52. Electronmicrograph of a kidney biopsy from a patient with post-streptococcal glomerulonephritis. Note the subepithelial deposit (*D*) "hump" along the border of the basement membrane. ×6000. (Courtesy of Dr. Leticia U. Tiña.)

exemplified in renal allograft rejection in which sensitized lymphoid cells attack the graft and result in immune renal injury (Chapter 20B). This type of immune reaction is diffusely distributed throughout the kidney and proceeds via the release of soluble substances by sensitized lymphoid cells (Chapter 9). These soluble lymphoid cell products, called lymphokines, are capable of propagating an inflammatory immune response and inducing immune injury (Chapter 9).

Another form of renal disease that may fall under the category of Type IV hypersensitivity is chronic glomerulonephritis. One hypothesis to explain this progressive destruction of renal tissue is that cell-mediated hypersensitivity to renal antigens occurs when injured renal tissue antigens are released after acute glomerulonephritis (e.g., poststreptococcal). Renal injury is then propagated by cell-mediated attack on renal tissue. Support of this pathogenesis of chronic glomerulonephritis has been provided by studies showing the release of migration inhibitory factor (MIF) on exposure to renal tissue antigens by lymphoid cells from patients with chronic glomerulonephritis.

Miscellaneous Forms of Immune Renal Disease

A number of renal diseases appear to have immunologic bases that do not fit precisely into one of the above categories. Two such diseases

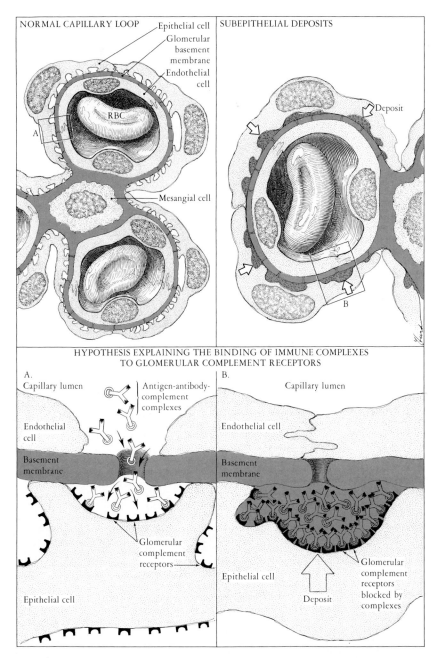

Figure 20–53. Hypothesis to explain development of subepithelial immune deposits as a result of binding of immune complexes to complement receptors on the visceral epithelial cell. Inset *A* shows the complexes, composed of antigen, antibody, and complement (C3), migrating through the basement membrane to come in contact with complement receptors on the surface of the visceral epithelial cell. Inset *B* depicts the accumulation of immune complexes to form a subepithelial deposit with the blocking of all available complement receptor sites that have migrated to the site of the deposit.

are IgG-IgA nephropathy (Berger's disease) and membranoproliferative or mesangiocapillary glomerulonephritis.

In IgG-IgA nephropathy, the patient may present with proteinuria and hematuria. The renal biopsy shows deposition of IgG and IgA immunoglobulin in mesangial areas of the glomerulus, with subsequent reactive mesangial cell hyperplasia. The precise cause of the immunoglobulin deposition in this disease in not known; however, in rabbits given repeated injections of bovine serum albumin (BSA) in amounts to balance antibody production, antibody deposition is predominantly localized to the mesangial region during the first few weeks of antigen administration. It is only subsequently that immune-complex deposition may be observed in the capillary wall or extraglomerular (tubulointerstitial) locations. These results suggest that the mesangium may function to clear small amounts of immune complexes early during antigen-antibody production or when the level of complexes is relatively small. Later perhaps, after saturation of other mononuclear phagocytic systems such as in the liver and spleen, complexes may begin to accumulate in capillary wall and extraglomerular sites.

Membranoproliferative glomerulonephritis is a very interesting form of renal disease that appears to result from deposition of activated complement components within the kidney. It is probable that in this form of renal disease, activation of the complement system proceeds predominantly via the alternative pathway (Chapter 6), i.e., as a result of direct activation of C3 to C3b. The direct activation of C3 is likely to be related to a factor in the serum known as nephritic factor, a 7S gamma globulin (MW 150,000) that is heat stable. Nephritic factor is capable of cleaving C3 to C3b directly. In this form of renal disease (although two variants have been described), C3 is deposited densely within the capillary wall of the glomerulus, possibly by fixation to GCR. It is of note that the membranoproliferative form of glomerulonephritis has been found clinically associated with other complement system abnormalities and susceptibility to infections in patients with partial lipodystrophy. Although membranoproliferative glomerulonephritis does not proceed to renal failure in all instances, patients who develop renal failure and receive a renal transplant are at very significant risk of experiencing the recurrence of the disease in the transplant.

MUSCLE

Myasthenia gravis is a disorder of voluntary muscles characterized by muscle weakness and fatigability. A transitory neonatal form has been described occurring in infants born of myasthenic mothers (Chapter 26). Rarely, it is congenital and persists. Juvenile and adult cases are chronic, although signs and symptoms may be variable. There are thymic abnormalities consisting of hyperplasia and plasma cell infiltration in at least 80 per cent of patients. Evidence suggests that there is a thymic polypeptide factor that acts to inhibit neuromuscular transmission at the myoneural junction. More recently, antibodies to neuromuscular receptors have been described.

Immunologic Factors.   Serum antibodies directed against muscle may be detected by a variety of tests, including direct and indirect immunofluorescence (Fig. 20–54), complement fixation, precipitation, and tanned-cell hemagglutination. Delayed hypersensitivity does not appear to be impaired in these patients.

The presence of these antibodies may be useful in diagnosis, prognosis, and therapy. If found, they may provide a differential point in distinguishing myasthenia gravis from other disorders characterized by muscle weakness. If they are detected, the physician is well advised to persist in a careful search for thymic abnormalities (e.g., thymoma), even if there is an absence of X-ray evidence of an enlarged gland. Antibodies may also serve in a prognostic way, aiding in the follow-up of the patient after surgery, since it is sometimes difficult to detect and remove aberrant thymic tissue.

Treatment of the disorder includes the use of anticholinergic drugs, thymectomy, and, in certain cases, the use of steroids and X-irradiation of the thymus.

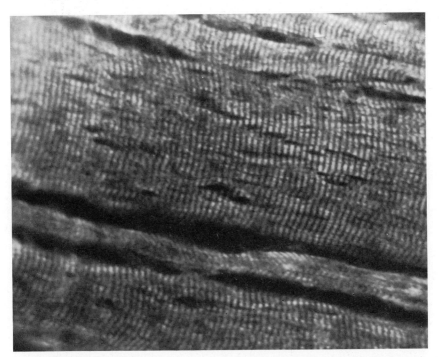

Figure 20–54.   The presence of serum antibody to cross-striations of skeletal muscle in a patient with myasthenia gravis demonstrated by indirect immunofluorescence. (Courtesy of Dr. Heinz Bauer.)

HEART

Antibodies directed against heart tissues are found in two clinical situations: (1) antibody produced to cardiac antigen released into the serum after damage or trauma and (2) antibody produced to a cross-reacting antigen, such as following Group A beta hemolytic streptococcal infections.

In the first situation, antigen may be released into the circulation after trauma, myocardial infection, myocardial infarction, or surgery. This is a normal reaction to the release of cardiac antigen. These antibodies have been implicated in the postcardiotomy syndrome and postmyocardial infarction syndrome in which the patient may have retrosternal pain, pleuritis, and pericarditis. In the second type, the antibody is directed primarily against antigens of the infecting microorganisms and secondarily against cardiac tissue because of its structural similarity to the microorganism. Rheumatic fever has been classified as an autoimmune disease and is thought to result as a consequence of these cross-reacting antibodies. Only a small percentage of patients with Group A beta hemolytic streptococcal infections develop rheumatic fever (from 2 to 3 per cent). However, once it has been initiated, the incidence of recurrence after a subsequent streptococcal infection increases to 50 to 60 per cent. Since there is no way of identifying individuals at risk for rheumatic fever and acute glomerulonephritis, the physician should promptly diagnose and adequately treat Group A beta hemolytic streptococcal infections in order to lower the risk of these sequelae.

SKIN

The diseases is which an autoimmunologic basis has been described include dermatitis herpetiformis, lupus erythematosus, bullous pemphigoid, and pemphigus vulgaris. Shown in Table 20–38 are typical immunologic fluorescent staining patterns seen in these various diseases.

Dermatitis herpetiformis is a disease characterized by grouped vesicles surmounted on an erythematous base involving predominantly the extensor surfaces of the back and arms (Fig. 20–55). The disease is characterized by an incapacitating burning pruritus, and patients have recently been shown to have a patchy duodenal-jejunal atrophy indistinguishable from that of adult celiac disease. However, this gastrointestinal lesion is generally asymptomatic and has not been associated with an increased incidence of steatorrhea or malabsorption. HLA-B8 antigen has been found in approximately 75 to 80 per cent of patients with dermatitis herpetiformis. The examination of the perilesional skin of patients with dermatitis herpetiformis has revealed a granular deposition of IgA in 95 per cent of patients thus far examined (Fig. 20–56). The

TABLE 20–38. Immunofluorescence Staining Pattern in Autoimmune Diseases of the Skin, Illustrating Demonstration of Immunoglobulins (Ig) and Complement (C)

| | DIRECT | | | | | | | INDIRECT | |
| | *Intercellular* | | *Basement Membrane* | | | | | *Intercellular* | *Basement Membrane* |
DISEASE	IgG	C	IgG	IgA	IgM	C			
Dermatitis herpetiformis	−	−	+	++++	0	+		0	0
Lupus erythematosus									
Systemic lupus (SLE)*	−	−	++++	++	++	++		0	0
Discoid lupus**	−	−	++++	++	++	++		0	0
Bullous pemphigoid	−	−	++++	−	++	++		0	+
Pemphigus vulgaris	++++	+	−	−	−	−		+	0

*involved and uninvolved skin
**uninvolved skin only

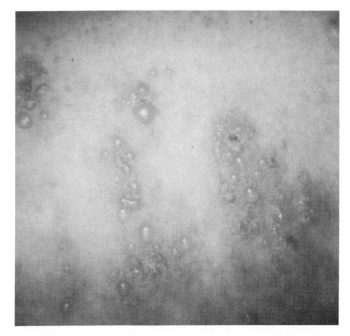

Figure 20-55. Characteristic lesions from a patient with dermatitis herpetiformis. Note the characteristic grouped vesicles surmounted on an erythematous base. (Courtesy of Dr. Thomas T. Provost.)

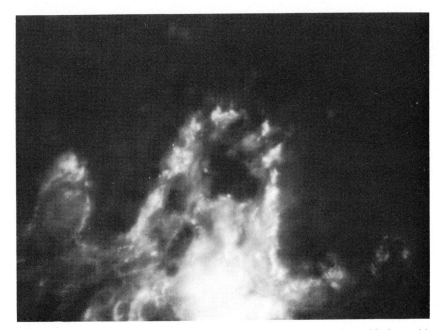

Figure 20-56. Photomicrograph of a biopsy of skin from a patient with dermatitis herpetiformis, illustrating the granular deposition of IgA that appears to be virtually pathognomonic for the disease. (Courtesy of Dr. Thomas T. Provost.)

IgA deposition is virtually pathognomonic for dermatitis herpetiformis (Table 20–38). In addition, C3, C5, properdin, and properdin factor B have been frequently noted in a granular deposition along the dermal-epidermal junction; IgG and early components of the complement system, i.e., C1q and C4, are infrequently noted (Table 20–38). These direct immunofluorescent findings suggest that the major activation of the complement system in dermatitis herpetiformis may be via the alternative complement pathway (Chapter 6). The disease is responsive to sulfapyridine and diaminodiphenylsulfone (dapsone). Within a short time after either of these two drugs is instituted, the patient's burning pruritus and lesions often disappear. Surprisingly, the examination of asymptomatic patients receiving these two drugs has consistently revealed the continued deposition of IgA and in some instances complement components. The precise pharmacologic mechanism of action of sulfapyridine and dapsone in this disease remains an intriguing mystery.

Skin manifestations of lupus erythematosus are seen in both the systemic and the chronic discoid forms of the disease. The clinical and immunologic manifestations of SLE have been described elsewhere in this chapter. The characteristic skin lesions of chronic discoid lupus consist of a sharply circumscribed scaling erythematous dermatitis (Fig. 20–57) in which follicular plugging, telangiectasia, and atrophy are

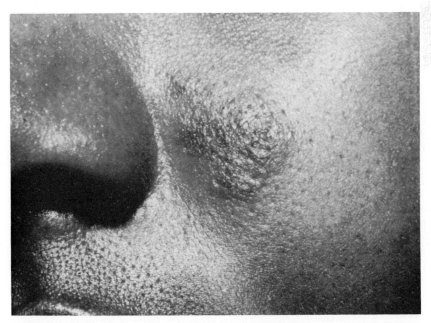

Figure 20–57. Photograph of a patient with chronic discoid lupus erythematosus, illustrating a sharply circumscribed scaly erythematous dermatitis. (Courtesy of Dr. Thomas T. Provost.)

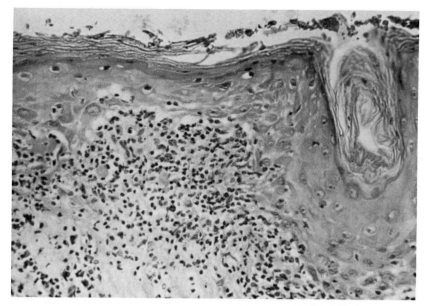

Figure 20–58. Photomicrograph of a skin lesion of chronic discoid lupus erythematosus showing the characteristic atrophy of skin, follicular plugging and cellular infiltrate. (Courtesy of Dr. Thomas T. Provost.)

common features (Fig. 20–58). In both SLE and discoid lupus, immunoglobulins and complement components are found in a granular deposition at the dermal-epidermal junction (Fig. 20–59). In SLE, however, the deposition is seen in both involved and uninvolved areas of skin, whereas in chronic discoid lupus, the deposition of the immune reactants appears to be confined to the involved areas of skin.

Bullous pemphigoid is a disease characterized by an onset in the fifth and sixth decades of life. The skin lesions are characterized by tense subepidermal blisters that may arise on normal as well as inflamed skin (Fig. 20–60). The lesions have a predilection for flexural areas of the body, including the neck, the axillae, and the inguinal area. The disease is a generally benign, self-limited entity that usually responds to steroid therapy within four to six months with complete resolution. Recurrences after therapy occur in approximately 10 to 15 per cent of cases. The characteristic immunopathologic findings in skin include a linear homogeneous IgG deposition along the basement membrane zone, detected by direct immunofluorescence (Fig. 20–61). All classes of immunoglobulins and early and late complement components are seen, as well as fibrin. Approximately 80 per cent of patients demonstrate in their serum an IgG anti–basement membrane antibody that can be detected by indirect immunofluorescence (Table 20–38). With treatment, the serum autoantibody and the tissue deposition of immunoglobulins and complement disappear.

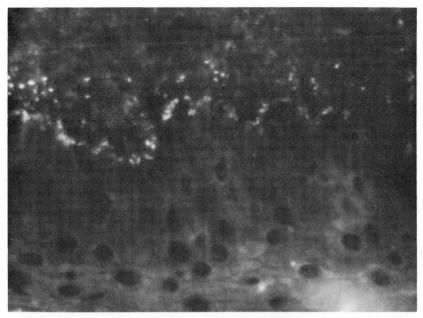

Figure 20–59. Photomicrograph of skin of a patient with chronic discoid lupus erythematosus, showing a characteristic lupus band with granular deposition of IgG at the dermal-epidermal junction involving only the affected skin. (Courtesy of Dr. Thomas T. Provost.)

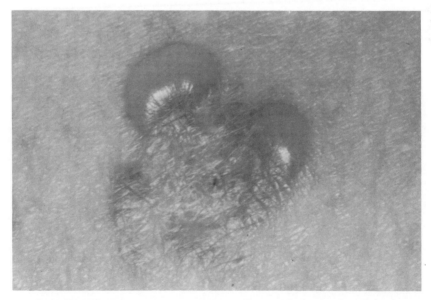

Figure 20–60. Photograph of a patient with pemphigus vulgaris, illustrating the large flaccid blisters characteristic of the disease. (Courtesy of Dr. Thomas T. Provost.)

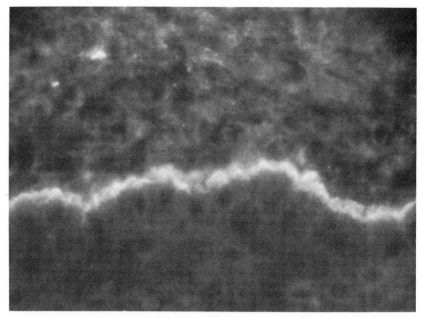

Figure 20–61. Photomicrograph of skin of a patient with bullous pemphigoid, illustrating the characteristic linear homogeneous IgG deposition along the basement membrane zone detected by direct immunofluorescence. (Courtesy of Dr. Thomas T. Provost.)

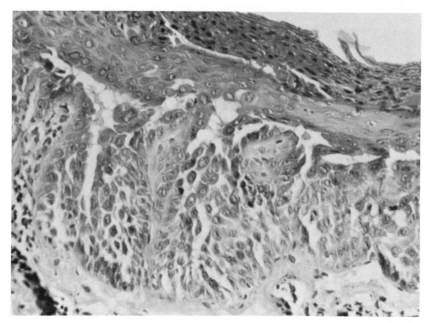

Figure 20–62. Photomicrograph of the skin lesion of pemphigus vulgaris, showing the characteristic interepidermal edema formation associated with destruction of normal intercellular bridges. (Courtesy of Dr. Thomas T. Provost.)

Pemphigus vulgaris is a blistering disease characterized by the presence of flaccid bullae arising in the mouth and scalp but rapidly disseminating over the entire body. Its striking feature is interepidermal blister formation that occurs with destruction of normal intercellular bridges (Fig. 20–62). Upon pressure, the lesions rapidly extend their margins (Nikolski's sign). Although previously associated with a predilection in the Jewish race, recent reports indicate that the disease occurs in all racial and ethnic groups. This serious blistering disease carried with it a significant mortality rate prior to the era of steroids, with approximately 50 per cent of patients dying within 12 to 15 months after initial diagnosis. The disease can be controlled with steroids or with a combination of steroids and immunosuppressive agents (e.g., cyclophosphamide) (Chapter 25). Direct immunofluorescence of perilesional skin lesions of patients with pemphigus vulgaris has demonstrated IgG, C1q, C3, properdin, and properdin factor B in the squamous intercellular spaces. In addition, in about 90 per cent of patients, the presence of circulating autoantibody to intercellular squamous epithelium has been demonstrated by indirect immunofluorescence (Table 20–38 and Fig. 20–63).

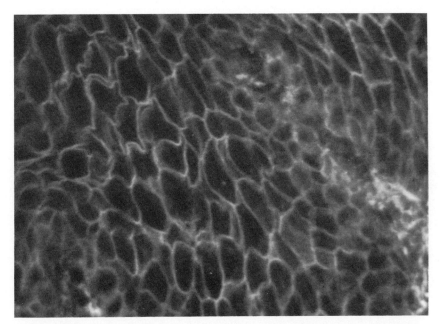

Figure 20–63. Photomicrograph of an indirect immunofluorescent examination of a monkey esophagus that has been layered with the serum of a patient with pemphigus vulgaris, illustrating the presence of circulating autoantibody to intercellular squamous epithelium detected by indirect immunofluorescence. (Courtesy of Dr. Thomas T. Provost.)

EYE

The eye is isolated anatomically and contains a variety of antigens that normally are not in contact with the circulation (sequestered antigens). Autoimmune phenomena have been implicated in three diseases of the eye: (1) phacogenic uveitis (lens), (2) sympathetic ophthalmia (uvea), and (3) autoimmune reaction involving the lacrimal gland (Sjögren's syndrome).

The release of lens protein into the circulation due to trauma or surgery may result in a sequence of immunologic events leading to inflammation and destruction of the lens. Both inflammatory and immunologic events are triggered. Inflammatory cells are found within the lesions and antilens antibody is found within the circulation and aqueous humor of the affected individual.

Sympathetic ophthalmia results from a perforating wound of the eye. Following trauma to one eye (exciting eye), there is secondary involvement of the other (sympathizing eye). Antiuveal antibodies have been detected in the serum.

SUMMARY

The autoimmune diseases represent a collection of poorly defined, incompletely understood groups of disorders that have in common the manifestation of antibody or delayed hypersensitivity to body constituents (autoimmune phenomena). They are commonly grouped into those disorders that involve multiple systems (multisystemic disorders) and those that are confined or restricted to one organ (organ-specific). The relationship of the autoimmune phenomena to the disease is not understood. A frequent finding in many of these disorders has been an abnormal sex ratio, usually with a female predominance. Although the cause of these diseases is unknown, recent evidence suggests that they are under genetic control and that they represent disorders of regulation (suppression) of the lymphoid system.

SUGGESTIONS FOR FURTHER READING

A. Immunologically Mediated Disease Involving Exogenous Antigens (Allergy)

Austen, K. F., and Lichtenstein, L. M.: Asthma: Physiology, Immunopharmacology and Treatment. New York, Academic Press, Inc., 1973.

Bates, D. V., Macklem, P. T., and Christie, R. V.: Respiratory Function in Disease. 2nd ed., Philadelphia, W. B. Saunders Co., 1971.

Bellanti, J. A.: Biologic significance of the secretory γA globulins. Pediatrics, *48*:715, 1971.

Claman, H. N.: How corticosteroids work. J. Allergy Clin. Immunol., *55*:145, 1975.

Dale, D. C., Fauci, A. S., and Wolff, S. M.: Alternate-day prednisone: Leukocyte kinetics and susceptibility to infections. N. Engl. J. Med., *291*:1154, 1974.

Fauci, A. S., Dale, D. C., and Balow, J. E.: Glucocorticosteroid therapy: Mechanisms of action and clinical considerations. Ann. Intern. Med., *84*:304, 1975.

Frank M. M., Gelfand, J. A., and Atkinson, J. P.: Hereditary angioedema: The clinical syndrome and its management. Ann. Intern. Med., *84*:580, 1976.

Gell, P. G. H., Coombs, R. R. A., and Lachmann, P. J.: Clinical Aspects of Immunology. Oxford, Blackwell Scientific Publications, Ltd., 1975.

Gleich, G. J., and Dunnette, S. L.: Comparison of procedures for measurement of IgE protein in serum and secretions. J. Allergy Clin. Immunol., *59*:377. 1977.

Hubscher, T. T.: Immune and biochemical mechanisms in the allergic disease of the upper respiratory tract; role of antibodies, target cells, mediators and eosinophils. Ann. Allergy, *38*:83, 1977.

Ishizaka, T., and Ishizaka, K.: Biology of immunoglobulin E: Molecular basis of reaginic hypersensitivity. Prog. Allergy, *19*:60, 1975.

Kaplan, A. P.,Gray, L., Shaff, R. E., Horakova, Z., and Beaven, M. A.: In vivo studies of mediator release in cold urticaria and cholinergic urticaria. J. Allergy Clin. Immunol., *55*:395, 1975.

Lefkowitz, R. J.: β-adrenergic receptors: Recognition and regulation. N. Engl. J. Med., *295*:323, 1976.

Levine, B. B.: Genetic factors in hypersensitivity reactions to drugs. Ann. N.Y. Acad. Sci., *151*:988, 1968.

Lichtenstein, L. M., Ishizaka, K., Norman, P. S., Sobotka, A. K., and Hill, B. M.: IgE antibody measurements in ragweed hayfever: Relationship to clinical severity and results of immunotherapy. J. Clin. Invest., *52*:472, 1973.

Lopez, M., and Salvaggio, J.: Hypersensitivity pneumonitis: Current concepts of etiology and pathogenesis. Ann. Rev. Med., *27*:453, 1976.

Middleton, E., Reed, C., and Ellis, E. (eds.): Allergy: Principles and Practice. St. Louis, C. V. Mosby, 1978 (in press).

Parker, C. W.: Drug allergy. N. Engl. J. Med., *292*:51, 732, 957, 1975.

Patterson, R.: Allergic Diseases: Diagnosis and Management. Philadelphia, J. B. Lippincott Co., 1972.

Patterson, R., Mellies, C. J., and Roberts, M.: Immunologic reactions against insulin: II. IgE anti-insulin, insulin allergy and combined IgE and IgG immunologic insulin resistance. J. Immunol., *110*:1135, 1973.

Pepys, J.: Hypersensitivity Diseases of the Lungs Due to Fungi and Organic Dusts. Basel, S. Karger, 1969.

Platts-Mills, T. A. E., von Mauer, R. K., Ishizaka, K., Norman, P. S., and Lichtenstein, L. M.: IgA and IgG anti-ragweed antibodies in nasal secretions. J. Clin. Invest.,*57*:1041, 1976.

Rosenow, E. C.: The spectrum of drug-induced pulmonary disease. Ann. Intern. Med., *77*:977, 1972.

Samter, M.: Immunological Diseases. Boston, Little, Brown and Co., 1971

Tada, T., Taniguchi, M., and Takemori, T.: Properties of primed suppressor T cells and their products. Transplant. Rev., *26*:106, 1975.

Zweiman, B., Mishkin, M. M., and Hildreth, E. A.: An approach to the performance of contrast studies in contrast material-reactive persons. Ann. Intern. Med., *83*:159, 1975.

B. Immunologically Mediated Disease Involving Homologous Antigens

Gell, P. G. H., Coombs, R. R. A., and Lachmann, P. J.: Clinical Aspects of Immunology, Oxford, Blackwell Scientific Publications, Ltd., 1975.

Mollison, P.: Blood Transfusion in Clinical Medicine. Philadelphia, F. A. Davis Company, 1968.

Race, R. R., and Sanger, R.: Blood Groups in Man. Philadelphia, F. A. Davis Company, 1969.

Rapaport, F. T., and Dausset, J.: Human Transplantation. New York, Grune & Stratton, Inc., 1968.

Russell, P. S.: Transplantation, I, II, III. N. Engl. J. Med., *282*:786, 848, 896, 1970.

Witebsky, E., Rubin, M. I., Engasser, L., and Blum,I.: Studies on erythroblastosis fetalis. II. Investigation on detection of sensitization of red blood cells of newborn infants with erythroblastosis fetalis. J. Lab. Clin. Med., *32*:1339, 1947.

Zmijewski, C. M.: Immunohematology. New York, Appleton-Century-Crofts, 1968.

Organ Transplantation

Belzer, F. O., et al.: Is HL-A typing of clinical significance in cadaver renal transplantation? Lancet, 775–777, 1976.

Braun, W. E., Banowsky, L. H., et al.: Lymphoceles associated with renal transplantation. Report of cases and review of the literature. Am. J. Med., 57:714–728, 1974.

Calne, R. Y., and Williams, R.: Orthotopic liver transplantation: The first 60 patients. Br. Med. J., 1:471–476, 1977.

Cochrum, S., et al.: Mixed lymphocyte reaction and graft survival. Ann. Surg., 1974.

Friedman, B. A., Wenglin, B. D., Hyland, R. N., and Rifkind, D.: Roentgenographically atypical Pneumocystis carinii pneumonia. Am. Rev. Resp. Dis., 111:89–95, 1975.

Gallis, H. A.: Fungal infections following renal transplantation. Arch. Intern. Med., 135:1163–1172, 1975.

Kiser, W. S., Hewitt, C. B., and Montie, J. E.: The surgical complications of renal transplantation. Surg. Clin. North Am., 51:1133, 1971.

Maher, J. F.: A logical approach to the diagnosis of renal transplant rejection. Immunologic, ischemic, and inflammatory impairment of renal function. Am. J. Med., 56:275–289, 1974.

Matthew, T. H., Mathews, D. C., Hobbs, J. B., and Kincaid-Smith, P.: Glomerular lesions after renal transplantation. Am. J. Med., 59:177–199, 1975.

Merrill, J. P.: New perspective on pathogenesis and treatment of rejection in kidney transplantation. Kidney Int., 7:S318–S322, 1976.

Myerowitz, R. L., Medeiros, A. A., and O'Brien, T. F.: Bacterial infection in renal homotransplantation recipients. A study of 53 bacteremic episodes. Am. J. Med., 53:308, 1972.

Rifkind, D., Marchioro, T. L., et al.: Infectious diseases associated with renal homotransplantation. J.A.M.A., 189:397, 402, 1964.

Suwansirikul, S., Ho, M., et al.: The transplanted kidney as a source of cytomegalovirus infection. N. Engl. J. Med., 293:1109–1112, 1975.

Van Bekkum, D. W., Fritz, H. B., et al.: A report from histocompatible allogeneic donors for aplastic anemia. A report from the ACS/NIH Bone Marrow Transplant Registry. J.A.M.A., 236(10):1131–1135, 1976.

C. Immunologically Mediated Disease Involving Autologous Antigens

Anderson, J. R., Buchanan, W. W., and Goudie, R. B.: Autoimmunity: Clinical and Experimental. Springfield, Illinois, Charles C Thomas, Publisher, 1967.

Asherson, G. L.: The role of microorganisms in autoimmune responses. Prog. Allergy, 12:192, 1968.

Burnet, F. M.: Autoimmune disease: Some general principles. Postgrad. Med., 30:91, 1961.

Carpenter, C. B.: Immunologic aspects of renal disease. Ann. Rev. Med., 21:1, 1970.

Churg, J., and Grishman, R.: Ultrastructure of glomerular disease: A review. Kidney Int., 7:254, 1975.

Dawson, R. B.: HLA Typing. Washington, D. C., Am. Assoc. Blood Banks, 1976.

Gelfand, M. C., Shin, M. L., Nagle, R. B., Green, I., and Frank, M. M.: The glomerular complement receptor in immunologically mediated renal glomerular injury. N. Engl. J. Med., 295:10, 1976.

Gell, P. G. H., Coombs, R. R., and Lachmann, P. J.: Cinical Aspects of Immunology. Oxford, Blackwell Scientific Publications, Ltd., 1975.

Humphrey, J. H., and White, R. G.: Immunology for Students of Medicine. 3rd ed., Oxford, Blackwell Scientific Publications, Ltd., 1970.

Koffler, D.: Immunopathologenesis of systemic lupus erythematosus. Ann. Rev. Med., 25:149, 1974.

Krakauer, R. S., Strober, W., Rippeon, D. L., and Waldmann, T. A.: Prevention of autoimmunity in experimental lupus erythematosus by soluble immune response suppressor. Science, 196:56, 1977.

Lehman, D. H., Wilson, C. B., and Dixon, F. J.: Extraglomerular immunoglobulin deposits in human nephritis. Am. J. Med., 58:765, 1975.

McLean, R. H., and Michael, A. F.: Activation of the complement system in renal conditions in animals and man. Prog. Immunol., 5:69, 1974.

Mikkelsen, W. M., Calabro, J. J., Castor, C. W., et al.: Twenty-second rheumatism review:

Review of the American and English literature for the years 1973 and 1974. Arthritis Rheum., *19*(Suppl. 6):973–1236, 1976.

Mullin, B. R., Levinson, R. E., Friedman, A., Henson, D. E., Winand, R. J., and Kohn, L. D.: Delayed hypersensitivity in Graves' disease and exophthalmos: Identification of thyroglobulin in normal human orbital muscle. Endocrinology, *100*:351, 1977.

Otaka, Y.: Immunopathology of Rheumatic Fever and Rheumatoid Arthritis. Tokyo, Igaku Shoin, Ltd., 1976.

Sell, S.: Immunology, Immunopathology and Immunity. Hagerstown, Md., Harper and Row, Publishers, 1975.

Sharp, G. C., Irwin, W. S., Tan, E. W., et al.: Mixed connective tissue disease. An apparent distinct rheumatic disease syndrome associated with a specific antibody to an extractable nuclear antigen (ENA). Am. J. Med., *52*:148–159, 1972.

Shearn, M.: Rheumatic diseases. Med. Clin. North Am., *61*:203–461, 1977.

Solomon, D. H., Chopra, I. J., Chopra, U., and Smith, F. J.: Identification of subgroups of euthyroid Graves' ophthalmopathy. N. Engl. J. Med., *296*:181, 1977.

Strober, W.: Gluten-sensitive enteropathy. Clin. Gastroenterol., *5*:429, 1976.

Volpé, R., Farid, N. R., von Westarp, C., and Rose, V. V.: The pathogenesis of Graves' disease and Hashimoto's thyroiditis. Clin. Endocrinol. (Oxf.), *3*:239, 1974.

Wilson, C. B., and Dixon, F. J.: Anti-glomerular basement membrane antibody induced glomerulonephritis. Kidney Int., *3*:74, 1973.

Wilson, C. B., and Dixon, F. J.: Renal response to immunological injury. *In* B. M. Brenner and F. C. Rector, Jr. (eds.): The Kidney, Philadelphia, W. B. Saunders Company, 1976.

PROLIFERATIVE DISORDERS OF THE IMMUNE SYSTEM

George M. Bernier, M.D.

Several diseases of man are characterized by abnormal proliferation of those cells that normally are the mediators of specific immunity: lymphocytes and plasma cells. When such proliferation involves cells that usually synthesize and secrete immunoglobulin, the disorder may be associated with excessive production of immunoglobulins. The nature of the immunoglobulins produced may indeed be characteristic of the disorder.

The immunoproliferative disorders discussed in this chapter are multiple myeloma, macroglobulinemia, and heavy-chain disease. These three disorders are often called the "monoclonal gammopathies" and will be described as a unit. The lymphomas and lymphatic leukemias will be considered as examples of lymphoproliferative diseases in which immunoglobulin aberration is less readily apparent. Under these conditions, distinctive features are often found in the proliferative cells themselves.

THE MONOCLONAL GAMMOPATHIES

CONCEPT

The immunoglobulins produced in response to the myriad antigens to which man is exposed are an extremely heterogeneous group of molecules. This heterogeneity undoubtedly reflects those variations in primary sequence related to antibody specificity and may be readily demonstrated by immunoelectrophoresis of serum (Fig. 21-1). The IgG globulin fraction of serum is dispersed over a wide electrophoretic range, in contrast to the albumin and transferrin that migrate as discrete components. In a similar fashion, but to a less striking degree, the other immunoglobulins (IgA, IgM, IgD, and IgE) are electrophoretically heterogeneous or polydisperse. An individual plasma cell appears to produce immunoglobulins that are homogeneous in terms of antibody specificity, light- and heavy-chain composition, genetic factors,

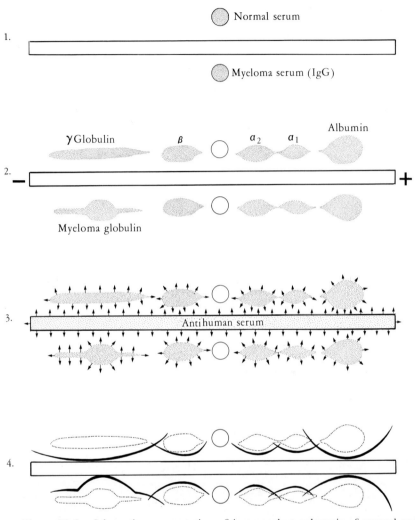

Figure 21-1. Schematic representation of immunoelectrophoresis of normal and myeloma serum.

Step 1: The sera are applied to wells punched out of agar slides.

Step 2: The agar slide is placed in an electric field, and the proteins migrate — albumin to the anode (+) and γ globulin to the cathode (−). Note that the myeloma globulin is restricted in its mobility to a portion of the γ globulin fraction.

Step 3: Antisera to human serum proteins are applied in the central trough and the antibodies diffuse into the agar toward the serum proteins which also diffuse into the agar.

Step 4: Where serum proteins and their homologous antibodies meet, precipitation arcs develop. The arc has a characteristic position and shape for the particular protein. In this diagram, the serum is depicted as being composed of only five components, whereas most antisera detect at least 25 components. The normal IgG forms a long sweeping arc. Note that the IgG arc formed by the myeloma serum is distorted with a localized antigenic excess forming a "blister" on the IgG arc.

and electrophoretic charge. The heterogeneity of immunoglobulins must therefore be the result of a heterogeneous cell population. Thus, for each of the 10^8 possible antibodies, there exists a different cell line or clone capable of producing that antibody. If one cell out of the many different cell lines or clones were selected for abnormal uncontrolled proliferation, and if it retained the ability to synthesize its immunoglobulin, a great excess of a homogeneous immunoglobulin could be expected to result (Fig. 21–2). When such situations occur, they are viewed as abnormalities of the immune, or gamma, system ("gammopathies"), arising in a single disordered clone of cells. They are called "monoclonal gammopathies" (Table 21–1). The protein elaborated is often called a monoclonal immunoglobulin or an "M-component." When monoclonal immunoglobulins occur, they may be of any class (IgG, IgA, IgM, IgD, or IgE) or type (κ or λ). They are usually recog-

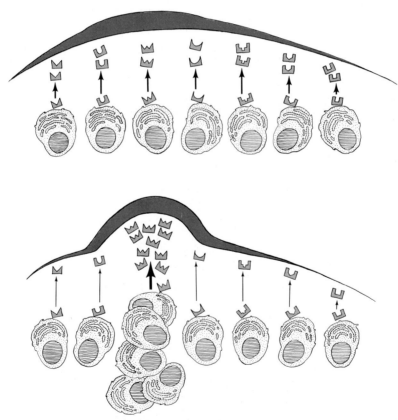

Figure 21–2. Diagrammatic illustration of the monoclonal immunoglobulin concept. Normal individuals (*top*) have many populations or clones of plasma cells, each producing immunoglobulins of differing electrophoretic mobility, indicated as molecules of differing shapes. The wide extremes of electrophoretic mobility give rise to a long, polydisperse immunoelectrophoretic arc. In contrast, if one clone or population were to be selected for proliferation (*bottom*), its product would be greatly increased. In association with this, the products of the other clones are decreased. This gives rise to an immunoglobulin of restricted mobility and the characteristically distorted immunoelectrophoretic arc.

TABLE 21-1. Monoclonal Gammopathies

DISORDER	CLASS OF PROTEIN	LIGHT CHAIN
Multiple myeloma	IgG, IgA, IgD or IgE	κ or λ
Macroglobulinemia	IgM	κ or λ
Heavy-chain disease	IgG, IgA or IgM	None

nized as an increased homogeneous serum globulin. In many instances, patients with serum monoclonal immunoglobulins also have detectable amounts of free light chains. Light chains of either κ- or λ-type may be produced in excess of heavy chains and may circulate as free homogeneous light chains. Because of their small size (a dimer of light chains has a molecular weight of 45,000 daltons), they are excreted rapidly in the urine. Free light chains in the monoclonal gammopathies are usually detected as electrophoretically homogeneous urinary proteins bearing the κ or λ antigenic determinants. Free light chains have unusual thermal solubility properties, which were first described by H. Bence Jones in 1847, and are often called Bence Jones proteins. They may be detected by appropriately heating the urine (see later). In approximately 20 per cent of myeloma patients, the affected clone of cells secretes only free light chains.

MULTIPLE MYELOMA

Multiple myeloma, a malignant proliferation of plasma cells, is the most common of the monoclonal gammopathies. In a pathophysiologic sense, the various features of the disorder may be viewed as consequences of the following: (1) the expansion of the cell mass; (2) the elaboration of the proteins by cells; and (3) the associated suppression of normal antibody synthesis. In its full-blown expression, the disease involves the skeletal system, the bone marrow, the kidneys, and the nervous system.

Bone

The skeletal problems are extraordinarily troublesome and range from multiple osteolytic lesions and pathologic fractures to diffuse osteoporosis and painful compression fractures (Fig. 21–3). As progressive vertebral collapse occurs, marked diminution in the patient's height may result. Spinal cord transection and paraplegia are uncommon tragic consequences of vertebral column compression fractures. The multiple individual osteolytic lesions of bone (myelomas) are readily explained as being due in part to plasma cell growth, but the mechanics of the diffuse osteoporosis is less well understood. Elaboration by myeloma cells of a low molecular weight factor that selectively stimulates *osteoclasts* has been demonstrated and this factor most likely

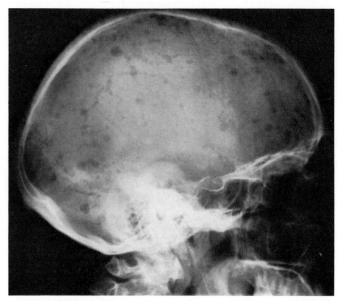

Figure 21–3. Skull x-ray of a myeloma patient showing many well-demarcated osteo-lytic lesions in the calvarium.

plays a role in both osteolytic and osteoporotic lesions. A direct con-sequence of the skeletal problems is disturbed calcium balance. During the course of their disease or even before it has been diagnosed, pa-tients with multiple myeloma may have hypercalcemia of life-threaten-ing degree. Symptoms of polyuria, constipation, lethargy, confusion, and stupor may occur. Unlike the case in hypercalcemia due to hyper-parathyroidism or metastatic carcinoma, serum alkaline phosphatase activity is usually normal. It is important to point out that the im-mobilization of a myeloma patient for any reason predisposes to the development of hypercalcemia. For this reason, activity is to be en-couraged to maintain the normal stress on the skeletal system.

Bone Marrow Effects

The effect upon the bone marrow is, in part, related to the replace-ment of normal marrow elements with malignant plasma cells (Fig. 21–4). Some depression of normal cellular development occurs in instances in which extensive replacement is not evident, however, and less direct mechanisms of bone marrow suppression have to be postulated.

Anemia of some degree is remarkably common in multiple mye-loma. In the early stages of the disease, the anemia may be slight. With progression of the disease, reduction of hematocrit to the 20 to 30 range is common. The anemia is usually normochromic and normocy-tic, but many instances of macrocytic anemia have been described.

Leukopenia and thrombocytopenia are less constant features. The anemia is the result of many factors, including infection, renal failure, blood loss, decrease in production due to bone marrow replacement by plasma cells, and a reduced red cell life span.

Bone marrow aspiration performed for the evaluation of anemia is sometimes the first clue to the presence of myeloma. Whereas normal bone marrow contains approximately 1 per cent plasma cells, myeloma is evidenced by increased numbers of plasma cells, often in clusters or sheets. In addition, myeloma cells appear to mature in an abnormal fashion; nuclear maturation lags behind that of the cytoplasm. For instance, when the cytoplasm has reached the developmental stage of synthesizing and secreting immunoglobulin, the nucleus may still be very primitive and retain its ability to divide (Fig. 21–5).

Occasionally, plasma cells are found in the circulating blood. In a form of plasmacytic proliferation called plasma cell leukemia, the number of plasma cells in the peripheral blood may reach 100,000 per mm^3.

Kidney Involvement

Renal failure is a common cause of death in multiple myeloma. This is often associated with marked Bence Jones proteinuria. The kidney appears to have a dual relationship with Bence Jones protein. Free light chains are normally catabolized by the kidney, probably after a process of glomerular filtration and reabsorption. Impaired renal function interferes with the ability of the kidney to catabolize free light chains, and therefore the serum and urinary concentrations of Bence Jones protein increase. In turn, the large amounts of Bence Jones protein appear to have deleterious effects on the kidney: proteinaceous casts may form, urine flow through the kidney may be impeded, and abnormalities of renal function, such as renal tubular acidosis, may occur.

Other ways in which the kidney may suffer in multiple myeloma are through plasma cell infiltration of the renal parenchyma, through associated amyloidosis of the kidney (which may produce a nephrotic syndrome picture), and through hypercalcemia and hyperuricemia. It is not surprising, therefore, that the diagnosis of multiple myeloma is frequently established through the investigation of unexplained proteinuria or azotemia in a patient.

Because a number of myeloma patients (mostly with Bence Jones proteinuria) have developed acute renal failure following intravenous pyelography, much caution must be exercised when using this procedure in patients with obscure renal failure. The dehydration that usually accompanies the procedure is surely responsible in part for the problem. Interaction between the x-ray contrast dye and light chains has been implicated in the production of intratubular deposits.

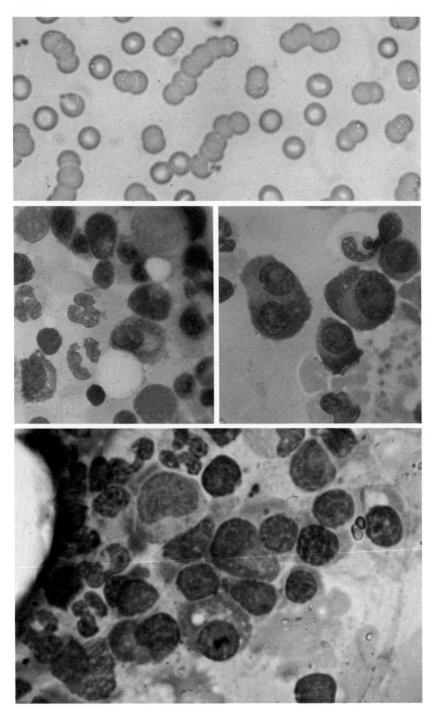

Figure 21–4. Photomicrographs of morphologic abnormalities in patients with monoclonal gammopathies. *Top,* Peripheral blood smear showing rouleaux (side to side stacking of red blood cells) and diffuse staining of the background, indicating high protein content. Smear is from a patient with IgA myeloma. *Middle,* Comparison of marrow from a patient with reactive plasmacytosis (left) and one with myeloma (right).

Legend continued on the following page

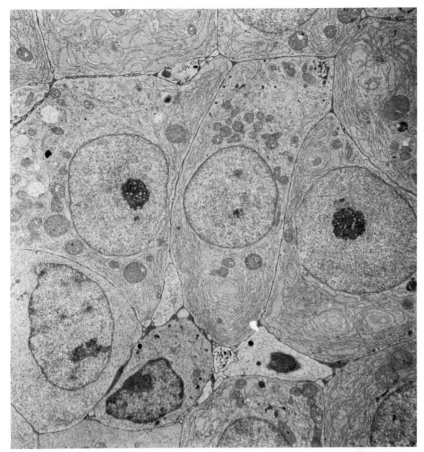

Figure 21-5. Electron micrograph of bone marrow plasma cells from a patient with advanced multiple myeloma. Shown are a cluster of asynchronous plasma cells showing primitive nuclei (little or no chromatin condensation) and very mature cytoplasms featuring well-developed endoplasmic reticulum (× 5000). (Courtesy of Dr. Richard C. Graham, Jr.)

Nervous System

The brain, spinal cord, and peripheral nerves may all be affected in myeloma. It is easiest to demonstrate a causal relationship when the spinal cord is involved. Plasmacytomas, or masses of extramedullary plasma cells, may surround the cord, constrict the blood supply to it, and thus produce the signs and symptoms of transection.

Figure 21-4 *Continued.* The reactive cells have condensed nuclear chromatin and mature cytoplasms, markers of developed cells. The myeloma cells show large, primitive nuclei in the presence of well-developed cytoplasms (nuclear-cytoplasmic asynchrony). *Bottom,* Bone marrow from patient with macroglobulinemia showing cells of the lymphocytic-plasmacytic type.

Unexplained peripheral neuropathies also occur in multiple myeloma and have been variously attributed to protein deposits in the peripheral neural sheaths and to small vessel occlusions. Amyloidosis may cause compression of the median nerve as it passes beneath the tenaculum at the wrist, resulting in a "carpal tunnel syndrome."

Central nervous system symptoms of lethargy, stupor, and coma may be brought on by extreme blood viscosity due to the massive amounts of protein in the serum, by hypercalcemia, or by advanced renal failure.

For all the varied manifestations of the disease, the most common presenting complaint is low back pain. The most common finding of routine laboratory tests is anemia. Since these symptoms are common to many diseases, a high degree of suspicion is necessary in establishing the diagnosis.

Proteins in Multiple Myeloma

M-Components.   A virtual hallmark of multiple myeloma is the monoclonal immunoglobulin, which is present in more than 99 per cent of myeloma patients (Fig. 21–6). This M-component abnormality may be either a serum myeloma globulin (IgG, IgA, IgD, or IgE), a Bence Jones protein (free κ chains or free λ chains), or both. The frequency of these manifestations in several large series of myeloma patients is indicated in Table 21–2. The most common finding is a serum myeloma globulin by itself. Bence Jones protein with a serum myeloma globulin and Bence Jones protein alone are less common. In somewhat less than 1 per cent of myeloma patients, a monoclonal gammopathy cannot be demonstrated, even though the rest of the clinical

Transferrin

γ globulin | Albumin

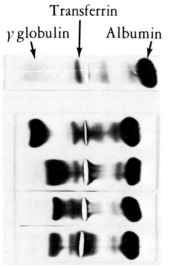

Normal

IgG myeloma

IgA myeloma

Macro-
globulinemia

IgD myeloma

Figure 21–6.   Agar gel electrophoresis of human sera. At the top is a normal serum with the albumin, transferrin, and gamma globulin fractions indicated. The four sera below are from patients with monoclonal gammopathy, and the type of monoclonal immunoglobulin is indicated at the right.

TABLE 21-2. Frequency of Various M-Components in Multiple Myeloma

FINDING	PER CENT OCCURRENCE
Serum myeloma globulin alone	48
Serum myeloma globulin plus Bence Jones protein	31
Bence Jones protein alone	20.5
No monoclonal immunoglobulin	0.5

picture is entirely consistent with multiple myeloma. In many cases, the cells synthesize an immunoglobulin but fail to secrete it. In other cases, neither extracellular nor intracellular immunoglobulin can be detected by the highly sensitive techniques used, and one must conclude that the cells are making "blanks." Great care must be taken to test for the presence of very small amounts of Bence Jones protein by concentration and electrophoresis of the urine. Methods of detection are described later.

Bence Jones Proteins. Bence Jones proteins, which are homogeneous free light chains, were first recognized 130 years ago and have provided a valuable tool in the diagnosis of multiple myeloma. These urinary proteins have peculiar heat precipitability properties. When the urine is heated at pH 5, most Bence Jones proteins will precipitate at temperatures in the range of 48° to 56° C, and will redissolve on boiling. When the urine is allowed to cool, the proteins reprecipitate.

Immunologic and electrophoretic techniques can be employed in the detection of Bence Jones protein and, at present, provide the definitive test for this entity. An electrophoretically homogeneous urinary protein that reacts with antiserum to κ chains or λ chains and does not react with antiserum to the heavy chain of any immunoglobulin is, by modern criteria, a Bence Jones protein.

Approximately 50 per cent of myeloma patients are found to have detectable Bence Jones proteinuria if the added precaution of concentrating the urine is taken. Under some conditions, particularly in the presence of renal failure, Bence Jones proteins may be found in the serum.

Immunoglobulin Deficiency in Multiple Myeloma

Quite commonly in multiple myeloma, the concentration of normal immunoglobulins is sharply reduced, and a functional hypogammaglobulinemia may be present. This can be seen when quantitative measures of serum immunoglobulins are made. Frequently, the concentrations of IgA and IgM globulins are subnormal when a IgG myeloma globulin is present, and IgG and IgM globulin levels are often low when IgA myeloma globulin is present. For practical purposes, if one could remove the monoclonal immunoglobulin from the electrophoretic pattern, a deficiency of its class would be present as well.

This phenomenon of paucity in the midst of plenty is a major contributor to defective antibody formation and repeated bacterial infections. At least two mechanisms for the decreased serum levels of immunoglobulin exist — a decrease in the number of normal immunoglobulin-producing cells and accelerated catabolism of normal antibodies. Decreased numbers of normal plasma cells may reflect an inhibitor substance (*chalone*) released by the myeloma cells or an increased number of suppressor cells (T-lymphocytes or monocytes). Hypercatabolism of nonmyelomatous IgG occurs in patients with large amounts of monoclonal IgG of the IgG1, IgG2, or IgG4 subclass. Whatever the mechanism, the patient with antibody deficiency is uniquely susceptible to repeated pneumonias, particularly of the pneumococcal type.

Frequency Distributions of Myeloma Globulins

As previously indicated, a myeloma globulin may be of either light-chain type or the IgG, IgA, IgD, or IgE globulin class. The IgM class by definition is associated with macroglobulinemia, but on rare occasion, patients with classic multiple myeloma have been found to have an IgM paraprotein. A close parallel exists between the serum concentration of an immunoglobulin class or type in normal individuals and the frequency of that class or type in a population of myeloma globulins. Of the many thousands of myeloma globulins that have been classified, IgG and IgA myeloma are the most common. IgD myeloma has been detected approximately 150 times, and IgE globulin only four times. The ratio of IgG to IgA myeloma globulins is approximately 3:1. A similar finding is true for light-chain type. In the normal individual, the ratio of κ chains to λ chains is 60:40, and the same distribution is observed in populations of myeloma globulins. As was indicated earlier, individual plasma cells appear to produce only a single kind of light chain. The ratio of κ-producing cells to λ-producing cells is the same ratio as is found in normal serum and in large surveys of myeloma globulins (approximately 60:40). Therefore, it seems reasonable to conclude that the cellular population at risk in the genesis of multiple myeloma is in proportion to its normal frequency distribution.

In terms of prognostic factors, it would appear that patients with "light-chain myeloma" do least well (those with λ type worse than κ type), and patients with IgA myeloma probably do poorer than those with IgG. IgD myeloma appears to occur in a younger age group than the other forms of myeloma and, curiously, is almost always of λ type and associated with excretion of Bence Jones protein.

Treatment

A number of therapeutic measures are used in the treatment of multiple myeloma. The need for ambulation, activity, braces, and other general supportive measures is stressed by many physicians in order to prevent acceleration of osteoporosis. Sodium fluoride has been used to increase the strength of bone. High fluid intake is important in forestalling renal complications and in treating hypercalcemia. Localized bone pain due to osteolytic lesions is often relieved by x-ray treatment. Testosterone has been used as an anabolic steroid and as a stimulator of erythropoiesis.

Chemotherapy. Use of the alkylating agents cyclophosphamide and phenylalanine mustard has produced subjective and objective signs of improvement in a significant percentage of myeloma patients. Improvement in some patients has been dramatic. Intermittent high doses of phenylalanine mustard combined with prednisone have had the best reported results, with as high as 60 per cent of patients so treated having a favorable response. More recently, Adriamycin and the nitrosoureas have been used with some success in treating patients who are refractory to alkylating agents. Major toxic side-effects of cyclophosphamide have been bone marrow depression, alopecia, and hemorrhagic cystitis. Phenylalanine mustard has bone marrow suppression, notably thrombocytopenia, as its major toxic effect. A significant number of myeloma patients treated for prolonged periods (years) with alkylating agents have developed acute granulocytic leukemia. Whether this is drug-induced or the "natural history" of myeloma remains conjectural.

MACROGLOBULINEMIA

In 1944, on the basis of ultracentrifugation studies, Waldenström identified a group of hyperglobulinemic patients as having excessive amounts of high molecular weight protein in their serum. The clinical picture could be distinguished from more classic multiple myeloma in symptomatology and pathologic findings. The protein was called "macroglobulin," and the condition has been known as "Waldenström's macroglobulinemia." The clinical disturbance seen in this disorder is in part a result of the abnormal cellular proliferation and in part a result of the abnormal protein produced by the cells.

Abnormality and Symptomatology

The abnormal protein in this condition is an electrophoretically homogeneous IgM globulin that is of high molecular weight (approximately 900,000) and has the chemical and immunochemical characteristics of the IgM globulin class. Because of the high intrinsic viscosity of the IgM globulin, large amounts of this protein may result in a marked increase in the viscosity of the patient's serum that in turn can lead to sluggish blood flow, thromboses, central nervous system disturbances, and bleeding. The most common bleeding sites are the skin, nasal mucosa, and gastrointestinal tract. Sluggish blood flow in the retinal vessels is particularly striking, with segmental disturbances in blood flow ("sausage linking"), and may eventuate in retinal vein thrombosis and blindness. Coating of the red blood cells, the polymorphonuclear leukocytes, and particularly the platelets may result in impaired survival or function of these elements. Frequently, the hyperproduction of IgM globulin is accompanied by a decreased production of the other immunoglobulins. This functional hypogammaglobulinemia, in concert with the impaired white cell function and granulocytopenia, leads to repeated severe bacterial infections. Approximately one in 10 macroglobulinemia patients has demonstrable Bence Jones proteinuria, and this may have adverse effects on the kidney, as described in the preceding section.

In addition to protein, the cells engaged in the synthesis of the macroglobulin produce abnormalities (Fig. 21–4). Proliferation of the lymphoid tissue in lymph nodes, liver, and spleen is often excessive and can result in enlargement of these organs, which is detectable clinically. On occasion, marked lymphocytosis may be present, and the condition may be indistinguishable from chronic lymphocytic leukemia. Total replacement of the bone marrow may occur. An increased number of tissue mast cells are often found in the bone marrow, but their significance is not known.

Many patients with macroglobulinemia produce detectable amounts of low molecular weight macroglobulin (7S IgM). This monomer IgM contains two heavy chains and two light chains that are not linked to form the usual pentamer of IgM globulin (see Chapter 5), and does not possess the viscosity properties of the pentamer.

If the monoclonal IgM has antibody activity, it may produce further symptoms by virtue of this property. Many cases are known in which monoclonal IgM protein is produced with an antibody specificity directed against the I antigen of the red blood cell. This results in a chronic hemolytic anemia and is often called "high-titer cold agglutinin syndrome." Another antibody activity that has been found for IgM globulins is that against IgG globulin, in which circulating antigen-antibody complexes occur and arthritis and glomerular lesions ensue. Such macroglobulins usually are cryoglobulins as well, and produce problems of local blood flow.

Treatment

The management of macroglobulinemia involves treatment of the cellular proliferation and treatment of the effects produced by the protein. Alkylating agents, particularly chlorambucil, have been useful in keeping the mass of lymphocytes reduced and the level of macroglobulin low. In the patient population we have treated, intermittent high-dose phenylalanine mustard and prednisone treatment for approximately one year has led to a substantial number of long-term stable remissions. In the acute treatment of the hyperviscosity syndrome, however, more immediate measures are necessary to remove the protein. In such instances, plasmapheresis (removal of whole blood with reinfusion of cells) may be life-saving.

HEAVY-CHAIN DISEASE

In 1965, a different kind of proliferative disorder of immunoglobulins was described by Franklin. The cardinal feature of this disorder was the elaboration of a monoclonal protein of relatively low molecular weight that was present in both serum and urine. By immunologic analysis, it was seen that the protein possessed the antigenic determinants of IgG globulin but lacked light-chain antigenic determinants. Chemical analysis (amino acid composition, peptide mapping, carbohydrate content) indicated that the protein was very similar to the Fc fragment of IgG that is produced by partial hydrolysis with papain (Chapter 5), and the disorder was termed "heavy-chain disease." Amino acid sequence analysis of heavy-chain disease proteins demonstrated that the sequence of the heavy chains began with a normal amino terminal sequence, followed by an extensive deletion of most of the Fd fragment, and resumption of the normal sequence at position 216 in the hinge region. The extent of the deletion has varied, but the place where the normal sequence is resumed appears rather constant.

The size of this protein (approximately 55,000 daltons) is somewhat greater than that of Bence Jones protein and accounts for the fact that appreciable concentrations of the protein have often been found in both serum and urine of affected patients. Since the same protein occurs in serum and in urine, the presence of a homogeneous protein of beta-globulin mobility in these body fluids should alert the clinician to the possibility of heavy-chain disease. The diagnosis of gamma heavy-chain disease generally rests upon the demonstration of a protein with the antigenic characteristics of IgG and no light-chain component.

To date, approximately 20 cases of this disorder have been recognized, and the common features (in addition to the protein elaborated) have been repeated bacterial infections, enlargement of the lymphoid organs, anemia, eosinophilia, and edema of the palate, secondary to involvement of Waldeyer's ring, the lymphoid tissue of the pharynx. A varied pathologic picture has been present, with histologic features of lymphoma, ranging from Hodgkin's disease to reticulum cell sarcoma. Bone marrow examination has shown mixtures of lymphocytes and plasma cells.

The most frequent cause of death has been infection, a direct consequence of the profound impairment of antibody production that appears to be an integral part of the disorder.

Heavy-chain disease of the IgA system has quite predictably involved the gastrointestinal tract and the respiratory tree. Most of the cases of alpha-chain disease have occurred in association with intestinal lymphoma in patients living in the Mediterranean area. Cases outside that area have been recorded and at least two instances of alpha heavy-chain disease have occurred in persons with lymphoma of the respiratory tract. The abnormal protein in alpha chain disease has not been characterized as extensively as the gamma heavy-chain disease proteins, but in general the protein is not detected in the urine. It has a tendency to polymerize and has a rapid and polydisperse electrophoretic mobility, usually in the alpha$_2$ globulin region.

IgM heavy-chain disease is quite rare, and has occurred in patients with chronic lymphocytic leukemia. Unlike the other heavy-chain diseases, free light chain has been produced as well as the heavy chain, and indeed both chains arise in the same cell — plasma cells with large vacuoles. Obviously, there is a failure of heavy and light chain link-up, and a defect in the hinge region has been postulated.

Although IgD and IgE heavy-chain diseases should be expected to occur, to date no cases have been observed. This is in keeping with the relative rarity of myelomas of these classes.

A few instances of other "defective" molecules have been observed in the malignant immunoproliferative disorders. Half molecules (one heavy, one light chain) of IgG and IgA have been described, and in at least one case of "Ig$\frac{A}{2}$," a deletion of the carboxyl-terminal domain has been observed. Similar deletions of the carboxyl-terminal domain have occurred in the IgM class.

As more unusual monoclonal proteins have been scrutinized, more and more "defective" molecules have been identified. Whether these molecules have "normal" counterparts has not been clearly established.

CRYOGLOBULINEMIA

A striking property of some monoclonal immunoglobulins is a markedly reduced solubility at temperatures lower than body temperature. When the insolubility is of such a degree that aggregation or precipitation may take place within the vascular space, severe impairment of normal physiologic processes may result. The term cryoglobulin is applied to those immunoglobulins that are very insoluble in the cold. The clinical condition that results from their presence is termed cryoglobulinemia.

The symptomatology of cryoglobulinemia is directly related to the abnormal protein. Blood with high concentrations of cryoglobulin will encounter severe restrictions in flow through those portions of the

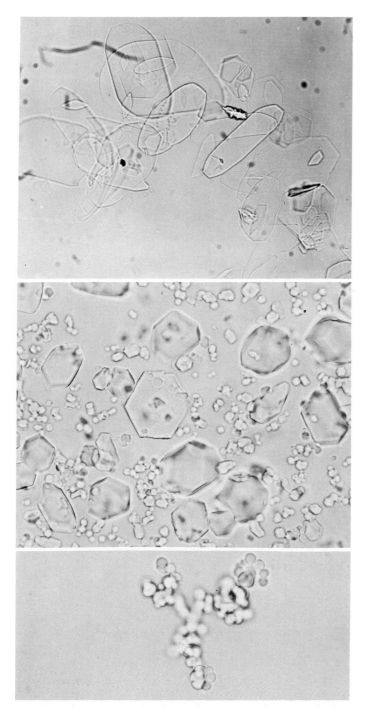

Figure 21–7. Photomicrographs of crystalline cryoglobulins (magnified ×250) from three patients with cryoglobulinemia. In each case, the protein is an IgG globulin with κ-type light chains. The protein at the bottom forms amorphous crystals, whereas the other two specimens have more definite structure.

skin where exposure to cold is high. The regions chiefly affected are the digits, shins, nose, and ears. Painful ischemia of these areas, even infarction of the tissues, may result from prolonged cold exposure; ulceration and purpura of the extremities can also occur.

At least three different mechanisms have been found to account for the protein abnormalities in cryoglobulinemia. IgM monoclonal proteins with an antibody specificity directed against IgG globulin may cause cryoprecipitation of serum. Similarly, IgG or IgA globulin molecules with such specificity may produce cryoprecipitation. A third mechanism, which is represented in Figure 21–7, is crystallization of the cryoglobulin. This has been seen to occur with a few IgG monoclonal gammopathy proteins.

PYROGLOBULINEMIA

As the name implies, pyroglobulins are proteins sensitive to heat. They are monoclonal serum immunoglobulins that are precipitated when the serum is heated to 56° C. Often the phenomenon is explained by the presence of significant amounts of Bence Jones protein in the serum. Since free light chains precipitate at temperatures of 56° C, they may confer this property to serum. However, some complete monoclonal immunoglobulins also possess this property. At the present state of our knowledge, this heat precipitability imparts no functional or pathologic significance to the protein, but is merely a laboratory curio.

AMYLOIDOSIS

One way products of the plasma cell tumor may affect the patient is seen in the disorder called primary amyloidosis. Amyloid is a proteinaceous substance that is deposited in tissues and exhibits birefringence when stained with dyes such as Congo Red. The so-called secondary form of the disease occurs in patients with chronic infectious processes such as tuberculosis and leprosy and affects chiefly liver, spleen, and kidneys. In primary amyloidosis, infiltration of organs such as skin, skeletal muscle, tongue, and heart causes severe compromise of these organs. This disorder is usually associated with the presence of monoclonal immunoglobulin (particularly free light chains). Elegant studies by Glenner and associates have shown a causal link between immunoglobulin and amyloidosis. They have demonstrated that free monoclonal immunoglobulin light chains from patients with amyloidosis can be cleaved by proteases or heat into variable and constant halves, and that the variable halves will undergo polymerization into amyloid substance. Hence, the protein by-product of plasma cell proliferation can and does cause problems by itself.

Benign Monoclonal Gammopathy

As serum protein electrophoresis has become an extremely common procedure in clinical laboratories, an increasing number of individuals have been found to have serum monoclonal immunoglobulins but none of the other stigmata of multiple myeloma. Although this condition is termed "benign monoclonal gammopathy," the true nature of the condition is not known. Some of these patients have been observed for at least 20 years without detectable change occurring in their clinical condition. In some instances, patients have died of unrelated causes, and at postmortem, no evidence of myeloma has been found in the tissues. On the other hand, occasional patients have developed classic pictures of multiple myeloma as long as 18 years after detection of the monoclonal immunoglobulin. More extensive follow-up of affected patients will be necessary before one can fully evaluate this entity, but present concepts would favor the current usage of the "benign" designation.

The Problems of Diagnosis of Myeloma

When the full spectrum of abnormalities associated with multiple myeloma is present, the diagnosis and the need for treatment are evident. A problem on both counts is presented by the patient with minimal evidence of multiple myeloma, since chemotherapy has been neither curative nor uniformly successful and has its own hazards. The difficulty can be illustrated by the three following case histories.

Case 1. A 49-year-old man presented with cough, fever, and signs of right upper lobe pneumonia. The etiologic organism was identified as pneumococcus and the patient improved after treatment with penicillin. He had a history of low back pain and generalized fatigue for the past six months. The hematocrit (28 per cent) and the white blood count (3700) were low, the blood calcium and urea nitrogen were elevated, and the serum phosphorus and alkaline phosphatase were normal. The urine showed 3+ protein, and the heat test for Bence Jones protein was positive. Total protein was 9 gm per 100 ml. Electrophoresis and immunoelectrophoresis of the serum showed a monoclonal IgG globulin to be present at a concentration of 6 gm per 100 ml. X-rays showed a right upper lobe infiltrate, collapse of the lumbar spine, and multiple osteolytic lesions of skull and long bones. Bone marrow aspirate revealed sheets of plasma cells.

Case 2. A 60-year-old woman was seen by her physician for mild low back pain. X-rays showed moderate diffuse osteoporosis but no other abnormality. The hematocrit was slightly reduced (34 per cent). Total serum protein was 7.8 gm per 100 ml and a monoclonal IgA globulin was present (concentration 1.5 gm per 100 ml). Other blood and urine studies were normal. Bone marrow aspirate showed 2 per cent plasma cells.

Case 3. An asymptomatic 52-year-old man was discovered to have a monoclonal gammopathy during the laboratory portion of a routine physical examination. The M-component was determined to be a IgG globulin (concentration 0.6 gm per 100 ml). X-rays, blood counts, blood chemistries, bone marrow examinations, and urine examinations were all within normal limits.

The first of the three patients presented with a great many symptoms and signs of multiple myeloma. He was severely ill and in need of treatment.

The third patient was asymptomatic and his disorder generally fit the criteria of benign monoclonal gammopathy. Few physicians would elect to do anything other than follow the patient.

The second case illustrates the problems associated with diagnosis and indication for therapy. A diversity of opinion would be encountered regarding whether the label "multiple myeloma" should be applied to this case at this time and whether chemotherapeutic measures should be begun. Until such time as uniformly successful therapy is available, such cases will probably remain a subject for disagreement and a problem for the physician involved in their care.

ETIOLOGY

As is the case with most forms of neoplasia, the cause of the malignant monoclonal gammopathies remains obscure, but several etiologic theories have been advanced. Separate lines of experimentation have suggested an environmental cause. In some instances, virus-like particles have been observed in myeloma cells and this has fostered a viral theory of the disease. An inbred strain of mice (Balb C) has been found to form plasmacytomas with paraprotein production in response to immunization with oil adjuvants. Such tumors are transplantable to other mice within the strain. Other species, including dogs and horses, less commonly and less constantly have been noted to develop monoclonal gammopathy. Of particular interest are monoclonal antibodies to streptococcal antigens arising in rabbits immunized with these proteins.

An ever-growing number of human monoclonal immunoglobulins have been found to possess antibody specificities against antigens ranging from such simple chemicals as dinitrophenol to such complex antigens as human lipoproteins. It is possible, therefore, that all human monoclonal immunoglobulins represent antibodies formed in response to antigenic stimulation and that the control of cellular proliferation is the major defect. Since monoclonal gammopathy is not an absolute requirement for myeloma (approximately 0.5 per cent of myeloma patients lack a monoclonal immunoglobulin), it is difficult to assign to it a central role in the pathogenesis of multiple myeloma.

CELLULAR BASIS OF DISEASE

The elegant studies of Salmon and coworkers have provided an example of how the basic information of immunology can be applied to an understanding of a human disease. They showed that very accurate estimates of tumor cell mass may be made in myeloma patients by measuring (1) the *in vitro* rate of synthesis of immunoglobulin per cultured myeloma cell; (2) the rate of catabolism of myeloma globulin *in vivo*; and (3) the total body mass of myeloma globulin. If the rate of catabolism of the myeloma protein and the rate at which cells produce myeloma globulin are known, the number of cells present in the patient may be calculated. Sequential measurements of the cell mass in myeloma patients have been used to provide objective estimates of rate of tumor growth and response to chemotherapeutic agents.

POLYCLONAL GAMMOPATHY

In contrast to the relatively few disorders characterized by homogeneous increases in immunoglobulins, many diseases of man are associated with heterogeneous increases of immunoglobulins. Such disorders are termed "polyclonal gammopathies," a term that implies that multiple cell lines are involved in the immunoglobulin increase. In most instances, increases occur in the three major classes of immunoglobulins and in both kinds of light chains. The disorders that are frequently associated with polyclonal gammopathies include inflammatory, infectious, and neoplastic diseases. Chief among these are rheumatoid arthritis, lupus erythematosus, cirrhosis of the liver, tuberculosis, leishmaniasis, some lymphomas, and metastatic carcinoma. A recently recognized pseudoneoplastic process, immunoblastic lymphadenopathy, is also associated with striking polyclonal increase in immunoglobulins. Although it is possible to demonstrate increases in the immunoglobulins in such diseases, it is impossible to identify an antibody role for a major percentage of the increase. For instance, many antibodies directed against normal tissue or serum antigens are found in lupus erythematosus, but these antibodies constitute only a small percentage of the immunoglobulin increase. In at least one instance (the original case of heavy-chain disease), transition from a polyclonal gammopathy to a monoclonal gammopathy has been observed.

LYMPHOPROLIFERATIVE DISEASES WITH INCONSTANT IMMUNOGLOBULIN ABERRATION

Increases in the mass of lymphocytes owing to abnormal proliferation occur in Hodgkin's and non-Hodgkin's lymphomas, acute and chronic lymphocytic leukemias, and several other neoplastic disorders. Profound impairment of the immune response may occur in these disorders. In non-Hodgkin's lymphoma and chronic lymphocytic leukemia, the proliferating cell is of the B-cell line. A marked accumulation of nonfunctional B-cells occurs and very often the normal B-cell populations are decreased in number, with concomitant hypogammaglobulinemia. In a large percentage of such B-lymphocyte neoplasms, monoclonal immunoglobulin is detected on the surface of the disordered lymphocytes. In a small percentage of patients, monoclonal immunoglobulin is also detectable in serum or urine. In many ways, it is convenient to think of these B-cell neoplasms as affecting the immediate precursor to the plasma cell line with a maturation block that prevents normal plasma cell formation and humoral immune function.

On the other hand, T-cell neoplasms include Sézary syndrome (Fig. 21–8), mycosis fungoides (lymphoproliferative disorders with significant involvement of skin), and at least some instances of acute childhood leukemia. Hodgkin's lymphoma behaves very much like a T-cell neoplasm, and the major functional deficit is in cellular immunity.

The most striking functional evidence of the immunologic difference between these diseases is seen in the kinds of infection that beset the patients. The patients with hypogammaglobulinemia associated with chronic lymphatic leukemia or non-Hodgkin's lymphoma have frequent bacterial pneumonias. Infections with fungi (Monilia,

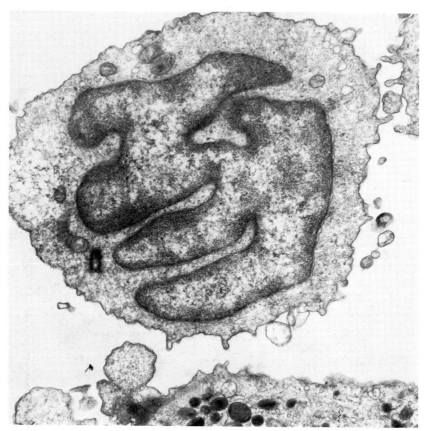

Figure 21–8. Electron micrograph of a lymphocyte from a patient with Sézary syndrome (× 14,000). (Courtesy of Dr. Richard C. Graham, Jr.)

Cryptococcus, Aspergillus) and unusual agents (*Pneumocystis carinii*) are seen more commonly in Hodgkin's disease and the skin-linked T-cell proliferative diseases. The association of Hodgkin's disease with defects in delayed hypersensitivity and of lymphocytic lymphoma or leukemia with defects in humoral immunity is by no means exclusive. In any individual patient, either one or both kinds of abnormality may occur. In advanced stages of all lymphocytic malignant disorders, functional impairment of both B- and T-cell populations occurs, and patients are susceptible to all forms of infection.

SUGGESTIONS FOR FURTHER READING

Graham, R. C., Jr., and Bernier, G. M.: The bone marrow in multiple myeloma: Correlation of plasma cell ultrastructure and clinical state. Medicine, 54:225–243, 1975.

Frangione, B., and Franklin, E. C.: Heavy-chain diseases: Clinical features and molecular significance of the disordered immunoglobulin structure. Semin. Hematol., 10:53–64, 1973.

Levin, W. C. (ed.): Symposium on myeloma. Arch. Intern. Med., 135:27–196, 1975. (*A collection of papers dealing with virtually every aspect of the myeloma problem.*)

Salmon, S. E.: Immunoglobulin synthesis and tumor kinetics of multiple myeloma. Semin. Hematol., 10:135–148, 1973.

IMMUNE DEFICIENCY DISEASES

Robert J. Schlegel, M.D.,
and Charles H. Kirkpatrick, M.D.

Immune deficiency disorders reflect an impairment in one or more of the major mechanisms of immunity, including (1) the defensive perimeter of the body (the skin or mucosal lining of the gastrointestinal or respiratory tracts); (2) phagocytosis and bactericidal activity; (3) the inflammatory response, including complement and other aspects of the biologic amplification system; (4) antibody responses; and (5) cell-mediated (delayed hypersensitivity) responses. Whereas the major congenital or inherited varieties are rare, the acquired disorders, secondary to other diseases or therapy, are not uncommon.

The study of such aberrant immunologic responses has unveiled important information concerning the function of normal immune processes. Just as the elucidation of immunoglobulin structure became possible only after multiple myeloma was described, other mechanisms of developmental immunobiology have been recognized from the study of immune deficiency disorders (Chapter 3).

The discovery of immune deficiency states is often made by clinical observations at the bedside or in the clinic. Every physician, therefore, should be alert to such possibilities when a patient presents with signs and symptoms suggesting defects in one of the major functions of the immune system—protection against infection (defense), preservation of uniformity of a given cell type (homeostasis), and the removal of malignant cells (surveillance) (Chapter 2).

CLINICAL SETTING

The concept of immune deficiency disorders was first introduced in 1952, when Colonel Ogden Bruton made the startling discovery that a child who presented with repeated bacterial infections had no detectable gamma globulin in his serum. Since then, defects in other humoral and cellular components of the immune system have been identified (Table 22–1). Although the cardinal feature in many has been a propensity to repeated infections, more recently other abnormalities in homeostasis and surveillance have signaled the underlying state of immune

644

TABLE 22–1. Lymphocyte Defects and Genetic Aspects of Selected Primary Immunodeficiency Syndromes

| | Affected Lymphocyte Populations | | | | |
| | T-Cells | | B-Cells | | Mode of |
Disorder	Stage 1*	Stage 2*	Stage 1	Stage 2	Inheritance
Disorders apparently affecting stem cells					
Reticular dysgenesis	yes	yes	yes	yes	unknown
SCID† (thymic alymphoplasia)	yes	yes	(yes)‡	(yes)	X-linked
SCID (Swiss type)	yes	yes	(yes)	(yes)	autosomal recessive
SCID with ADA deficiency	yes	yes	(yes)	(yes)	autosomal recessive
SCID with ectodermal dysplasia and dwarfism	yes	yes	yes	yes	? autosomal recessive
SCID (sporadic)	yes	yes	yes	yes	unknown
Disorders mainly affecting B-cells					
Congenital hypogammaglobulinemia (Bruton type)	no	no	yes	yes§	X-linked
Congenital hypogammaglobulinemia	no	no	yes	yes	autosomal recessive
Common variable immunodeficiency	no	(no)	no	yes§	? autosomal recessive
IgA deficiency	no	(no)	no	no§	variable
IgM deficiency	no	no	no	?	unknown
IgG subclass deficiency	no	no	no	?	X-linked
Immunodeficiency with elevated IgM	no	no	no	(yes)	X-linked
X-linked immunodeficiency with normal globulin count or hyperglobulinemia	no	no	(no)	(yes)	X-linked
Hypogammaglobulinemia with thymoma	no	no	no	yes§	unknown
Disorders mainly affecting T-cells					
Thymus hypoplasia (Nezelof's syndrome)	yes	yes	(no)	(no)	variable
DiGeorge's syndrome	yes	yes	no	no	variable
Nucleoside phosphorylase deficiency	yes	yes	no	no	? autosomal recessive
Chronic mucocutaneous candidiasis with endocrinopathy	no	yes	no	no	? autosomal recessive
Complex immunodeficiencies					
Wiskott-Aldrich syndrome	yes	yes	no	(yes)	X-linked
Ataxia-telangiectasia	(yes)	yes	no	(no)	autosomal recessive
Hyper-IgE syndrome	no	yes	no	no	unknown
Cartilage-hair hypoplasia	?	yes	no	(no)	autosomal recessive

*Indicates first or second stages of lymphoid cell differentiation (see text)
†SCID = severe combined immunodeficiency
‡Statements enclosed in parentheses indicate defects that are variable in severity or expression
§Recent evidence indicates the presence of excessive suppressor cell activity (see text)

deficiency. It is now clear that many of these disorders are associated with direct or familial predispositions to autoimmunity and neoplasia.

Today, as in Bruton's day, the clinician identifies patients to be studied for immune deficiency by first separating cases that are due to "parasite-related" causes from those in which there is an intrinsic "host-related" deficit. Some children in underprivileged communities (e.g., Indian reservations) or in other group settings (e.g., day nurseries) are exposed to an unusual number of pathogens. Only after examining the life setting of the patient does it become important

TABLE 22–2. Secondary Host-Related Defects of Immunity

Type	Examples
Integumental disorders	Burns
Malnutrition	Kwashiorkor
Neoplasia	Leukemia
Congenital defects	Congenital heart disease
Congenital infections	Rubella
Metabolic derangements	Diabetes mellitus

to consider either primary immune deficiency or secondary immune deficiency. Instances of secondary immune deficiency include burns, eczema and other cutaneous disorders, congenital defects of the heart and vessels with pulmonary edema, diabetes, and a variety of other metabolic disorders and are far more common than primary immunologic deficiencies (Table 22–2).

Once parasite-related and other host-related defects have been excluded, the clinician turns to the primary immune deficiency disorders (Table 22–1). Even here, however, another set of considerations comes into play. In all individuals, there is a variable rate of maturation of the specific mediators of immune responses. In some, there occurs a physiologic delay in development of one or more of the cells or molecules of immunity. This imposes the need to view immune responsiveness against a developmental backdrop and to consider states of pathologic but transitory delay in the development of immune competence.

DEVELOPMENTAL BACKGROUND

Because many of the congenital immunodeficiency syndromes result from abnormalities in lymphoid cell maturation, a brief résumé of the development of this immune system is in order. In postnatal life, the bone marrow provides stem cells that migrate and differentiate into three types of immunologically significant cells: (1) those of the phagocytic system, (2) those of the thymic-dependent lymphoid tissues, and (3) those of the thymic-independent lymphoid tissues (Fig. 22–1). The cells of the lymphoid series populate peripheral tissues and carry out humoral and cell-mediated processes.

The humoral and cell-mediated compartmentalization is illustrated by the architecture of lymph nodes in which cortex and medulla have been shown to possess separate and discrete functions (Fig. 22–2) (Chapter 2). The peripheral cortical regions contain germinal centers and, together with the medullary cords, are responsible for antibody synthesis. These regions are referred to as thymic-independent regions. Interposed between these two areas is the deep cortical or paracortical region, the thymic-dependent region that controls cell-mediated immunologic events. Although these compartments appear to be anatomically distinct, there are important interactions between B-lymphocytes of the thymus-independent regions and subsets of T-lymphocytes in the thymus-dependent regions that are essential for optimal immune responses. In newly hatched chickens, if the organ responsible for differentiation of the cells that populate either of these regions is extirpated and the bird is irradiated to eradicate previously differentiated cells, the result is profound immunologic deficiency. For example, the bursa of Fabricius provides the environment for differentiation of precursors of antibody-forming B-cells (Fig. 22–1). Removal of the bursa produces deficient antibody production. If the thymus is removed, profound deficiencies in cell-mediated immunity occur. If both differentiative organs are removed, deficiencies in both immune mechanisms result. Many immunologic deficiency states of man may be viewed as human counterparts of these experimentally induced deficiencies.

The maturation of cell-mediated immunity and phagocytosis are currently subjects of intensive investigation. More is known of the developmental aspects of antibody-mediated functions. Normally, the

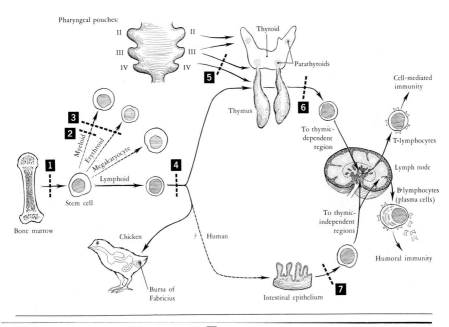

1 RETICULAR DYSGENESIS

2 CGD

3 FANCONI'S SYNDROME

4 SEVERE COMBINED IMMUNODEFICIENCY

5 THYMIC APLASIA (DiGeorge) (III-IV)

6 THYMIC DYSPLASIA (normal gg)

7 AGAMMAGLOBULINEMIA

Figure 22–1. Schematic representation of points in immunologic development at which blocks leading to immune deficiency might occur.

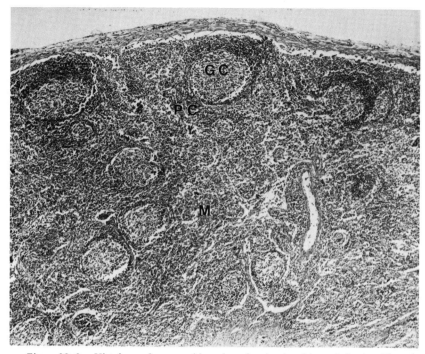

Figure 22–2. Histology of a normal lymph node stimulated by an infection. Note the germinal centers (GC) in the cortex and the medullary (M) cords, regions that contain B-cells; the paracortical (PC) region, interposed between these regions, contains T-cells. Hematoxylin and eosin stain, × 120.

fetus does not synthesize antibodies unless exposed to antigenic stimuli. Those cells that are capable of synthesizing immunoglobulins, however, differentiate during the first trimester (Chapter 2). The first cells that appear produce IgM; cells capable of producing other immunoglobulins develop later, probably from the IgM-producing cells. These differentiative events occur in the absence of antigenic stimulation and are referred to as Stage 1 in Table 22–1. Later, these Ig-bearing B-cells mature into antigen-responsive cells that differentiate into plasma cells and antibody-secreting lymphoid cells. Differentiation and replication of these cells is driven by antigenic stimulation and is designated Stage 2 (Table 22–1).

A major source of protection for the newborn is the maternal IgG antibody that is passively transferred across the placenta. At three months of age, the normal infant manifests a temporary hypogammaglobulinemia referred to as "physiologic" hypogammaglobulinemia. In some infants, this condition is prolonged until the age of 18 to 21 months, a state referred to as transient hypogammaglobulinemia. Usually, though, by the age of three months, independent synthesis of immunoglobulins is initiated, and serum levels gradually increase, reaching adult levels during adolescence (Chapter 2, Fig. 2–25).

Cellular immunity also develops during embryonic life. By the seventh to twelfth week of gestation, the fetus possesses cells that can recognize and respond to alloantigens. By the end of the first trimester, fetal lymphoid organs contain E-rosette-forming T-lymphocytes that are responsive to polyclonal mitogens such as phytohemagglutinin and concanavalin-A. Differentiation of these responses is antigen-independent (analogous to differentiation of Ig-bearing B-cells) and is referred to as Stage 1 in Table 22–1. Maturation of the ability to respond to specific antigens occurs later in fetal life, but there is comparatively little information on the appearance of specific antigen-responsive T-cells in man. These responses are antigen-dependent, just as with the B-cell system (Stage 2, Table 22–1) (Chapter 2).

From a practical standpoint, the immunologic deficiency syndromes may be divided into those that primarily affect (1) B-cells (e.g., hypogammaglobulinemias), (2) T-cells (e.g., DiGeorge syndrome), or (3) combinations of both thymic-dependent and thymic-independent tissues (e.g., combined immunodeficiency).

PRIMARY DISORDERS OF THE B-CELL (ANTIBODY-SYNTHESIZING) SYSTEM

Although diseases have been described in which there is disjunction between the cells (B-cells) and molecules (immunoglobulins) that mediate antibody responses on the one hand and the effective function of those cells and molecules in response to antigens on the other, most of the antibody deficiency states are associated with demonstrable abnormalities of the B-cells or secretion of immunoglobulins, or both. The rare exceptions can be identified by studying specific antibody responses following immunization of the patient who has normal serum immunoglobulin levels but clinical evidence of immunodeficiency. Typhoid vaccine, tetanus toxoid, keyhole-limpet hemocyanin, and blood group substances may be used for this purpose. Wedgwood and his associates have used ΦX-174, a bacteriophage that is not infectious for humans, to study immune responses and have found defects in primary and secondary antibody responses and defects in the rate of clearance of phage from the circulation that suggest impairment of reticuloendothelial function.

Caution is important, however. The immunization of immunologically deficient individuals, particularly with live vaccines, is potentially hazardous. It should also be noted that whole blood transfusions may be unsafe in certain types of immune deficiency because of the possibility of graft-versus-host reactions.

THE PRIMARY HYPOGAMMAGLOBULINEMIAS

Congenital Hypogammaglobulinemia

Hypogammaglobulinemia was the first recognized immunodeficiency disease. The clinical history of the remarkable child discovered by Bruton (Fig. 22–3) before initiation of replacement therapy is typical of the infectious illnesses of these patients. It is now recognized that the disorder is of several genetic types, including an X-linked recessive type (the Bruton type), an autosomal recessive type, and a sporadic type.

Clinical Features. Typically, infants with this disorder do well during the first few months of life. The maternally acquired IgG provides adequate protection during this time. After the maternal immunoglobulin is catabolized, the child begins to experience repeated

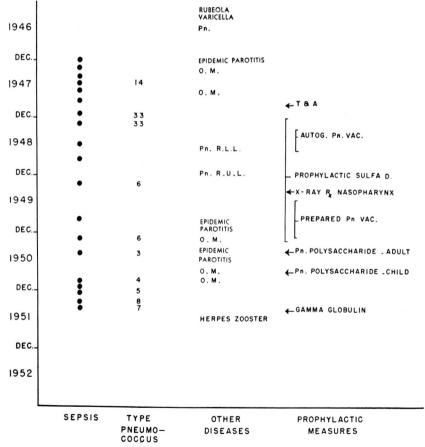

Figure 22–3. Chart published by Bruton showing his original observations of infection due to the same type of pneumococcus in his case of agammaglobulinemia. (From Bruton, O. C.: Agammaglobulinemia. Pediatrics, *9*:722, 1952.)

infections. In exceptional cases, predisposition to infection may not occur until the child is five or six years of age.

An important clinical clue in the recognition of the hypogammaglobulinemias is the unique susceptibility to an extremely narrow range of bacterial agents. These include the encapsulated pyogenic organisms, *Micrococcus pyogenes, Diplococcus pneumoniae, Haemophilus influenzae,* and *Streptococcus pyogenes.* This phenomenon probably traces its origin to the ability of polymorphonuclear leukocytes to ingest and digest successfully the nonencapsulated organisms without participation of the opsonins that are lacking in these patients. In contrast, with the possible exception of infectious hepatitis, these patients show no impairment in recovery from viral infections such as rubeola, rubella, mumps, or varicella, and they are not unusually susceptible to chronic superficial fungal infections. They do, however, have a predisposition for "autoimmune" diseases such as dermatomyositis and rheumatoid-like arthritis and for a spruelike malabsorption syndrome.

Diagnosis. The diagnosis is suggested by immunoelectrophoresis that shows that the patient's serum is deficient in one or more of the major immunoglobulin classes (Fig. 22–4) and is confirmed by quantitative radial immunodiffusion or a similar test. In most instances, the patients have IgG levels of less than 200 mg per deciliter and undetectable IgM, IgA, IgE, and IgD. The serum contains no isohemagglutinin activity. These patients produce essentially no antibody in response to antigenic stimulation. In the first year of life, the major diagnostic consideration is transient hypogammaglobulinemia, and it may be necessary to study a patient over several months to determine with certainty his capacity to synthesize immunoglobulins.

Immunology. Most, but not all, patients with congenital hypogammaglobulinemia lack immunoglobulin-bearing B-lymphocytes, and their lymphoid tissues do not contain plasma cells. From the maturational scheme presented in Figure 22–1, it appears that they lack the

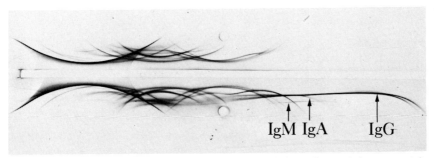

Figure 22–4. Immunoelectrophoresis of serum (*A*). *Top,* Congenital agammaglobulinemia. Note complete absence of IgM, IgA and IgG bands. *Bottom,* Normal serum showing normal amounts of IgM, IgA and IgG. (Courtesy of Dr. Fred S. Rosen.)

mammalian equivalent of the bursa of Fabricius, the organ responsible for B-cell maturation in the chicken. It should be emphasized that there are still many unanswered questions concerning maturation and function of B-lymphocytes, and current models should be regarded as tentative.

Treatment. Intramuscular injections of 0.025 gm (0.15 ml) of commercial globulin (immune serum globulin) per kilogram are given once every three to four weeks (Chapter 24). In some patients this dosage is inadequate, but larger volumes of injected material cannot be tolerated. In these cases, transfusions of plasma from compatible donors have been used successfully. The usual dosage is 10 ml of plasma per kilogram every three to four weeks. Infusion of this dosage of plasma into a 50-kg patient would provide IgG equal to approximately 30 ml of commercial gamma globulin. The major risk to the patient is hepatitis. To minimize this, the size of donor pool is restricted to as few persons as possible.

Common Variable Immunodeficiency

The cardinal feature of this syndrome is development of recurrent pyogenic infections, especially of the sinopulmonary system, during adult life. Typically, the patient has no history of unusual susceptibility to infections during childhood or teenage years. The onset of immunodeficiency is insidious, and often the diagnosis is not made until the patient has suffered severe and irreversible damage to the pulmonary tissues. Other components of the syndrome may include spruelike malabsorption that may be associated with hyperplasia of the intestinal lymphoid tissues and giardiasis.

Diagnosis. As with the congenital hypogammaglobulinemias, the diagnosis is made by quantification of the serum immunoglobulins and antibody responses. Most patients are deficient in all of the immunoglobulins, although IgG levels may not be as low as in congenital hypogammaglobulinemia. Some patients are able to synthesize IgE antibodies, and these may be related to anaphylactic-type reactions to gamma globulin therapy.

Immunology. Many patients with common variable immunodeficiency have immunoglobulin-bearing B-cells in their blood and lymphoid tissues, but plasma cells are not present. In contrast to B-cells from normal subjects, these cells do not respond to *in vitro* stimulation with pokeweed mitogen by secreting immunoglobulins into the cytoplasm or into the culture fluid. Thus, a component of this disorder is the inability of lymphoid cells to differentiate into plasma cells or to secrete immunoglobulins or antibodies even though the cells contain the genetic capacity to synthesize immunoglobulin molecules. In this regard, there are a few instances in which serum samples collected prior to the onset of clinical immunodeficiency were studied and normal immunoglobulin concentrations were found. This observation suggests an abnormality in the processes that regulate immunoglobulin synthesis and secretion.

It has been reported that some patients with common variable immunodeficiency have lymphocytes that are deficient in 5'-nucleotidase, an enzyme involved in purine catabolism. If confirmed, this would be the third instance in which enzymatic defects in these pathways have been associated with immunodeficiency (Fig. 22–5).

T-cell functions in common variable immunodeficiency vary from patient to patient. In some cases they are normal, but other patients may have severe defects in T-cell function. An especially important recent observation is that some patients with either congenital or common variable hypogammaglobulinemia have T-lymphocytes with "suppressor" activity. These cells, when added to cultures of normal lymphocytes, inhibit the normal pokeweed mitogen–induced immunoglobulin synthesis and secretion. At this time, it is uncertain whether these suppressor T-cells are related to the pathogenesis of the hypogammaglobulinemic syndromes or are secondary to the immunodeficiency.

Treatment.   Treatment consists of replacement of immunoglobulin by injections of gamma globulin or transfusions of plasma.

THE DYSGAMMAGLOBULINEMIAS

This term is applied to a variety of syndromes in which there are selective deficiencies of one or more but not all of the immunoglobulin classes in patients whose responses to antigenic stimulation are subnormal. There are two general groups of disorders: (1) those disorders in which the patients are unable to synthesize or secrete immunoglobulin molecules and (2) those in which functionally deficient proteins are produced. The cellular basis and the role of suppressor cell activity in these syndromes is still under study. The patients typically have recurrent infections, and the clinical manifestations in many respects resemble those of hypogammaglobulinemia. Cell-mediated responses are often normal but vary from case to case. Although a multitude of dysgammaglobulinemias have been reported, only the most frequent and clinically significant will be described in detail.

Selective IgA Deficiency

This is the most common of the "dysgammaglobulinemias"; the overall incidence is estimated to be from 1:700 to 1:500. It is important to realize that many persons with this abnormality lead completely normal lives and have normal longevity. In other cases, however, it may be associated with repeated infections, autoimmunity, and increased risk of neoplasia. The mode of inheritance of IgA deficiency is variable;

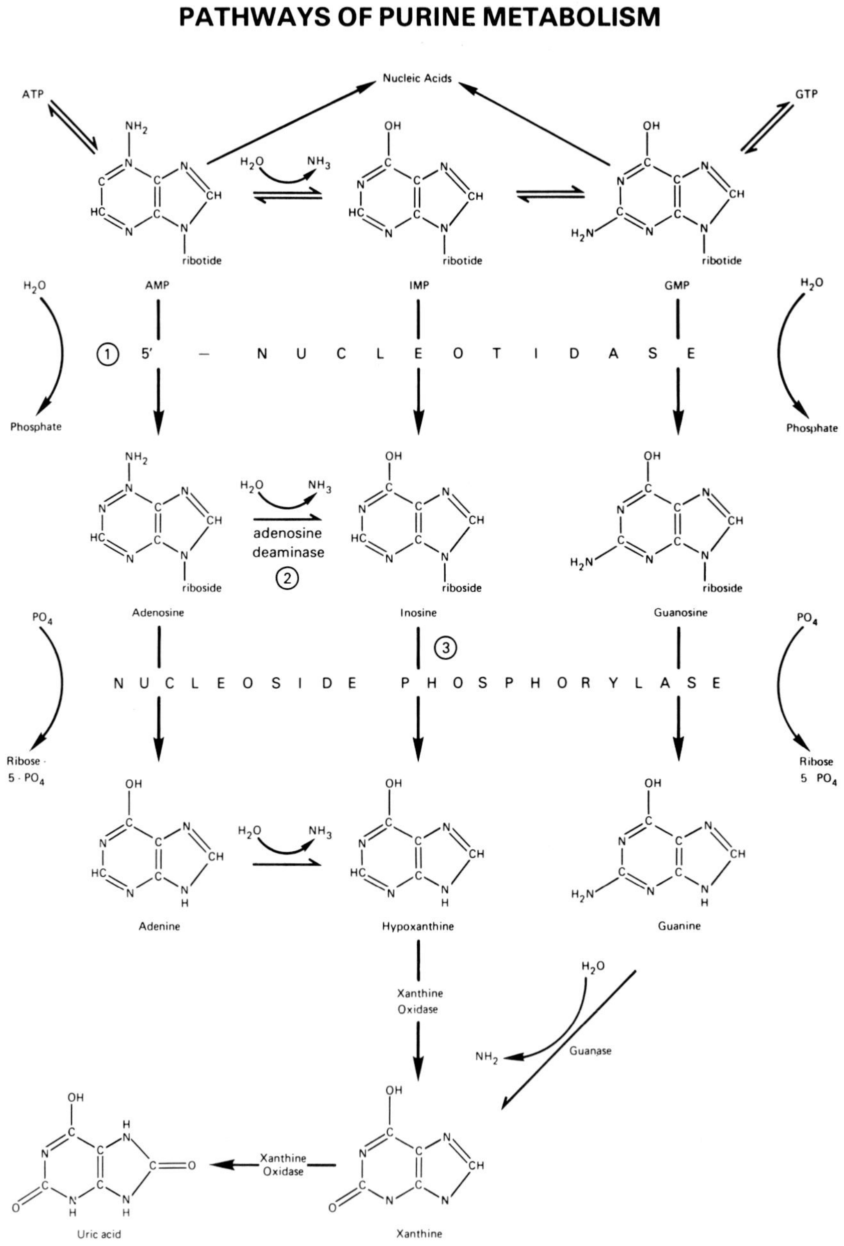

PATHWAYS OF PURINE METABOLISM

Figure 22–5.   Pathways of purine catabolism in humans. Three immune deficiency syndromes have been associated with enzymatic defects in these pathways. ① Lymphocytes from patients with common variable immunodeficiency may be deficient in 5'-nucleotidase. ② Deficiency of adenosine deaminase occurs in some cases of combined immunodeficiency. ③ Nucleoside phosphorylase deficiency has been found in some patients with deficient T-cell functions.

pedigrees showing either autosomal dominant or autosomal recessive inheritance have been recorded.

Clinical Features. In the respiratory tract, recurrent pneumonia, chronic bronchitis, and sinusitis are the common manifestations. In addition, allergic symptoms are common, and the incidence of IgA deficiency in atopic populations has been reported to be as high as 1:200. Among the mechanisms proposed for development of IgE-mediated symptoms in IgA-deficient patients is an imbalance in the competition between secretory IgA and IgE antibodies for antigens. Presumably, deficiency of IgA in the intestinal tract would allow absorption of intact allergenic proteins. In support of this, bovine immunoglobulin has been found in sera from many IgA-deficient individuals.

Transfusion reactions of the anaphylactoid type have also been reported. It has been found that as many as 40 per cent of IgA-deficient patients have antibodies directed against IgA. Most of them have not received blood products and are suspected of developing these antibodies as a consequence of breast-milk feeding or absorption of bovine IgA.

The gastrointestinal disorders in IgA deficiency include chronic diarrhea, gluten-sensitive enteropathy, ulcerative colitis, regional enteritis, and pernicious anemia. Some patients with IgA deficiency and celiac disease have an antibody that reacts with intestinal basement membranes; this antibody is not present in celiac patients who are not IgA-deficient.

IgA deficiency has been described in association with almost all of the major varieties of autoimmune disease, and the incidence in systemic lupus erythematosus and rheumatoid arthritis (reported to be as much as 1:100) seems too high to be merely coincidental.

Diagnosis. The diagnosis is confirmed by demonstrating serum levels of less than 5 mg of IgA per deciliter. Since IgA is thought to play a role in local immunity of the respiratory and gastrointestinal mucosa, it is also helpful to demonstrate the absence of IgA in respiratory secretions. As a matter of fact, cases have been described in which secretory IgA and normal numbers of IgA-containing plasma cells were found in the gastrointestinal tract, although serum levels were diagnostically low.

Immunology. At one time, it was believed that isolated IgA deficiency was not accompanied by abnormalities of other immunoglobulins or of T-cell function. Subsequently, a considerable body of evidence has accumulated indicating varying degrees of impaired T-cell function. Patients have been described in whom there were deficient numbers of E-rosette-forming T-cells or deficient responses to PHA. In other IgA-deficient disorders, such as ataxia-telangiectasia or the candidiasis patient reported by Schlegel and coworkers, blatant abnormalities of T-cell function are observed.

Most patients with IgA deficiency have B-lymphocytes with α-chains on their surface membranes. Stimulation of these cells with pokeweed mitogen causes immunoglobulin to appear in the cytoplasm, but not in the culture fluid. Thus, these patients can synthesize but not secrete IgA. In one case, addition of normal T-cells to the reaction mixture resulted in IgA secretion and suggested that in this patient there was a deficiency of helper T-cells.

A special instance of deficient IgA function has been described in a patient with chronic diarrhea and chronic intestinal candidiasis. This patient was able to synthesize IgA but was unable to make transport piece, the portion that allows IgA to be secreted onto mucosal surfaces, i.e., secretory component.

Treatment.   Treatment with gamma globulin is of no value because these preparations contain little or no IgA. Moreover, IgA given parenterally does not enter the secretions and could stimulate production of anti-IgA antibodies in IgA-deficient individuals. Should blood transfusions be required, the chance of a reaction can be minimized in one of three ways: (1) the patient's own red cells can be frozen for future use; (2) blood from a matched IgA-deficient donor can be used; or (3) packed washed red cells can be given.

Bacterial complications of respiratory infections can be minimized by early and aggressive antibiotic treatment in those who have recurrent sinopulmonary infections. There is no information on the efficacy of a vegetarian diet in those who have gastrointestinal disease or complications possibly traceable to antibovine antibodies.

Selective IgM Deficiency

This disorder is defined as serum IgM levels of less than two standard deviations below the normal mean. The incidence is about 1 per 1000, so it is the second most common selective deficiency.

Clinical Features.   The usual infection in these patients is sudden, overwhelming sepsis. Other associated disorders include splenomegaly, atopy, and hemolytic anemia. The disorder may cluster in families, but a pattern of inheritance has not been defined. The differential diagnosis should include the Wiskott-Aldrich syndrome because these patients are also deficient in IgM. The absence of eczema, thrombocytopenia, a hemorrhagic tendency, and X-linked inheritance, however, would exclude this diagnosis.

Immunology.   In animals, it is possible to create panhypogammaglobulinemia by eradicating IgM-bearing precursor cells with anti-μ serum. However, patients with isolated IgM deficiency have normal concentrations of other immunoglobulins and normal numbers of μ-bearing B-cells. Thus, the underlying defect in this disorder occurs after development of the IgA, IgG, and IgE cell lines.

Treatment.   There is no effective replacement therapy for this disorder. Acute episodes require prompt antibiotic therapy.

Selective IgG Subclass Deficiency

Deficiencies have been described in one or more of the four sub-classes of IgG (IgGl, IgG2, IgG3, IgG4). These patients have repeated infections of the lungs, ears, and upper respiratory tract due to high-grade encapsulated bacterial pathogens (e.g., *Diplococcus pneumoniae, Haemophilus influenzae*). Usually, the clinical state is less severe than that of congenital hypogammaglobulinemia. Diagnosis is made by quantifying the subclasses of IgG. This requires highly specific antisera that are not generally available. Sometimes the total IgG levels are within normal limits. Treatment with commercial gamma globulin is successful.

PRIMARY DEFICIENCIES IN T-CELL-DEPENDENT IMMUNITY

Just as the hypogammaglobulinemias are disorders of B-cell dysfunction, there is another category of diseases in which the primary lesion is maldevelopment or malfunction of the T-cell system. Patients having defective T-cell function may or may not have abnormalities of antibody synthesis. This is somewhat unexpected from the current evidence of cooperative interplay between T- and B-cells in mounting optimal immune responses. In the most severe examples of combined deficiency, neither B-cell nor T-cell function is detectable, and these disorders appear to result from failure to differentiate both cell types from precursor cells, from deficiencies of essential metabolic enzymes, or from deficient function of the thymus. The treatments themselves are experimental and not always successful.

Whereas the most common infectious pathogens in antibody deficiency states are encapsulated bacteria, patients with cellular immunodeficiency are unusually susceptible to infections with viruses such as cytomegalovirus, fungi such as *Candida albicans*, and low-grade pathogens such as *Pneumocystis carinii*. Attenuated live virus or bacterial vaccines can produce fatal infections and are contraindicated. Blood transfusions may cause graft-versus-host reactions and should be given only under controlled circumstances or for therapy of the immune deficiency state, and then only after irradiation of the cells to destroy the leukocytes.

COMBINED ANTIBODY (B-CELL) AND CELL-MEDIATED (T-CELL) IMMUNE DEFICIENCY (SCID)

Severe combined immunodeficiency disease (SCID) represents a heterogeneous group of disorders that have a variety of underlying lesions, occur in several genetic forms, and vary in the extent of the immunologic dysfunction (Table 22–1). Hong writes of two general groups: patients in whom there are severe deficiencies of both cellular and humoral responses with lymphopenia and virtual absence of T-cells and B-cells, and patients with cellular immunodeficiency and circulating immunoglobulins. In the latter group, the immunoglobulins may be structurally abnormal, such as monomeric IgM, and they are usually devoid of antibody activity. These patients may have immunoglobulin-bearing B-cells.

Clinical Features

Often the first evidence of immunodeficiency is oral candidiasis that resists treatment. This infection may appear during the first weeks of life and may spread to the circumoral and perineal tissues and then over the skin. The patients are susceptible to pneumonias caused by viruses such as cytomegalovirus, low-grade pathogenic bacteria, and parasites such as *P. carinii.* Chronic, resistant diarrhea and failure to thrive are regular occurrences. In the severe form of combined immunodeficiency, death usually occurs during the first two years unless successful reconstitution is achieved.

Diagnosis

In most cases, there is marked reduction in the absolute lymphocyte counts, and both B- and T-cells are very few in or absent from the peripheral blood and lymphoid tissues. Immunoglobulin levels are markedly reduced, although during the first six months of life the serum contains maternally derived IgG. Peripheral blood lymphocytes fail to respond to antigens, mitogens, or allogeneic cells with either lymphocyte transformation or lymphokine production. Antibody responses are feeble or nonexistent.

Genetic Types

Combined immunodeficiency occurs in X-linked recessive, autosomal recessive, and sporadic forms. One of the autosomal recessive forms is associated with deficiency of adenosine deaminase (ADA), another enzyme that participates in catabolism of purines (Fig. 22–5). This is the first immunodeficiency that was associated with an enzyme deficiency. The mechanism through which the enzyme deficiency impairs lymphoid cell function is not clear, although there is evidence that the cells accumulate excessive quantities of adenosine triphosphate and that adenosine derivatives may inhibit cell replication. Addition of adenosine deaminase to lymphoid cells from an ADA-deficient patient has caused improvement (but not normalization) of *in vitro* responses to PHA and allogeneic cells. A few patients have been treated with repeated transfusions of ADA-containing erythrocytes, and at least one patient has developed essentially normal immune functions. The findings indicate that the enzyme deficiency is an integral part of the syndrome and not just an epiphenomenon.

Immunology

In addition to ADA deficiency, there is evidence that two other developmental defects of the lymphoid system can produce combined immunodeficiency. The original suggestion that the disease was due to a defect in generation of lymphoid stem cells is supported by the reports of successful reconstitution of immune functions with grafts of stem cells from fetal liver and, in some cases, from bone marrow. Recently, a considerable body of evidence has accumulated indicating that some forms of combined immunodeficiency may result from deficient thymus function. Bone marrow cells from an SCID patient, when cultured on normal thymus epithelium, have matured into E-rosette-forming T-cells and have supported generation of antibody-producing cells *in vitro*. Other SCID patients have shown significant immunologic reconstitution after receiving grafts of fetal thymus or cultured thymic epithelium.

Cases in which detailed studies of cellular immune functions have been conducted have shown the heterogeneity of cell functions that may occur in SCID. Although most patients are devoid of all immune responses, some have T-cells that are able to respond to allogeneic antigens, but not mitogens or environmental antigens, or that can provide helper functions for *in vitro* immunoglobulin synthesis. As mentioned earlier, some patients may have immunoglobulin-bearing B-cells.

The lymph nodes of SCID patients show poor organization. They are composed of stromal tissues and histocytes but are devoid of lymphoid elements. The thymus, in contrast to that of normal subjects (Fig. 22–6), shows few lymphoid elements, poor differentiation of cortical and medullary regions, and no Hassall's corpuscles (Fig. 22–7).

Treatment

The goal of treatment is to replace the missing component of the immune system. Transplantation of bone marrow or fetal liver from genotypically matched donors offers hope for patients with this disorder (Table 22–3). The risk of graft-versus-host disease, however, even with apparently ideal matches, is high enough to prompt trials of other therapies. Currently, thymus transplantation, especially the use of cultured thymic epithelium, injections of thymosin, and replacement of deficient enzymes, is being evaluated.

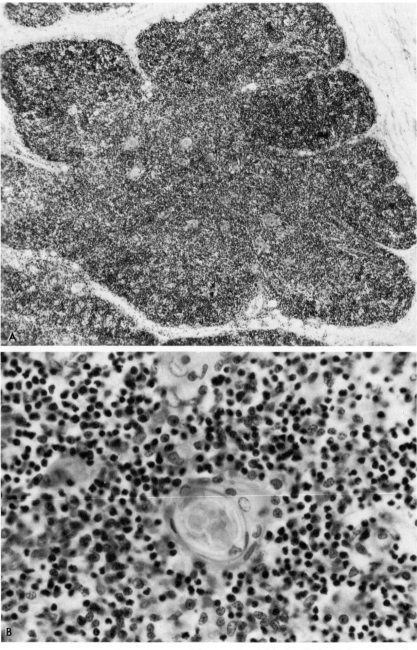

Figure 22–6. Histology of a normal thymus of a child who died with herpes simplex encephalitis. *A*, Note the clearly defined structure of the thymus gland with numerous Hassall's corpuscles and the clear delineation of cortex and medulla of thymic lobules. *B*, A higher magnification of the thymus gland showing a Hassall's corpuscle.

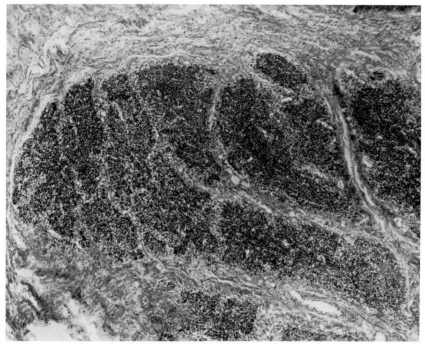

Figure 22–7. Histology of a thymus gland from a child with thymic dysgenesis and chronic mucocutaneous candidiasis. Note the dysplasia of the gland, the absence of Hassall's corpuscles and the lack of clear delineation between cortex and medulla.

TABLE 22–3. Results of Reconstitutive Therapy of SCID

Histocompatibility Group	Number of Patients	Survivors: 6 months	Moderate or Severe GVH Disease*
Genotypic identity of HLA-A, HLA-B, and HLA-D	16	10 (63%)	5/14
Identity at HLA-D; HLA-A, and HLA-B are either identical or nonidentical	13	5 (38%)	6/11
Nonidentity at HLA-D; HLA-A and HLA-B are either identical or nonidentical	19	1 (5%)	7/10
Fetal tissues (liver or thymus)	21	9 (21%)	4/13

*Not every patient could be scored for GVH. Data from Bortin, M. M. and Rihm, A. A.: J.A.M.A., in press.

IMMUNODEFICIENCY WITH SHORT-LIMBED DWARFISM

There are several immune deficiencies associated with short-limbed dwarfism. Some involve both B- and T-cell responses; in others only B-cell or T-cell abnormalities are evident. One of the best characterized of these syndromes is cartilage-hair hypoplasia. In this disorder, the T-cell dysfunction may be progressive, and the patients seem to be especially susceptible to viral infections, especially varicella, but not to other organisms.

Clinical Features

All patients with these syndromes are short, have pudgy hands and feet, with redundant skin folds over the wrists, ankles, knees, and elbows; and have short arms and legs. Unlike achondroplastic or thanatophoric dwarfs, the head is not disproportionately large. X-rays of the bones show irregular, scalloped metaphyseal ends of the long bones. In cartilage-hair hypoplasia, the hair is fine and light-colored and lacks a central pigmented core.

Immunology

Patients with cartilage-hair hypoplasia have normal numbers of B-lymphocytes, normal or supranormal levels of serum immunoglobulins, and good antibody responses. In contrast, there is lymphopenia of the T-cell population; subnormal responses of lymphocytes to T-cell mitogens, antigens, and allogeneic cells; and cutaneous anergy. Some patients also have chronic neutropenia.

Treatment

Treatment of the immune deficiency state is tailored to the functional abnormalities demonstrated. One patient with cartilage-hair hypoplasia responded to thymus transplantation but then developed aplastic anemia that was corrected by bone marrow transplantation.

DEFICIENT CELL-MEDIATED (T-CELL) IMMUNITY WITH VARIABLE ANTIBODY (B-CELL) DEFICIENCY (NEZELOF'S SYNDROME)

This is a variant form of combined immunodeficiency in which immunoglobulins are produced. The profile of serum immunoglobulins is variable, with some patients having normal concentrations of all immunoglobulins while others may produce only one immunoglobulin (usually IgM). In most cases, there is a poor response to antigenic stimulation. Thus, even though they have immunoglobulins, the patients have functional defects of both the T-cell and B-cell systems.

Clinical Features

The clinical features are generally similar to those of other combined immunodeficiencies, with repeated infections, chronic diarrhea, and failure to thrive occurring during infancy. Survivals of several years have been reported, however. The disorder occurs in both X-linked and autosomal recessive forms.

Diagnosis

The patients have deficient numbers of T-lymphocytes and impaired T-cell-mediated immune responses. It is important to do studies of antibody responses to determine whether functional immunoglobulins can be synthesized.

Treatment

Experience is limited, but bone marrow and thymus transplantations have provided benefits to some patients.

ISOLATED T-CELL DEFICIENCY

THE DIGEORGE SYNDROME

In the fully expressed form, this disorder is characterized by neonatal hypocalcemia with tetany and aplasia of the thymus. In addition, there are other abnormalities of facial and midline structures including low-set, notched, or folded ears; hypertelorism; an antimongoloid slant to the eyes; a small fishlike mouth; absence of the philtrum (Fig. 22–8); and abnormalities of the aortic arches and heart, including tetralogy of Fallot.

Clinical Features

The clinical expression of immune deficiency is similar to that of other syndromes with subnormal T-cell function. The patients usually develop oral candidiasis, chronic diarrhea, and failure to thrive during the first year of life. In some cases, there are also cutaneous candidiasis and chronic interstitial pneumonia. The overall health of the patient is also affected by the severity of the cardiovascular malformations and by the control of hypocalcemia.

Diagnosis

T-cell functions are variable, but in the fully expressed syndrome the patients have lymphopenia, deficient numbers of E-rosette-forming

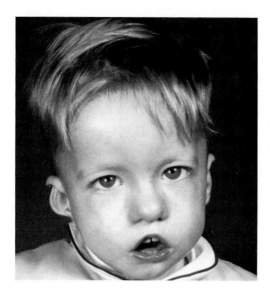

Figure 22–8. Photograph of a child with DiGeorge syndrome. Note the dysplasia of the ears and mouth and the hypertelorism. (Courtesy of Dr. Fred S. Rosen; from Kretschmer, R., et al.: Congenital aplasia of the thymus gland. N. Engl. J. Med., 279:1295, 1968.)

T-cells, and deficient responses to antigens and mitogens *in vitro.* Cutaneous anergy is common. Hypoparathyroidism is expressed by hypocalcemia and hyperphosphatemia.

Immunology

This disorder is the consequence of deficient differentiative activity from the thymus gland. One would anticipate that such profound T-cell deficiencies would also involve the helper cells and cause deficient antibody responses. Surprisingly, immunoglobulins and antibody responses by these patients are normal. Whether this is a reflection of the sensitivity of the assays or of the complexity of the antigens employed is unclear.

Treatment

There are instances in which patients with the DiGeorge syndrome have developed normal T-cell function apparently spontaneously. Injections of thymosin or thymus transplantation with either naked thymus or thymus tissue enclosed in Millipore chambers has also been effective in several cases.

NUCLEOSIDE PHOSPHORYLASE DEFICIENCY

During the past few years, a small number of patients with isolated defects in T-cell function have been found to be deficient in the enzyme nucleoside phosphorylase. After adenosine deaminase, this is the next enzyme in the sequential degradation of purines to hypoxanthine and eventually to uric acid (Fig. 22–5).

Clinical Features

The patients have recurrent or chronic pneumonias and diarrhea and may have chronic candidiasis. In one family, autosomal recessive inheritance was suggested.

Immunology

The patients are deficient in T-cells and their functions. Physiologically, this is expressed as cutaneous anergy and failure of lymphocytes to respond to antigens, mitogens, or allogeneic cells. A low serum uric acid may suggest this diagnosis.

Treatment

Experience is limited. Presumably, thymus transplantation or thymosin would be beneficial. There is no reported experience with enzyme replacement therapy.

CHRONIC MUCOCUTANEOUS CANDIDIASIS

This disorder is characterized by chronic, treatment-resistant infections of the skin, nails, and mucous membranes with *Candida* species, usually *C. albicans*. Although it is often referred to as a specific disorder, it is preferable to consider it as a syndrome that is a hallmark of defective cell-mediated immunity.

Clinical Features

The infection may present as resistant thrush or diaper rash within the first months of life. Typically, the infections spread from the perineal and circumoral areas over the extremities, the scalp and facial skin (Fig. 22–9), and the nails. Cultures and KOH preparations reveal the organisms. Aside from esophageal candidiasis, which may produce significant dysphagia and esophageal stricture, most patients have essentially no predisposition to development of *Candida* infections of parenchymal organs or *Candida* sepsis.

There is a distinct subset of patients with candidiasis in whom endocrine failure is common. The organs most often affected are the adrenals, parathyroids, thyroid, and gonads. The endocrinopathies may appear at any age, although they usually begin during childhood. In some patients, there is sequential loss of multiple endocrine functions. This form of candidiasis often occurs in siblings, and an autosomal

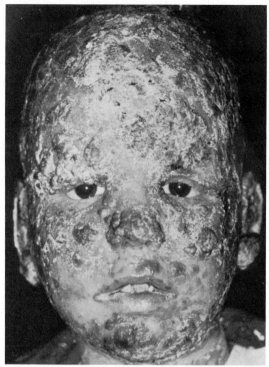

Figure 22-9. Photograph of a nine-year-old boy with chronic mucocutaneous candidiasis who was found to be deficient in cell-mediated immunity. (From Schlegel, R. J., et al.: Severe candidiasis associated with thymic dysplasia, IgA deficiency, and plasma anti-lymphocyte effects. Pediatrics, *45*:926, 1970.)

recessive form of inheritance has been proposed. Since, in most cases, the mucocutaneous candidiasis is an expression of the underlying defect in T-lymphocyte function, the genetics of the primary disease determine the familial occurrence.

Immunology

It is important to understand that clinically similar candidiasis may appear in patients with quite different cellular immune defects. This includes patients with combined immunodeficiency, primary defects of the thymus-dependent system, and thymoma. The most common immunologic profile in patients with chronic candidiasis indicates failure of the secondary stage of T-cell function (Chapter 9). The patients usually have normal numbers of T-cells and normal lymphocyte responses to T-cell mitogens and allogeneic cells. In contrast, their cells fail to respond to specific antigens by producing lymphokines. In some cases, there is total anergy, that is, failure to respond to any of the test antigens. In other patients, the deficit is limited to *Candida* antigens.

Antibody responses to *Candida* antigens are normal or supranormal. The patients have high concentrations of precipitins and agglutininins in the serum, and scratch tests with *Candida* extracts usually disclose marked wheal and flare reactions, indicating IgE antibodies. A few patients with candidiasis have IgA deficiency, but the significance of this is unclear. Presumably, these antibodies and the complement system prevent dissemination of the organisms.

In addition, patients with the candidiasis-endocrinopathy syndrome often have serum antibodies that react with endocrine tissues. There is no evidence that these antibodies mediate injury to the tissues; it is more likely that they are secondary to injury produced by other, perhaps cellular, immune mechanisms. The antibodies may also indicate impairment of the suppressive mechanisms that normally prevent production of autoantibodies.

Treatment

In general, successful therapy depends upon identification and correction of the underlying immunodeficiency. Patients with combined immunodeficiency may respond to reconstitution with grafts of thymus or bone marrow; patients with the DiGeorge syndrome respond to thymus transplantation. Many patients with the most common form of chronic mucocutaneous candidiasis, in which there are normal numbers of T-lymphocytes, normal responses to T-cell mitogens and allogeneic cells, but deficient responses to antigens, have achieved long-lasting remissions after treatment with amphotericin B and transfer factor.

COMPLEX IMMUNODEFICIENCIES

WISKOTT-ALDRICH SYNDROME

This is an X-linked disorder characterized by thrombocytopenia, with a hemorrhagic tendency, eczema, and immunodeficiency with recurrent infections.

Clinical Features

Thrombocytopenia with a bleeding tendency may be the first manifestation and may appear during infancy. Eczema appears later and is indistinguishable from typical atopic eczema (Fig. 22–10). The infections involve the middle ears and often lead to chronic otitis media. In addition, the patients are susceptible to infections with herpes viruses and the wart virus. Finally, as with many immunodeficiency syndromes, the incidence of lymphoreticular malignancies, especially of the central

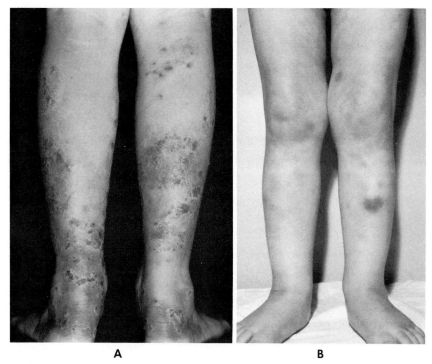

A   **B**

Figure 22–10. Wiskott-Aldrich syndrome. *A*, Eczematoid lesions in a four-year-old boy. *B*, Purpuric lesions in a six-year-old boy.

nervous system, is very high in patients who survive the infectious illnesses (Chapter 19).

Diagnosis

It is imperative to recognize the triad of thrombocytopenia, eczema, and recurrent otitis in male children as a specific syndrome with a poor prognosis. Measurement of the serum immunoglobulins discloses low levels of IgM, normal or elevated levels of IgA and IgG, and extreme elevations of IgE. Antibody responses to polysaccharide antigens such as blood group substances and pneumococcal polysaccharides are feeble. Thus, the patients have low titers of isohemagglutinins. In contrast, antibody responses to protein antigens are essentially normal.

Cellular immune responses are also abnormal. There is usually a reduction in the absolute number of E-rosette-forming T-cells. *In vitro* responses to mitogens such as PHA may be normal, but antigens and allogeneic cells do not stimulate normal increments of DNA synthesis. Cutaneous anergy is common.

Immunology

Although the abnormalities described above reveal the complexity of immunodeficiencies in this syndrome, the underlying mechanisms have not been defined. The inability to respond to polysaccharide antigens has prompted the suggestion that the defect is in the afferent limb of the immune response, perhaps at the level of the macrophage. Thus far, with the exception of impaired responses of monocytes to chemotactic molecules, it has not been possible to identify a macrophage defect. Another factor that contributes to the low levels of immunoglobulins is hypercatabolism. There is also evidence that the Wiskott-Aldrich syndrome is characterized by progressive attrition of immune responses. Young patients may have normal immunoglobulin levels but abnormalities appear with age. The evidence of T-cell dysfunction (anergy, impaired responses to antigens and allogeneic cells) may indicate abnormalities in T-cell-dependent immunoregulatory processes.

Treatment

Eczema responds to topical steroid therapy and local skin care. Severe thrombocytopenia may require platelet transfusions, but splenectomy is contraindicated because it may predispose the patient to sepsis.

There is less experience with treatment of the immunodeficiency. A few patients have received grafts of thymus or bone marrow, and in some cases, there have been definite and long-lasting benefits. Dialyzable transfer factor has been used in a number of patients with this syndrome, and somewhat over 50 per cent of the patients have shown improvement of susceptibility to infections and the chronic eczema and reduction of splenomegaly. These responses appear to occur most frequently in patients whose monocytes lack receptors for IgG.

ATAXIA-TELANGIECTASIA

This autosomal recessive syndrome is characterized by severe cerebellar ataxia, multiple telangiectases of the skin and ocular mucosa (Fig. 22–11), recurrent sinopulmonary infections, and endocrine abnormalities.

Clinical Features

Ataxic symptoms may not be recognized until the child attempts to ambulate but then are progressive and lead to essentially total incapacitation by adolescence. Mentation is not seriously affected.

The immunodeficiency is expressed as recurring and chronic

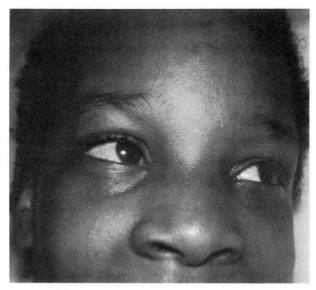

Figure 22–11. Photograph of a 12-year-old girl with ataxia-telangiectasia showing the ocular telangiectasia of the conjunctivae. (Courtesy of Dr. Sanford Leiken.)

infections of the lungs, bronchi, and sinuses. The patients do not develop the meningitis, osteomyelitis, or sepsis that is common in hypogammaglobulinemia.

In adolescent years, endocrine abnormalities including gonadal dysgenesis, insulin-resistant diabetes, and hepatic abnormalities may occur. Finally, patients with ataxia-telangiectasia have a marked predilection to malignant tumors, especially lymphomas, and these are a common cause of death (Chapter 19).

Diagnosis

In addition to studying clinical features, one should determine serum IgA and IgE, often deficient in these patients. T-cell dysfunction is common and is revealed by both *in vivo* and *in vitro* tests.

Immunology

It is not clear whether this disorder is due to a single defect in maturation that is concomitantly expressed in the nervous, cutaneous, endocrine, and immunologic systems thereby producing the syndrome or whether there are multiple defects that occur independently. It seems clear that the neurologic and gonadal lesions are not secondary to infection or ischemia. In support of a common basis for the abnormalities, Waldmann and McIntyre found elevated levels of alpha-fetoprotein in all of 20 patients studied and proposed that the underlying defect was in the entodermal component of the mesodermal-entodermal interface. IgA deficiency could thereby be due to failure of the inductive influences in the gastrointestinal tract. On the other hand, the patients may have autoantibodies, which could indicate an imbalance in the immune system that could be expressed as tissue injury. In this regard, the proposed defect would be similar to that in the candidiasis-endocrinopathy syndrome.

Other than the deficiency of IgA and IgE that occurs in the majority of patients, the concentrations of the other immunoglobulins are usually normal. It is well known that hypercatabolism, possibly due to anti-IgA antibodies, is a component of the IgA deficiency. T-cell abnormalities are expressed as quantitative reductions in the number of T-cells and impaired *in vivo* and *in vitro* T-cell responses. At autopsy, the thymus is often dysplastic, and some have suspected neoplastic degeneration.

Treatment

Thus far, a variety of treatments including transplantation of bone marrow and thymus, thymosin, and transfer factor have been used, but with little sustained success.

HYPERIMMUNOGLOBULINEMIA E WITH RECURRENT INFECTIONS

The original descriptions of this disorder were probably designated Job's syndrome. These patients were red-haired girls who had eczema and recurrent cold abscesses due to staphylococci. It was subsequently shown that patients with this syndrome had elevated serum concentrations of IgE. Buckley et al. reported two boys with similar infections, eczema, and extreme elevations of IgE who had cutaneous anergy and deficient antibody responses. Shortly thereafter, Hill and Quie reported that a similar, if not identical, disorder was associated with defective granulocyte chemotaxis. The patient reported by Clark et al. had defects in chemotaxis and cell-mediated immunity, hyperimmunoglobulinemia E, and recurrent pyogenic infections and may have represented all of the components of the syndrome. It is now recognized that this syndrome occurs in adults as well as in children and is not restricted by sex or race.

Diagnosis

Recurrent pyogenic infections often affecting the skin but without associated marked inflammatory responses are the clinical hallmark of this disorder. Appropriate studies reveal high levels of serum IgE and usually disclose defective chemotactic responses by monocytes and granulocytes. Cellular immunodeficiencies are often present.

Immunology

At this time, it is not clear what, if anything, is the common denominator in this syndrome. Hill and Quie have postulated that the high IgE levels may predispose one to histamine release. Histamine, in turn, could interfere with directed cell migration (chemotaxis) and, through its effect on cyclic AMP, could cause impairment of lymphocyte functions. Alternatively, the presence of anergy, impaired *in vitro* lymphocyte responses, and elevated IgE suggests an abnormality in integration of T-cell-dependent phenomena.

Treatment

It is important to treat the acute infections aggressively with the appropriate antibiotics and drainage procedures. Recently, it has been shown that levamisole, a common antihelminthic drug, may improve or even normalize the chemotactic responses in these patients. It has not been conclusively demonstrated that this treatment is clinically efficacious.

DEFICIENCIES OF THE COMPLEMENT SYSTEM

The complement system is a complex array of highly integrated enzymatic reactions. Activation of this system may occur through the classic pathway involving C1, C4, and C2 or through the alternative pathway involving the properdin system. Both pathways result in cleavage of C3 and subsequent activation of the late components (C5 to C9) with production of chemotactic factors, anaphylatoxins, and tissue injury (Chapter 6). There are many diseases that are due to or associated with abnormalities of the complement system, and most of these are genetically determined (Table 22–4). Only the disorders of major clinical importance are included in this review.

HEREDITARY ANGIOEDEMA (HAE)

This disorder is due to an inborn deficiency of activity of an α_2-globulin that is the normal inhibitor of C1 esterase (Fig. 22–12). Two genetic variants exist: one in which no protein is produced and another in which a protein is made but is not functional.

The disorder may be seen at any age but usually appears during late adolescence or early adult life. It is characterized by recurrent attacks of edema confined to the skin (Fig. 22–13), gastrointestinal tract, or respiratory mucosa. The edema is nonpitting and nonpruritic. Episodes last for 48 to 72 hours. The involvement of the larynx may be life-threatening, and approximately one third of the patients die from

TABLE 22-4. Deficiencies of the Complement System in Man

Component	Associated Abnormalities	Inheritance
C1q	SCID and other immunodeficiency diseases	unknown
C1r	SLE-like skin lesions, glomerulonephritis, arthralgia	autosomal recessive
C1s	SLE-like syndrome	unknown
C4	SLE-like syndrome	unknown (autosomal recessive in guinea pigs)
C2	SLE-like syndrome, glomerulonephritis, dermatomyositis, may occur in normal persons	autosomal recessive
C3	recurrent infections	autosomal recessive
C5	recurrent infections, SLE-like syndrome	autosomal recessive
C6	probably none	autosomal recessive
C7	none	unknown
C8	deficient serum bactericidal activity for *Neisseria gonorrhoeae*	autosomal recessive
C1 esterase inhibitor	hereditary angioedema	autosomal dominant
C3 inhibitor	recurrent infections	unknown

this complication. It is diagnosed by the characteristic hereditary pattern and by quantitation of the levels of the inhibitor activity, C2, or C4.

Recently, considerable success has been achieved in treating this potentially life-threatening disease. Epsilon-aminocaproic acid (EACA) and tranexamic acid are antifibrinolytic agents that are effective in reducing the frequency of attacks. Danazol, a derivative of ethinyltestosterone, has also been effective in preventing attacks; of particular interest is the finding that serum levels of the inhibitor and the complement components increase into the normal range during danazol therapy.

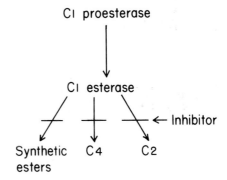

Figure 22-12. Schematic representation of activation of C1 showing the block in hereditary angioedema. (Courtesy of Dr. Fred S. Rosen.)

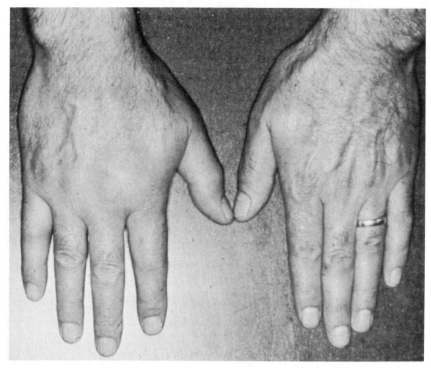

Figure 22–13. Photograph of the hands of a patient with hereditary angioedema, showing swelling of the dorsum of the right hand during an attack. (Courtesy of Dr. Fred S. Rosen.)

C1 DEFICIENCIES

Some individuals with C1 deficiency are clinically normal. Others having C1r deficiency, however, have an increased susceptibility to respiratory infections and autoimmune phenomena such as necrotizing vasculitis, dermatitis, and renal disease. The disorder is probably inherited in an autosomal recessive fashion. C1s deficiency has been found in patients having a lupus erythematosus-like illness.

C2 DEFICIENCY

This abnormality has been observed in patients with an SLE-like disorder, glomerulonephritis, and dermatomyositis, as well as in normal persons. It is transmitted as an autosomal recessive trait.

C3 DEFICIENCIES

Four clinical conditions involving deficiency of this complement component have been described. In the first, an autosomal recessive disorder, there was a defect in synthesis of C3, and the one known patient with this syndrome had recurrent, severe pyogenic infections of skin and lungs. In addition, there are two instances of hypercatabolism of C3 associated with recurrent infections. In one case, the disorder was inherited as an autosomal recessive trait; the second case was sporadic. Finally, in sickle cell disease, there is deficient activation of C3 through the alternate pathway.

C4 Deficiency

This disorder occurs as an autosomal recessive trait in guinea pigs; the affected animals are not unusually susceptible to infection. In man, C4 deficiency has been observed in a few patients with SLE-like syndromes.

C5 Deficiency

This deficiency has occurred in two settings. In one family, C5 deficiency was found in several members, one of whom had an SLE-like illness. The inheritance is unclear but probably autosomal recessive. The other instance is somewhat less clear. The patient was an infant with recurrent infections, chronic diarrhea, and seborrhea whose serum failed to opsonize yeast and staphylococci. This dysfunction was corrected by addition of C5 to the patient's serum, and transfusions of plasma (presumably providing C5) provided clinical benefits.

C6 Deficiency

This autosomal recessive trait has not been associated with clinical abnormalities.

C7 Deficiency

Two examples have been recorded: one in a healthy male and the second in a patient with scleroderma. Neither was susceptible to infections.

C8 Deficiency

This deficiency has been recognized only rarely and may be associated with susceptibility to *Neisseria* infections.

ABNORMALITIES OF LEUKOCYTE FUNCTION

Disorders of Phagocytes

The primary cells of the phagocytic system include the fixed and circulating cells of the mononuclear phagocyte system (MPS) and neutrophils (Chapter 2). Little is known of inborn diseases affecting the macrophages. Certain disorders of the spleen, however, may be associated with an undue susceptibility to infection and reflect defects of the macrophage system (Table 22–5).

Defective function of the spleen occurs in congenital aplasia, surgical removal, or asplenia secondary to hemolytic states. Splenectomy in children less than two or three years of age has been associated with severe and sometimes fatal bacterial septicemias. Deficits in pneumococcal opsonins have been described in sickle cell disease, in which functional asplenia may also occur. Evidence is accumulating that indicates that the spleen plays an important role in antibody responses. Splenic defects that occur prior to acquisition of immunologic competence may predispose to serious bacterial infection by a failure of adequate opsonin production.

DISORDERS OF NEUTROPHILS

More is known of disorders affecting the polymorphonuclear leukocytes (Table 22–6). Clinical entities affecting these cells fall into two broad classes: (1) quantitative — those in which the total numbers of neutrophils are decreased (e.g., neutropenias) and (2) qualitative — those in which the total number of phagocytes is normal but the cells are functionally defective.

NEUTROPENIAS

In the neutropenias, impaired immunity results from a breach in the first line of defense provided by neutrophils. Some neutropenias are associated with decreased production, others with increased destruction, and in others both causes operate simultaneously. There are acquired and inherited forms of neutropenia.

Acquired Neutropenias

Acquired neutropenias are caused by drugs, pollutants, radiation, overwhelming infections, endotoxins, autoimmune disorders, hypersensitivity states, neoplasms, and other myelophthisic processes and

TABLE 22–5. Disorders of the Spleen Associated with Immune Defects

TYPE	EXAMPLE
Congenital	Congenital absence of the spleen
Acquired	Splenectomy
	Functional splenectomy with hemolytic diseases (sickle cell disease)

TABLE 22–6. Disorders of the Phagocytic-Bactericidal System

DISEASE	DEFICIENCY	INHERITANCE
Leukocyte Defects		
Neutropenia	Inadequate numbers of responsive cells	Variable
Chédiak-Higashi syndrome	Defective migration, possibly due to reduced deformability	Autosomal recessive
Lazy leukocyte syndrome	Deficient random migration and chemotactic responses	Unknown
Hyper-IgE syndrome	Deficiency cellular chemotaxis	Unknown
Disorders of Microbicidal Activity		
Chronic granulomatous disease	Complex disorder with impaired activity of the hexose monophosphate shunt, oxygen utilization, and hydrogen peroxide generation	Usually X-linked, but females may be affected
Myeloperoxidase deficiency	Impaired halogenation of ingested organisms	Autosomal recessive
Chédiak-Higashi syndrome	Impaired degranulation	Autosomal recessive
Glucose-6-phosphate dehydrogenase deficiency	Probably similar to CGD	X-linked
Disorders of Chemotaxis		
Complement component deficiencies		
C3	Impaired generation of chemotactic factors	Autosomal recessive
C5	Impaired generation of chemotactic factors	Autosomal recessive
C1r	Delayed generation of chemotactic factors	Autosomal recessive
C2	Delayed generation of chemotactic factors	Autosomal recessive
Antibody deficiency syndromes	Impaired generation of chemotactic factors	
Cellular immunodeficiencies		
Wiskott-Aldrich syndrome	Impaired generation of chemotactic lymphokines, abnormal monocyte chemotaxis	X-linked
Chronic mucocutaneous candidiasis	Impaired generation of chemotactic lymphokines	Autosomal recessive
Impaired Opsonization		
Newborn	Impaired opsonic capacity of serum (IgM and complement)	—
Antibody deficiency syndromes	Impaired opsonic capacity of serum (immunoglobulins)	See Table 22–1
Complement deficiencies	Impaired opsonic capacity of serum	See Table 22–4
Sickle cell disease	Impaired opsonic capacity of serum	Autosomal intermediate
Disorders of Phagocytosis		
Occur in a variety of syndromes in which the opsonic properties of the complement or serum immunoglobulin systems are impaired		Variable

disorders of the spleen. Ionizing radiation appears to be a dose-related phenomenon leading to diminution in bone marrow production of neutrophils. Drugs, on the other hand, act in a variety of ways (Chapter 20). Some drugs lead to bone marrow depression; others act as haptens that in combination with tissue protein induce the formation of antibody. The list of drugs associated with neutropenia is ever increasing and includes analgesics, antithyroid drugs, anticonvulsants, sulfonamides, antihistamines, antimicrobial agents, and tranquilizers. Furthermore, it might be expected that the increased pollution of man's environment will give rise to new and more numerous causes of neutropenia.

Neutropenia occurs during infection with a variety of gram-negative and gram-positive bacteria and viruses such as influenza, rubella, measles, and infectious hepatitis. In some cases, it may be difficult to decide whether an infection is caused by underlying neutropenia or whether the neutropenia is the result of the infection. In the latter, the white cell concentration returns to normal following recovery from infection. Transient neutropenia is also seen during severe infections associated with immune deficiency disorders. An additional mechanism in infections caused by gram-negative organisms is dependent on the peripheral destruction of neutrophils and bone marrow depression by endotoxin produced by these organisms.

Neutropenia occurs in autoimmune diseases, e.g., lupus erythematosus, juvenile rheumatoid arthritis, and Felty's syndrome (neutropenia, splenomegaly, and arthritis). Bone marrow production of neutrophils appears to be diminished in these conditions. A transient neonatal neutropenia is associated with maternal isoimmunization, and the mechanism is believed to be analogous to that seen in maternal-fetal Rh incompatibility (Chapter 20).

Neutropenia may result from bone marrow replacement by neoplastic tissue (myelophthisis) and is a common complication of leukemia. In certain cases, neoplastic involvement of the spleen is associated with increased destruction of neutrophils (hypersplenism). A number of diseases associated with splenomegaly may cause neutropenia, and these include Banti's syndrome, Gaucher's disease, primary splenic neutropenia, and cirrhosis of the liver with splenomegaly.

Inherited Neutropenia

Inherited forms of neutropenia compose a second major group. Some are associated with stigmata of congenital syndromes; others occur as isolated defects. Neutropenias occurring in episodic fashion are referred to as cyclic; those that are more protracted are referred to as noncyclic. Cyclic neutropenia is typically manifested by episodes of neutropenia, fever, malaise, and aphthous stomatitis occurring at approximately three-week intervals. The late myeloid precursors of neutrophilic leukocytes are absent in bone marrow during periods of neutropenia, suggesting a defect in neutrophil maturation (maturational arrest). In some cases, leukocyte agglutinins are present in the serum, and the pathogenesis may involve both diminished production and increased immune destruction. Severe infections may be seen in cyclic neutropenias, particularly when they coexist with immunoglobulin deficiency states.

Noncyclic neutropenias differ from cyclic varieties in etiology, clinical features, and prognosis. Most are inherited and associated with diminished production of neutrophils by bone marrow. Some follow a benign course with possible spontaneous cure in later childhood. Others are characterized by more severe infections, and many children die in the first year of life. A syndrome of neutropenia, pancreatic insufficiency, and malabsorption has been described. Neutropenia is also seen in congenital aplastic anemias, or it may occur as an isolated defect. An autosomal recessive mode of transmission has been described in one condition that occurs with high frequency in geographic regions of Sweden where consanguineous marriages are common. There are also X-linked recessive and autosomal dominant types.

Clinical Features

Infections are the hallmark of both acquired and inherited forms of neutropenia. Bacteria causing infection are of many varieties, the most common being *Micrococcus pyogenes*, *Streptococcus pyogenes*, and *Diplococcus pneumoniae*. Many patients with noncyclic hereditary neutropenia die early in infancy from omphalitis and sepsis. Rapidly spreading cellulitis and bacteremia are common. Terminally, perforation of the cecum and peritonitis are typical. During neonatal life, the common infectious agent is *M. pyogenes*.

Resistance to bacterial infections improves if the children survive infancy, presumably reflecting compensatory development of other components of immunity. Antibody synthesis and cell-mediated responses are functionally intact in most of the hereditary neutropenias. It is difficult to manage infections during early childhood since the smallest skin abrasions may result in cellulitis and sepsis. Bacterial infections of the upper respiratory tract are rapidly progressive and difficult to clear, often leading to peritonsillar abscess, retropharyngeal abscess, otitis media, or mastoiditis.

Diagnosis

It is usually possible to distinguish inherited from acquired cases by considering the age of onset; the history of exposure to toxic substances and drugs; the pedigree, including parental consanguinity; and the hematologic studies (e.g., bone marrow analysis). Rarely, leukokinetic studies with radioactive tracers may be useful in distinguishing disorders of leukocyte production from disorders of leukocyte destruction. Tests for circulating leukoagglutinins may be performed, although these antibodies may be found in otherwise normal individuals.

It is sometimes difficult to distinguish hereditary inborn neutropenias from the transient neonatal neutropenias. In the latter, the neutrophil count begins to rise after the first month of life. This reflects the turnover of the maternally derived IgG antileukocyte antibody, which has a half-life of 20 to 30 days.

Treatment

There is no specific treatment for the neutropenias per se. Discontinuance of drugs is indicated in the case of drug-induced neutropenia. Treatment is directed toward preventing infections, since the most trivial abrasion may lead to microbial invasion and sepsis. In recent years, white cell transfusions have been a useful adjunct in the treatment of severe infections in patients with neutropenia. Diagnostic blood studies should be minimized, since skin puncture can result in severe cellulitis. It is worthwhile in some cases to isolate patients for protection against common bacterial pathogens, especially during the early phases of the disease.

Long-term prophylaxis with antimicrobial drugs is not indicated, but antibiotic management may be tailored to an individual patient. Parenteral antibiotic treatment with bactericidal drugs is recommended for upper respiratory infections or skin abrasions during early childhood. In older children and adults, it is advisable to await the results of bacterial cultures before instituting antimicrobial therapy. Effective prevention of the hereditary neutropenias rests on genetic counseling.

QUALITATIVE DEFECTS OF NEUTROPHILS (NEUTROPHIL DYSFUNCTION SYNDROMES)

A clinical picture of recurrent sepsis and disseminated pyogenic lesions is characteristic of the neutrophil dysfunction syndromes. A number of different disorders make up these syndromes; each of them is characterized by normal numbers of polymorphonuclear leukocytes that are qualitatively defective. There are abnormalities of the movement of cells toward foreign matter (defective chemotaxis); preparation of substances for cell ingestion (opsonization); or intracellular destruction of molecules, pathogens, or cells (ingestion and digestion). Many of these disorders are inherited; some are acquired. Defects affecting phagocytosis may occur in systems intrinsic to the neutrophil leukocyte itself (intracellular) or in systems extrinsic to it (extracellular) (Chapter 2) (Table 22–6).

INTRACELLULAR DEFECTS

Chronic Granulomatous Disease (CGD)

This is the prototype of the syndrome of defective bactericidal activity. In most cases, the disorder is X-linked. The underlying defect is impaired generation of hydrogen peroxide and metabolism of oxygen presumably resulting from a deficiency of the enzyme NADPH oxidase, although this has not been established with certainty and there may be different defects in different cases.

Clinical Features. The onset of symptoms is usually at about the age of one year, when the first of recurrent and severe episodes of sepsis and disseminated abscesses occurs. Etiologic bacterial agents are commensal microorganisms normally found on the skin and in the gut (Staphylococci, *Escherichia coli*, *Klebsiella*, *Enterobacter*, *Serratia marcescens*, *Proteus vulgaris*, and *Actinomyces* species). In contrast to other immune deficiencies, these causative agents of infection are restricted to bacteria of low-grade virulence that are catalase-positive and peroxide-negative. Organisms that are catalase-negative and peroxide-positive do not cause serious infection in these children. It has been postulated that these latter organisms can provide an alternate source of the H_2O_2, thereby partially correcting the defect (Chapter 2). Affected infants develop pneumonia, hepatosplenomegaly, suppurative lymph nodes that occasionally rupture through the skin and drain, and, less frequently, brain or retinal abscesses (Fig. 22–14).

The characteristic suppurative granulomas are scattered throughout the body in bone, lung, and liver. The granuloma consists of inflammatory cells surrounding a necrotic central core (Fig. 22–15). Similarities exist between these granulomata and those resulting from infectious granulomatoses. In infectious granulomatoses, the microorganisms possess properties enabling them to resist phagocytic digestion by normal cells. In CGD, the metabolic abnormality of host cells allows persistence of organisms.

Diagnosis. The diagnosis should be suspected in a newborn when such a diagnosis has previously been made in a maternal cousin or uncle or male sibling. The disease is difficult to diagnose during neonatal life, since the spectrum of organisms normally causing infection closely resembles that of CGD. In an older child, the characteristically restricted group of infectious agents and the clinical picture should suggest the diagnosis. There is less diagnostic confusion in adults, since these organisms are uncommon causes of disease. Also, in the adult, there exist clear differences in the metabolism of normal and CGD leukocytes. This is not true in the neonate, whose leukocytes normally reduce nitroblue tetrazolium (NBT) dye less effectively following phagocytic stimulation and have relatively labile glucose-6-phosphate dehydrogenase (G-6-PD) activity.

The most useful test is the NBT dye reduction test in which, because of the block in the hexose monophosphate pathway and impaired peroxide metabolism, there is a subnormal capacity of the activated neutrophils to reduce the colorless dye to a blue formazan. Genetic carrier females can be detected by demonstration of intermediate levels of reduction.

The inflammatory lesions of neonatal sepsis, meningitis, and pneumonia are granulomatous in nature and may also resemble those seen in CGD. It is possible to accurately diagnose CGD in newborn infants by bioassay for phagocytic bactericidal capacity. Although normal leukocytes show quantitatively similar defects in phagocytic killing when suspended in newborn serum, suspensions of normal newborn leukocytes in adult serum show only slightly diminished killing even in the most sensitive available bioassays. The bactericidal activity of CGD leukocytes is not restored by normal adult serum.

Infections are frequently heralded by prolonged fevers of unknown etiology without local signs of infection. Blood cultures are often negative, even when the patient has not received antibiotics. An anemia

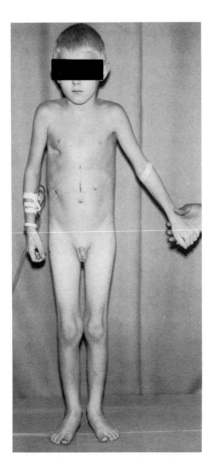

Figure 22–14. Photograph of a nine-year-old boy with chronic granulomatous disease. Note thoracotomy and laparotomy scars at sites of prior therapeutic procedures to drain abscesses of lung and liver.

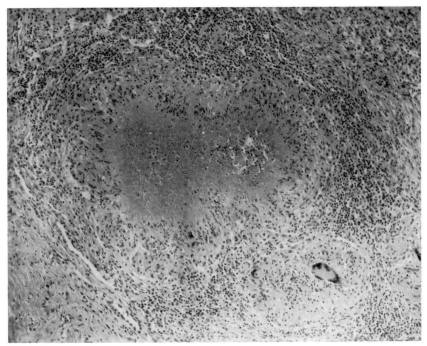

Figure 22–15. Photomicrograph of a granuloma seen in chronic granulomatous disease. Note the central area of necrosis surrounded by inflammatory cells and a multinucleated giant cell to the lower right. Hematoxylin and eosin stain, ×120.

occurs that is exacerbated during hyperpyrexia. It is usually normochromic and associated with low serum iron values and high total iron-binding capacity. There is no reticulocytosis and no indication of a relationship between erythrocyte G-6-PD lability and the anemia.

Cytologically, the neutrophils appear normal by light and electron microscopy. Specific immune reactions of cell-mediated and antibody types are normal. Characteristically, there occurs hypergammaglobulinemia with elevated levels of all immunoglobulins, presumably reflecting the high frequency of pyogenic infections.

A combination of clinical findings and laboratory tests is required for accurate diagnosis. These may be supported by biopsy evidence of typical granulomata, although it is infrequently necessary to biopsy infectious lesions.

Differential Diagnosis. The diagnostic possibilities include infectious granulomatous diseases and other neutrophil dysfunction disorders. Prolonged fevers of unknown origin may also cause one to suspect rheumatoid disease. Infectious granulomatoses do not usually produce either the large liver abscesses or the impetigo characteristic of CGD. Patients with CGD have a marked polymorphonuclear leukocytosis with a shift to the left, in contrast to nonsuppurative infectious granulomatoses in which there may be a lymphocytosis. Negative skin tests and negative bacterial smears and cultures from infectious lesions, urine, or gastric juice lend further support to the diagnosis of CGD by making the diagnosis of infectious granulomatoses less likely.

Abnormal Physiology. The metabolic adjustments of neutrophils to particle ingestion have been described in Chapter 2. Intracellular killing is accompanied by a respiratory burst and increased hexose monophosphate pathway (HMP) activity. In CGD there is a failure to generate increased HMP activity. Lability of glucose-6-phosphate dehydrogenase (G-6-PD) has been demonstrated in the leukocytes of affected patients. The cause of the lability is unknown, although the recent description of NADPH oxidase deficiency appears to best explain this phenomenon owing to lack of NADP. NADPH synthesis in leukocytes depends on the first two steps of the HMP. Since NADPH plays a necessary role in the biosynthesis of membrane phospholipids, defects may also exist in the complex membrane-related phenomena of intracellular lysosomal killing of bacteria. Other more distal links in the causal chain leading to defective intracellular killing have been uncovered. CGD leukocytes fail to generate hydrogen peroxide for halide fixation of ingested bacteria. The relative importance of this mechanism of bacterial killing is not completely understood, but it may be of significance in infections caused by the catalase-producing (peroxide negative) organisms that cause infections in CGD.

Treatment. Treatment has improved in recent years owing to better understanding of the disease. Most infections are successfully eradicated through early intervention with high doses of bactericidal antibiotics. Since blood cultures are often negative, antimicrobials are frequently selected according to the known spectrum of causative bacteria. There is a place for genetic counseling, and the determination of risk is defined in some instances by prenatal determination of fetal chromosomal sex. The prognosis is better than it used to be, and survival into the later years of childhood, or even into early adult years, is more frequent.

Other Enzyme Deficiency States With Impaired Bactericidal Activity

Following the description of X-linked chronic granulomatous disease, a series of other inborn errors of metabolism were discovered in which there was subnormal interference of bacterial killing by neutrophils and susceptibility to infection with commensal microorganisms. A syndrome identical to X-linked chronic granulomatous disease has been described in females having deficient glutathione peroxidase activity. Complete absence of glucose-6-phosphate dehydrogenase activity leads to a similar predisposition to infection. Myeloperoxidase deficiency is associated with increased susceptibility to deep *Candida* and to staphylococcal infections. In these conditions, the diagnosis is made by demonstrating the deficiency in enzyme activity (Table 22–6).

The Chédiak-Higashi Syndrome

This is an autosomal recessive disorder characterized by oculocutaneous albinism, neurologic abnormalities, a high incidence of lymphoreticular neoplasms, and recurrent pyogenic infections due to both commensal and pathogenic bacteria. The defective pigment metabolism, abnormal neutrophil function, and possibly other abnormalities appear to be related to the presence of abnormal lysosomes in many cell types including the skin and peripheral blood neutrophils. These appear as giant cytoplasmic granules. Deficient bactericidal activity is demonstrated in neutrophils, and there is delayed degranulation following stimulation of phagocytosis. Neutrophil chemotaxis is impaired in some patients, and there is often neutropenia.

Recent data suggest that the impairments in neutrophil function in these patients may be related to abnormalities of cyclic nucleotide metabolism, either as deficient production of cyclic guanosine monophosphate (cGMP) or as excessive accumulation of cyclic adenosine monophosphate (cAMP). It has also been found that some of the abnormalities of leukocyte function can be corrected with ascorbic acid, an agent that promotes cGMP accumulation in leukocytes.

Deficiencies of Neutrophil Chemotaxis

These conditions are sometimes due to causes extrinsic to the neutrophil and sometimes due to intrinsic cellular defects. Examples of the former have already been discussed (e.g., C5 dysfunction). A number of children have been described who have circulating inhibitors of neutrophil chemotaxis in their serum or plasma. The latter sometimes respond favorably to plasma therapy.

Intrinsic defects of neutrophil chemotaxis have also been identified. In the lazy leukocyte syndrome, there is also deficient random mobility of neutrophils and failure to mobilize a leukocyte response to epinephrine or endotoxin stimulation, suggesting a possible relationship between bone marrow release and random mobility of the cell. Job's syndrome is a familial state in which eczema and atypical light skin is associated with recurrent cold abscesses and defective neutrophil chemotaxis. Its relationship to the hyper-IgE syndrome has been described above. As mentioned, impaired cellular chemotaxis is a component of the Chédiak-Higashi syndrome (Table 22–6).

Deficient Phagocytosis

The phagocytic barrier to infection is lowered by inadequate numbers of polymorphonuclear leukocytes or by qualitative defects in their function. The latter are in some cases intrinsic and in others due to the lack of factors necessary for chemotaxis, random mobility, or opsonization or to the presence of abnormal factors that interfere with one or more of those functions. Intrinsic defects affect any of the aforementioned processes necessary for phagocytosis or result in deficient bacterial killing by the neutrophil (Table 22–6).

CONCLUSIONS

Since the first edition of this book seven years ago, there have been a number of newly discovered diseases. However, most have been variations on established themes of dysfunction. Hence, the thrust of research has turned away from descriptive accounts of alterations in the form and structure of cells and tissues and toward elucidation of the molecular bases of the various disease states, diagnosis, and treatment.

Clinical identification of the primary immune disorders is usually based on evidence of chronic, repetitious, or bizarre infection. These evidences are usually so flagrant that there is little difficulty in ruling out mere overexposure to communicable disease. Infections due to encapsulated bacteria suggest B-cell abnormalities; infections due to fungi and viruses suggest T-cell disorders; and those due to commensal bacteria suggest neutrophil dysfunction. In addition, a compatible pedigree is helpful in some cases and associated congenital abnormalities in others.

Laboratory diagnosis of antibody deficiency disorders is usually made on the basis of abnormal quantification of immunoglobulins by radial diffusion (Chapter 26). Lymph node biopsies are less frequently required nowadays. The diagnosis of deficient cell-mediated immunity has been immeasurably enhanced by the discovery of T-cell rosette formation, and current research is directed at definition of the roles of subsets of T-lymphocytes in disease. Complement deficiency of C1q, C1r, C1s, and C2 is usually diagnosed by means of the total hemolytic complement assay. Moreover, specific assay for C4 and C3 proteins is now generally available. The NBT reduction test is still the most useful way to screen for chronic granulomatous disease, and the total neutrophil and lymphocyte counts in peripheral blood continue to be valuable, but often overlooked, tools in diagnosing immune deficiency.

Diagnosis yields a host of fruitful consequences for medical management in addition to the possibility of definitively correcting the underlying defect. In most instances, early diagnosis allows avoidance of harmful blood transfusions or standard immunizations. Furthermore, a known spectrum of infectious agents peculiar to each of the various disease entities permits a more appropriate initial selection of antimicrobial drugs. Family counseling is improved by the increased security of prognostication and by the more accurate ascertainment of genetic risk.

Numerous experimental advances have occurred in specific treatment of immune deficiency states since the initial discovery that commercial gamma globulin prevented serious infections in the IgG deficiencies. Bone marrow transplantation with allogeneically identical donor cells has been successful in restoring immune responses in patients having combined immunodeficiency. Transplants of fetal thymus have been successful in some cases of isolated T-cell deficiency (e.g., DiGeorge syndrome). Both thymosin (an extract of bovine thymus) and transfer factor (a dialyzable factor from leukocytes) have been used with some success in treating deficiencies of cell-mediated immunity, but the results are not always satisfactory. Plasma infusions have been beneficial in C5 dysfunction, hypogammaglobulinemias and in some cases of defective neutrophil chemotaxis caused by circulating serum or plasma inhibitors.

In the individual case, it is equally important to attend to the psychologic consequences of chronic disease and medical dependence on the child and family. The preoccupation with complicated technology can lead to neglect of the risks of emotional depression and impaired prospects for a fulfilling life.

SUGGESTIONS FOR FURTHER READING

General

Bergsma, D., Good, R. A., Finstad, J., and Paul, N. W.: Immunodeficiency in Man and Animals. National Foundation—March of Dimes Original Article Series, Sunderland, Mass., Sinauer Associates, 1975.
Cline, M. J.: The White Cell. Cambridge, Harvard University Press, 1975.
Fudenberg, H. H., Stites, D. P., Caldwell, J. L., and Wells, J. V.: Basic and Clinical Immunology. Los Altos, California, Lange, 1976.

Clinical Setting

Bellanti, J. A., and Schlegel, R. J.: The diagnosis of immune deficiency diseases. Pediatr. Clin. North Am., *18*:49, 1971.
Janeway, C. A.: Syndromes of diminished resistance to infection. J. Pediatr., *72*:885, 1968.

Development

Adinolfi, M., and Wood, C. B. S.: Ontogenesis of immunoglobulins and components of complement in man. *In* M. Adinolfi (ed.): Immunology and Development. London, William Heinemann Medical Books Ltd., 1969.
Fudenberg, H., Good, R. A., Goodman, H. C., Hitzig, W., Kunkel, H. G., Roitt, I. M., Rosen, F. S. Rowe, D. S., Seligmann, M., and Soothill, J. R.: Primary immunodeficiencies. Pediatrics, *47*:927, 1971.

Disorders of Phagocytosis

Alper, C. A., Abramson, N., Johnston, R. B., Jr., Jandl, J. H., and Rosen, F. S.: Complement defect associated with increased susceptibility to infection. N. Engl. J. Med., *282*:349, 1970.

Baehner, R. L., and Nathan, D. G.: Quantitative nitroblue tetrazolium test in chronic granulomatous disease. N. Engl. J. Med., *278*:971, 1968.

Bellanti, J. A., Cantz, B. E., and Schlegel, R. J.: Enhanced degradation of leukocyte glucose-6-phosphate dehydrogenase activity in chronic granulomatous disease. Pediatr. Res., *4*:405, 1970.

Douglas, S. D., Davis, W. C., and Fudenberg, H. H.: Granulocytopathies: Pleomorphism of neutrophil dysfunction. Am. J. Med., *46*:901, 1969.

Kander, E., and Mauer, A. M.: Neutropenias of childhood. J. Pediatr., *69*:147, 1966.

Kaplan, E. L., Laxdal, T., and Quie, P. G.: Studies of polymorphonuclear leukocytes from patients with chronic granulomatous disease of childhood: Bactericidal capacity for streptococci. Pediatrics, *41*:591, 1968.

Kevy, S. U., Tefft, M., Vawter, G. F., and Rosen, F. S.: Hereditary splenic hypoplasia. Pediatrics, *42*:752, 1968.

Klebanoff, S. J., and White, L. R.: Iodination defect in the leukocytes of a patient with chronic granulomatous disease of childhood. N. Engl. J. Med., *280*:460, 1969.

Lehrer, R. I., and Cline, M. J.: Leukocyte myeloperoxidase deficiency and disseminated candidiasis: The role of myeloperoxidase in resistance to candida infection. J. Clin. Invest., *48*:1478, 1969.

Miller, M. E., and Nilsson, V. R.: Complement dysfunction with deficient phagocytosis enhancement by serum. N. Engl. J. Med., *282*:354, 1970.

Ward, P. A., and Schlegel, R. J.: Impaired leukotactic responsiveness in a child with recurrent infections. Lancet, *2*:344, 1969.

Antibody Deficiency Disorders

Bruton, O. C.: Agammaglobulinemia. Pediatrics, *9*:722, 1952.

Cooper, M. D., Chase, H. P., Lowman, J. T., Krivit, W., and Good, R. A.: Wiskott-Aldrich syndrome: An immunologic disease involving the afferent limb of immunity. Am. J. Med., *44*:499, 1968.

Schlegel, R. J., and Miller, M. M.: Immunogenetics. *In* Lytt I. Gardner (ed.): Endocrine and Genetic Disorders of Childhood and Adolescence. 2nd ed. Philadelphia, W. B. Saunders Co., 1975.

Yount, W. J.: Imbalance of IgG subclasses and gene defects in patients with primary hypogammaglobulinemia. *In* D. Bergsma (ed.): Immunodeficiency in Man and Animals. Sunderland, Mass., Sinauer, 1975, pp. 99–107.

Deficiencies of Cell-Mediated Immunity

Ammann A. J., Sutleff, W., and Millinchick, E: Antibody mediated immunodeficiency in short-limbed dwarfism. J. Pediatr., *84*:200, 1974.

Blaese, R. M., Oppenheim, J. J., Seeger, R. C., and Waldmann, T. A.: Lymphocyte-macrophage interaction in antigen induced in vitro lymphocyte transformation in patients with the Wiskott-Aldrich syndrome and other diseases with anergy. Cell. Immunol., *4*:228, 1972.

Giblett, E., Anderson, J., Cohen, F., Pollara, B., and Newissen, H. J.: Adenosine-deaminase deficiency in two patients with severely impaired cellular immunity. Lancet, *2*:1067, 1972.

Giblett, E. R., Ammann, A. J., Sandman, R., Wara, D. W., and Diamond, L. K.: Nucleoside-phosphorylase deficiency in a child with severely defective T-cell immunity and normal B-cell immunity. Lancet, *1*:1010, 1975.

Hitzig, W. H.: Congenital thymic and lymphocyte deficiency disorders. *In* E. R. Stiehm and V. Fulginiti (eds.): Immunologic Disorders in Infants and Children. Philadelphia, W. B. Saunders Co., 1973.

Kirkpatrick, C. H., and Montes, L. F.: Chronic mucocutaneous candidiasis. J. Cutan. Pathol., *1*:211, 1974.

Lischner, H. W., and DiGeorge, A. M.: Role of the thymus in humoral immunity. Lancet, *2*:1044, 1969.

Peterson, R. D. A., Cooper, M. D., and Good, R. A.: Lymphoid tissue abnormalities associated with ataxia-telangiectasia. Am. J. Med., *41*:342, 1966.

Schlegel, R. J., Bernier, G. M., Bellanti, J. A., Maybee, D. A., Osborne, G. B., Steward, J. C., Pearlman, D. S., Ovelette, J., and Biehusen, F. C.: Severe candidiasis associated with thymic dysplasia, IgA deficiency and plasma antilymphocyte effects. Pediatrics, *45*:926, 1970.

Complement Deficiency Disorders

Johnston, R. B., and Stroud, R. M.: Complement and host defense against infection. J. Pediatr., *90*, 169, 1977.

Phagocyte Deficiency Disorders

Bellanti, J. A., and Dayton, D. H.: The Phagocytic Cell in Host Resistance. New York, Raven, 1975.

McPhail, L. C., DeChatelet, L. R., Shirley, P. S., Wilfert, C., Johnson, R. B., Jr., and McCall, C. E.: Deficiency of NADPH oxidase activity in chronic granulomatous disease. J. Pediatr., *90*:213, 1977.

Greenberg, P. L., Box, I., Levin, J., and Andrews, T. M.: Alteration of colony-stimulating factor output, endotoxemia, and granulopoiesis in cyclic neutropenia. Am. J. Hematol., *1*:375, 1976.

Kander, E., and Mauer, A. M.: Neutropenias of childhood. J. Pediatr., *69*:147, 1966.

Therapy

Buckley, R. H.: Replacement therapy for prevention and treatment of pulmonary infections. *In* C. H. Kirkpatrick and H. Y. Reynolds (eds.): Immunologic and Infectious Reactions in the Lung. New York, M. Dekker, 1976, pp. 335–353.

Kirkpatrick, C. H.: The nature of transfer factor and its clinical efficacy in the management of cutaneous disorders. J. Invest. Dermatol., *67*:425, 1976.

Goldstein, A. L., et al.: Use of thymosin in the treatment of primary immunodeficiency diseases and cancer. Med. Clin. North Am., *60*:591, 1976.

Gelfand, J. A., et al.: Treatment of hereditary angioedema with danazol. N. Engl. J. Med., *295*:1444, 1976.

Chapter 23

IMMUNOPROPHYLAXIS: THE USE OF VACCINES

Joseph A. Bellanti, M.D.,
and John B. Robbins, M.D.

The use of vaccines, or immunoprophylaxis, began as a result of the realization that individuals recovering from a specific infectious disease did not contract that disease again. The use of killed or attenuated organisms or their products has been shown to be an effective method for increasing host resistance to infectious diseases. As Edsall so aptly put it, "Never in the history of human progress has a better and cheaper method of preventing illness been developed than immunization at its best" (Fig. 23–1).

Since Jenner's discovery of the resistance to smallpox after cowpox infection (vaccination) (Fig. 23–2), many other vaccines and various modes of application have been developed that are based on the principles and mechanisms of immunology described in Sections One and Two. During the last century, increasing emphasis was placed on the development of both viral and bacterial vaccines in the hope of eliminating disease (Figs. 23–3, 23–4, and 23–5).

During the 1930's, however, the effective use of chemotherapy and antibiotics seemed to diminish the necessity for the further development of bacterial vaccines. Since these therapeutic agents were not effective against viral diseases, the major emphasis of vaccine development centered on antiviral vaccines. However, the slow emergence of antibiotic-resistant bacteria gradually assumed widespread clinical significance. This resistance to antibiotics resulted in a resurgence of interest in the development of new bacterial vaccines. Lessons from previous experiences (some of them unfortunate) demonstrate the need for an understanding of the basic mechanisms of immunology so that new approaches to immunoprophylaxis can be used effectively.

The most significant use of vaccines has been in the prevention of viral diseases; one of immunology's greatest triumphs has been the eradication of certain fatal and crippling diseases of man, such as poliomyelitis. This overall progress in vaccine development has not been without cost, however. For almost every new vaccine that has been developed, an adverse reaction has been described. Moreover, several

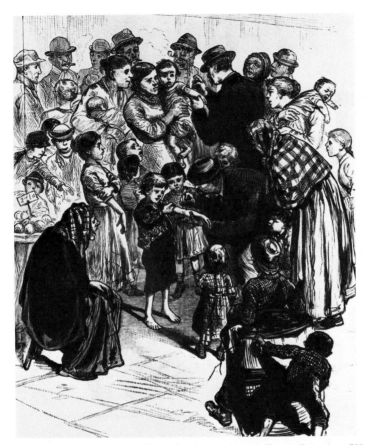

Figure 23–1. Compulsory public vaccination against smallpox. (Courtesy of National Library of Medicine.)

new problems surround the development and use of new vaccines, e.g., swine influenza virus vaccine, as well as vaccines currently available, e.g., measles vaccine. These problems include a wide range of complex issues that require a much broader dialogue among groups such as the government, health personnel, vaccine manufacturers, lawyers, social scientists, ethicists, and the public. Thus, the physician must be ever cognizant not only of the principles of immunology that are the basis of vaccines and their adverse effects but also of the broader social issues surrounding their use.

PRINCIPLES OF ACTIVE IMMUNIZATION

The use of vaccines is based on the stimulation of an immune response within a host (active immunization), in contrast to the transfer

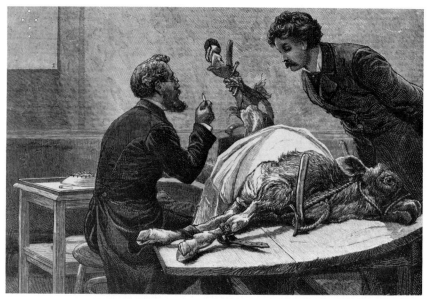

Figure 23-2.   Early scene showing preparation of smallpox vaccine. (Courtesy of National Library of Medicine.)

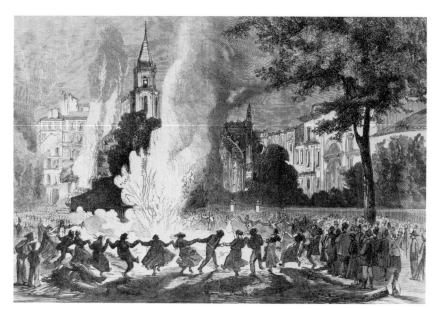

Figure 23-3.   Early scene at Marseilles showing folklore ritual in an attempt at cholera eradication by dancing and fire. (From Harper's Weekly, 9:724, 1865; courtesy of National Library of Medicine.)

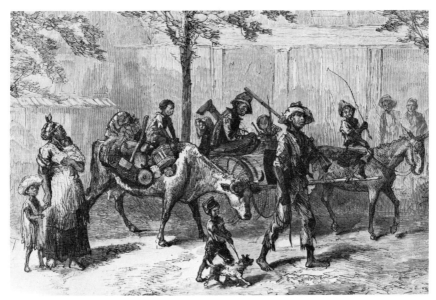

Figure 23-4. Scene of flight from yellow fever epidemic in Kansas. (From Harper's Weekly, *23*:652, 1879; courtesy of National Library of Medicine.)

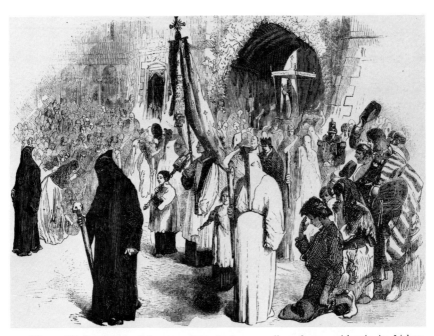

Figure 23-5. Penitential procession during a yellow fever epidemic in Lisbon, Portugal. (From Harper's Weekly, *2*:109, 1858; courtesy of National Library of Medicine.)

of preformed antibody or products of the immune response (passive immunization) (Chapter 7). The meaning of the term vaccine (*vacca:* L., cow), referring to jennerian vaccination with cowpox, has been broadened to include any biologic product prepared from micro-organisms that is useful in the prevention of disease. The term *toxoid* refers to a toxin preparation that has been rendered nontoxic but that still retains its immunogenic properties and is therefore useful as a vaccine. Although active and passive immunization procedures have been applied for the most part to infectious diseases, their application is being tested in other areas, such as the prevention and treatment of malignant disorders (Chapter 19).

GENERAL PRINCIPLES

The ultimate effectiveness or efficacy of a vaccine depends on the degree of protection induced in the immunized host after challenge and is generally determined by instituting a field study in which vaccinated and unvaccinated individuals selected at random are exposed to the same disease risk. The assessment of protection is made by calculating the incidence of disease in both groups. A vaccine is considered effective if it significantly reduces the disease incidence in the immunized group compared to that in the control group. *It should be stressed that the effectiveness of a vaccine is not determined by the induction of serum antibody alone, but rather this determination is made by the demonstration of enhanced protection against disease.*

A knowledge of the pathogenesis of the disease in question is essential in the use of vaccines. Infections may be divided into two major groups: (1) *localized,* which exert their effects at the portal of entry by local replication and inflammatory changes, and (2) *generalized,* which after a limited period of replication at a local site disperse either the organism (bacteria or virus) or its products (toxin) via blood-borne dissemination (Table 23–1).

Localized infections, as illustrated by those produced by the respiratory viruses, are surface infections involving primarily the tissues

TABLE 23–1. Characteristics of Infectious Diseases

	GROUP 1 (localized)	GROUP 2 (generalized)
Site of Pathology	Portal of entry	Systemic
Examples	Respiratory viral infections (influenza)	Diphtheria, measles, poliomyelitis
Incubation Period	Relatively short	Relatively long
Presence of Blood-Borne Phase	Negative	Positive
Duration of Immunity	Short or unknown	Usually lifelong
Immunity Mechanism	Local antibody (IgA); local CMI	Humoral antibody (IgG, IgM); systemic CMI

at the portal of entry. In general, the latent period between exposure and appearance of symptoms is short (days). Blood-borne dissemination of organisms or toxin is unusual, in spite of any generalized symptoms. Since the local tissues seem to be the primary sites of inflammation, local factors of immunity appear to be of major importance, e.g., local IgA and local cell-mediated immunity (CMI).

Systemic infections include diseases such as diphtheria and the childhood exanthems that are associated with relatively longer incubation periods. Since these diseases involve a more complex pathogenesis, with passage of the organisms or toxins through the bloodstream, the primary immunity mechanism appears to be effected by serum antibody of the IgG, IgM, and IgA varieties, as well as systemic cell-mediated immunity (CMI).

In general, the most effective vaccines are those that most closely simulate the recovery of protective mechanisms seen in the natural disease. For example, protection in many respiratory infections, such as parainfluenza type 1, has been shown to correlate better with the presence of IgA-associated antibody in the respiratory tract than with that of serum IgG antibody. Vaccines effective in localized viral infections are those that stimulate the local immune responses. On the other hand, the presence of serum IgG antidiphtheria antitoxin following active immunization has been shown to be correlated with clinical protection from this generalized disease.

DURATION OF PROTECTION

Perhaps the most important advantage of active immunization over passive immunization is its longer duration of protection. The host is protected after an appropriate time lapse (latent period), following which immunity is detected (Chapter 7). This protection is associated with many of the factors of immunity (cellular and humoral) but is usually measured *in vitro* by the presence of serum antibody. Unlike the case in passive immunity, in which the duration of serum antibody is relatively short, levels of antibody after active immunization are detected for several months and, in some cases, for years.

The response associated with the initial encounter with vaccine is referred to as *primary immunization*. The initial immunoglobulin responses detected in serum are of the IgM class; later, IgG antibody is found. The IgA class of antibody seems to appear as an intermediate phase between IgM and IgG (Chapters 7 and 16).

Following subsequent exposure of the immunized host to the same or a similar antigen in the form of a vaccine or natural disease, there is a rapid recall of antibody production that occurs much sooner, involves a shorter latent period, and attains much higher levels of antibody. This response is referred to as an *anamnestic, secondary,* or *booster response* (Chapter 7). During this secondary response, the major antibody component in serum is of the IgG variety; the IgM is present, but in diminished amount.

It is important to stress that the ability to demonstrate this recall phenomenon occurs after stimulation not only with the same antigen but also with closely related antigens. For example, certain strains of influenza change antigenically and are responsible for recurring epidemics (Chapter 16). This changed antigenicity may involve new antigenic specificities while retaining antigens found in earlier strains. Thus, upon encounter with an influenza variant, an individual may elicit a primary response to the new antigenic determinants along with a booster effect to the older antigenic specificities of previous strains, i.e., the doctrine of "original antigenic sin" proposed by Francis. This booster effect is one explanation of enhanced resistance seen in older persons who have had prior antigenic experience with related strains.

STATUS OF ANTIGEN

Another principle underlying the use of active immunization is the status of the immunogen itself (Chapter 4). In general, vaccines that contain virulent, attenuated, or "live," organisms are more effective than inactivated or killed preparations. This enhanced effect is manifested by a greater degree of initial protection and a longer duration of immunity. After the use of inactivated influenza vaccine, for example, protection may be noted, but influenza can occur in immunized individuals. Infections with yellow fever, on the other hand, are generally prevented in individuals receiving the live yellow fever vaccine. The reasons for this enhanced efficacy of live vaccines are unclear but may be related to destruction of critical antigens during the preparation of inactivated vaccine, e.g., neuraminidase of swine influenza virus vaccine. Another explanation is that duration of immunity seems to be favored by antigens that persist. Live vaccines contain antigens capable of sustained persistence and prolonged immunogenic effect.

Immunization with certain types of inactivated vaccines (measles and respiratory syncytial virus vaccines) can also be followed by serious untoward responses seen after subsequent exposure to virus in nature. These reactions are tertiary manifestations of the immune response due to prior sensitization with killed vaccine that result in hypersensitivity rather than protective immunity and are described in detail below.

SIMULTANEOUS ADMINISTRATION OF VACCINES

Another principle that has practical relevance to whether vaccines may be administered simultaneously is the phenomenon of interference. If a live viral vaccine is given and a different live vaccine is administered thereafter, the second immunization may be inhibited. This effect appears to be mediated by the antiviral mechanism of interferon

(Chapter 16). Interference has been demonstrated in the human with measles, smallpox, and poliovirus vaccines. For example, if one administers smallpox vaccine to an individual immediately after administering measles vaccine, there will be a reduction in the number of successful immunizations. Similarly, successful immunization with live oral poliovirus vaccine may be inhibited if immunization is carried out during community epidemics of enterovirus infections. Because of this problem of interference, immunization with live viral vaccines should be postponed if significant intercurrent infections exist. Although the simultaneous administration of live virus vaccines was not recommended previously because of this problem of virus interference, more recent studies have indicated that combined virus vaccines given at the same or separate sites are as effective as administration of individual vaccines. From a practical standpoint, therefore, the phenomenon of interference does not appear to present a major obstacle in the design of vaccine programs, and several viral vaccines may be administered simultaneously with good efficacy, e.g., measles, mumps, and rubella (MMR) vaccine. In addition, inactivated vaccines (e.g., bacterial vaccines) can be administered simultaneously at different sites. It should be pointed out, however, that when vaccines that individually have side-effects are combined, the adverse effects of the combination may be accentuated.

ROUTES OF ADMINISTRATION

Most vaccines are administered by the parenteral route regardless of their natural portal of entry (Table 23–2). There are notable exceptions to this general statement. For example, live, oral poliovirus vaccine is given via the enteric route and yellow fever vaccine is given by the parenteral route—the natural portal of entry of the respective pathogens.

In addition to those listed in Table 23–2, there are new approaches

TABLE 23–2. Route of Administration of Vaccine

EXAMPLE OF VACCINE	VACCINE ROUTE*	NATURAL PORTAL OF ENTRY
Rubeola	I.M.	Respiratory Tract
Rubella	I.M.	
Influenza	I.M.	
Poliovirus (Sabin)	P.O.	Gastrointestinal Tract
Poliovirus (Salk)	I.M.	
Smallpox	I.D.	Respiratory Tract
Rabies	I.M.	Skin (neural)
Yellow fever	I.M.	Skin (blood-borne)

*I.M. = intramuscular
I.D. = intradermal
P.O. = oral

to immunoprophylaxis being introduced, such as the local application of antigen in the respiratory tract. Intranasal immunization has been shown to stimulate local IgA immune mechanisms. These applications are currently being investigated in the case of influenza, rubella, and respiratory syncytial virus vaccines. Thus, a more durable immunity that is similar to the responses seen following natural infection may be attained.

IMMUNOLOGIC STATUS OF THE HOST

Another important principle guiding immunization procedures is the immunologic competence and reactivity of the host. The significance is apparent when the developmental immaturity of the young infant and the clinical entities in which underlying immunologic or physiological deficiencies exist (Chapter 22) are considered.

Previously, infants were believed to be incapable of eliciting an immune response; this was attributed to physiological or immunologic immaturity of the young host. This widely held view led to the tacit assumption that small infants could not be immunized successfully. Fortunately, this fallacy was corrected as a result of many studies that clearly demonstrated the immunologic responsiveness of the young infant (Fig. 23–6). There are, however, quantitative and qualitative differences from adult responses. A pattern of prolonged or exclusive macroglobulin synthesis was shown to be the hallmark of the immature

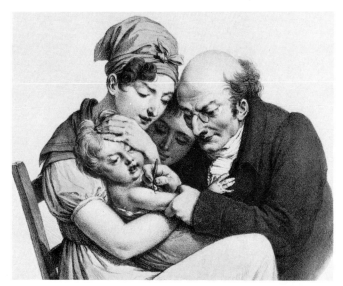

Figure 23–6. Vaccination of an infant with smallpox vaccine. (From L. L. Boilly, 1827; courtesy of National Library of Medicine.)

immunologic response and is seen after immunization of the young infant and after intrauterine infections of the fetus (rubella, cytomegalovirus infection, toxoplasmosis, and syphilis). This pattern of prolonged IgM antibody synthesis lasts for varying intervals and is different from the IgG response characteristic of the adult.

The inhibitory effect of passively acquired antibody is another example of the effect of the host's immunologic reactivity to subsequent immunization procedures (Chapter 10). Passively acquired antibody can be obtained through (1) transplacental transfer of maternal IgG antibody, (2) passive immunization by serum gamma globulin through immunoprophylaxis, or (3) transfer of antibody in breast milk.

The placental transfer of maternal IgG globulins to the infant occurs readily and provides the newborn with a rich source of preformed antibodies from the maternal circulation. There is great variability, however, in the types of antibodies obtained in this manner (Table 23–3). This is in part reflective of the quantity and molecular size of antibody in the maternal circulation. For example, the low molecular weight IgG antibodies (e.g., rubeola antibody) present in high concentration in maternal serum are readily transferred; IgG antibodies present in lower concentration (e.g., antibody to *Bordetella pertussis*) are poorly transferred; and macroglobulin antibodies (e.g., Wassermann antibody) are excluded.

In addition to providing the newborn with protection, these passively acquired IgG antibodies may interfere with active antibody synthesis following certain immunization procedures. This observation is relevant to the design of immunization schedules for infants, particularly with regard to certain live viral vaccines. From a practical standpoint, the effectiveness of beginning immunization procedures with killed vaccines, e.g., diphtheria, pertussis, and tetanus (DPT), in infants two to three months old does not appear to be appreciably inhibited by passive antibody. The passively acquired antibody can

TABLE 23–3.   Relationship of Antibody Type with
Transplacental Transfer

Good Passive Transfer	Poor Passive Transfer	No Passive Transfer
Diphtheria antitoxin	*Hemophilus influenzae*	Enteric somatic (0) antibodies
Tetanus antitoxin	*Bacillus pertussis*	(salmonella, shigella, *E. coli*)
Antierythrogenic toxin	Dysentery	Skin-sensitizing antibody
Antistaphylococcal antibody	Streptococcus MG	Heterophil antibody
Salmonella flagella (H) antibody		Wassermann antibody
Antistreptolysin		
All the antiviral antibodies present in maternal circulation (rubeola, rubella, mumps, poliovirus)		

inhibit successful immunization of infants with parenteral live virus vaccines; therefore, such live virus immunization procedures should be delayed until the age of 15 months. Since oral poliovirus vaccines are given by the enteric route, they are not inhibited by serum IgG poliovirus antibody and therefore can be effectively administered to infants at two to four months of age.

Another situation in which passively acquired antibody may interfere with active antibody synthesis is in the case of "natural" immunity acquired by the newborn from breast milk. Although not absorbed, this IgA antibody may provide local immunity to many enteric pathogens. Large quantities of this local antibody present in the gastrointestinal tract may neutralize virus; however, breast-fed infants have recently been shown to be capable of successful immunization with oral poliovirus vaccines while receiving breast milk.

The status of the immune response not only affects the success of the primary immunization procedures but also may contribute to adverse effects. These adverse effects are seen primarily following the use of live vaccines and predominantly in those individuals with depressed immune function, and are described below.

PHYSICOCHEMICAL STATE OF THE ANTIGEN

There are several other factors that determine the overall immunogenicity of a vaccine, including the size and complexity of the antigen and its physical state (Chapter 4). The larger and more complex the molecule is, the greater is its immunogenicity. In general, soluble proteins are poorer immunogens than those rendered insoluble or those enhanced through the use of adjuvants (Chapter 10).

THE USE OF VACCINES

INDICATIONS FOR USE

Immunization should be instituted in those population groups that have (1) the least protection, (2) the highest rates of exposure to a given pathogen, and (3) the greatest risk of disease or its complications. For the most part, immunization procedures are used to prevent diseases in situations for which there are no other satisfactory means of treatment, e.g., viral diseases. The population groups at greatest risk to disease are determined by the following factors.

Age

In general, the population groups that are at greatest risk and have the least protection are at either end of the age spectrum—the very young and the very old. The very young are susceptible by virtue of their immunologic immaturity; the old are vulnerable because of waning immunity or secondary degenerative diseases that predispose them to illness, e.g., cardiac disease.

Ecology

Certain population groups are at greater risk by virtue of their environment. These groups include (1) *institutionalized individuals* in whom there is greater risk of hepatitis, influenza, and respiratory diseases, and (2) *military recruits,* who are predisposed to acute respiratory diseases. Individuals are also placed at increased risk by virtue of travel to foreign countries where they may have a greater exposure to new and exotic pathogens such as those producing cholera, plague, and dysentery. Environmental pollutants that are directly deleterious or function as chronic irritants (e.g., smog) also place the host at greater risk of infection.

Status of the Host

Physiological states, such as pregnancy, increase the risk of contracting diseases such as influenza and poliomyelitis. Individuals with chronic diseases of the lungs or heart (e.g., cystic fibrosis or congenital heart disease) are predisposed to serious complications of respiratory viral infections. Because of their increased risk, these groups should be adequately immunized.

PREPARATIONS AND IMMUNIZATION SCHEDULES

The commonly used vaccines and their optimal time of administration are listed in Table 23–4; the primary immunization of infants and children is given in Table 23–5. Broadly speaking, the currently available vaccines comprise two major categories: (1) nonreplicative and (2) replicative vaccines (Table 23–6).

Nonreplicative Vaccines

The nonreplicative vaccines are killed or "inactivated" and contain microorganisms or their products (Table 23–6). They include most of the currently used bacterial vaccines, e.g., diphtheria, pertussis (whooping cough), and tetanus vaccines (DPT) and also some viral vaccines, e.g., inactivated poliovirus (IPV). Recently, capsular polysaccharide

TABLE 23–4. Commonly Used Vaccines

	PREPARATION	COMMENTS
Bacterial		
Diphtheria		
Pertussis	Inactivated	Infancy and childhood
Tetanus		
Pneumococcal	Polysaccharide	
Meningococcal		
H. influenzae		
BCG	Live	Used only under certain circumstances
Cholera		
Salmonella	Inactivated	
Plague		
Viral		
Smallpox	Live—calf lymph	
Poliomyelitis	Live—Sabin (OPV); Salk (IPV)	Recommended in infancy and children
Rubeola	Live	
Rubella	Live	
Mumps	Live	
Rabies	Inactivated	
Influenza	Inactivated	
Yellow fever	Live	Used only under special circumstances
Adenovirus	Inactivated	
	Live (not licensed, used only in military)	
Rickettsial		
Typhus	Inactivated	Used only under special circumstances
Rocky Mountain spotted fever	Inactivated	

TABLE 23–5. Recommended Schedule for Active Immunization and Tuberculin Testing for Normal Infants and Children*

2 months	DTP—Trivalent OPV
4 months	DTP—Trivalent OPV
6 months	DTP—Trivalent OPV
15 months	Tuberculin test—live measles, mumps, rubella vaccine
18 months	DTP—Trivalent OPV
4–6 years	DTP—Trivalent OPV
14–16 years	Td
Thereafter	Td every 10 years

*Recommendations of the Committee on Infectious Diseases, American Academy of Pediatrics, J.A.M.A., *237*:2228–2230, 1977.

TABLE 23–6. Classification of Vaccines

	NONREPLICATIVE (Killed or Inactivated Vaccines)	REPLICATIVE (Live, Attenuated Vaccines)
Example	Bacterial (DPT) Some viral (poliovirus, measles, influenza)	Viral (yellow fever, vaccinia, rubeola, rubella, mumps, and poliovirus)
Immunization principle	Preformed antigenic mass	Self-replicative
Effect of passive antibody	No inhibitory effect	May prevent successful immunization
Duration of immunity	Relatively short; requires "boosters"	Relatively long (mimic natural infection); do not usually require boosters
Prime immunity mechanism	Humoral IgG	Humoral IgG; local IgA

vaccines have been investigated for use in specialized circumstances of exposure and include pneumococcal, meningococcal, and *Haemophilus influenzae* polysaccharide vaccines; these are described below. These nonreplicative vaccines rely on the ability of a preformed antigenic mass to stimulate serum antibody. There is no further increase of the antigen through replication; the duration of vaccine effect may be prolonged by use of adjuvants. Because a large antigenic mass is delivered, these vaccines appear to be unaffected by the presence of circulating antibody. The duration of immunity is relatively short, however, and boosters of additional vaccine are required to maintain adequate levels of serum antibody. The primary immunity mechanism that appears to be stimulated is antibody of the serum IgG variety, the type of immunity mechanism shown to be most effective in those infections whose pathogenesis involves a blood-borne phase. Since these vaccines are inactivated, they do not possess the hazards of the live vaccines. They do, however, have certain undesirable properties, including toxic and hypersensitivity reactions, described below.

Capsular Polysaccharide Vaccines.

Encapsulated bacteria, including *Diplococcus pneumoniae, Neisseria meningitidis, Haemophilus influenzae* type b, *Escherichia coli*, and Group B beta hemolytic streptococci, cause disease primarily because of their invasive properties (Chapter 14). This invasive property is due to their polysaccharide capsule. Although the overall physical and chemical properties of capsular polysaccharides are similar, there is a high degree of specificity related to this property of invasiveness. Thus, although there are 83 different pneumococcal types, most disease is caused by 15 to 20 types. Similarly for meningococci, most disease is caused by Groups A, B, and C (each denotes a capsular polysaccharide). The mechanism by which the capsular polysaccharide exerts its activity is interference with effective phagocytosis. A direct effect on leukocyte opsonization and an interference with the C1 complement component have been demonstrated. However, in the presence of specific anticapsular antibodies of the IgM and IgG immunoglobulin classes, effective opsonization can occur. The remarkable susceptibility of individuals with X-linked hypogammaglobulinemia to repeated infection with encapsulated bacteria and the successful treatment of such patients with passive immunization with pooled immunoglobulin provide evidence for the protective activity of serum antibody (Chapter 22). Also, the recently reported susceptibility of individuals with C3 deficiency to repeated disease with encapsulated bacteria and individuals with C7 and C8 deficiencies to repeated neisserial infections, including meningococcal meningitis, emphasizes the critical protective role of these immune components.

Success in preventing serious disease, including meningitis and pneumonia, has been achieved by immunization of children and adults with pneumococcal and meningococcal capsular polysaccharides. Preliminary evidence indicates the efficacy of multivalent pneumococcal vaccines in prevention of the sepsis in patients with sickle cell anemia. Currently, both Group A and Group C meningococcal polysaccharide vaccines are licensed for limited use in individuals over the age of two years in the United States. Their use has been confined to case contacts in outbreaks and individuals traveling to high-risk areas. Group C vaccine is used for routine immunization of U.S. Armed Forces recruits. Efficacy for *Haemophilus influenzae* type b vaccine has been verified in individuals over the age of 18 months. Unfortunately, the highest attack rate of this common childhood disease (about two-thirds of the cases) occurs in infants less than 18 months of age.

The immune response to purified capsular polysaccharide may be characterized in general terms, with several exceptions. Capsular polysaccharides are simple polymers of one or as many as five monosaccharides. This property of a simple repeating polymer is most likely related to its property of a T-cell-independent antigen (Chapters 4 and 7). Thus, the T-cell activities of memory and helper effect upon rechallenge are not induced by the capsular polysaccharide. Subcutaneous injection of older children or adults with a wide dosage range of these capsular polysaccharide antigens results in a rapid rise in serum antibodies of all immunoglobulin classes to a maximal level in about two to four weeks. Thereafter, this level declines slowly so that at least one half of the original maximum is detected many years later. Reinjection may bring this lower level to the maximum observed after primary immunization. One explanation for this prolonged synthesis is the observation that most capsular polysaccharides are poorly or not entirely degraded by mammalian enzymes. In animal experiments, some polysaccharides are demonstrable in the tissues for the life of the animal. This lack of a booster response poses a difficult problem for scientists concerned with the induction of protective immunity in infants, those individuals with the highest attack rate.

There are several exceptions to these principles. The first is that meningococcal Group B and *Escherichia coli* K1 polysaccharides, both homopolymers of N-acetyl α 2,8–linked sialic acid, are nonimmunogenic in adults. Second are the curious observations concerning the immune response of young infants to meningococcal Group A and Group C polysaccharides. For meningococcal Group A, reinjection provides a booster response that is demonstrable up to the age of two years. This vaccine has been shown to be effective against Group A meningitis in this age group. For meningococcal Group C, a primary injection may result in suppression of the secondary injection in children up to two years. The precise basis for this is not clear, but animal work suggests that these capsular polysaccharide immunogens may interact with T-cells to release suppressor substances, and this may be dominant early in development.

Replicative Vaccines

The replicative vaccines in current use are live or attenuated viruses and include yellow fever, smallpox, trivalent oral poliovirus (TOPV),

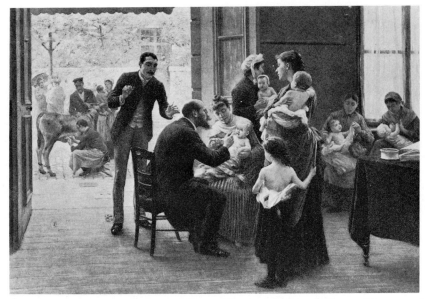

Figure 23-7. Administration of live smallpox vaccine by Scalbert. (Courtesy of National Library of Medicine.)

rubeola, rubella, and mumps vaccines. They also include some of the live, attenuated bacterial vaccines, such as the BCG. In general, these vaccines have been shown to mimic the immunologic events that follow natural infection and lead to a more durable immunity than the nonreplicative vaccines. Normally, they do not require subsequent booster immunizations. The immunogenic potential of these live vaccines is related to their ability to be self-replicative, so that even small infective doses still obtain satisfactory immunogenic responses. Most live vaccines are given by the parenteral route, either by intramuscular injection (rubeola, rubella, and mumps) or by intradermal scarification (smallpox) (Fig. 23-7). Some are given by their natural portal of entry, e.g., oral poliovirus. The serious drawbacks of the replicative vaccines are that they are living and are subject to mutation to more virulent forms or production of devastating effects, particularly in hosts with underlying diseases or altered immunity.

COMPLICATIONS OF ACTIVE IMMUNIZATION

It has become apparent that a number of vaccine side-effects are being seen with increasing frequency (Fig. 23-8). This is due to the increase in number of vaccines available to the physician; also, the complications of a vaccine can be adequately evaluated only after several years have lapsed. The decision to use a vaccine must be made therefore

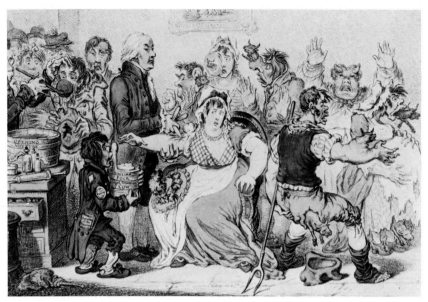

Figure 23–8. Fantasy depicting the side-effects of vaccination with cowpox by John Gillray. (Courtesy of National Library of Medicine.)

by weighing the risk of complications from the vaccine against the morbidity and mortality of the disease itself. Routine smallpox vaccination has been discontinued in the United States because it now appears that the disease is virtually eradicated here; moreover, the incidence of complications from the vaccine is higher than the risk of contracting smallpox. The wisdom of this decision will require the passage of time.

Many vaccines that have been introduced are accompanied by both *immunologic* and *nonimmunologic* complications. These are given in Table 23–7.

NONIMMUNOLOGIC COMPLICATIONS

Nonimmunologic complications are related to *host response* or to properties of the *vaccine.*

Host Response

Perhaps the most common complication seen following immunization is a local reaction occurring at the site of inoculation. It consists of localized swelling and tenderness and may be accompanied by systemic symptoms (fever) that are usually seen within the first 24 hours and seem to be related to the toxic properties of the vaccine itself. In the case of a small infant, these signs may be associated with high fever and sometimes with convulsions. Febrile convulsions occur so frequently in

TABLE 23–7.   Adverse Effects of Vaccines

Type	Example	Example of Vaccine	Pathogenetic Mechanism(s)
Nonimmunologic effects			
Host response	Localized reactions: swelling	DPT	
	Generalized reactions: Pyrogenic or febrile reactions	DPT	Toxins and other contaminating materials
	Eczema vaccinatum	Smallpox	Break in integrity of skin; (?) T-cell defect
Vaccine response	Adventitious agents; potential oncogenic effect of SV-40	Salk (IPV)	Constituents of vaccine
	Paralytic poliomyelitis	Sabin (OPV)	Reversion of virulence; lack of sufficient attenuation; higher incidence in children with hypogammaglobulinemia
Immunologic effects			
Immunologically compromised hosts	Progressive vaccinia	Smallpox	Primary or secondary immunodeficiency, e.g., T-cell
	Disseminated BCG	Bacille Calmette-Guérin (BCG)	
	Infection of fetal tissues following immunization in pregnancy	Smallpox Rubella (?not proved)	Diminished CMI during pregnancy; greater susceptibility of fetal tissues to infection; immunologic immaturity of the fetus
Allergic (atopic) hosts	Anaphylaxis due to egg sensitivity	Influenza	Contamination of vaccine with egg proteins leading to Type I immunologic injury
Normal hosts (effects related to nature of antigen or route of administration)	Postinfectious or postvaccinal encephalomyelitis	Rabies, smallpox, mumps, measles	Type IV (cell-mediated ?)
	Urticaria or Arthus reaction	Tetanus toxoid	Type I or III
Normal hosts (?)	Atypical measles	Killed measles	Type III, Type IV (?) injury
	RSV bronchiolitis	Killed RSV vaccine	Type I, III, IV
	Arthritis	Rubella	Unknown
	Thrombocytopenia	Rubella, rubeola	Unknown
	SSPE	Rubeola, rubella (?)	Unknown
	Stevens-Johnson syndrome	Smallpox	Unknown
	Erythema multiforme	Smallpox	Unknown
	Guillain-Barré syndrome	Swine influenza	Unknown

infants with cerebral damage that immunization procedures should be postponed for one year.

Rarely, in infants under one year of age, a poorly understood encephalopathy occurs following the use of pertussis vaccine. This is usually seen within a few days after the first inoculation and is manifested by convulsions and coma. The precise mechanism of this entity is not understood, but it does not appear to be mediated by any of the known mechanisms of immunologic injury. Thus, when an infant requires a second DPT inoculation the volume of the next injection should be reduced if fever, somnolence, or adverse local reactions occurred after the initial immunization. If a convulsion occurred, no further injections of pertussis vaccine should be given.

Another type of nonimmunologic complication related to host response is that of vaccinial spread to the lesions of eczema (eczema vaccinatum). Infants with eczema or other breaks in the continuity of the skin (burns) should not be immunized with smallpox vaccine because of the danger of spread. Furthermore, siblings of infants with eczema should not be vaccinated unless they can be physically removed from the patient for several days. The use of vaccinia immune globulin (VIG) has been recommended for this complication of eczema vaccinatum (Chapter 24).

Properties of the Vaccine

Other complications of a nonimmunologic nature appear to be related to the properties of the vaccine itself (Table 23–7). Since viral vaccines are grown in tissue culture or eggs, there is an opportunity for viruses indigenous to the tissue to contaminate the vaccine. Such an occurrence was described in 1960 when a monkey virus (simian virus-40 [SV-40]) was found to contaminate many lots of monkey kidney tissue used to produce inactivated and attenuated poliovirus vaccines. Since SV-40 had been shown to induce tumors in newborn hamsters, potential danger lay in the fact that millions of people in the United States and abroad had received this virus during the course of poliovirus vaccination. Fortunately, there have been no recognized problems with human neoplasms to date. This experience, however, has caused a greater awareness of the potential complications related to vaccine quality.

A more serious problem was observed in 1962, shortly after the licensure of Type III oral poliovirus vaccine, when a number of cases of paralytic poliomyelitis occurred in temporal association with administration of live poliovirus vaccine. A formal report issued by the Surgeon General of the Public Health Service, based on the finding of his advisory committee, revealed that a small but significant number of cases were due to the vaccine itself. The mechanism of this response appeared to be related to a reversion of the attenuated virus vaccine to a more neurovirulent form. This complication continues to occur in both the immunized subject and the household contacts of infants fed oral poliovirus vaccines. Most of the cases occurred in older individuals. It is currently recommended, therefore, that immunization with live oral poliovirus vaccines not be routinely performed in individuals over the age of 18 years. Recently, infants and children with hypogammaglobu-linemia were shown to be at particular risk of developing vaccine-associated paralytic disease with an incidence estimated to be 10,000 times greater than that of normal children (Chapter 22).

IMMUNOLOGIC COMPLICATIONS

The immunologic complications that follow the use of vaccines are those occurring in either immunologically deficient hosts or those with normal immune mechanisms in whom immunologic factors play a role (Table 23–7). For ease of discussion, the adverse effects to vaccines may be divided into (1) those effects that are seen in immunologically compromised hosts, (2) those hypersensitivity reactions that are seen predominantly in allergic (atopic) individuals, (3) those effects that are seen in normal hosts and appear to be related to the nature of the antigen or the route of administration, and (4) those effects that are seen in normal hosts and whose pathogenesis is unclear but may have an immunologic basis.

Adverse Effects Seen in Immunologically Compromised Hosts

Not only does the status of the immune response affect the success of primary immunization, but it also may contribute to its adverse effects. These are usually seen after the use of live vaccines and predominantly in individuals with depressed immune function. For example, progressive vaccinia (vaccinia necrosum or vaccinia gangren-osa) has been observed in children with defects in the thymic-dependent limb of immunity, such as severe combined immunodeficiency (Fig. 23–9A). This rare, but highly fatal complication of smallpox immuniza-tion consists of a failure of the primary lesion to heal normally, with progressive spread to adjacent areas of skin (Fig. 23–9B and C). With necrosis of tissue, new lesions develop over a period of months, often involving metastatic lesions to other parts of the body, such as bone and viscera. This complication carries a high mortality and has been observed predominantly in children with immunologic deficiency of the thymic- (T-) dependent type (Chapter 22). It has also been seen in secondary immunologic deficiency, e.g., in leukemia, in lymphoma, and in patients receiving immunosuppressive therapy. The basis for this tragic complication appears to be a specific deficiency of the immune

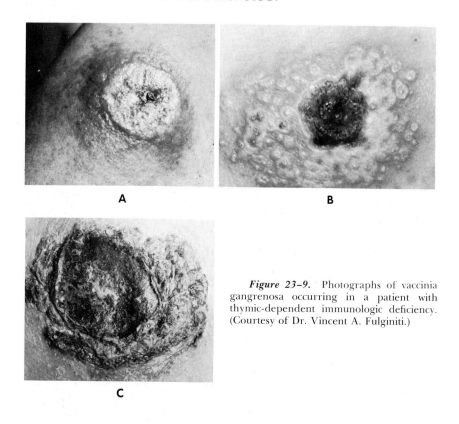

A   B

C

Figure 23-9. Photographs of vaccinia gangrenosa occurring in a patient with thymic-dependent immunologic deficiency. (Courtesy of Dr. Vincent A. Fulginiti.)

system, particularly of cell-mediated immunity. The recommended treatment with vaccinia immune globulin (VIG) alone, therefore, is not totally satisfactory, and immunologic reconstitution through transplantation of immunocompetent cells or transfer factor may be more effective (Chapter 24).

Another example of a vaccine complication related to an underlying immunologic deficiency is the fatal giant cell (Hecht cell) pneumonia reported in children exposed to measles or receiving live measles vaccine. This has been described in children with primary immunodeficiency diseases and in malnourished children, particularly in the developing countries of the world. These children fail to develop the rash of measles and specific measles-neutralizing antibody and subsequently die. Although these children appear to be deficient in both cell-mediated and humoral immunity, the deficiency in cellular immunity appears to be of more frequent occurrence and of greater import in these reactions.

Pregnancy also constitutes an altered physiologic state in which the use of certain live vaccines, such as smallpox or rubella, is contraindicated because of the possibilities of infection of the fetus and a more severe spread of virus. In the case of rubella immunization, exposure of the immunized pregnant woman to wild virus has been associated with the finding of wild virus shedding in the recipient, but no reports of congenital rubella syndrome in infants delivered by a previously vaccinated woman have been verified. The general status of cell-mediated immunity has recently been shown to decrease during pregnancy, particularly with respect to certain viruses, such as rubella and cytomegalovirus, which may account for the increased susceptibility of the pregnant female to certain live viral vaccines.

It is apparent from these unfortunate experiences that individuals with impaired immunologic reactivity, on the basis of either *primary* or *acquired* causes, should not receive live vaccines. Recent descriptions of overwhelming viral infections in patients receiving antilymphocyte serum add another example to the list of the "right treatment for the wrong patient."

Adverse Hypersensitivity Reactions Seen Predominantly in Allergic (Atopic) Individuals

Since many vaccines are grown in tissue culture or eggs, e.g., viral vaccines, there is an opportunity for them to be contaminated with heterologous tissues, proteins, or other foreign substances that can lead to immunologically mediated reactions.

The possible allergens in viral vaccines that could give rise to allergic reactions include (1) those of the host cells in which the virus is grown, (2) those of the medium or its additive, and (3) those foreign antigens that may be added during the preparation and purification of the vaccine, e.g., antibiotics. Most hypersensitivity reactions are seen in atopic individuals and are associated with egg proteins or antibiotics, e.g., penicillin.

Newer techniques in vaccine preparation, such as zonal centrifugation and the use of avian tissue cell culture, appear to have reduced the incidence of severe anaphylactic reactions. Nonetheless, allergic reactions continue to occur, and the physician should be aware of the tissue cultures in which vaccines are grown in order to prevent certain allergic reactions in atopic individuals. Table 23–8 contains a listing of commercially available viral vaccines and the tissue cultures in which they are prepared. Individuals sensitive to eggs may also be allergic to vaccines grown in chick embryo. Screening by history of ability to eat eggs without adverse effects is a reasonable way to identify those individuals possibly at risk of reaction to egg-grown vaccines. Furthermore, if individuals who are allergic to eggs need protection against influenza, for example, a scratch test with the vaccine as antigen can be used as a screening procedure.

TABLE 23–8. Commercially Available Viral Vaccines

Vaccine	Strain	Source	Manufacturer	Brand Name
Influenza	A/Port Chalmers/1/73(H3N2) B/Hong Kong/5/72 A/New Jersey/76 (swine influenza)	chick embryo	Parke-Davis Eli Lilly Wyeth	Fluogen Zonomune
Mumps	Jeryl Lynn	chick embryo cell culture	Lederle Merck, Sharp & Dohme	
Rabies		duck embryo	Eli Lilly	
Rubella	Cenderhill	rabbit kidney cell culture	Dow Smith, Kline & French	Cendevax
	HPV-77, DE-5	duck embryo	Merck, Sharp & Dohme	Meruvax
Rubeola (measles)	Schwartz	chick embryo cell culture	Dow	Lirugen
	Enders-Edmonston (Moralen)	chick embryo cell culture	Merck, Sharp & Dohme	Attenuvax
Vaccinia		chick embryo	Lederle	
		calf lymph tissue	Wyeth Lincoln	Dryvax Monovac
		monkey kidney cell culture	Lederle	Orimune
Poliovirus	Sabin	human diploid (WI-38) cell culture	Pfizer Laboratories	Deplovax

Adverse Effects of Vaccines Seen in Normal Hosts that Appear to be Related to the Nature of the Antigen or the Route of Administration

Postinfectious or postvaccinal encephalomyelitis is the classic example of a disease mediated by cell-mediated hypersensitivity resulting from the use of vaccines or natural infection (Chapter 20C). This disease was originally shown to follow the use of rabies vaccine (Pasteur vaccine), and later was seen following the use of smallpox, measles, and mumps vaccines. Natural viral infections have also been associated with postinfectious encephalitis. The pathogenesis of the encephalitis is believed to be similar to that of experimental allergic encephalitis (EAE) (Chapter 20C). Evidence now supports the view that this type of reaction is related to a delayed-hypersensitivity phenomenon mediated by sensitized T-lymphocytes. Sensitization by these viral vaccines may occur because most viruses associated with this complication contain a lipid envelope. During maturation these viruses are released from infected tissues at cell surfaces (steady-state viruses) (Chapter 16). This virus-host interaction may provide a pathogenetic mechanism of "alteration of self" at the host's cell surface, with the resulting induction of a delayed-hypersensitivity reaction. With rare exceptions, efforts to recover virus from the brain of an individual with postvaccinal encephalitis have been unsuccessful. However, in light of the recent recovery of measles virus from the brain biopsy material from patients with subacute sclerosing panencephalitis (SSPE), the possibility of the so-called "slow viruses" being present in masked form in other entities exists. This possibility may prove to be of importance in the pathogenesis of postvaccinal encephalitis.

Immunologic complications associated with hypersensitivity phenomena mediated by humoral factors occurring in otherwise normal individuals represent another category (Table 23–7). These reactions range from immediate Type I (reaginic) hypersensitivity phenomena, associated with localized urticaria occurring within a few minutes after immunization, to the Arthus or immune-complex type of hypersensitivities (Type III), seen after a more prolonged interval. For example, localized reactions at the site of immunization have been noted in individuals receiving tetanus toxoid. These reactions consist of localized tenderness, redness, and swelling and are believed to be of the Arthus type, induced by antigen-antibody complexes (Chapter 13). Because of these adverse reactions and because protective serum tetanus antitoxin is detectable for as long as 10 years after immunization, it is now recommended that booster injections of tetanus toxoid not be given more often than every 10 years.

Another more serious complication of killed virus vaccines is the atypical responses seen in children who have received inactivated viral vaccines, such as killed measles virus vaccine (Chapters 16 and 20A).

When these children are later exposed to wild virus in nature, an atypical illness is observed that is significantly more severe and more toxic than the disease that occurs in unimmunized children. Following immunization with inactivated vaccine, there appears to be a selective stimulation of serum antibody but little IgA antibody in the respiratory tract (Fig. 23–10). Immunization with either live vaccine or natural infection, however, stimulates both serum and local antibody levels (Fig. 23–10). Following immunization with inactivated measles virus vaccine, therefore, the respiratory tract is not fully immunized. There is produced the anomalous situation of compartmentalization with selective immunization of the humoral compartment without immunization of the secretory IgA antibody (immunologic imbalance) (Chapter 2). After this compartmentalized immunization, natural infection leads to replication of virus in the respiratory tract and an accelerated response of serum antibody (Fig. 23–11). Thus, favorable conditions exist for immune-complex formation within the lung, with subsequent tissue injury mediated by an immune-complex reaction. Similar mechanisms have been proposed (1) for the altered reactivity to respiratory syncytial virus (RSV) seen in children previously immunized with inactivated RSV

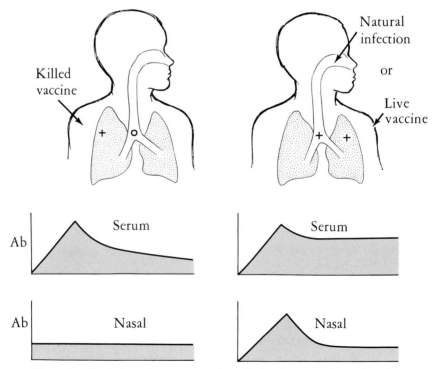

Figure 23–10. Schematic representation of development of nasal and serum antibody after immunization with live and killed measles vaccine and natural infection. Note the absence of development of nasal antibody after administration of killed vaccine.

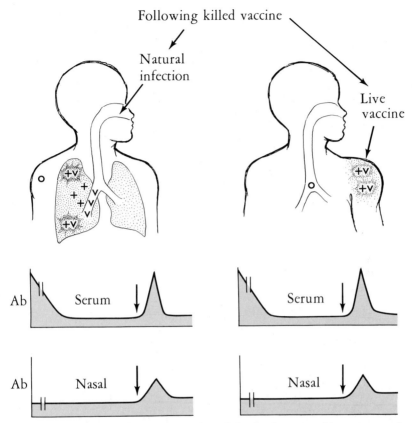

Figure 23–11. Schematic representation of the development of immune-complex–type injury due to deposition of virus-antibody complexes in the respiratory tract (generalized) after exposure to natural measles and in the skin (localized) after subsequent immunization with live measles vaccine.

vaccine and (2) in the pathogenesis of respiratory tract disease of early infancy due to RSV in immunized infants. It is believed that in both situations a compartmentalization occurs in which there is a selective serum IgG antibody in the absence of respiratory tract IgA antibody. After the individual is exposed to wild virus, conditions for the resultant complex formation between serum antibody and RSV antigen in the lungs occur with immunologic injury as the result.

Localized Arthus-type reactions have been observed in children who were previously immunized with killed measles vaccine and who subsequently receive live measles virus immunization. Swelling, tenderness, and erythema occur at the site of the live measles virus vaccination (Fig. 23–12). Recently, histopathologic and immunofluorescent evidence has been obtained for an Arthus-type hypersensitivity in the pathogenesis of these lesions (Figs. 23–13 through 23–18). In addition to Type III

Text continued on page 719

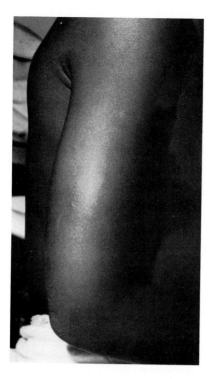

Figure 23–12. Arthus reaction occurring at the site of a subsequent live measles vaccination in a child previously immunized with inactivated measles vaccine.

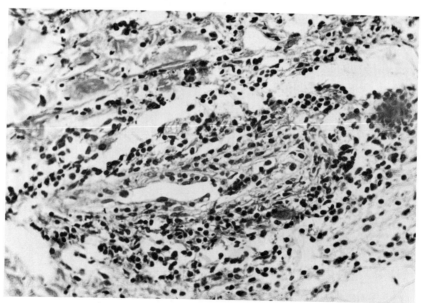

Figure 23–13. Histologic section of localized measles reaction (24 hours) showing a mixed cellular infiltration consisting of lymphocytes, monocytes, and neutrophils. Hematoxylin and eosin stain, × 100. (From Bellanti, J. A.: Biologic significance of the secretory γA immunoglobulins. Pediatrics, *48*:715, 1971.) (Courtesy of Dr. Peter A. Ward.)

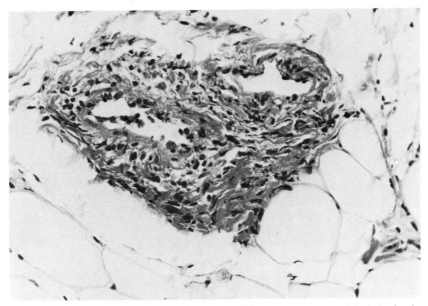

Figure 23–14.   Histologic section of localized measles reaction consisting predominantly of neutrophils. Hematoxylin and eosin stain, × 100. (From Bellanti, J. A.: Biologic significance of the secretory γA immunoglobulins. Pediatrics, *48*:715, 1971.) (Courtesy of Dr. Peter A. Ward.)

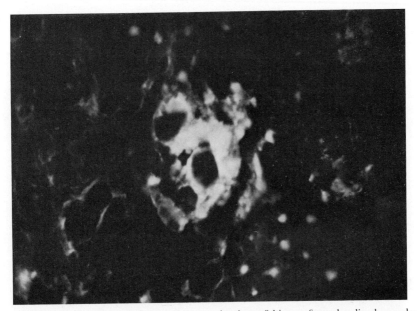

Figure 23–15.   Immunofluorescent examination of biopsy from localized measles reaction showing deposition of IgG globulin. (From Bellanti, J. A.: Biologic significance of the secretory γA immunoglobulins. Pediatrics, *48*:715, 1971.) (Courtesy of Dr. Peter A. Ward.)

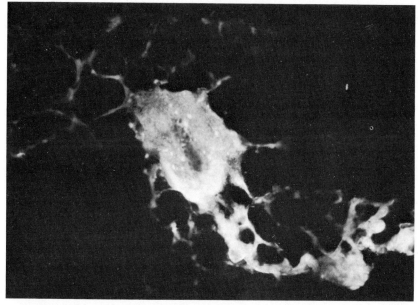

Figure 23–16. Immunofluorescent examination of biopsy from localized measles reaction showing C3 deposition within blood vessel wall. (From Bellanti, J. A.: Biologic significance of the secretory γA immunoglobulins. Pediatrics, *48*:715, 1971.) (Courtesy of Dr. Peter A. Ward.)

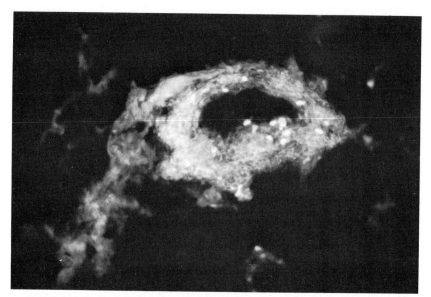

Figure 23–17. Immunofluorescent examination of biopsy from localized measles reaction showing fluorescence of measles antigen. (From Bellanti, J. A.: Biologic significance of the secretory γA immunoglobulins. Pediatrics, *48*:715, 1971.) (Courtesy of Dr. Peter A. Ward.)

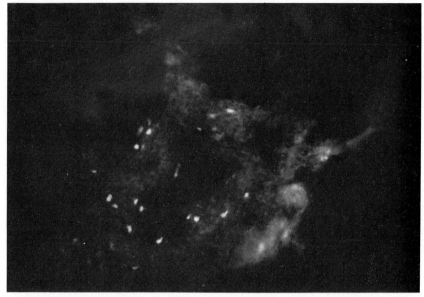

Figure 23-18. Immunofluorescent examination of biopsy from localized measles reaction showing negative fluorescence for IgA globulin. (From Bellanti, J. A.: Biologic significance of the secretory γA immunoglobulins. Pediatrics, 48:715, 1971.) (Courtesy of Dr. Peter A. Ward.)

mechanisms have also been implicated in the pathogenesis of these re-injury, IgE-mediated (Type I) and delayed-hypersensitivity (Type IV) actions (Table 23-7).

Adverse Effects of Viral Vaccines Seen in Normal Hosts Whose Pathogenesis is Unclear but that are Thought to Have an Immunologic Basis

A number of other adverse effects of vaccines have been described that are similar to those seen after natural disease and whose pathogenesis may be immunologic in nature. These complications include the occurrence of joint manifestations and neuropathy observed in association with natural rubella infection and, to a lesser extent, with rubella vaccines. In 20 to 40 per cent of adults receiving the live rubella vaccine, arthralgia and arthritis have been observed. The implications of these responses in immunologically mediated disease were described in Chapter 20C. In addition, thrombocytopenia has been observed following the use of rubella or rubeola vaccines, sometimes severe enough to be associated with purpura. Of perhaps greater clinical significance are recent reports of the possible association of subacute sclerosing panencephalitis (SSPE) with rubeola vaccine. The number of cases of SSPE associated with natural rubeola virus disease has been decreasing, and an upward trend has been observed in association with rubeola vaccine. However, recent reports suggest no significant increase in the number of SSPE cases associated with rubeola vaccine. Other complications are listed in Table 23–7, the most recent being the occurrence of the Guillain-Barré syndrome in recipients of the swine influenza virus vaccine.

Thus, in using vaccines for the stimulation of protective immunity, the physician must be constantly aware of the undesirable complications. These may take the form of nonimmunologic as well as immunologic reactions. Since more vaccines will be developed and undoubtedly introduced in the future, the physician must be alert to known complications as well as future, as yet unknown, complications. All physicians would be well advised to keep in mind the warning "Primum non nocere!" ("First do no harm!")

PROJECTIONS FOR FUTURE USES OF IMMUNOPROPHYLAXIS

Vaccines against varicella virus, herpes virus, cytomegalovirus and hepatitis virus are possibilities for future development. Work is in progress on a further attenuated strain of vaccinia virus for smallpox immunization in children with eczema and on vaccines for the prevention of varicella and hepatitis B (HB$_S$Ag). In addition, new approaches utilizing different routes of administration may promote better vaccine efficacy. With recognition of the importance of local IgA antibody in protection against certain types of localized infections, encouraging results have been obtained with local application of virus vaccines directly into the respiratory tract to stimulate local IgA antibody and local cell-mediated immunity, e.g., temperature-sensitive influenza vaccines.

Another area for vaccine development is that of bacterial vaccines. This has become increasingly important in recent years because of the problems of antibiotic resistance and the carrier state. These include not only the pneumococcal, meningococcal, and *H. influenzae type b* vaccines that are now available for use in certain high risk susceptible groups but also others that are undergoing investigation, e.g., *Neisseria gonorrhea.*

The effective use of vaccines may provide the long-sought answer to some of the problems of human malignant disease (Chapter 19). Such vaccines, employing purified viruses or tumor-specific antigens, may find clinical application in the future.

SUGGESTIONS FOR FURTHER READING

Asano, Y., Nakayama, H., Yazaki, T., Ito, S., Isomura, S., and Takahashi, M.: Protective efficacy of vaccination in children in four episodes of natural varicella and zoster in the ward. Pediatrics, 59:8, 1977.

Asano, Y., Nakayama, H., Yazaki, T., Kato, R., Hirose, S., Tsuzuki, K., Ito, S., Isomura, S., and Takahashi, M.: Protection against varicella in family contacts by immediate inoculation with live varicella vaccine. Pediatrics, 59:3, 1977.

Bellanti, J. A.: The biologic significance of the secretory γ A immunoglobulin. Pediatrics, 48:715, 1971.

Bellanti, J. A., and Frenkel, L. D.: Adverse reactions to immunizing agents. In F. Middleton, C. Reed, and E. Ellis (eds): Allergy: Principles and Practice. St. Louis, C. V. Mosby Co., 1978.

Fulginiti, V. A., and Clyde, W. A. (eds.): Workshop on bronchiolitis. Pediatric Res., 11:209, 1977.

Gold, R., and Lepow, M. L.: Present status of polysaccharide vaccines in the prevention of meningococcal disease. Adv. Pediatr., 23:71, 1976.

Immunization Against Disease. United States Department of Health, Education and Welfare, Public Health Service, October 1970.

John, T. J., Devarajan, L. V., Luther, L., and Vijayarathnam, P.: Effect of breast-feeding on seroresponse of infants to oral poliovirus vaccination. Pediatrics, 57:47, 1976.

Krugman, S.: Present status of measles and rubella immunization in the United States: A medical progress report. J. Pediatr., 90:1, 1977.

Modlin, J. F., Jabbour, J. T., Witte, J. J., and Halsey, N. A.: Epidemiologic studies of measles, measles vaccine, and subacute sclerosing panencephalitis. Pediatrics, 59:505, 1977.

Report on the Control of Infectious Diseases. American Academy of Pediatrics, 1974.

Reports and Recommendations of the National Immunization Work Groups, submitted to the Office of the Assistant Secretary for Health, Department of Health, Education and Welfare, Public Health Service, March 15, 1977.

Chapter 24

IMMUNOTHERAPY: THE USE OF PASSIVE IMMUNIZATION

Joseph A. Bellanti, M.D.
and John B. Robbins, M.D.

Classically, immunotherapy referred to passive immunization through the use of serum or gamma globulin that confers temporary protection by transferring to one host antibodies actively produced in another. A specialized application of immunotherapy is its use in immunosuppression and prevention of isoimmunization (Chapter 10). Recently, the meaning of immunotherapy has been broadened to include the use of immunopotentiators, agents used in the treatment of cancer (Chapter 10) and in hyposensitization therapy of allergy (Chapter 20A). The complexity of the term has been increased by the extension of its meaning to include the replacement not only of antibody but also of immunocompetent lymphoid tissues, e.g., bone marrow and thymus, or their products, e.g., thymosin and transfer factor (Chapters 10 and 22). This chapter will deal primarily with those applications of immunotherapy that pertain to the more classic uses of serum or gamma globulin therapy.

The first uses of antitoxin in the therapy of infectious diseases, such as diphtheria and tetanus, were seen during the early part of this century (Fig. 24–1). The early dramatic successes obscured the preferable clinical situation of prevention of infectious diseases by active immunization through the use of vaccines (Chapter 23). Today, the use of antitoxin in these same diseases would mean a failure of community or private medical practice, which has the alternative of active immunization during childhood and later life. Nevertheless, passive immunization is still needed for protection against those diseases for which vaccines are not available, e.g., botulism, and in the treatment of individuals incompletely immunized. Newer applications of immunotherapy include the prevention of Rh_0 sensitization and immunosuppression during tissue transplantation. In some situations, such as severe burns, the patients may have a limited period of severe acquired immune deficiency that requires immunotherapy to prevent serious and sometimes life-threatening infection. A fundamental understanding of the princi-

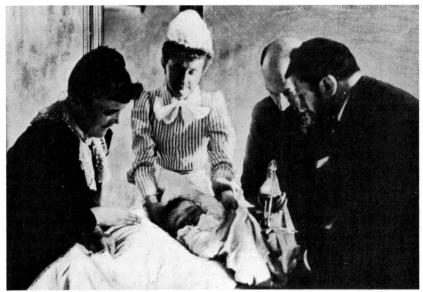

Figure 24-1. Photograph showing early use of diphtheria antitoxin in immunotherapy of diphtheria. (Courtesy of National Library of Medicine.)

ples underlying immunotherapy is, therefore, necessary for the student and for the modern-day practitioner so that they can use passive immunization properly and evaluate applications that will inevitably appear in the future.

PRINCIPLES OF PASSIVE IMMUNIZATION

GENERAL PRINCIPLES

There has been some confusion of terminology in the areas of active and passive immunization. The term *vaccine* should be reserved solely for those antigenic substances that result in a state of active immunity; such terms as serum, antitoxin, and gamma globulin refer to *antibody preparations.* The uses of antibody preparations in immunotherapy are shown schematically in Figure 24–2 and include such antimicrobial activity as *toxin neutralization, viral neutralization,* and *antibacterial* effects due to lysis or opsonization and phagocytosis. In addition, immunosuppressive activity with antibody preparations has been successful in the prevention of maternal Rh_0 isoimmunization and in immunosuppression during tissue transplantation.

Antibody preparations may be derived from (1) whole sera from individuals recovering from a specific disease, (2) gamma globulin from

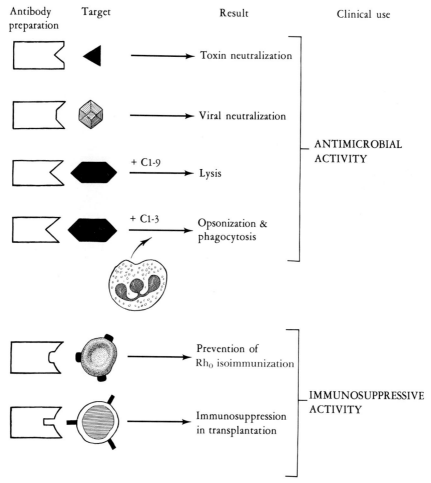

Figure 24-2. Schematic representation of the uses of antibody preparations in immunotherapy.

sera having high specific antibody content (special immune serum globulins [SIG]), (3) gamma globulin from pooled sera (immune serum globulin [ISG]), and (4) whole serum from an animal hyperimmunized against a specific pathogen (antitoxin or therapeutic immune sera).

IMMEDIACY OF ACTION

The most important reason for the use of passive immunization is its "immediacy of action"—the ability of preformed antibody to exert its effect immediately on interaction with an antigen (Fig. 24–2). The delay of the *latent period* required by an active immune response is thereby avoided. The obvious advantage, therefore, is that passive immunization procedures can be used in emergency situations in which there is insufficient time to achieve an active immune response or vaccine is unavailable. In general, the efficacy of passive immunization is related to the length of time between exposure to the pathogen and administration of the antibody, i.e., the shorter the interval, the greater the likelihood of prevention of the disease or of its successful treatment. In some instances, the antibody may be given prior to exposure, as in the use of gamma globulin for prevention of hepatitis A (infectious hepatitis) in individuals traveling to high-risk areas.

METABOLISM OF GAMMA GLOBULIN

Also important in the use of passive immunization are the factors that govern the metabolism of the antibody preparation (Chapter 7). It is now generally accepted that once antibody molecules are synthesized, they, like all other protein molecules, have a limited biologic half-life. There is a continual loss and replacement of these molecules in a dynamic state that is referred to as *turnover*. By the very nature of the passive immunization procedure, the introduction of preformed antibody into a host ensures that in the absence of any active synthesis the duration of antibody activity will be finite. For example, if human (homologous) IgG immunoglobulin is administered to a healthy human, the biologic half-life will be 20 to 30 days. The half-life of horse (heterologous) immunoglobulin administered to humans, on the other hand, is considerably shorter. In the latter case, in addition to the degradation governed by the biologic properties of the preparation, the recognition of foreign horse gamma globulin by the human results in an active immune response leading to antibody-mediated enhanced catabolism or immune elimination (Chapter 7). These events are represented schematically in Figure 24–3.

The pattern of elimination of gamma globulin (antibody) administered intravenously to an animal occurs in three phases (Fig. 24–3). Phase 1 is a period of redistribution or equalization between vascular and extravascular spaces that results in a striking drop in peak titer shortly after administration of the antibody. Phase 2 is a slower, steady drop in serum levels due to the metabolic (catabolic) half-life of the gamma globulin. These diminutions in serum levels apply to both homologous and heterologous gamma globulins. Phase 3 is an accelerated period of degradation, occurring only in the case of heterologous gamma globulin, that takes place simultaneously with the development of antibody of the foreign gamma globulin. This third phase is referred to as *immune elimination.*

These metabolic properties of gamma globulin also have relevance to the passive immunization that occurs as a natural event in every human—the transplacental transfer of homologous IgG immunoglobulins from mother to fetus (Chapter 2). There is a gradual de-

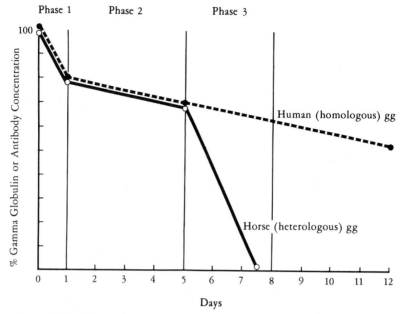

Figure 24–3. Schematic comparison of the catabolism of homologous and heterologous antibody (gg) preparations in the human.

gradation and diminished concentration of IgG immunoglobulins following birth (physiologic hypogammaglobulinemia).

VARIABILITY OF PREPARATIONS

A third principle governing the use of passive immunization is the great variability of biologic effectiveness seen with different preparations of gamma globulin. The use of immunotherapy is highly effective for some diseases, particularly when antibody is called on to neutralize the effect of extracellular toxin, e.g., tetanus toxin, or in certain viral diseases, e.g., measles. In other instances, the effectiveness of immunotherapy is less than optimal, but its use continues nevertheless. For example, the use of immunotherapy in hepatitis A does not necessarily prevent the disease, but it may convert a clinical disease into a subclinical one. In still other situations, the value of passive immunization is uncertain, highly questionable, and often controversial. For example, administering gamma globulin to a pregnant female exposed to rubella in the first trimester may prevent clinical rubella in the mother, but a subclinical disease may occur. This may be followed by the full-blown congenital rubella syndrome in the infant.

The reason for the disparity in efficacy between various gamma globulin preparations employed in immunotherapy is not entirely apparent. The following factors appear to be of importance: (1) The *time of administration* of the preparation. Optimally, an antibody preparation should be given immediately after exposure to an infectious agent. (2) The *differences in pathogenesis* of the various disease entities. Those infectious agents that have a blood-borne phase will be more effectively neutralized by the use of gamma-globulin than those that are localized. (3) The *content of specific antibody* in any given preparation. Because of variations in antibody content in serum and to ensure an adequate level of antibody, gamma globulin preparations are obtained preferably from hyperimmune sera.

INHIBITION OF PRIMARY IMMUNE RESPONSE

A fourth important principle is the application of immunotherapy in the suppression of the immune response (Chapter 10). The passive administration of specific antibody will inhibit active production of antibody by means of negative feedback inhibition. Thus, if red cells from an Rh_0-positive individual are coated with incomplete anti-Rh_0 antibody prior to injection into an Rh_0-negative individual, the formation of anti-Rh_0 antibodies is prevented. This use of antibody immunosuppression apparently affects the "afferent" limb of the immune system by preventing the production of antibody (Fig. 24–4). The use of antilymphocyte sera (ALS), on the other hand, appears to inhibit the primary immune response by interfering with the "efferent" limb of immunity (Fig. 24–4).

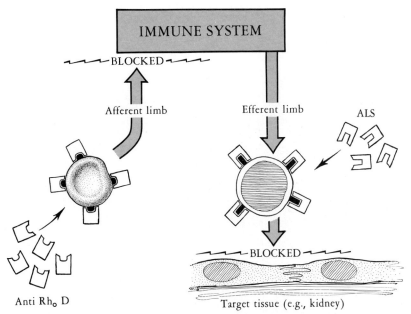

Figure 24–4. Schematic representation of the modes of immunosuppression by specific anti-Rh_0 antibody and by antilymphocyte sera (ALS).

TYPES OF PREPARATIONS

The various preparations commonly available for use in immunotherapy are listed in Table 24–1. The official titles of these products are taken from the Code of Federal Regulations, Title 21, Parts 600–1299, April 1, 1977, Bureau of Biologies, Food and Drug Administration.

IMMUNE SERUM GLOBULIN (ISG)

Immune serum globulin (human), also called "gamma globulin," is derived from the blood, plasma, or serum of human donors and contains most of the antibodies found in whole blood. The amounts of specific antibody vary in different preparations. The ISG preparation (usually derived from placental blood) contains a concentration of antibodies approximately 25 times that found in blood. Final concentration of the preparation contains 165 mg of gamma globulin per milliliter. Each lot of immune serum globulin represents a pooling of not

TABLE 24–1.   Preparations in Common Use for Immunotherapy

PREPARATION	SOURCE	COMMENTS
Immune serum globulin (ISG)	Human	Rubeola, hepatitis A, congenital agammaglobulinemia
Specific immune serum globulin (SIG)	Human	Prepared from hyperimmune sera; use established
Measles immune globulin		
Mumps immune globulin		
Pertussis immune globulin		
Tetanus immune globulin		
Vaccinia immune globulin		
Rh$_0$(D) immune globulin		
Therapeutic immune sera		
Antirabies serum	Animal	
Chickenpox immune serum	Human	
Measles immune serum	Human	
Mumps immune serum	Human	
Pertussis immune serum	Human	Not established or produce untoward complications, e.g., serum hepatitis or sensitization
Antitoxins (animal)		
Botulism	Animal	
Diphtheria	Animal	
Dysentery	Animal	
Gas gangrene	Animal	
Perfringens	Animal	
Tetanus	Animal	
Recommended by WHO		
Diphtheria	Human	
Varicella	Human	
Botulism	Human	
Rabies	Human	
Malaria	Human	

less than 1000 donors, which provides a wide spectrum of antibody but also increases the risk of sensitization after prolonged usage. These preparations contain primarily IgG immunoglobulins, with lesser amounts of IgM antibodies important in bacterial defense. Although there are IgA immunoglobulins in commercial gamma globulin, these proteins are poorly transmitted to mucosal surfaces, sites where the secretory IgA globulins normally provide defense.

The advantages of gamma globulin preparations over whole serum are as follows: (1) gamma globulin is free from hepatitis virus B; (2) it is concentrated, permitting the administration of a large amount of antibody in a small volume; and (3) it is stable during long-term storage.

There are disadvantages to the use of concentrated ISG preparations. All preparations have a tendency to aggregate into large 11S polymers. These aggregates account for the occasional anaphylactic reactions seen following prolonged usage. The frequency of these reactions is far too high for ISG to be administered via the intravenous route; therefore, the intact preparation should not be given intravenously. Since each lot represents a pool of many donors, the likelihood of sensitization is increased with continued usage. Isoimmunization against the Gm factors of gamma globulin has been reported after prolonged administration in immunologically normal individuals and in children with acquired agammaglobulinemia.

The value of immune serum globulin (human) has been demonstrated unequivocally in only three situations: (1) prevention of rubeola, (2) prevention of hepatitis A and (3) replacement therapy in congenital agammaglobulinemia of the Bruton type. Although it has not been proved, ISG may be useful in preventing three other infectious diseases: (1) rubella in the first trimester of pregnancy, (2) varicella in exposed patients on immunosuppressive therapy, and (3) post-transfusion hepatitis. One reason for the lack of effectiveness in these latter diseases may be the lack of sufficient specific antibody in ordinary ISG preparations.

Any uses of immune serum globulin other than those listed previously constitute misuses or abuses of the preparation. There is no justification for the use of gamma globulin in children with repeated upper respiratory tract infections due to viruses. Similarly, there is no indication for its use in asthma, tonsillitis, or chronic pyelonephritis. In the interpretation of possible immunoglobulin deficiencies in children, the level of serum gamma globulin must be age-adjusted because of the developmental immunologic immaturity of the young infant and child (Chapters 22 and 26).

SPECIFIC IMMUNE SERUM GLOBULIN (SIG)

Specific immune serum globulins (SIG) are prepared from the sera of convalescent individuals or those who are hyperimmunized to a given material (Table 24–1). Since such preparations contain a higher content of specific antibody to the agent in question than that found in ISG, they are preferable to the latter.

The more commonly used specific immune globulins are listed in Table 24–1. The World Health Organization has also recommended human sources for specific immune globulins that are currently unavailable or in short supply. e.g., zoster immune globulin (ZIG).

THERAPEUTIC IMMUNE SERUMS AND ANTITOXINS

The antisera and antitoxins listed in Table 24–1 are produced in animals and should be used only in clinical situations in which human sources of immune globulin are not available because they present the problem of possible hypersensitivity reactions (serum sickness) (Chapter 20A).

$Rh_0(D)$ IMMUNE GLOBULIN

This material consists of IgG–anti-Rh_0(D) prepared from pooled human sera. This preparation has been used in the prevention of Rh_0 isosensitization and has received several thousand clinical trials.

ANTILYMPHOCYTE SERA (HORSE)

This material is produced by active immunization of horses with human lymphocytes for use in immunosuppression in transplantation. At present, this is an experimental and nonlicensed product, and its use in humans is not well established.

USES OF PASSIVE IMMUNIZATION

The classic use of passive immunization has been and continues to be its application in the prevention or treatment of infectious diseases, including those associated with bacteria or their products (toxins), viruses, and certain protozoa (malaria). However, new applications of passive immunization in the suppression of the primary immune response are now being included. Applications of passive immunization are given in Table 24–2. The uses of passive immunization form two major categories: *replacement therapy* and *suppression* of the primary immune response. Replacement therapy is used in cases in which gamma globulin is congenitally deficient, e.g., agammaglobulinemia, or in which there is an absence of specific antibody, e.g., unimmunized individuals. The use of passive immunization in suppressing the

TABLE 24-2.   Applications of Passive Immunization

Indication	Application	Type of Preparation
Replacement therapy	Immunologic deficiency syndrome	Immune serum globulin (ISG)
	Prevention or treatment of certain infectious diseases (rubeola, mumps, hepatitis, and tetanus)	ISG, Serum immune globulin (SIG)
Suppression of primary immune response	Prevention of Rh_0 isoimmunization	Rh_0 (D) immunoglobulin
	Immunosuppression in transplantation	Antilymphocyte sera (ALS)

immune response includes the prevention of Rh_0 isoimmunization and immunosuppression in tissue transplantation.

Replacement Therapy

This type of therapy employs either immune serum globulin (ISG) or specific immune globulins (SIG).

Immunologic Deficiency Syndromes

The use of gamma globulin therapy in the immunologic deficiency syndrome is described in Chapter 22. Its greatest efficacy is seen in the disorders involving the thymic-independent types of immune deficiency, such as the Bruton type of congenital agammaglobulinemia and acquired types of hypogammaglobulinemia. Since ISG has a high content of specific antibody against those organisms that commonly infect agammaglobulinemic patients, this type of replacement therapy is highly effective. However, since immune serum globulin contains predominantly IgG antibodies, these patients may continue to have localized infections, particularly of the respiratory and gastrointestinal tracts.

Prevention of Certain Infectious Diseases

Hepatitis (Types A and B).   The use of immune serum globulin has been shown to be highly effective in reducing the frequency of overt clinical disease, although inapparent infection still occurs. The uses of immune serum globulin for preventing hepatitis A are based on guidelines suggested by recommendations of the Public Health Service Advisory Committee on Immunization Practices (Table 24-3). Under most conditions of exposure, protection has been afforded by giving 0.01 ml of ISG per pound of body weight.

TABLE 24-3.   Guidelines for Prophylaxis of Hepatitis A

WEIGHT (lbs)	ISG DOSE (ml)
Up to 50	0.5
50–100	1.0
>100	2.0

ISG should be given as soon as possible after exposure, since its prophylactic value decreases with time after exposure. Its use after five to six weeks after exposure is not indicated. ISG is used when there is (1) definite exposure to a known case or (2) anticipated continuous or intermittent exposure.

Travelers to foreign countries appear to be at no greater risk than they are in the United States when their travel involves ordinary tourist activities. For these travelers, ISG is not recommended. For travelers who are exposed to infected persons or contaminated food and water while visiting areas where hepatitis is a major health problem, there is increased risk. A single dose of ISG is recommended for them, and, if the risk continues, this dose should be repeated every six months.

Transfusion-associated hepatitis constitutes another form of a serious and continuing problem; the risk increases as the number of transfusions increases. Previous evidence was advanced both for and against the use of ISG in prophylaxis against transfusion-associated hepatitis. Although earlier claims have reported that the administration of ISG at the time of transfusion reduces the number of cases of hepatitis, other equally well-controlled studies have not substantiated this claim. Recently, high-titered anti-hepatitis B surface antigen (HBAg) has been licensed for its specific immunoprophylactic effect. Preliminary results indicate efficacy against transfusion-associated hepatitis virus B. Other means of effectively lowering the incidence of transfusion-associated hepatitis include the careful selection of donors, the development of central registry, and the use of blood and potentially icterogenic blood products only when necessary. Moreover, the screening of all blood donors for hepatitis B antigen and the institution of a voluntary-donor transfusion have provided a significant lowering of this viral disease.

Measles (Rubeola).   Immune serum globulin is also useful in the prevention of rubeola, in which even small amounts of ISG (0.1 ml per pound) can prevent the disease. A second preparation that is useful in the prevention of rubeola is measles immune globulin (human), which differs from ISG in that it contains a titrated amount of specific measles antibody. It is given simultaneously with the Edmonston live measles vaccine in a dose of 0.02 ml per kilogram to modify the undesirable effects of the vaccine, e.g., fever and rash. The use of gamma globulin is not necessary in the case of further attenuated measles vaccines, e.g.,

Schwarz strain. The second use of measles immune globulin is in the prevention of disease after the known exposure of nonimmunized children under the age of three years and in the prevention of measles in high-risk groups, such as institutionalized children with chronic illnesses. A dose of 0.25 mg per kilogram of the preparation should be given intramuscularly as soon as possible after exposure. In older children and adults with no past history of measles, a smaller dose of 0.05 mg per kilogram is recommended for modification of the disease. With the widespread effective use of live, attenuated measles vaccines in the immunoprophylaxis of measles, the use of measles immune globulin should become increasingly infrequent in the future.

Mumps. The effectiveness of mumps immune globulin (human) has not been demonstrated clinically in preventing either the disease or its complications. The recommended dose for adults is 2.5 to 7.5 ml intramuscularly. The problem of prophylaxis, however, should decrease in the future with the availability of live, attenuated mumps vaccine.

Pertussis. Because of the high mortality of pertussis in infancy, the use of immunotherapy has been proposed for both prophylaxis and treatment of the disease in young infants. There are three preparations available for general use: (1) antipertussis serum, (2) human hyperimmune serum, and (3) pertussis immune globulin. Only the pertussis immune globulin is recommended for general use because of its freedom from hepatitis virus B and its reduced rate of hypersensitivity reactions. The efficacy of pertussis immunoglobulin in prophylaxis or therapy of whooping cough has not been established. The recommended dosage, when used, is 1.25 ml intramuscularly, repeated every other day for three to four doses.

Tetanus. One of the most significant recent advances in passive immunization was the development of a human source of tetanus immune globulin. This preparation is obtained from donors who are hyperimmunized with tetanus toxoid. It has all the advantages cited previously, and protective levels are detected for at least 21 days after administration of the immune globulin. For treatment of tetanus, 3000 to 6000 units are given intramuscularly. In the unlikely possibility that human globulin is unavailable, 100,000 units of horse tetanus antitoxin should be given but only after appropriate tests for sensitivity to horse serum are conducted. For the prevention of disease in individuals not actively immunized, 250 to 500 units may be injected intramuscularly.

Vaccinia. The production of a vaccinia immune globulin (VIG) has been made possible through the American National Red Cross and the Armed Forces. It is prepared from the pooled plasma of 1000 or more volunteers. This material has been recommended for use in the catastrophic complications of smallpox vaccination, including those that occur in eczema (eczema vaccinatum) and certain of the immunologic deficiency syndromes (Chapters 22 and 23). It is recommended in infants suffering from eczema who have been inadvertently vaccinated or exposed to recently vaccinated individuals, in infants with other breaks in the continuity of the skin, e.g., burns, and in infants with eczema who are required to have a smallpox vaccination prior to overseas travel. The use of VIG has not been shown to be beneficial in the prevention or treatment of postvaccinial encephalitis. The use of the preparation is also recommended in the prevention of smallpox in close contacts of patients with the disease. The dose for prophylaxis is 0.3 ml per kilogram and the dose for treatment is 0.6 ml per kilogram intramuscularly. Although the use of VIG is recommended in the treatment of progressive vaccinia, its efficacy is doubtful, since many of these children have been shown to be deficient predominantly in the thymic-dependent, cell-mediated limb of immunity. The basic defect, therefore, does not appear to be correctable by VIG alone.

Diphtheria. The serious and permanent manifestations of diphtheria are mediated by a toxic protein having a molecular weight of approximately 45,000 daltons. Inactivation of the toxic properties of this protein with formaldehyde without interference with its immunogenic properties was one of the greatest advances in clinical immunology and in all medicine. When used as recommended, immunization with diphtheria toxoid provides protective immunity to virtually all vaccine recipients. However, physicians are occasionally required to treat diphtheria in individuals who have not been immunized or who have not been "boosted" and whose serum antidiphtheria antibodies decrease to nonprotective levels. Therapy with antidiphtheria antibodies has several considerations. First is that only equine antidiphtheria antibodies are available for passive immunization. Thus, the problem of acute hypersensitivity reactions, such as anaphylactoid reactions, must be avoided, and the possibility of late complications, such as serum sickness, should be anticipated. Second, the dosage of equine antidiphtheria antibodies is related to the duration of the clinical disease. Thus, an estimation must be made each day of clinical diphtheria. There is a substantial increase in the recommended dose based on this estimated number of days. Third is that active immunization with vaccine should commence as passive therapy is administered. Although passive immunization is an effective therapy in that it reduces the mortality and morbidity of diphtheria, serum antibody is an ineffective method for neutralization of tissue-fixed and presumably injurious toxin. It is a general principle without a recorded exception that *prevention* is the most effective method of control for all disease, including diphtheria.

Zoster Immune Globulin (ZIG). An innovative approach and specialized series of immunologic events have permitted the preparation of a useful immunoprophylactic and therapeutic reagent called ZIG (zoster immune globulin). Individuals who have recovered from herpes zoster neuritis (shingles) have a brief period of high-titered antibodies to it and varicella virus (chickenpox). Plasma extracted from such convalescent patients has been prepared (ZIG) for use in the prevention or treatment of varicella in susceptible or infected individuals, such as those with acquired immunodeficiency states. Especially susceptible are adults with treated or advanced chronic lymphatic leukemia or Hodgkin's disease. At this time, the availability of this material is conditioned by the availability of donors (convalescent patients) and funds for the manufacture of ZIG.

Other Infectious Diseases

Passive immunization with serum antibodies is also a useful therapy for rarely encountered infectious diseases, such as botulism, rabies, Lassa fever, and laboratory-acquired infections. In these instances, specific high-titered antibody preparations are available from the Center for Disease Control and other national agencies in other countries for the treatment of these diseases. Obviously, routine immunization against these diseases is not indicated. Thus, passive immunotherapy will be a useful therapeutic adjunct for these specialized situations.

Digoxin Intoxication.   It is a medical emergency when digoxin is taken in an excessive dose, either by deliberate action of a patient or by inadvertent administration to a patient. By a clever combination of the properties of this commonly used compound with our new knowledge of immunoglobulins, a therapeutic preparation of antidigoxin antibodies has been successfully used for treatment of overdosage with this agent. Digoxin is a glycone trisaccharide and is not immunogenic by itself. By chemical attachment to a protein, specific antibodies to this compound may be raised in rabbits and goats. These digoxin-specific antibodies may be purified from the antisera by use of affinity resins. The specific antibody is further treated with pepsin to selectively remove the Fc fragment without loss of antibody activity. The Fab fragment has two unusual properties that give it greater therapeutic effectiveness than that of the intact antidigoxin antibodies. The first is that the catabolic rate of the Fab fragments is markedly greater than that of the intact immunoglobulin. Thus, the almost instantaneous combination of the Fab fragment with the hapten (digoxin) results in inactivation of the cardiotoxicity and rapid excretion of the antigen-antibody complex in the urine. Second is the decreased immunogenicity of the Fab fragment as compared to the intact immunoglobulin. Thus, the Fab anti-intoxicant has the specificity and combining activity of the intact antibody but has a more rapid excretion and lesser immunogenicity. The limitations of this therapeutic approach are the need for the immunochemist to produce high-binding antibodies and the relation between the amount of hapten (potential toxin) and the amount of antibody-derived Fab protein required for a therapeutic effect. The success of this approach for intoxication with digoxin and related molecules will inspire scientists to seek preparations for the treatment of other conditions caused by small molecules with intoxicant activities at comparatively low concentrations.

IMMUNOSUPPRESSION

Rh₀ Prevention

The use of specific anti-Rh₀(D) globulin has been shown to be effective in preventing Rh₀ isoimmunization by preventing transplacentally acquired fetal erythrocytes from reacting with maternal immunologically competent cells. The production of anti-Rh₀ antibody is therefore "blocked" (Fig. 24–4). The recommended dose of the preparation is 1.0 ml administered within 72 hours of delivery in cases in which an Rh₀-positive baby is born to an Rh₀-negative mother (Chapter 10). The use of this preparation represents one of the most exciting new applications of immunotherapy.

Immunosuppression by ALS

Recently, the administration of antilymphocyte sera has been shown to be effective in immunosuppression in animals. Similar immunosuppressive approaches using this preparation have been used in man. The sera are produced in animals such as the horse by the injection of suspensions of lymphocytes with Freund's adjuvant. The sera are then administered to recipients of transplants, usually in conjunction with other forms of immunosuppressive therapy (Chapter 25). The precise mechanism of action of ALS is unknown. The most plausible theory is that the preparation is reacting with critical receptors on the surface of lymphocytes, coating them, and making the lymphocyte unavailable for its interaction with target cells (Fig. 24–4). ALS has been shown to be a potent inhibitor of cell-mediated immunologic events and may be a possible adjunct in transplantation immunology. However, there are several undesirable features of ALS: (1) the lack of standardized preparations, (2) the problem of reactions with heterologous horse sera, (3) the recent demonstration that ALS enhances viral replication *in vitro* and *in vivo*, leading to overwhelming viral infections in man, and (4) the enhancement of tumor development following its use (Chapter 19).

THE HAZARDS OF IMMUNOGLOBULIN THERAPY

Millions of doses of gamma globulin have been administered to humans over the past 25 years. With this increased usage and experience, a number of reactions and hazards have become apparent. Prior to considering immunotherapy, therefore, the physician must critically evaluate the indications for its use. The problems associated with immunoglobulin therapy are related to properties of the *preparation* as well as to the *host's response* to the gamma globulin.

The properties of the preparation that are of clinical importance include the following: (1) commercial gamma globulin is prepared from many foreign genetic types of gamma globulin, and therefore the likelihood of sensitization is great, particularly after prolonged usage; (2) the preparation contains mainly IgG, and (3) preparations from placental sources are contaminated with A and B blood group substances. Another important property of the gamma globulin is that all commercial preparations have a tendency to aggregate into large 11S biopolymers. These aggregates are of clinical importance, since they may be responsible for severe reactions, particularly when given intravenously. These polymers can also lead to sensitization and upon standing tend to fragment, with subsequent loss of antibody content (Table 24–4).

The clinical reactions to gamma globulin are given in Table 24–4. Standard gamma globulin cannot be given intravenously, since severe pyrogenic and cardiovascular reactions have occurred that are believed to be related to the presence of aggregates in the preparation. The reactions are believed to be nonimmunologic in nature and can occur in individuals receiving intravenous gamma globulin for the first time. The use of plasmin digests of gamma globulin has been shown recently to be clinically effective, and plasmin digests appear to eliminate the problem of aggregates. These preparations are still biologically active and can be given intravenously.

In addition to this type of reaction, the repeated use of gamma globulin can lead to sensitization in normal persons and even in patients with various types of immunologic deficiencies. At least three types of sensitization have been described (Table 24–4). The first of these is caused by antibody to the Gm determinant and is seen after prolonged gamma globulin usage. A second type of sensitization to the aggregated gamma globulin itself may occur. The development of precipitating antibody to aggregated but not native gamma globulin was demonstrated in children with acquired agammaglobulinemia who had been receiving gamma globulin. This was associated with "anaphylactic shock" after intramuscular administration. A third type of sensitization to

TABLE 24–4. Clinical Reactions After Immunoglobulin Therapy

Reaction	Mechanism
Cardiovascular shock, fever after intravenous use	Aggregates
Loss of antibody activity	Fragmentation
Sensitization	Sensitization due to:
	(1) Anti-Gm
	(2) Antibody to aggregates
	(3) Anti-IgA antibody
Development of anti-A and anti-B	A and B contamination of placental sources

gamma globulin is the development of anti-IgA antibodies. This was first described in patients with ataxia-telangiectasia with IgA deficiency but has been subsequently described in normal persons with normal IgA levels. Patients with IgA deficiency develop anti-IgA with broad class specificity; normal persons develop anti-IgA of a more restricted specificity (Chapter 5).

All these antigammaglobulin antibodies of the IgG class are able to fix complement and may be associated with hypersensitivity reactions mediated by antibody (Chapter 13). They all appear to be important in nonhemolytic transfusion reactions, particularly the anti-IgA antibodies (Chapter 20B).

A final complication of the use of gamma globulin is the development of isohemagglutinins of anti-A and anti-B specificity in individuals receiving gamma globulin. This is primarily true of gamma globulin prepared from placental sources that appears to be contaminated by the blood group substances. This complication may be of particular significance in women receiving anti-$Rh_0(D)$ globulin for the prevention of Rh_0 disease.

PROJECTIONS FOR THE FUTURE USE OF IMMUNOTHERAPY

The use of immunotherapy in medicine is perhaps one of the oldest forms of treatment for the specific infectious diseases. In spite of its early expectations, it never has come into the wide use that was originally intended, except in the toxin-dependent diseases and certain of the viral diseases. The initial drawbacks arose from the hazards of allergic reactions to foreign sera; however, with the introduction of human sources of antibody, these hazards have been decreasing significantly. There continues to be a need for the use of hyperimmune sera, particularly for those virus diseases for which no active immunization procedures exist. The interesting work of Brunell and his associates has shown that the development of varicella immune globulin is feasible by preparing material from patients with herpes zoster (zoster immune globulin [ZIG]). Fatal varicella has been seen in individuals who are at risk from underlying diseases of the lymphoreticular tissues or who are receiving immunosuppressant therapy. The use of ZIG may prevent this fatal disease. Better preparations for other infectious diseases, such as rubella, infectious hepatitis, and malaria, and a human source of globulin for diphtheria should be obtained in the future.

The interesting and challenging data obtained from studies of the prevention of Rh_0 sensitization by use of Rh_0-specific immune globulin offer approaches for the prevention of other disease entities that are acquired prenatally. Such an approach may eventually pave the way for the prevention of neoplasms, particularly those induced by viruses

(Chapter 19). The use of antilymphocyte sera, though suffering from a number of drawbacks, offers another possible approach for the suppression of the cell-mediated responses. The use of plasmin digest fragments, which retain antibody activity but have minimal problems of sensitivity, offers still another approach in immunotherapy.

Finally, an extension of immunotherapy is the replacement not of gamma globulin but of the immunocompetent lymphoid tissues. The transplantation of thymus or bone marrow has now been successfully accomplished in restoring immunocompetence to children with immune deficiencies involving the thymic-dependent limb (Chapters 20B and 22). Recently, the successful use of transfer factor in the reconstitution of such individuals has been reported. This form of immunotherapy has the obvious advantage over gamma globulin replacement of permanency. As better methods of histocompatibility matching become available, this form of immunotherapy will become increasingly useful in the restoration of immunologic function.

SUGGESTIONS FOR FURTHER READING

Brunell, P. A., Ross, A., Miller, L. H., and Kuo, B.: Prevention of varicella by zoster immune globulin. N. Engl. J. Med., *280*:1191, 1969.

Edsall, G.: Passive immunization. Pediatrics, *32*:599, 1963.

Fudenberg, H., Good, R. A., Goodman, H. C., Hitzig, W., Kunkel, H. G., Roitt, I. M., Rosen, F. S., Rowe, D. S., Seligmann, M., and Soothill, J. R.: Primary immunodeficiencies. Pediatrics, *47*:927, 1971.

Krugman, S.: The clinical uses of gamma globulin. N. Engl. J. Med., *269*:195, 1963.

Merler, E. (ed.): Immunoglobulins: Biologic Aspects and Clinical Usage. Washington, D.C., National Academy of Sciences, 1970.

Pollack, W., Gorman, J. G., and Freda, V. J.: Prevention of Rh_0 hemolytic disease. Progr. Hematol., *6*:121, 1969.

Chapter 25

CLINICAL ASPECTS OF IMMUNOSUPPRESSION: USE OF CYTOTOXIC AGENTS AND CORTICOSTEROIDS

Anthony S. Fauci, M.D.

Immunosuppression is the negative control or regulation of immunologic reactivity (Chapter 10). There are several major categories of immunosuppressive agents, including x-irradiation, antilymphocyte globulin, cytotoxic agents, and corticosteroids. Radiation therapy is used predominantly for its cytocidal effects on certain types of neoplastic cells; the major use of antilymphocyte globulin has been in the prevention of organ transplant rejection. Certain categories of cytotoxic agents (usually in very high doses) have been used in a variety of neoplasms. As with radiation therapy, the desired effect has been cytocidal for tumor cells. However, in recent years cytotoxic agents have been used with increasing frequency solely for their immunosuppressive effects in immunologically mediated diseases. Although corticosteroids are used in certain neoplasms, particularly of the lymphoid, reticuloendothelial, and hematopoietic organs, their major use has been as anti-inflammatory or immunosuppressive agents.

In this chapter we will not attempt to encompass the entire scope of immunosuppression but will be concerned predominantly with the mechanisms of action and clinical considerations in the use of cytotoxic agents and corticosteroids in man. We will focus on the use of these agents in the treatment of diseases characterized by inflammatory or immunologically mediated phenomena (Chapter 20).

CYTOTOXIC AGENTS

CLINICAL USAGE

Although a variety of classes of cytotoxic agents have been used in immunologically mediated diseases, the most commonly used agents have been cyclophosphamide (an alkylating agent), azathioprine (a

740

purine analog antimetabolite), and methotrexate (a folic acid antagonist). These agents have been used mainly in diseases in which corticosteroid therapy was attempted but was unsuccessful in controlling the
aberrant inflammatory or immunologic reactivity.

Depending on the disease in question, cyclophosphamide generally
appears to be the most efficacious of these agents for chronic use in
man because it results in a high degree of immunosuppression without
great cost in adverse side-effects. For example, it results in striking
remissions in certain diseases, such as Wegener's granulomatosis and
corticosteroid-resistant nephrotic syndrome, at doses that cause relatively few side-effects. Cyclophosphamide therapy may also be efficacious in certain collagen vascular diseases and hypersensitivity vasculitides, although further clinical trials are clearly needed in these areas.
It is for this reason that cyclophosphamide and, to a lesser extent,
azathioprine are often considered the prototypes in discussions of
mechanisms of action and clinical effects of cytotoxic agents in immunologically mediated diseases.

However, regardless of the cytotoxic agents employed or the
disease in question, it is essential that one understand the general
mechanisms of the immunosuppressive effects of these agents and appreciate the delicate balance between the therapeutically desirable
suppression of aberrant immune reactivity and the potentially dangerous suppression of normal host defense mechanisms against infections,
in addition to being aware of the spectrum of other adverse side-effects
of these agents.

MECHANISMS OF ACTION OF CYTOTOXIC AGENTS

Since the pathogenesis of many of the immunologically mediated
diseases that are treated with cytotoxic agents is unclear, it is difficult to
delineate the precise mechanisms whereby cytotoxic agents cause clinical improvement in a particular disease. It is possible that clones of autoreactive or aberrantly reactive lymphoid cells are selectively eliminated by the drug. In a less specific manner, the general
anti-inflammatory and immunosuppressive effects may control the abnormal immune reactivity until the stimulus is removed or until a state
of tolerance ensues naturally. It is also possible that the drug directly
induces a state of tolerance to the stimulus in question. These potential
mechanisms are outlined in Table 25–1.

TABLE 25–1. Potential Mechanisms Whereby Cytotoxic Agents Are
Efficacious in Immunologically Mediated Diseases

Elimination of autoreactive or aberrantly reactive lymphoid clones
General suppression of aberrant immunologic reactivity
Nonspecific anti-inflammatory effects
Induction of tolerance to the underlying stimulus

Cytotoxic agents, particularly cyclophosphamide at extremely high doses, have been shown to have profound effects on practically every aspect of cell-mediated and humoral immune responses. These effects vary with the immunizing antigen, the dose of administered drug, and the temporal relationship between drug administration and immunization. Different cytotoxic agents have been shown in one study or another to suppress all parameters of immune reactivity, to selectively inhibit one or more limbs of the immune response, to cause enhancement of responses by selectively eliminating suppressor cells, and to induce tolerance by eliminating immune-reactive clones of cells. Although these studies are important in elucidating the scope of the mechanisms of action of these agents and in providing information regarding cellular requirements and interactions in different stages of the immune response, they may not all be directly applicable to the clinical situation. In the treatment of immunologically mediated diseases, cytotoxic agents are almost always administered to suppress an ongoing immunologic process. Low to moderate doses are usually administered over long periods of time (up to several years). Under these circumstances, it appears that the major mechanism of the immunosuppressive effect of these agents is a quantitative one of absolute lymphocytopenia. The mechanism of cell death varies with the particular cytotoxic agent used. For example, cyclophosphamide causes cross-linkage of DNA, and although it is most effective in depleting rapidly dividing cells, it is also effective against resting cells. Hence, a dramatic absolute lymphocytopenia of all identifiable lymphocyte populations occurs, despite the fact that several subpopulations of lymphocytes have relatively long half-lives. In this regard, it has been demonstrated in animal studies that cyclophosphamide has a selective effect against B-lymphocytes, which in general have shorter half-lives than T-lymphocytes. This selective effect on B-cells occurs with brief courses of high-dose therapy. In chronic drug reigmens used in human immunologically mediated diseases, there may indeed be an early but briefly selective effect on B-cells. However, as therapy continues, one gradually sees a depletion of all lymphocyte classes.

There is some debate regarding the degree to which cytotoxic agents suppress the functional capabilities of lymphocytes remaining in the circulation during drug-induced lymphocytopenia. The question arises whether the effect of drug on lymphoid cells is an all-or-none phenomenon. In other words, is the effect on lymphocytes merely one of elimination, with resulting lymphocytopenia, or are otherwise healthy-appearing cells that survive suppressed in their functional capabilities? Some studies have shown that *in vitro* blastogenic responses of lymphocytes to mitogenic stimuli such as phytohemagglutinin (PHA) are suppressed by cyclophosphamide therapy. The majority of studies, however, demonstrate that although *in vitro* responses to antigenic stimuli such as tetanus toxoid are suppressed, responses to mitogenic stimuli remain intact during chronic cyclophosphamide administration. This may be due to the greater relative strength of mitogenic stimuli or perhaps to the greater sensitivity of antigen-reactive cells to drug administration. The well-documented immunosuppressive effects of cyclophosphamide administered chronically to man in dosages of 1 to 2 mg per kilogram per day are listed in Table 25–2. It should be pointed out that many of the tests of cell functional capability are carried out *in vitro* in the absence of drug. In addition, these tests are often relatively unsophisticated and most likely do not truly reflect the complex functional interactions occurring *in vivo*. Hence, to what degree functional impairment of *in vivo* immunologic parameters occurs is still unclear.

In recent years, a wide range of lymphocyte functional capabilities has been delineated in connection with both the afferent and efferent limbs of immunologic reactivity. More detailed discussions of the mechanisms of tissue injury resulting from immunologic reactions and in immunologically mediated disease states are found in Chapters 13 and 20. Although immunologic reactions in their final manifestations are often attributed to a single type or class of lymphoid cell, it is clear that practically all reactions in either their inductive or effector phases require complex interactions with other cell types and various mediators. Cytotoxic agents can potentially exert their immunosuppressive effects by a direct functional impairment of one or more of these cell types, by an actual depletion of the cells, or by a combination of these two mechanisms. These effects are illustrated in Figure 25–1. The clinical situation in which both of these effects are clearly seen is during massive dose therapy, usually in neoplastic diseases and usually with combined chemotherapy. The major goal in this setting is to eliminate neoplastic cells. Severe leukopenia and even bone marrow aplasia, which are usually reversible, ensue. The functional capabilities of lymphoid cells during these inductions of therapy are almost always severely suppressed, either because the cells are dying and will soon be cleared from the circulation or because their metabolic capabilities are severely compromised. As mentioned previously, however, the most obvious effect of cytotoxic agents used chronically in relatively low doses that can be correlated with therapeutic efficacy is absolute lymphocytopenia and not a dramatic impairment of the functional capabilities of surviving

TABLE 25–2. Immunosuppressive Effects of Chronic Cyclophosphamide Therapy

Absolute lymphocytopenia of both T- and B-cells with early preferential depletion of B-cells
Suppression of *in vitro* lymphocyte blastogenic responses to specific antigenic stimuli
Reduction of elevated serum immunoglobulin levels
Suppression of antibody response and cutaneous delayed hypersensitivity to a new antigen with relative sparing of established cutaneous delayed hypersensitivity

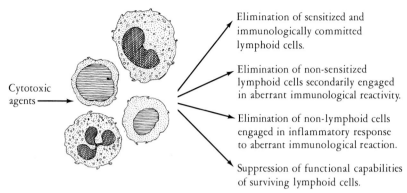

Cytotoxic agents ⟶

Elimination of sensitized and immunologically committed lymphoid cells.

Elimination of non-sensitized lymphoid cells secondarily engaged in aberrant immunological reactivity.

Elimination of non-lymphoid cells engaged in inflammatory response to aberrant immunological reaction.

Suppression of functional capabilities of surviving lymphoid cells.

Figure 25–1.   Various mechanisms of action of cytotoxic agents on inflammatory and immunological responses.

cells. This has obvious practical clinical relevance since lymphocyte counts can easily be monitored.

It is desirable to reduce the lymphocyte count as much as possible while maintaining the total leukocyte count (particularly the neutrophil count) above a certain critical level, which in effect is that level above which there is no significant risk of infection. It is often erroneously assumed that patients receiving cytotoxic agents are at an extremely high risk of infection because of their immunosuppressed state, regardless of the level of their granulocyte count. Indeed, it has been demonstrated in patients treated solely with cytotoxic agents such as cyclophosphamide that there is virtually no increased risk of bacterial infection if the drug dosage is carefully monitored to maintain the leukocyte count at a level no lower than 3000 per mm^3. This point deserves emphasis since such therapeutic regimens can thus lend themselves not only to close monitoring of the immunosuppressive effects but also to a realistic appraisal of the general host defense status of the patients.

A point should be made regarding the kinetics of the leukopenia associated with administration of cytotoxic agents such as cyclophosphamide. When using the drug regimens described above, specifically chronic administration of 1 to 2 mg per kilogram per day, a significant decrease in lymphocyte count is usually seen at approximately the fourteenth day of therapy. About this time a noticeable clinical response usually occurs; a decrease in neutrophil count occurs almost simultaneously with the lymphocytopenia. At this point the slope of decline of the leukocyte count must be determined and the drug dose eventually adjusted so that the total leukocyte count "levels off" at more than 3000 per mm^3. The neutrophil count is usually 1500 per mm^3 or greater at this point and the lymphocyte count will probably be as low as it feasibly can be. Any attempt to further decrease the lymphocyte count or to further suppress the functional capabilities of the remaining cells usually results only in a disproportionately greater decrease in the neutrophil count. A typical kinetic pattern of leukopenia with cyclophosphamide administration is shown in Figure 25–2.

Another important observation made with cytotoxic regimens is the progressive decrease in bone marrow reserve that occurs with chronic administration of these agents. In other words, most patients can tolerate progressively less drug while maintaining an adequate leukocyte count after months or years of therapy. The same degree of leukopenia (of all leukocyte classes) can be maintained with lower doses of drug. Therefore, reasonably frequent monitoring of the leukocyte count must be done, despite the fact that the disease is stable and the count appears stable.

COMPLICATIONS OF TREATMENT WITH CYTOTOXIC AGENTS

As mentioned above, one of the most important complications of treatment with cytotoxic agents is increased risk of infection, which is usually directly related to neutropenia. As a rule, the infections are bacterial and the organisms frequently are gram-negative rods such as *Pseudomonas aeruginosa*, which is the most common bacterial infection associated with the neutropenic state. For patients who are mildly neutropenic owing to cytotoxic agents, but whose leukocyte counts are within the range recommended above, there is relatively little increased risk of mycobacterial, fungal, parasitic, or viral infection unless there

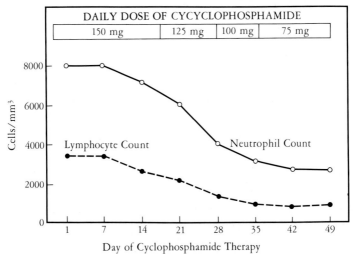

Figure 25–2. Kinetics of cyclophosphamide-induced leukopenia. This patient with Wegener's granulomatosis was started on 1½ mg per kg per day of cyclophosphamide. A typical kinetic pattern of drug-induced leukopenia is shown. Within 10 to 14 days of initiation of therapy, a gradual but progressive leukopenia of neutrophils and lymphocytes ensues that requires adjustment of dosage until a plateau is reached. Maintenance of high dose therapy during leukopenia usually results in a disproportionate further decrease, more in neutrophils than lymphocytes.

are other factors involved such as corticosteroid therapy or some underlying host defense defect.

Another complication of cytotoxic therapy is decreased immune surveillance and subsequent development of malignant disorders. This has been seen most commonly in renal transplant patients receiving chronic azathioprine therapy. In this group there has been a strikingly large percentage of histiocytic lymphomas involving the central nervous system.

There are other complications with cytotoxic agents that are too numerous to list and beyond the scope of this discussion, since many of them are specific for a given agent. However, the immunosuppressive doses of a cytotoxic agent such as cyclophosphamide that are commonly used in immunologically mediated diseases only infrequently result in serious or life-threatening side-effects. Gonadal dysfunction and variable degrees of alopecia are rather consistent findings with chronic cyclophosphamide therapy. Hemorrhagic cystitis and bladder fibrosis also occur. In addition, other less well documented findings such as pulmonary fibrosis have been reported.

Cytotoxic drugs clearly hold an important place as immunosuppressive agents in the treatment of immunologically mediated diseases. No doubt new agents will be developed with even greater efficacy and specificity, and thus their use will increase. It must be re-emphasized that at doses commonly employed clinically, most of the effects of cytotoxic agents related to immunosuppression and suppression of host defenses are predictable and quantifiable. Appreciation of this will allow intelligent and confident use of these agents when indicated, with appropriate respect for the hazards involved.

Finally, it should be pointed out that, above all, controlled clinical trials of these agents are mandatory in order to firmly establish their degree of efficacy in various diseases and to ensure their appropriate clinical use, guided by the principles outlined above.

CORTICOSTEROIDS

CLINICAL USAGE

Corticosteroids are clearly the most widely used agents in the treatment of inflammatory and immunologically mediated diseases. Their beneficial effects are often dramatic and their efficacy has been clearly established in several disease states. A partial list of diseases in which corticosteroid therapy frequently results in clinical improvement is shown in Table 25–3. However, the hazards and side-effects of these agents are numerous and must always be considered when embarking on therapeutic regimens.

Corticosteroids, as anti-inflammatory and immunosuppressive

TABLE 25–3. Diseases Commonly Treated with Corticosteroid Therapy

---

Connective tissue diseases: systemic lupus erythematosus, rheumatoid arthritis, acute rheumatic fever, polymyositis, dermatomyositis, scleroderma, and so forth
Inflammatory bowel disease: ulcerative colitis and regional enteritis
Hypersensitivity or allergic states: allergic vasculitis and severe drug reactions
Renal disease: idiopathic nephrotic syndrome and various nephritides
Immunologically mediated hematologic diseases: autoimmune hemolytic anemia
Organ transplantation rejection
Severe asthma
Noninfectious granulomatous diseases: sarcoidosis
Dermatologic diseases: contact dermatitis, pemphigus, and so forth
Ophthalmologic diseases: uveitis, allergic blepharitis, and so forth

---

agents, differ greatly from the cytotoxic drugs discussed previously. The prototype of corticosteroids is cortisol, an endogenous hormone in man essential for proper physiologic and metabolic function of virtually every organ system. Administration of this hormone or its analogs in pharmacologic doses not only results in anti-inflammatory and immunosuppressive effects, but also has profound effects on a variety of metabolic functions. The mechanisms of action of these agents are also clearly quite different from those of cytotoxic drugs. In order to gain maximal therapeutic benefit from the use of these agents, it is essential to appreciate their real and potential mechanisms of action in suppressing the inflammatory and immune responses, as well as understanding the delicate interrelationships between the pharmacologic concentrations of these agents and the normal physiologic and endocrinologic functions of the patient.

MECHANISMS OF ACTION OF CORTICOSTEROIDS

It has been known for many years that corticosteroid administration results in the destruction of lymphoid tissue in certain animal species, with subsequent shrinkage of spleen and lymph nodes and reduction in thymic weight and circulating lymphocytopenia.

The precise mechanisms whereby corticosteroids cause destruction of lymphoid tissue in these animal species is uncertain at present. However, it is felt that most of the tissue and cellular responses to corticosteroids are mediated by intracellular corticosteroid receptors. In a series of complex events, hormone binds to intracytoplasmic corticosteroid receptors and forms steroid-receptor complexes that migrate to and become associated with the cell nucleus. Synthesis of specific mRNA, which directs new protein synthesis, follows. This new protein may be inhibitory. Indeed, it has been shown that corticosteroid-induced RNA and protein synthesis is associated with the earliest detectable inhibitory effect on lymphoid cells, which is inhibition of glucose uptake. This is followed by inhibition of protein and nucleic acid metabolism, inhibition of growth, and cell lysis.

There is a fundamental difference between man and several animal species with regard to lymphoid-cell lysis as a major mechanism of immunosuppression. Certain animal species, such as the mouse, rat, and rabbit, are "corticosteroid-sensitive"; destruction of lymphoid tissue as described above is a major mechanism of action of this hormone on the immune system. On the other hand, man, as well as the monkey and guinea pig, is "corticosteroid-resistant." Pharmacologic concentrations of corticosteroids *in vivo* and even suprapharmacologic concentrations *in vitro* do not result in lysis of normal lymphocytes in man. It is true that in certain malignancies of lymphoid tissue in man, corticosteroid administration results in rapid shrinkage of enlarged nodes. This is most likely due, at least in part, to cell lysis. However, it should be pointed out that these lymphocytes are abnormal, and in certain lymphoid neoplasms they have been shown to contain a high density of corticosteroid receptors that are not found on normal lymphocytes and that render them susceptible to corticosteroid-induced lysis. Hence, cell lysis is not a major mechanism of corticosteroid-induced immunosuppression in inflammatory or immunologically mediated diseases in man. The mechanisms of action in man involve an overlap of pure anti-inflammatory effects with true immunosuppressive effects.

It is very difficult to clearly and distinctly separate anti-inflammatory from immunosuppressive effects, since the inflammatory response can function in both the afferent and the efferent limbs of the immune response. However, it has recently been possible to separate some of these effects while maintaining an appreciation of the natural overlap. Table 25–4 lists some of these effects, several of which will be described in detail below.

It is important to emphasize again that much of the information regarding the effect of corticosteroids on various cell types originates from animal studies in which the species employed was not comparable to man in degree of corticosteroid sensitivity. In addition, in most *in vitro* studies with human cells, the concentrations of *in vitro* corticosteroids used are clearly suprapharmacologic and unattainable *in vivo*.

TABLE 25–4. Anti-inflammatory and Immunosuppressive Effects of Corticosteroids

---

I. Anti-inflammatory effects
    1. Stabilization of vascular bed with decrease in leakage of fluid and cells into inflammatory sites
    2. Decreased granulocyte and monocyte accumulation in inflammatory loci
    3. Impairment of various granulocyte and monocyte functional capabilities
    4. Suppression of various steps in immediate hypersensitivity reactions

II. Immunosuppressive effects
    1. Decrease in circulating lymphocytes and monocytes
    2. Decrease in certain lymphocyte and particularly monocyte functional capabilities
    3. Decrease in immunoglobulin and complement levels

Practically every functional capability of leukocytes can be suppressed if a high enough concentration of corticosteroids is added to cultures. It is important to separate laboratory phenomena from true anti-inflammatory and immunosuppressive effects of *in vivo* corticosteroids in concentrations that can feasibly be administered to patients. This will be pointed out in the following discussions.

It is convenient to divide the effects of corticosteroids on various leukocyte classes into effects on (1) cell movement (traffic, kinetics, and circulatory capabilities), and (2) cell functional capabilities.

Effects on Cell Movement

Perhaps the major mechanism whereby corticosteroids exert their anti-inflammatory effects in man is simply by preventing the accumulation of neutrophils at inflammatory sites. This can be accomplished with reasonable pharmacologic doses of drug, whereas suppression of such functional capabilities as phagocytosis, enzyme release, and intracellular killing of microbes require concentrations of drug that for all practical purposes are unattainable *in vivo*. The effects of corticosteroids on neutrophil movement are complex and multifaceted. They cause a release of young neutrophils from the bone marrow into the circulation; this is the basis for the use of these agents to determine bone marrow reserves. In addition, they cause an increase in neutrophil circulating half-life. The combination of these two effects results in the well-recognized corticosteroid-induced neutrophilia. Finally, these agents cause a decrease in migration and accumulation of neutrophils in inflammatory sites. Neutrophils adhere to vascular endothelium following an inflammatory stimulus and subsequently migrate into the inflammatory site. Corticosteroids prevent this action by impeding the initial adherence. In this regard, it has been clearly demonstrated that corticosteroid administration significantly decreases the normal neutrophil adherence to nylon-wool columns. Similar phenomena have recently been demonstrated with eosinophil adherence. The various effects of corticosteroids on neutrophil kinetics are illustrated in Figure 25–3.

The striking degree of eosinopenia seen following corticosteroid administration is felt to be due not to a destruction of cells, but to a redistribution of circulating eosinophils from the intravascular space into other body compartments. Hence, the effect of corticosteroids on circulating eosinophils is at least twofold: they impede cell adherence and subsequent migration into inflammatory sites, and they cause an eosinopenia by redistribution of cells.

Corticosteroid administration also has profound effects on lymphocyte and monocyte traffic and circulatory kinetics. There is a marked but transient lymphocytopenia and monocytopenia that is maximal at four to six hours after oral or parenteral administration of the drug,

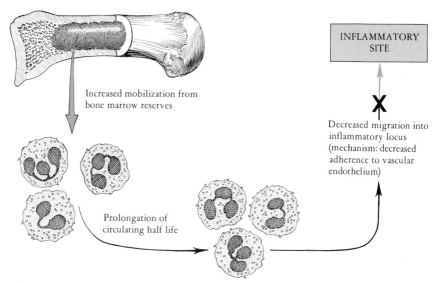

Increased mobilization from
bone marrow reserves

INFLAMMATORY
SITE

X

Decreased migration into
inflammatory locus
(mechanism: decreased
adherence to vascular
endothelium)

Prolongation of
circulating half life

Figure 25–3.   Effect of corticosteroid therapy on neutrophil kinetics. Corticosteroids
effect neutrophil kinetics by increasing mobilization of cells from bone marrow reserves,
by prolonging the circulating half-life of the neutrophil and by decreasing migration of
neutrophils into inflammatory loci.

with a return to normal counts by 24 hours. This phenomenon is
reproducible after each dose of corticosteroids (Figure 25–4). In addition, the effects are not cumulative over months and years of drug administration. This is particularly evident in patients who are receiving a
single daily dose or a single dose on alternate days of a corticosteroid
preparation such as prednisone. Before each dose the lymphocyte
count returns to a normal level, only to decrease dramatically four to
six hours after drug administration.

It is noteworthy that the lymphocytopenia is selective; i.e., T-
lymphocytes are preferentially depleted from the circulation to a
greater extent than are B-lymphocytes. In addition, there is a selective
depletion of certain functional T-cell subpopulations, as determined by
in vitro responsiveness to some mitogens and antigens. Of interest is the
fact that at the point of maximal lymphocytopenia, after doses of prednisone in the range of 60 to 80 mg, there is very little, if any, suppression of the functional capabilities of the lymphocytes left in the circulation, as measured by various *in vitro* functional parameters. In other
words, one of the major effects of corticosteroids on lymphoid cells in
doses commonly used in inflammatory and immunologically mediated
diseases is not a qualitative functional suppression but a quantitative
depletion of lymphocytes from the circulation, thus making them less
readily available to the tissue involved in the immunologic reaction.
There also appears to be a lower limit of lymphocytopenia beneath
which even massive doses of corticosteroids cannot push the lympho-

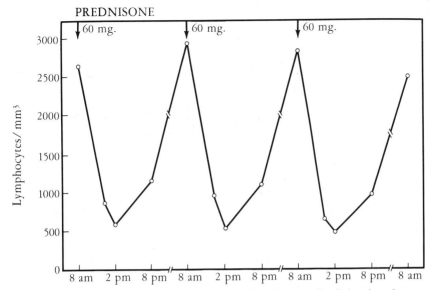

Figure 25-4. Effect of corticosteroid administration on circulating lymphocytes. This patient was given 60 mg per day of prednisone orally in a single dose. A marked, but transient, lymphocytopenia was seen 4 to 6 hours after each dose of drug, with a return to normal counts by the next morning.

cyte count. In fact, the degree and kinetics of lymphocytopenia that follows a wide range of doses of corticosteroids from approximately 20 mg of prednisone to as high as 1 gm of methylprednisolone are strikingly similar. The increase in immunosuppressive effects at these higher doses of corticosteroid are due much less to a quantitative effect of a greater degree of lymphocytopenia than to a qualitative effect on functional capabilities of cells, which will be discussed below. The effects of corticosteroid administration on leukocyte movement and kinetics in man are summarized in Table 25–5.

One can best understand the mechanisms whereby corticosteroid administration causes a lymphocytopenia in man by appreciating the

TABLE 25–5.   Effects of Corticosteroid Administration on Leukocyte Movement and Kinetics in Man

1. Neutrophilia resulting from a mobilization of bone marrow reserves and prolongation of circulating half-life
2. Decrease in accumulation of neutrophils in inflammatory loci by a decrease in cell adherence to vascular endothelium
3. Eosinopenia by redistribution of cells out of the circulation and decrease in accumulation of eosinophils in inflammatory loci by decrease in adherence to vascular endothelium
4. Circulating lymphocytopenia with a selectively greater depletion of T-lymphocytes than of B-lymphocytes by a redistribution of cells out of the circulation
5. Circulating monocytopenia, probably resulting from a redistribution phenomenon, and decrease in accumulation of monocytes in inflammatory loci

TABLE 25–6. Intravascular Pools of Circulating Lymphocytes

1. *Recirculating Pool:* makes up approximately 70 per cent of intravascular lymphocyte pool; comprises mostly long-lived T-lymphocytes; in constant equilibrium with and has free access to the vastly larger extravascular portion of the recirculating lymphocyte pool contained in the lymph nodes, spleen, thoracic duct, and bone marrow
2. *Nonrecirculating Pool:* makes up approximately 30 per cent of intravascular lymphocyte pool; comprises mostly short-lived non-T-lymphocytes; cells do not normally have free access into and out of the circulation; either live out their life span and become effete or are activated and leave the intravascular space

fact that intravascular lymphocytes comprise two major pools, as summarized in Table 25–6. Corticosteroids cause a depletion of cells predominantly from the intravascular recirculating pool. The depletion is caused by a redistribution of cells out of the circulation from the intravascular to the extravascular recirculating pool. This phenomenon is illustrated schematically in Figure 25–5. Corticosteroids thus cause a depletion in the intravascular space of predominantly long-lived T-cells, which are part of a large total-body recirculating pool of cells that under normal circumstances have relatively free access into and

INTRAVASCULAR LYMPHOCYTE POOL

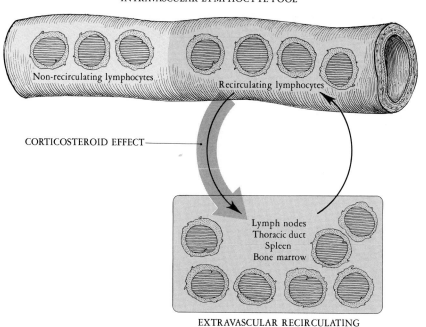

EXTRAVASCULAR RECIRCULATING
LYMPHOCYTE POOL

Figure 25–5. Corticosteroid-induced redistribution of recirculating lymphocytes from the intravascular to the extravascular pool. Recirculating lymphocytes are normally in equilibrium between these pools, and corticosteroids redirect traffic of these cells in the direction of the extravascular pool, resulting in a transient lymphocytopenia.

out of the intravascular space. The drug acts by affecting the traffic of these cells and temporarily altering this constant equilibrium in the direction of the lymphocytopenic state.

The precise mechanisms whereby corticosteroids cause this redistribution are unclear at present. The drug may act directly or indirectly on the microvasculature, or it may affect the lymphocyte itself, or a combination of the two may occur. *In vitro* treatment of lymphocytes with various enzymes that affect the cell-surface molecular configuration cause modifications of circulation patterns upon reinfusion similar to that seen with *in vivo* corticosteroids. Thus, it is likely that corticosteroid-induced modification of the lymphocyte surface plays a major role in the mechanisms of redistribution. Similar effects on cell-surface molecular configuration may explain the corticosteroid effects on monocyte circulation and on adherence properties of neutrophils and eosinophils.

Effects on Cell Function

As mentioned previously, it is possible to interfere with virtually every functional capability of the different classes of leukocytes by using sufficiently high concentrations of *in vitro* corticosteroids. Probably very few of these suppressive effects are relevant with pharmacologic concentrations of *in vivo* corticosteroids used in patients, however. For example, *in vitro* corticosteroids have been shown to suppress phagocytosis and microbicidal functions of neutrophils. When used in suprapharmacologic concentrations they stabilize granulocyte lysosomal membranes and can potentially alter all functional capabilities, as well as decreasing inflammatory responses by blocking the release of lysosomal enzymes. In addition, the responses of granulocytes to chemotactic factors have been suppressed by high concentrations of *in vitro* corticosteroids. However, it appears that the major neutrophil-related effect of corticosteroids at pharmacologic *in vivo* concentrations is a blockage of cells from reaching the inflammatory site, with a relative sparing of actual functional capabilities.

It is noteworthy that monocytes are more sensitive to the effects of corticosteroids than are neutrophils. Corticosteroids not only cause monocytopenia and decreased migration of monocytes into inflammatory sites, but also inhibit microbicidal activity of human monocytes at concentrations of drug that are attainable *in vivo*. The inability of monocytes to respond normally to macrophage migration inhibitory factor (MIF) produced by sensitized lymphocytes may well explain the suppression of cutaneous delayed hypersensitivity seen during daily corticosteroid therapy.

Monocyte-macrophages are the cells that are transformed into epithelioid cells and multinucleated giant cells in the formation of granulomatous reactions. Thus, this high degree of monocyte sensitivity to corticosteroids may explain the dramatic response of certain hypersensitivity granulomatous diseases to corticosteroid therapy as well as the breakdown of granulomas that contain dormant mycobacteria leading to the reactivation of tuberculosis in some patients receiving corticosteroid therapy.

Practically all aspects of lymphocyte function, ranging from antigen processing and lymphocyte activation, through proliferation, differentiation, and a whole host of effector functions, can be suppressed by high enough concentrations of *in vitro* corticosteroids. There is much conflicting evidence in the area of corticosteroids and lymphocyte function, relating partially to the fact that in some studies drug was given *in vivo* and *in vitro* functions were measured, and in other studies drug was placed *in vitro* and the cell suspension was assayed. Moreover, most phenomena related to cell-mediated, as well as humoral, immunity represent a complexity of cellular interactions and cooperations ranging from a balance of helper and suppressor effects to the cumulative effects of multiple cooperating cell types involved in the effector limb of the immune response. Interference with the functions or availability of a given cell type may impede the entire immunologic reaction. Corticosteroids have the potential to directly suppress the functional capability of lymphocytes and monocytes or interfere with their availability to the immunologic reaction, or both. As mentioned previously, certain monocyte functions are quite sensitive to corticosteroids. From a practical standpoint, however, most of the lymphocyte functional capabilities, such as mediator production and release, cytotoxic effector activity, and even proliferative responses, are relatively resistant to pharmacologically attainable concentrations of corticosteroids. It should be mentioned that although immunoglobulin production in man can be suppressed somewhat by high doses of corticosteroids, specific antibody production, particularly in secondary IgG responses, is quite resistant to corticosteroid therapy. Thus, it appears that the major mechanism whereby pharmacologic concentrations of corticosteroids exert their effects on lymphoid cells is by interfering with their availability to the immunologic reaction.

THERAPEUTIC REGIMENS

The major goal in designing or choosing a therapeutic regimen is to obtain the maximal anti-inflammatory and immunosuppressive effects balanced with the least adverse side-effects. It is clear, however, that the most effective immunosuppressive regimen, namely high-dose, divided-dose, daily therapy, is associated with the most severe side-effects. A list of some of the adverse side-effects associated with corticosteroid therapy is given in Table 25–7. As the total dose of drug is lowered, and more importantly as one goes from divided daily doses to a single daily dose or preferably to a single dose on alternate days,

TABLE 25-7.   Adverse Side-Effects Associated with Daily
Corticosteroid Therapy

Diabetes mellitus
Osteoporosis
Psychologic disorders
Hypertension
Electrolyte disturbances
Increased susceptibility to infections
Suppression of normal hypothalamic-pituitary-adrenal axis
Cushingoid body habitus
Retardation of growth in children
Cataracts
Glaucoma
Aseptic necrosis of bone
Pancreatitis
Intracranial hypertension
Panniculitis
Poor wound healing
Exacerbation of peptic ulcer
Hypercatabolism

there are relatively few side-effects. It has been shown that alternate-day corticosteroid regimens cause significantly less growth retardation in children and result in relatively little suppression of the normal pituitary-adrenal axis. In addition, there is a marked reduction, if not disappearance, of most of the other adverse side-effects listed in Table 25–7.

The preferable approach in serious active inflammatory or immunologically mediated diseases is to initiate therapy with high (45 to 80 mg of prednisone) divided daily doses until the disease activity is brought under control. At this point, attempts should be made to convert to a single daily dose of drug and then gradually to a single-dose alternate-day regimen.

With alternate-day corticosteroid regimens, for the entire "off day" and part of the "on day," monocyte and lymphocyte counts, proportions of lymphocyte subpopulations, various functional capabilities of cells, and all other measurable parameters are normal. This explains the intact cutaneous delayed hypersensitivity and the lack of increased susceptibility to infections in patients receiving alternate-day corticosteroid regimens. Such regimens are quite effective, in certain diseases, in maintaining a state of remission, despite the fact that inflammatory and immunologic reactivity are normal for at least half the time. This is due to the fact that full expression of inflammatory activity in most immunologically mediated diseases requires several days to accelerate in order to be clinically detectable. The intermittent suppression of the mechanisms of inflammatory or immunologic reactivity are sufficient to keep the disease process from reaccelerating, and hence it remains at a subclinical level. However, as mentioned above, induction of disease

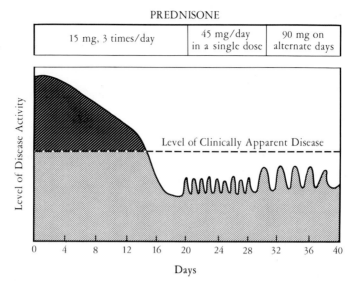

PREDNISONE

15 mg, 3 times/day	45 mg/day in a single dose	90 mg on alternate days

Figure 25-6.   Effect of various regimens of corticosteroid therapy on disease activity in inflammatory and immunologically mediated diseases. During flagrant disease activity, daily divided dose therapy is usually necessary to bring the disease process under control and to a state of clinically inapparent activity. Once this is achieved, one can gradually convert to a single daily dose or alternate-day dose. This type of regimen can usually maintain the disease process in remission with slight fluctuations in activity related to the drug administration but within the subclinical or clinically inapparent area.

remission usually requires "semi-continuous" administration of drug in daily divided doses until disease activity is brought to the clinically inapparent level, where it can be maintained with alternate-day therapy. This therapeutic approach is illustrated in Figure 25-6. Likewise, when a disease relapses on alternate-day therapy, it is usually necessary to revert back temporarily to daily single-dose or divided-dose therapy until the disease activity is brought to a point where it can again be maintained in remission by an alternate-day regimen. Such an approach should provide the optimal necessary immunosuppressive effect with minimal adverse side-effects, which is the major objective in the treatment of immunologically mediated diseases with corticosteroids.

SUGGESTIONS FOR FURTHER READING

Baxter, J. D., and Forsham, P. H.: Tissue effects of glucocorticoids. Am. J. Med., 53:573–589, 1972.

Baxter, J. D., and Harris, A. W.: Mechanisms of glucocorticoid action: General features with reference to steroid-mediated immunosuppression. Transplant. Proc., 7:55–65, 1975.

Calabresi, P., and Parks, R. E., Jr.: Alkylating agents, antimetabolites, hormones, and other antiproliferative agents. *In* L. S. Goodman, and A. Gilman (eds.), *The Pharmacological Basis of Therapeutics.* 4th ed., London, The Macmillan Co., 1971.

Claman, H. N.: Corticosteroids and lymphoid cells. N. Engl. J. Med.,*287*:388–397, 1972.

David, D. S., Grieco, M. H., and Cushman, P., Jr.: Adrenal glucocorticoids after twenty years. A review of their clinically relevant consequences. J. Chronic Dis., *22*:637–711, 1970.

Fauci, A. S., Dale, D. C., and Balow, J. E.: Glucocorticosteroid therapy: Mechanisms of action and clinical considerations. Ann. Intern. Med., *84*:304–315, 1976.

Fauci, A. S., Dale, D. C., and Wolff, S. M.: Cyclophosphamide and lymphocyte subpopulations in Wegener's granulomatosis. Arthritis Rheum., *17*:355–362, 1974.

Gabrielsen, A. E., and Good, R. A.: Chemical suppression of adaptive immunity. Adv. Immunol., *6*:91–229, 1967.

Steinberg, A. D., Plotz, P. H., Wolff, S. M., Wong, V. G., Agus, S. G., and Decker, J. L.: Cytotoxic drugs in treatment of nonmalignant diseases. Ann. Intern. Med., *76*:619–642, 1972.

Thompson, E. B., and Lippman, M. E.: Mechanisms of action of glucocorticoids. Metabolism, *23*:159–202, 1974.

Thorn, G. W.: Clinical considerations in the use of corticosteroids. N. Engl. J. Med., *274*:775–781, 1966.

_____

Chapter 26

DIAGNOSTIC APPLICATIONS
OF IMMUNOLOGY

Joseph A. Bellanti, M.D.

Immunologic testing is used in conjunction with other laboratory procedures in the diagnosis of disease states and in the assessment of immunologic function. The following series of appendices is grouped into two major categories: (1) *immunologic techniques used in the assessment of normal immune competence or in the diagnosis of diseases in which altered immunologic function occurs* and (2) *immunologic techniques employed in the diagnosis of nonimmunologic diseases.*

In this section, it is not possible to describe in detail the numerous tests useful in clinical immunology. Through the monumental efforts of the American Society for Microbiology, however, a comprehensive *Manual of Clinical Immunology* has been published recently, and the reader is referred to this excellent source for further details of the procedures.*

TESTS OF IMMUNOLOGIC FUNCTION

The tests that may be used in assessing immunologic function are shown in Table 26–1. For ease of discussion, these are classified according to an arbitrary scheme (presented in Chapter 20) as *nonspecific (primary)*, *specific (secondary)*, and *tissue-damaging (tertiary)* immune responses.

TESTS OF NONSPECIFIC (PRIMARY) IMMUNE FUNCTION

The tests of nonspecific immune function measure one or more aspects of the *inflammatory response* and *phagocytosis* and reflect the body's nonspecific responses to encounter with a foreign configuration (Chapter 2).

_____

*Rose, N. R., and Friedman, H. (eds.): Manual of Clinical Immunology. Washington, D.C., American Society of Microbiology, 1976.

TABLE 26–1.   Tests of Immunologic Function

Nonspecific (Primary) Immune Response	Specific (Secondary) Immune Response	Tissue-Damaging (Tertiary) Immune Response
Tests of Inflammatory Response WBC count and differential Sedimentation rate C-reactive protein Complement activity Rebuck skin window technique Chemotactic assay *Tests of Phagocytic Function* Phagocytic index Bactericidal activity Quantitative or histochemical NBT test Measurement of specific WBC enzymes	*Enumeration of B- and T-lymphocytes (EA, EAC, and E rosettes)* *Tests of Humoral (Antibody) Function* Quantification of immuno-globulins Specific antibody responses: prior sensitization, isohemag-glutinins (IgM), DPT, polio-virus, or measles (IgG) Shick and Dick tests (IgG) Specific antibody responses: *de novo* sensitization, Sal-monella O (IgM); H (IgG) *Tests of Cell-Mediated (Delayed Hypersensitivity) Function* *In vivo* Skin tests (prior sensitization), Candida, Trichophyton, streptokinase-strepto-dornase (SKSD) Skin tests (*de novo* sensitiza-tion): DNCB Skin grafts *In vitro* Lymphocyte stimulation: nonspecific (PHA); specific (antigen) Measurement of effector molecules (MIF) *Lymph node biopsy*	*Tests of Reagin (IgE) Hyper-sensitivity* Direct measurement of IgE globulins (RIST, PRIST); IgE antibody (RAST) Immediate hypersensitivity skin tests Histamine release *Tests of Cytotoxic Injury* Red cell agglutinins Antiglobulin test (Coombs) *Tests of Ag-Ab Complex Injury* Rheumatoid factor (RF) Antinuclear factor (ANF) or LE prep Serum complement (C1q, C3, C5) Tissue biopsy (localization of IgG and C components by immunofluorescence) *Tests of Injury Due to Delayed Hypersensitivity* Tissue biopsy, infiltration of lymphocytes in areas of injury Skin tests (patch) in contact hypersensitivity

Tests of Inflammatory Response

The white blood cell count and differential, sedimentation rate, C-reactive protein, complement activity, Rebuck skin window technique, and chemotactic assay are all useful in assessing whether an inflammatory response is in progress and in determining the functional integrity of the *afferent* limb of the immune response. In general, they all are increased during the phase of acute inflammation, and the sedimentation rate is elevated in more protracted (chronic) inflammatory responses.

Complement. Measurement of serum complement activity is a useful test in several clinical situations. Either total serum complement or individual complement components may be measured (Chapter 6). C3 (β_1C globulin) is the major component of complement in serum and is easily measured by radial immunodiffusion. The complement system is evaluated to detect deficiencies resulting from (1) inborn deficiencies of the complement components, e.g., hereditary angioedema (HAE), or the presence of inhibitors of complement activity (Chapters 6 and 22) or (2) increased complement utilization resulting from ongoing immunologic processes, e.g., acute glomerulonephritis (Chapter 20C).

The primary role of the inflammatory response and phagocytosis in the body economy is the localization and removal or destruction of foreign substances, such as bacteria. For ease of discussion, the tests of inflammatory response and phagocytic function can be divided into the sequential steps described in Chapter 2 that measure (1) cell movement (motility), (2) phagocytosis (attachment and ingestion), (3) metabolic events associated with phagocytosis, and (4) antimicrobial mechanisms.

Tests of Cell Movement

Rebuck Skin Window Technique. A widely used *in vivo* method for the study of inflammation is the "skin window" technique of Rebuck. A sterile cover slip is placed over a superficially abraded area of skin; several hours later, the cover slip is removed and the number of leukocytes is counted. Within three to four hours, over 90 per cent of the cellular composition consists of polymorphonuclear leukocytes. After 12 hours, they are replaced by mononuclear cells, and at 24 hours, well over 50 per cent of the cells are monocytes and macrophages. The technique may also be used to study the response to both antigenic and nonantigenic stimuli. Its use is indicated in defects of chemotaxis (e.g., complement deficiencies) and in other conditions. An impairment of the inflammatory response is seen in a variety of clinical conditions, such as alcoholism, steroid administration, and diabetes, and as a developmental immaturity. Although the technique is semiquantitative and may not be truly measuring chemotaxis, it provides some useful information regarding *in vivo* cell movement.

In Vitro Tests of Cell Movement. The movement of phagocytic cells can be either *random* or *directed* (chemotaxis). A test for the random motility of leukocytes developed by Miller is performed by the vertical migration of white blood cells in a capillary tube. Patients with the lazy leukocyte syndrome have been described as demonstrating abnormalities of random migration in conjunction with defective chemotaxis and neutropenia (Chapter 22).

The technique most widely used today for *in vitro* examination of chemotaxis is that introduced by Boyden and employs a plastic chamber separated into two parts by a filter of known porosity, e.g., Millipore filter. A leukocyte suspension is introduced on one side of the chamber and fluid containing a chemoattractant is placed on the other side. After a variable interval of time, the filter is removed and stained and the number of leukocytes that have migrated through is determined (Fig. 26–1). Attractants used in this assay can be derived from several sources,

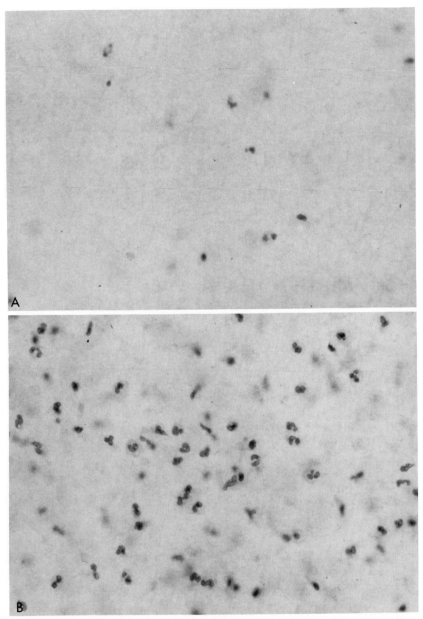

Figure 26–1. Millipore filter stained with Wright-Giemsa stain (magnification approximately × 500) after 30 minutes' incubation in the presence of control medium (*A*) or a chemoattractant (*B*). Note the paucity of leukocytes in the control preparation (*A*) as compared to the large number of cells, predominantly polymorphonuclear leukocytes, that have emigrated through the filter toward the attractant.

including bacterial extracts, products of the complement system (Chapter 6), or products of the lymphocytic cells, e.g., lymphokines (Chapter 9). Moreover, chemoattractants have been described not only for phagocytic cells e.g., monocytes, neutrophils, and eosinophils, but also for basophils, and lymphocytes. Assays of chemotaxis most frequently involve the functional assessment of blood neutrophils, however, since these cells are the most importantly involved.

Chemotactic defects are found most commonly in patients with chronic recurrent bacterial infections that can be due to either *intracellular defects*, e.g., Chédiak-Higashi syndrome or diabetes mellitus, or defects in the generation of *extracellular* chemotactic factors, e.g., C3 deficiency (Chapter 22).

Tests of Phagocytosis (Attachment and Ingestion)

These tests of phagocytosis measure the capacity of the phagocytic cell to take up inert particles, e.g., polystyrene, or microorganisms, e.g., bacteria. Since internalization of these particles may require the presence of opsonins (complement or antibody), the tests are usually performed in the presence of fresh serum, either the patient's serum, which will test its opsonic ability, or pooled human serum. After an appropriate incubation under specified conditions, the average number of particles ingested per phagocytic cell is determined, as well as the percentage of phagocytic cells or cells that have phagocytosed the particles. These tests measure the ability of the phagocyte to ingest particles but not necessarily its ability to degrade them intracellularly. However, recent modifications of these tests, employing either supravital stains or fluorochromes, have made it possible to combine tests of phagocytic function with those measuring intracellular killing. Tests of phagocytosis are performed in patients suspected of having disorders of the phagocytes, such as the neutrophil dysfunction syndrome, or defects in complement or antibody-mediated opsonization (Chapter 22).

Tests Measuring Metabolic Events Associated with Phagocytosis

After the uptake of a particle by a phagocytic cell, a series of biochemical events is initiated. Primarily, these events include the stimulation of the glycolytic pathway and the hexose monophosphate (HMP) shunt ("respiratory burst"), the release of lysosomal enzymes into the phagosome ("degranulation"), and the generation of H_2O_2 and several activated forms of oxygen, e.g., superoxide radical and singlet oxygen, that can be measured by chemiluminescence (Chapter 2). Although a number of sophisticated biochemical reactions can be measured, two assays have received attention in clinical immunology laboratories, i.e., the nitroblue tetrazolium dye reduction (NBT) test and a test for degranulation (the "frustrated phagocytosis test").

A quantitative NBT test has been developed that is based on the increased metabolic activity of the phagocyte that occurs with particle uptake and intracellular digestion. The increased flow of protons through the hexose monophosphate shunt during phagocytosis and intracellular digestion is measured colorimetrically by the reduction of the nitroblue tetrazolium dye to a blue formazan pigment. The results are expressed as an increase in optical density (ΔOD), the difference between resting and phagocytosing states. The quantitative NBT test is markedly depressed in cases in which there is an impairment in metabolic activity of leukocytes, such as in chronic granulomatous disease (CGD).

A number of histochemical tests for NBT dye reduction that measure the number of cells reducing the dye *in situ* have been developed. These tests may also measure the relative degree of dye reduction by resting (unstimulated) leukocytes as well as those that have been stimulated by the ingestion of particles or by exposure to endotoxin. Since young infants have relatively high numbers of neutrophils that reduce dye in this "resting" state, this test has not been found to be useful in diagnostic screening for neutrophil dysfunction in the newborn. Furthermore, since there is an increase in quantitative NBT function with age, interpretations of this test must be age-adjusted. Table 26–2 gives the values of quantitative NBT function by age level. Although the NBT test has been suggested as an aid in differentiating viral from bacterial febrile disorders, this application is not generally accepted owing to a number of variables that affect the interpretation of the test.

A test for *degranulation* has also been developed that has been called a test of frustrated phagocytosis. The assay measures degranulation independent of ingestion of particles and employs the release of lysosomal enzymes from the phagocyte following exposure to heat-aggregated gamma globulin or immune complexes that are fixed to a solid surface. The rate of release of lysosomal enzymes, e.g., β-glucuronidase and acid phosphatase, is taken as an estimate of the rate of

TABLE 26–2. Quantitative NBT Values with Maturation

Age	Number Tested	Quantitative NBT Test ΔOD $\pm$ S.E.
Newborn	23	0.127 $\pm$ 0.011
1–6 months	13	0.090 $\pm$ 0.008
6–12 months	21	0.098 $\pm$ 0.008
12–18 months	18	0.123 $\pm$ 0.011
1.5–4 years	20	0.148 $\pm$ 0.013
4–10 years	19	0.139 $\pm$ 0.007
10–14 years	8	0.175 $\pm$ 0.024
Adults	18	0.206 $\pm$ 0.025

degranulation. The assay has been employed in the study of the neutrophil dysfunction syndrome. Neutrophils from patients with CGD have a delayed release of lysosomal enzymes.

Tests Measuring Antimicrobial Mechanisms

The ultimate test of the phagocyte's function is its microbicidal activity. These tests are usually performed with bacteria and measure the ability of the phagocytic cell to ingest (phagocytose) and subsequently kill the organism. Phagocytic activity involves a multiphasic act requiring the integrity of both extracellular factors (complement and antibody) and intracellular factors (intact metabolic integrity of the cell). The test is usually performed by mixing a suspension of leukocytes with bacteria in the presence of fresh serum. After an appropriate length of time, the amount of viable bacteria remaining within the cells is measured by direct culture technique, fluorescence, or supravital stains. Although *Staphylococcus aureus* is commonly used, the test should also include the infectious organism found in the patient (Fig. 26–2). These tests are indicated in the diagnosis of neutrophil dysfunction and in deficiencies of specific antibody or complement.

Quantitative Measurement of Specific Leukocyte Enzymes

It is now apparent that a number of causes of recurrent infections are related to selective enzyme deficiencies, as seen in the neutrophil dysfunction syndrome. These specific enzyme deficiencies include leukocyte NADH-oxidase, NADPH-oxidase, glucose-6-phosphate dehydrogenase (G-6-PD), glutathione peroxidase, and leukocyte myeloperoxidase (MPO) (Chapter 22). Although these assays are not currently performed in most clinical laboratories, it is conceivable that they will become more readily available within the near future.

TESTS OF SPECIFIC (SECONDARY) IMMUNE FUNCTION

Tests of specific immune function measure those functions associated with humoral (B-lymphocyte-mediated) immunity or with cell-mediated (T-lymphocyte-mediated) immunity (Table 26–1).

Enumeration of Lymphocyte Populations

Diagnostic studies should begin with a white blood cell and differential count to assess the total and the relative number of lymphocytes in the peripheral blood. The absolute lymphocyte count is usually greater than 2500 cells per cubic millimeter, and a count below 1500 per cubic millimeter is suggestive of a *primary* immune deficiency that could occur at the stem cell, B-cell, or T-cell level or any of a

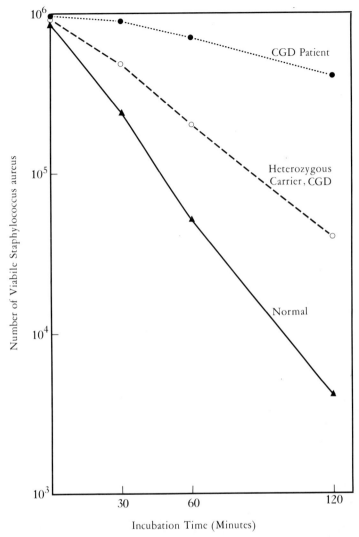

Figure 26–2. Schematic representation of microbicidal activity of phagocytes from normal subjects, carriers, and patients with CGD.

number of *secondary* immune deficiencies that result in the diminution of the total numbers of circulating lymphocytes (Chapter 22). The next step in the process is the determination of the relative numbers of B- and T-lymphocytes. These tests are recent, valuable additions to the armamentarium of the physician and are based on the surface properties of lymphocytes, described in Chapter 7. Shown in Table 26–3 are five types of lymphocyte markers commonly measured, together with the method employed, their significance, and the values obtained.

TABLE 26–3. Values of Lymphoid Cell Populations by Various Methods of Enumeration*

Marker	Method	Significance	Values (%) Range	Values (%) Mean
Membrane Ig (mIg)	Immunofluorescence	B-cell, plus	1–18	5.9
Fc receptor	Immune complexes	B-cell, plus	8–30	20
	EA			
	$E_{ox}A$		8–36	22
Complement receptor	EAC rosettes	B-cell, plus	10–25	18
B-cell antigens	Immunofluorescence	B-cell, plus	10–30	18
E rosette	E_{sheep} rosette	T-cell	85–93	89

*After Winchester, R. J., and Ross, G.: Methods for enumerating lymphocyte populations. *In* N. R. Rose, and H. Friedman (eds.): Manual of Clinical Immunology. Washington, D.C., American Society for Microbiology, 1976.

B-Lymphocyte Assays. The typical B-lymphocyte is recognized by the presence of readily detectable membrane immunoglobulin (mIg) and receptors for the Fc region of IgG and for complement Chapter 7).

Membrane immunoglobulin (mIg). Lymphocytes bearing surface immunoglobulins are detected by antibody tagged with fluorochrome. It is important in these determinations that the surface immunoglobulin be shown to be synthesized by the lymphocyte and not exogenously adsorbed. The predominant immunoglobulins on the surface of the peripheral blood B-lymphocyte are the IgD and IgM (Table 26–4). These values are considerably lower than those previously reported, which were factitiously in error owing to nonspecific responses, adsorption of immune complexes, and the use of anti–whole Ig rather than anti-Fab'2.

Tests for Fc receptor (Immune complex–binding assay and EA assay). B-lymphocytes can also be detected by the presence of a receptor for the Fc region of IgG. This receptor, which is also present on K-cells, is capable

TABLE 26–4. Membrane Immunoglobulin (mIg)–Bearing B-Lymphocytes in Normal Adult Blood*

Class	Range (%)	Mean (%)
IgG	0–1	<1
IgA	0–1	<1
IgD	1–14	4.6
IgM	1–16	4.8
IgD, IgM	1–18	5.9
κ and λ	1–18	6.0

*After Winchester, R. J., and Ross, G.: Methods for enumerating lymphocyte populations. *In* N. R. Rose, and H. Friedman (eds.): Manual of Clinical Immunology. Washington, D.C., American Society for Microbiology, 1976.

of binding antigen-antibody complexes but not the Fc regions of native immunoglobulin. The tests commonly employ immune complexes tagged with fluorochrome or rosette formation with IgG antibody–coated erythrocytes (EA rosette test). Recently, an ox erythrocyte assay $E_{ox}A$ test) for the detection of the Fc receptor has been developed and offers several additional advantages of specificity. The mean value for immune complex–binding assay is 20 per cent, with a range of 8 to 30 per cent; the mean value for the EA test employing sheep cells or ox cells is 22 per cent, with a range of 8 to 36 per cent.

Tests for complement receptor (EAC assay). Human lymphocytes also contain two types of complement receptors, including (1) the immune adherence receptor, C3b, and (2) the C3d receptor. These are found predominantly on B-cells but also to a lesser extent on some lymphoid elements in the "third" compartment. Complement receptor–bearing lymphocytes are detected by rosette formation with sheep erythrocytes coated with IgM-associated antibody and complement (EAC). The mean value for EAC rosette–forming cells is 18 per cent, with a range of 10 to 25 per cent. Since monocytes and polymorphonuclear leukocytes also contain Fc receptors, these must be taken into account in interpreting tests that are performed in the presence of elevated numbers of these cells.

T-Lymphocyte Assays

E-rosette-forming cells. One of the most important recent discoveries was that T-lymphocytes form spontaneous but weak rosettes with sheep erythrocytes, providing one of the simplest biologic markers for identifying T-lymphocytes. Although several modifications of the test have appeared in the literature, some purporting to measure "active" E rosettes that correlate better with cell-mediated immunity, the major use of the test is for enumerating total numbers of T-lymphocytes. The mean value of E rosettes is 89 per cent, with a range of 85 to 93 per cent (Table 26–3).

Specific T- and B-Cell Antisera. Antisera specific for T- and B-lymphocyte antigens have been generated by immunization of animals with either human T- or human B-lymphocytes followed by extensive adsorption with appropriate cells (Table 26–3). Recently, subsets of T-lymphocytes have been described with Fc receptors for μ and γ heavy chains, which show helper (T_m) or suppressor (T_g) activities.

Interpretation and Significance of Test Results. According to the results of these tests, B-lymphocytes account for 1 to 15 per cent of the circulating blood lymphocytes and the T-cells account for 75 to 85 per cent of peripheral blood lymphocytes. The nature of the cell population composing the remainder is unclear but it appears to represent a heterogeneous collection of lymphocytes, including killer (K-) cells (mIg–, C-receptor+, Fc-receptor+) that participate in antibody-dependent cellular cytotoxicity (ADCC) reactions, null cells that contain no detectable surface markers, and possibly the natural killer (NK-) cells (Chapter 9).

Clinical Indications for Performing Tests of Lymphocyte Enumeration. Currently, the enumeration of B- and T-lymphocytes by surface markers is receiving widespread application in clinical medicine for both the diagnosis and the management of many disease processes with immunologic features. Shown in Table 26–5 are some examples of current applications of the tests in clinical medicine, including their use in the diagnosis of the lymphoproliferative diseases in which abnormal collections of B-cells e.g., CLL, or of T-cells, e.g., Sezary syndrome, are seen (Chapter 21); their use in the immune deficiencies in which there are deficiencies of B-cells, e.g., X-linked agammaglobulinemia, or of T-cells, e.g., DiGeorge syndrome (Chapter 22); and the most exciting applications that may continue to appear in the area of immunologically mediated diseases, e.g., allergy, autoimmune disease (Chapter 20), or immune deficiencies associated with malignant disorders (Chapter 19).

It should be stressed that in performing these tests errors of interpretation may occur owing to differences in techniques and reagents employed, e.g., the nonspecific reactions of anti–whole Ig but not anti-Fab'2 on non-B-cell lymphocytes. In addition, a number of intrinsic factors may contribute to errors, e.g., the presence of Fc receptors and complement receptors on macrophages that might affect the interpretation of these tests.

Functional Tests of Lymphocytes

Tests of Humoral (B-Lymphocyte-Mediated) Immune Function. The most commonly used test is the quantification of the

TABLE 26–5.   Clinical Indications for Enumeration of Lymphocyte Subpopulations

INDICATION	EXAMPLE	FINDING
Lymphoproliferative disease	CLL, multiple myeloma	B-cell proliferation
	Sezary syndrome	T-cell proliferation
Immune deficiency	X-linked agamma-globulinemia	B-cell—low to absent, compensatory increase in T-cells
	DiGeorge syndrome	T-cell—low to absent, compensatory increase in B-cell number
Immunologically mediated disease	Allergy (atopy)	T-cell decrease (?)
	Autoimmune disease, e.g., RA	Suppressor T-cell dysfunction (?)
	Immune deficiency with malignant disease	T-cell decrease (?) or blockage

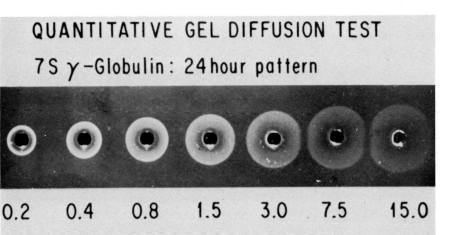

QUANTITATIVE GEL DIFFUSION TEST

7S γ-Globulin: 24 hour pattern

0.2   0.4   0.8   1.5   3.0   7.5   15.0

Protein Concentration (mg/ml)

Figure 26–3. Photograph of radial-immunodiffusion method of quantification of the immunoglobulins. Note the gradually increasing diameters of rings of precipitation, which are proportional to the concentration of gamma globulin. (Courtesy of Dr. John L. Fahey; from Fahey, J. L., and McKelvey, E. M.: Quantitative determination of serum immunoglobulins in antibody-agar plates. J. Immunol., *94*:84, 1965.)

individual gamma globulins. The test is available in most clinical laboratories and is most commonly performed by radial immunodiffusion in agar, using plates impregnated with specific antisera to each of the individual immunoglobulins (Fig. 26–3). It is preferred to quantification by paper or cellulose acetate electrophoresis, which lacks the sensitivity and specificity of the immunochemical techniques. Immunoelectrophoresis of immunoglobulins in serum or urine frequently provides additional information, e.g., multiple myeloma. In addition, newer and more sensitive techniques have been developed for the quantification of immunoglobulins, including (1) automated immune precipitation (AIP), (2) electroimmunoassay (EIA), also called the Laurell rocket technique, and (3) a wide variety of methods based on antigen-antibody interactions employing fluorescent, enzymatic, or radioactive markers (Chapter 8). These tests are indicated in the assessment of patients with immunologically mediated diseases (Chapter 20), and with immunoproliferative diseases (Chapter 21), and in the immunologic deficiency states (Chapter 22).

The postnatal development of the individual gamma globulins proceeds at different rates, and interpretations of gamma globulin deficiency must be made with reference to age-adjusted normal values (Chapter 2). This is particularly important in the diagnosis of immunologic deficiency in infancy and childhood. Because of difficulty in standardizing normal values between laboratories, it has been suggested that control values be established for each laboratory before immunoglobulin concentrations are assessed. Currently, through the WHO and the IUIS, standards and reference sera are available for the quantification of immunoglobulins. In addition, since prior gamma globulin administration may alter the results of these studies, gamma globulin administration therapy should be withheld for at least six to eight weeks before the true levels of gamma globulin are determined. Shown in Tables 26–6 and 26–7 are age-adjusted values for immunoglobulins.

Tests of specific antibody responses: prior sensitization. The patient's ability to produce specific antibody is measured in one of two ways: (1) measurement of antibody that occurred as a consequence of natural exposure or prior immunization, e.g., isohemagglutinins, poliovirus, and measles antibody, or (2) measurement of *de novo* antibody synthesis following the use of specific vaccines, e.g., tetanus toxoid and salmonella vaccines. These functional tests of antibody are sometimes used in the assessment of immune deficiencies involving the humoral limb of immunity, e.g., hypogammaglobulinemia (Chapter 22).

In addition to these *in vitro* studies, the Schick and Dick tests are *in vivo* procedures that·measure circulating IgG–associated diphtheria and erythrogenic antitoxin activity, respectively.

Tests of Cell-Mediated (T-Lymphocyte-Mediated) Immune Function. The patient's ability to elicit cell-mediated immunity can be measured by *in vivo* or *in vitro* tests (Table 26–1). The *in vivo* tests, i.e., delayed-hypersensitivity skin testing, measure either prior sensitization or *de novo* sensitization. Since it is known that over 80 per cent of individuals have delayed-hypersensitivity responses to Candida, Trichophyton, and streptokinase-streptodornase, these skin antigens provide convenient *in vivo* test vehicles for delayed hypersensitivity. In addition, if it is known that a patient has had prior fungal infection or tuberculosis, delayed-hypersensitivity reactions to these organisms can be tested. Furthermore, in a patient known to be previously reactive to these antigens who no longer displays this reactivity (anergy), suspicion of underlying diseases, such as sarcoidosis or lymphoma, is aroused.

In vivo tests that demonstrate *de novo* sensitization include the use of dinitrochlorobenzene (DNCB) sensitization in which delayed responses are tested by applying a challenging dose that is followed 10 to 14 days later by a sensitizing dose. This test measures not only the ability of an individual to manifest a cell-mediated (delayed-hypersensitivity) phenomenon but also the afferent and efferent limbs of the thymic-dependent (T-lymphocyte) system. Although allogeneic skin grafts have been used to test this phenomenon, their use is rare. They may lead to isoimmunization and carry the additional hazard of graft-versus-host reactions in immunologically deficient individuals, as well as the problem of transmission of the hepatitis virus B.

With the increasing use of immunopotentiators, e.g., *C. parvum* and levamisole (Chapter 10), the delayed-hypersensitivity skin testing has

TABLE 26-6. Levels of Immune Globulins in Sera of Normal Subjects at Different Ages*

Age	Number of Subjects	Level of IgG†		Level of IgM†		Level of IgA†		Level of Total Ig-Globulin†	
		mg/dl (Range)	% of Adult Level	mg/dl (Range)	% of Adult Level	mg/dl (Range)	% of Adult Level	mg/dl (Range)	% of Adult Level
Newborn	22	1031±200 (645–1244)	89±17	11±5 (5–30)	11±5	2±3 (0–11)	1±2	1044±201 (660–1439)	67±13
1–3 months	29	430±119 (272–762)	37±10	30±11 (16–67)	30±11	21±13 (6–56)	11±7	481±127 (324–699)	31±9
4–6 months	33	427±186 (206–1125)	37±16	43±17 (10–83)	43±17	28±18 (8–93)	14±9	498±204 (228–1232)	32±13
7–12 months	56	661±219 (279–1533)	58±19	54±23 (22–147)	55±23	37±18 (16–98)	19±9	752±242 (327–1687)	48±15
13–24 months	59	762±209 (258–1393)	66±18	58±23 (14–114)	59±23	50±24 (19–119)	25±12	870±258 (398–1586)	56±16
25–36 months	33	892±183 (419–1274)	77±16	61±19 (28–113)	62±19	71±37 (19–235)	36±19	1024±205 (499–1418)	65±14
3–5 years	28	929±228 (569–1597)	80±20	56±18 (22–100)	57±18	93±27 (55–152)	47±14	1078±245 (730–1771)	69±17
6–8 years	18	923±256 (559–1492)	80±22	65±25 (27–118)	66±25	124±45 (54–221)	62±23	1112±293 (640–1725)	71±20
9–11 years	9	1124±235 (779–1456)	97±20	79±33 (35–132)	80±33	131±60 (12–208)	66±30	1334±254 (966–1639)	85±17
12–16 years	9	946±124 (726–1085)	82±11	59±20 (35–72)	60±20	148±63 (70–229)	74±32	1153±169 (833–1284)	74±12
Adults	30	1158±305 (569–1919)	100±26	99±27 (47–147)	100±27	200±61 (61–330)	100±31	1457±353 (730–2365)	100±24

*From Stiehm, E. R., and Fudenberg, H. H.: Serum levels of immune globulins in health and disease: A survey. Pediatrics, 37:715–727, 1966.

†Mean ± 1 SD.

TABLE 26–7. Normal Serum IgE Values as Determined by Two Radioimmunoassay Methods

		RIST		PRIST	
		Geometric Mean	+1 SD (+2 SD)*	Geometric Mean	+1 SD (+2 SD)*
Age	Number of Patients	U/ml	U/ml	U/ml	U/ml
1 year	12	7	21	3	7
2 years	18	11	26	3	9
3 years	6	11	21	2	6
4 years	7	20	37	9	24
7 years	19	26	75	13	46
10 years	17	39	115	24	116
14 years	19	32	78	20	63
Adults	175	25	65/150*	14	41/122*

64 per cent of nonatopics < 20 U/ml
1.7 per cent of nonatopics > 100 U/ml
0 per cent of atopics < 20 U/ml
63 per cent of atopics > 100 U/ml

*Modified from Johansson, S. G. O., Berglund, A., and Kjellman, N. I. M., 1976.

been of assistance in monitoring the efficacy of these agents. In addition, changes in the course of a disease process can be assessed by means of delayed-hypersensitivity skin testing.

Lymphocyte stimulation. These tests are based on the transformation, proliferation, and replication responses of normal lymphocytes to stimulation *in vitro* by either nonspecific stimulants (e.g., phytohemagglutinin [PHA]), foreign cells, or specific antigen. Although most of the mitogens stimulate both B- and T-lymphocytes, some exhibit a selectivity (Chapter 7) for certain classes of lymphocytes. The end point of the reaction is measured by blast transformation, a mitotic index, or the incorporation of radioactive precursors into DNA (tritiated thymidine) or RNA (tritiated uridine). It is believed that these techniques measure one parameter of the cell-mediated response, i.e., the afferent limb. Other parameters may be measured by the release of effector molecules, such as migration inhibitory factor (MIF) (Chapter 9). It should be pointed out that there are dissociations of lymphoproliferative responses and elaboration of lymphokines. For example, a normal MIF response can be seen with a deficient response to PHA. A number of other immunologic tests of T-cell activity have been described, e.g., leukocyte inhibition factor (LIF) and lymphocytotoxicity. Nonetheless, their clinical significance is poorly understood at present. The tests of effector molecules will undoubtedly assume greater clinical significance when the complete array has been identified. The procedures covered in this section are helpful in diagnosing the primary and secondary deficiencies in cell-mediated immunity (Chapter 22).

Measurement of lymphocyte enzymes.   It is now apparent that several enzyme deficiencies have been associated with certain forms of immune deficiency in the human, e.g., severe combined immune deficiency (SCID). These enzyme deficiencies include adenine deaminase (ADA) deficiency and nucleoside phosphorylase deficiency (Chapter 22). Tests are currently available to measure these enzymes in the erythrocytes of patients and have been developed for screening in the newborn.

TESTS OF TISSUE-DAMAGING (TERTIARY) IMMUNE FUNCTION

Tests of tissue-damaging immune function measure immune responses that cause disease manifestations through immunologic injury (Chapters 13 and 20). Examples of these are shown in Table 26–1 and are grouped according to four mechanisms of tissue injury. These include (1) measurement of specific reagins (IgE) by *in vivo* immediate-hypersensitivity skin testing and *in vitro* testing by RAST or histamine release or direct measurement of IgE globulins by RIST or PRIST (Chapters 8 and 22), (2) Coomb's test, (3) rheumatoid factor (RF) test, and (4) LE cell phenomenon and tissue biopsy (Chapter 20C). These are indicated when manifestations of immunologically mediated diseases are present (Chapter 20).

SUGGESTIONS FOR FURTHER READING

Tests of Nonspecific (Primary) Immune Function

Baehner, R. L.: The growth and development of our understanding of chronic granulomatous disease. *In* J. A. Bellanti, and D. H. Dayton: The Phagocytic Cell in Host Resistance. New York, Raven Press, 1975, p. 173.

Baehner, R. L., and Karnovsky, M. L.: Deficiency of reduced nicotinamide-adenine dinucleotide oxidase in chronic granulomatous disease. Science, *162*:1277, 1968.

Baehner, R. L., and Nathan, D. G.: Quantitative nitroblue tetrazolium test in chronic granulomatous disease. N. Engl. J. Med., *278*:971, 1968.

Bellanti, J. A., Cantz, B. E., and Schlegel, R. J.: Accelerated decay of glucose-6-phosphate dehydrogenase activity in chronic granulomatous disease. Pediat. Res., *4*:405, 1970.

Bellanti, J. A., and Dayton, D. H.: The Phagocytic Cell in Host Resistance. New York, Raven Press, 1975.

Boyden, S.: The chemotactic effects of antibody and antigen on polymorphonuclear leukocytes. J. Exp. Med., *115*:453, 1962.

Fudenberg, H. H., Stites, D. P., Caldwell, J. L., and Wells, J. V. (eds.): Basic and Clinical Immunology. Los Altos, California, Lange Medical Publications, 1976.

Gallin, J. I.: Abnormal chemotaxis, cellular and humoral components. *In* J. A. Bellanti, and D. H. Dayton (eds.): The Phagocytic Cell in Host Resistance. New York, Raven Press, 1975, pp. 227–249.

Gallin, J. I., and Wolff, S. M.: Leucocyte chemotaxis: Physiological considerations and abnormalities. Clin. Haematol., *4*:567, 1975.

Gewurz, H., and Suyehira, L. A.: Complement. *In* N. R. Rose, and H. Friedman (eds.): Manual of Clinical Immunology. Washington, D.C., American Society of Microbiology, 1976, p. 36.

Hohn, D. C., and Lehrer, R. I.: NADPH oxidase deficiency in X-linked chronic granulomatous disease. J. Clin. Invest., *55*:707, 1975.

Holmes, B., Park, B. H., and Malawista, S. E.: Chronic granulomatous disease in females. N. Engl. J. Med., *283*:217, 1970.

Matsuda, I., Oka, Y., Taniguchi, N., Feruyama, M., Kodama, S., Aroshima, S., and Matsuyama, T.: Leukocyte glutathione peroxidase deficiency with chronic granulomatous disease. J. Pediatr., *88*:581, 1976.

Ochs, H. G., and Igo, R. P.: The NBT slide test: A simple screening method for detecting chronic granulomatous disease and female carriers. J. Pediatr., *83*:77, 1973.

Quie, P. G., White, J. G., and Holmes, B.: *In vitro* bactericidal capacity of human polymorphonuclear leukocytes: Diminished activity in chronic granulomatous disease of childhood. J. Clin. Invest., *46*:668, 1967.

Ruddy, S., and Austen, K. F.: Complement and its components. *In* A. S. Cohen (ed.): Laboratory Diagnostic Procedures in the Rheumatic Diseases. Boston, Little, Brown and Company, 1974, p. 131.

Rutenberg, W. D., Yang, M. C., Doberstyn, B. D., and Bellanti, J. A.: Multiple leukocyte abnormalities in chronic granulomatous disease: A familial study. Pediatr. Res., *11*:158, 1977.

Southam, C. M., and Levin, A. G.: A quantitative Rebuck technique. Blood, *27*:734, 1966.

Stossel, T. P., and Taylor, M.: Phagocytosis. *In* N. R. Rose, and H. Friedman (eds.): Manual of Clinical Immunology. Washington, D.C., American Society for Microbiology, 1976, p. 148.

Ward, P. A.: Chemotaxis. *In* N. R. Rose, and H. Friedman (eds.): Manual of Clinical Immunology. Washington, D.C., American Society for Microbiology, 1976, p. 106.

Tests of Specific (Secondary) Immune Function

Aisenberg, A. C.: Studies on delayed hypersensitivity in Hodgkin's disease. J. Clin. Invest., *41*:1964, 1962.

Alford, C. A.: Immunoglobulin determinations in the diagnosis of fetal infection. Pediatr. Clin. North Am., *18*:99, 1971.

Davis, N. C., and Ho, M.: Quantitation of immunoglobulins. *In* N. R. Rose, and H. Friedman (eds.): Manual of Clinical Immunology. Washington, D.C., American Society for Microbiology, 1976, p. 4.

Fahey, J. L., and McKelvey, E. N.: Quantitative determination of serum immunoglobulins in antibody-agar plates. J. Immunol., *94*:84, 1965.

Fudenberg, H., Good, R. A., Goodman, H. C., Hitzig, W., Kunkel, H. G., Roitt, I. M., Rosen, F. S., Rowe, D. S., Seligmann, M., and Soothill, J. R.: Primary immunodeficiencies. Pediatrics, *47*:927, 1971.

Hobbs, J. R.: Primary immune paresis. *In* Adinolfi, M. (ed.): Immunology and Development. London, William Heinemann Medical Books Ltd., 1969.

Hong, R.: Immunodeficiency. *In* N. R. Rose, and H. Friedman (eds.): Manual of Clinical Immunology. Washington, D. C., American Society for Microbiology, 1976, p. 620.

Johnston, R. B., Jr., and Janeway, C. A.: The child with frequent infections: Diagnostic considerations. Pediatrics, *43*:596, 1969.

Kochwa, S.: Immunoelectrophoresis (including zone electrophoresis). *In* N. R. Rose, and H. Friedman (eds.): Manual of Clinical Immunology. Washington, D.C., American Society for Microbiology, 1976, p. 17.

Mancini, G., Vaerman, J. P., Carbonara, A. O., and Heremans, J. F: A single-radial diffusion method for the immunological quantitation of proteins. *In* H. Peeters (ed.): XI Colloquium on Protides of the Biological Fluids. Amsterdam, Elsevier, 1964, p. 370.

Spitler, L. E.: Delayed hypersensitivity skin testing. *In* N. R. Rose, and H. Friedman (eds.): Manual of Clinical Immunology. Washington, D.C., American Society for Microbiology, 1976, p. 53.

Stiehm, E. R., and Fulginiti, V. A. (eds.): Immunologic Disorders in Infants and Children. Philadelphia, W. B. Saunders Co., 1973.

Winchester, R. J., and Ross, G.: Methods for enumerating lymphocyte populations. *In* N. R. Rose, and H. Friedman (eds.): Manual of Clinical Immunology. Washington, D.C., American Society for Microbiology, 1976.

Tests of Tissue-Damaging (Tertiary) Immune Function

Adkinson, N. F., Jr.: Measurement of total serum immunoglobulin E and allergen specific immunoglobulin E antibody. *In* N. R. Rose, and H. Friedman (eds.): Manual of

Clinical Immunology. Washington, D.C., American Society for Microbiology, 1976, p. 590.

Norman, P. S.: Skin testing. *In* N. R. Rose, and H. Friedman (eds.): Manual of Clinical Immunology. Washington, D.C., American Society for Microbiology, 1976, p. 585.

Siraganian, R. P.: Histamine release and assay methods for the study of human allergy. *In* N. R. Rose, and H. Friedman (eds.): Manual of Clinical Immunology. Washington, D.C., American Society for Microbiology, 1976, p. 603.

Theofilopoulos, A. N., and Dixon, F. J.: Complement receptors on Raji cells as *in vitro* detectors of immune complexes in human sera. *In* N. R. Rose, and H. Friedman (eds.): Manual of Clinical Immunology. Washington, D.C., American Society for Microbiology, 1976, p. 676.

Winchester, R.: Tests for detection of the rheumatoid factors. *In* N. R. Rose, and H. Friedman (eds.): Manual of Clinical Immunology. Washington, D.C., American Society for Microbiology, 1976, p. 665.

APPROACH TO THE PATIENT WITH IMMUNOLOGIC DISEASE

———————————————————————————— Appendix   1

PROBLEM: REPEATED INFECTIONS IN THE YOUNG INFANT

CLINICAL EVALUATION

A. History

Age of onset (the earlier the onset, the more severe the defect)
Site of infection (pyodermas, otitis media, pneumonia, abscesses, sepsis, meningitis)
Type of organism (viruses and fungi: consider thymic-dependent defects; bacteria, high-grade virulence: consider agammaglobulinemia; bacteria, low-grade virulence: consider neutrophil dysfunction [e.g., chronic granulomatous disease]; protozoa [*Pneumocystis carinii*] common in all immunologic deficiencies)
Family history (similar familial infections; other infant deaths, particularly males; polyendocrinopathy: thyroid, parathyroid, adrenal; allergies; collagen-vascular diseases; malignant diseases; diabetes; *draw pedigree*)
Dietary history (unusual reactions to foods or other ingestants)
History of medications (prior gamma globulin administration, antibiotics)
History of unusual reactions to vaccines (vaccinia necrosum) or to allergens (if patient had poison ivy dermatitis, his cell-mediated responses are probably intact)
Associated findings (spruelike disorders)

B. Physical Examination

Growth and development (severe defects, e.g., thymic dysplasia, produce physical underdevelopment)
Skin and appendages (evaluate skin and subcutaneous tissues for signs of infection: staphylococcal, monilial; eczema [Wiskott-Aldrich syndrome, hyper-IgE syndrome]; telangiectasis [e.g, ataxia-telangiectasia]; clubbing; cyanosis [chronic pulmonary or cardiac disease])

777

Ears (otitis media; shape of ears, e.g., notching in DiGeorge syndrome)

Chest (chronic emphysematous changes; bronchiectasis)

Cardiovascular (murmurs, cardiomegaly; congenital heart disease can also present with repeated infections)

Abdomen (hepatomegaly, splenomegaly)

Lymph nodes (evaluate for lymphadenopathy)

Neurologic (ataxia: consider ataxia-telangiectasia)

UNDERLYING IMMUNOLOGIC PROBLEM

In the evaluation of the child with repeated infections, the physician must decide whether an immunologic problem exists. In general, there are four cardinal features suggestive of an immunologic defect: (1) repeated infections caused by bacteria of high-grade virulence, e.g., *D. pneumoniae*, (2) recurrent infections caused by bacteria of low-grade virulence, e.g., paracolon and bizarre organisms (Serratia), (3) recurrent fungal infections, e.g., Candida, and (4) unusual reactions to live vaccines (e.g., progressive vaccinia). The history of repeated respiratory viral infections commonly seen in clinical practice does not usually constitute an indication of underlying immunologic deficiency but rather results from increased exposure to infected individuals (e.g., common colds).

Other conditions that predispose to repeated infections must be considered and are easily excluded by appropriate testing. Examples of these include congenital cardiac disease, asthma, and cystic fibrosis. In those situations in which derangement of an underlying immunologic mechanism is suspected, specialized tests are required, e.g., sweat test.

LABORATORY TESTS

A rational approach to the diagnosis of immune deficiency is given in Figure 26–4. In this scheme, the history and physical findings are crucial in establishing the diagnosis. Although it is apparent that many of these procedures can be performed only in specialized centers, the provisional diagnosis can be established in most cases by procedures that are performed in the physician's office.

The choice of laboratory procedure will depend on the clinical expression of the recurrent infection and the availability of the test. The first step in identifying the underlying disorder rests with the identification of the infecting organism. The physician is well advised to identify the organism by appropriate cultures in order to determine the nature of the infection.

For example, patients with impaired phagocytic function will present with recurrent infections owing to bacterial organisms of low-grade

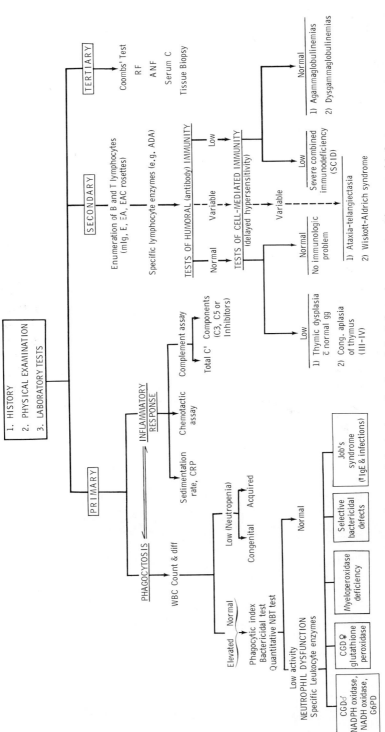

Figure 26–4. Scheme of approach in the investigation of the infant who presents with repeated infections.

virulence, such as *Serratia marcescens*. The tests indicated include a complete blood count and differential, which may show an elevated white count with leukocytosis. Impaired bactericidal activity and a low quantitative NBT test will establish the diagnosis of neutrophil dysfunction syndrome, e.g., chronic granulomatous disease. The use of pedigree and leukocyte enzyme tests can further differentiate one dysfunction from another.

Recurrent infections may also be a manifestation of impaired inflammatory response resulting from a lack or inhibition of certain complement components (Fig. 26–4). These children present with recurrent infections caused by gram-negative organisms or *Staphylococcus aureus*. Determination of chemotactic activity and the individual complement components would be indicated. If the infecting organism is identified as one producing high-grade fulminating infections, e.g., *D. pneumoniae*, the physician must differentiate between a quantitative lack of phagocytes (neutropenia) and a lack of opsonizing antibody (e.g., agammaglobulinemia). The former can be established by history and complete blood count. Enumeration of lymphocyte populations together with tests of humoral (antibody function) and quantitative immunoglobulin determination will establish the diagnosis of humoral deficiency or dysgammaglobulinemia (see Table 26–1 and Fig. 26–4).

Repeated infections due to certain viruses, e.g., vaccinia, and fungi, e.g., *Candida albicans*, may indicate a thymic-dependent lesion. Affected children will have normal primary immune functions (phagocytosis and inflammatory response) but will show striking deficiencies in tests of cell-mediated function. Tests of humoral immunity would differentiate severe combined immunodeficiency (SCID) from those defects restricted to the thymus. The associated finding of hypocalcemic tetany should raise a consideration of the III-IV pharyngeal pouch syndrome (DiGeorge syndrome).

Appropriate tests of tertiary function are indicated when hemolytic anemia, rheumatoid arthritis, or systemic lupus erythematosus is present.

PROBLEM: REPEATED INFECTIONS IN THE ADULT PATIENT

CLINICAL EVALUATION

A. History

Age of onset (the expression of recurrent infections in the adult varies with underlying disorders)
Site of infection (similar to those seen in the child)
Type of organism (viruses, fungi, bacteria, protozoa)
Occupation (certain pneumoconioses predispose to infection)
Family history (allergy, diabetes mellitus, autoimmune diseases)
History of medications (immunosuppressive drugs, steroids, gamma globulin, antibiotics)
Associated findings (weight loss, malaise, polydypsia, bone pain, spruelike illnesses)

B. Physical Examination

General appearance
Skin (pallor, purpura, and cyanosis)
Extremities (clubbing)
Eyes (retinopathy, e.g., diabetes)
Chest (emphysema)
Cardiovascular (murmurs, cardiomegaly)
Abdomen (hepatosplenomegaly seen in lymphomas, chronic liver disease that may present with frequency of infections)
Lymph nodes (node enlargement, e.g., lymphoma)
Neurologic (paraplegia, muscular weakness)

UNDERLYING IMMUNOLOGIC PROBLEM

The causes of repeated infections in the adult include the many etiologies of immunologic deficiency seen in the child (Appendix 1). In general, the severe primary immune defects are seen much earlier. The most frequent causes of increased susceptibility to infections in the adult are those related to underlying diseases, e.g., cardiac disease, respiratory

781

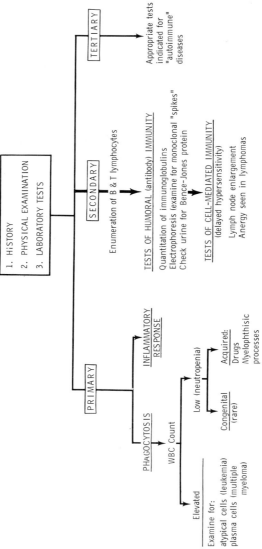

Figure 26–5.   Scheme of approach in the investigation of an adult who presents with repeated infections.

disease, allergy, and diabetes. The immunologic causes for repeated infections in the adult are mainly secondary immunologic deficiencies, including those secondary to lymphoproliferative diseases, the autoimmune diseases, immunosuppressive therapy, and malignant diseases.

LABORATORY TESTS

The laboratory tests used in the diagnosis of recurrent infections in the adult are shown in Figure 26–5. The choice of laboratory tests will be determined by the history and clinical presentation of the disease.

Although the underlying cause may differ from that seen in children, the same general approach should be used. For example, neutropenia that is drug-induced would require the same diagnostic test of primary immune function described in Appendix 1. In the adult, the most useful procedures include tests of secondary immune function: enumeration of lymphocyte populations, quantification of immunoglobulins, examination of serum electrophoresis for monoclonal peaks, and analysis of the urine for Bence Jones protein. These would substantiate the diagnosis of lymphoproliferative disease, e.g., multiple myeloma. Lymph node enlargement with loss of delayed hypersensitivity (anergy) would suggest a diagnosis of lymphoma. Those tertiary tests of immune function should be performed in cases in which autoimmune disease is suspected (Table 26–1).

Appendix 3 _____

PROBLEM: APPROACH TO PATIENT WITH "ALLERGIC" (HYPERSENSITIVITY) DISEASE

CLINICAL EVALUATION

A. History

Age of onset (can occur at any age)

History of environmental exposure and occupational hazards (foods, contactants, inhalants, pets, and other environmental exposures)

Site of involvement (skin, gastrointestinal tract, respiratory tract)

Type of disease expression (atopic eczema, contact dermatitis, hives, diarrhea and vomiting, rhinitis, wheezing)

Family history (obtain a pedigree because of the marked tendency of atopy to occur within families)

History of medication (important in the assessment of drug hypersensitivity)

Associated findings (anemia, weight loss, malaise)

B. Physical Findings

Growth and development (physical underdevelopment may occur in certain forms of chronic allergic diseases in children)

Skin (evaluate the type of eruption, its distribution, and its localization)

Mucous membranes (evaluate the extent and degree of congestion or pallor of the mucous membranes polyps)

Chest (evaluate emphysema, respiratory distress)

Extremities (evaluate clubbing and cyanosis)

Cardiovascular (evaluate the heart for murmurs, cardiomegaly; i.e., rheumatic fever can present with skin and other hypersensitivity manifestations)

Neurologic (parasthesias and muscle weakness are sometimes seen in hypersensitivity diseases of the CNS)

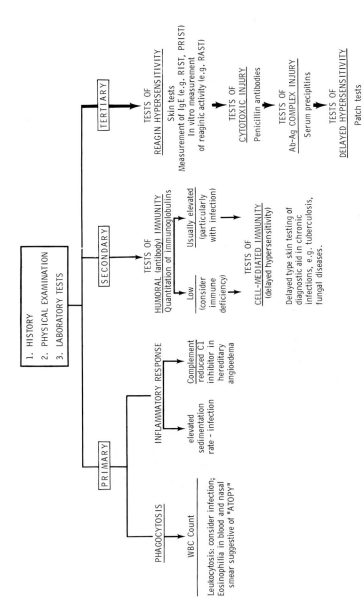

Figure 26–6. Scheme of approach in the investigation of the patient who presents with allergic (hypersensitivity) diseases.

UNDERLYING IMMUNOLOGIC PROBLEM

The IgE reagin–mediated (Type I) responses form the basis of most allergic diseases of man and are characterized by heightened responses to many exogenous antigens (Chapter 20A). In addition, cytotoxic (Type II) responses, immune-complex (Type III) hypersensitivity (serum sickness reactions), and delayed hypersensitivity (Type IV) (contact dermatitis) may also be present. In many cases of hypersensitivity, infection commonly enters into the differential diagnosis. At times it may be the precipitating event, and at other times it may complicate the clinical picture.

The diagnosis of hypersensitivity disease is made after a careful history has been taken and a thorough physical examination has been done. After this, a combined regimen of antigen elimination and appropriate immunologic testing should be performed to establish the diagnosis.

LABORATORY TESTS

The laboratory tests that are commonly used in the diagnosis of hypersensitivity diseases of man are listed in Figure 26–6. An elevated leukocyte count and leukocytosis may provide important clues to bacterial infection. Blood eosinophilia and nasal eosinophilia are commonly seen in atopic diseases. In the pulmonary hypersensitivity diseases, the examination of sputum for eosinophils or aspergillus and of serum for precipitins and IgE may be helpful (Chapter 20A). Other tests of primary immune function include the measurement of complement activity, which would help to establish some of the other hereditary causes of allergy, e.g., hereditary angioedema (Chapter 20A).

The measurement of total gamma globulins is often indicated to exclude underlying immunologic deficiency. Tests of delayed hypersensitivity may be helpful in cases in which chronic infection is suspected, e.g., tuberculosis. Since most of the allergic diseases are mediated through the IgE reaginic response, most test procedures center on measurement of these activities (Table 26–1). These include tests of immediate hypersensitivity, skin testing, the RIST, PRIST, and RAST tests, and *in vitro* tests of histamine release. In certain cytotoxicity-mediated reactions, such as pencillin hypersensitivity, antibodies to penicillin may be measured. In cases in which a Type III immune complex reaction is suspected (e.g., extrinsic allergic alveolitis, milk allergy), the measurement of serum-precipitating antibody can be performed. Finally, in cases of contact hypersensitivity, the mechanism of delayed hypersensitivity can be detected through the use of patch tests.

PROBLEM: APPROACH TO IMMUNOLOGIC DISEASES IN THE NEWBORN (ISOIMMUNIZATION AND IMMUNOLOGIC PROBLEMS IN THE MOTHER AFFECTING THE INFANT)

CLINICAL EVALUATION

A. History

Previous isoimmunization in mother (due to pregnancy or transfusions [Rh_0, ABO] or gamma globulin administration)

Previous diseases in the mother (autoimmune diseases, e.g., SLE, thyroiditis, myasthenia gravis, idiopathic thrombocytopenic purpura)

History of medications in mother (quinine, quinidine, apronalide [Sedormid])

History of infections during pregnancy (rubella, cytomegalic inclusion disease, toxoplasmosis, syphilis, herpes simplex; although nonimmunologic, these intrauterine infections must be considered, since they may occur because of immunodeficiency of the fetus or mother)

B. Physical Examination

General appearance (assess degree of activity: hyperactivity, consider hyperthyroidism, passive transfer of LATS; hypoactivity or muscle weakness, consider myasthenia gravis with transfer of antibodies to muscle; purpura, consider thrombocytopenia due to the passive transfer of antibodies to platelets)

Skin (jaundice in the first 24 hours; petechiae are characteristic of isoimmunization, e.g., erythroblastosis fetalis)

Eyes (exophthalmos due to LATS)

Chest (pneumonitis seen in many intrauterine infections)

Cardiovascular (evaluate murmurs for congenital heart disease)

Abdomen (hepatosplenomegaly: seen in severe erythroblastosis fetalis and in congenital intrauterine infections)

Extremities (note deformities and other birth defects)

Neurologic (convulsions, weakness)

787

UNDERLYING IMMUNOLOGIC PROBLEMS

Several clinical conditions must be evaluated in the assessment of the newborn, including congenital infections and congenital abnormalities, all of which could present with similar clinical expressions of immunologic disease. However, it is the laboratory findings that will reveal the immunologic basis of these diseases.

In all these entities, the newborn is affected by the passive transfer of maternal IgG antibody, which is deleterious to the infant (Fig. 26–7). These antibodies arise in the mother either as a consequence of isoimmunization due to previous pregnancies or transfusions or through diseases in which antibodies are found in the maternal circulation (Chapters 2 and 20B). Listed in Table 26–8 are some examples of the harmful effects of transplacentally acquired antibodies that have been associated with disease in the infant.

On the basis of the history and physical examination, the physician should be alerted to the possibilities of these abnormal immunologic responses in the newborn infant and order appropriate tests.

LABORATORY TESTS

Since the basic mechanism of injury involves the transfer of IgG antibody, detection is readily made by measurement of these antibodies

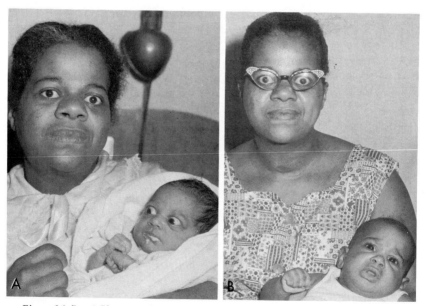

Figure 26–7. *A*, Photograph of a mother and her three-day-old daughter, illustrating exophthalmos in both due to transplacental transfer of LATS. *B*, Photograph of the same mother and her five-month-old daughter, showing exophthalmos only in the mother. (From Martin, M. M., and Matus, R. N.: Neonatal exophthalmos with maternal thyrotoxicosis. Am. J. Dis. Child., *111*:545, 1966.)

TABLE 26–8.   Maternal Antibodies That Can Lead to Harmful Effects in the Infant

MATERNAL DISEASE	ANTIBODIES	EFFECT ON NEWBORN
Hyperthyroidism	LATS	Transient hyperthyroidism (exophthalmos)
Idiopathic thrombo-cytopenia	Platelet antibodies	Transient thrombocytopenia
Isoimmunization (platelets, neutrophils, red blood cells)	Platelet, neutrophil, isohemagglutinins, or $Rh_0(D)$ antibodies	Transient thrombocyto-penia, neutropenia, anemia
Lupus erythematosus	Autoantibodies to blood elements (LE cell factor, Coombs' test, platelet)	Transient LE cell phenom-enon, neutropenia, thrombocytopenia

in maternal and infant sera (Table 26–8). Congenital intrauterine infections can also be excluded by appropriate history, physical examination, and cultures and through the use of tests that measure IgM responses characteristic of intrauterine infections (Appendix 6).

PROBLEM: APPROACH TO PATIENT WITH MUSCULOSKELETAL ("AUTOIMMUNE") DISORDERS

CLINICAL EVALUATION

A. History

Age of onset (usually occur in young adults and in children, e.g., juvenile rheumatoid arthritis)

Site of involvement (skin rashes, malar eminences, joints [arthralgia], muscle complaints [myalgia], kidney [hematuria])

Type of involvement (transient and migratory [e.g., SLE] or protracted and crippling [e.g., rheumatoid arthritis]; also assess degree of inflammation)

History of medications (drugs giving rise to serum sickness–like illnesses, e.g., penicillin; drugs giving rise to false positive LE phenomena, e.g., hydralazine)

Associated findings (malaise, weakness, fever)

B. Physical Findings

Growth and development (physical underdevelopment in childhood, e.g., juvenile rheumatoid arthritis)

Skin (rashes, malar eminence on pressure points, dystrophic changes)

Hair (alopecia)

Eyes (episcleritis, keratitis, funduscopic changes in many of the multisystem diseases)

Nails (periungual necrotic lesions)

Muscle (define areas of weakness, tenderness, or swelling)

Joints (localize and identify areas of joint involvement, degree of inflammation, joint effusions. If present, joint fluid should be withdrawn and tested)

Neurologic (evaluate neuropathies; footdrop)

UNDERLYING IMMUNOLOGIC PROBLEMS

Vasculitis seems to form the backbone of this group of multisystem disorders (Chapter 20C). In rheumatoid arthritis, synovial proliferation may occur with or without vasculitis. The presence of immune complexes may contribute to the pathologic changes in the joints. In systemic lupus erythematosus, immune-complex injury due to DNA–anti-DNA complexes is believed to account for the vasculitis and the kidney involvement.

On the basis of the history and physical examination, the physician must decide whether a multisystem disease is present. Since many of these entities are preceded by infection, the physician should decide whether an infectious disease is also present. The degree of multisystem involvement, together with the chronicity of the clinical course, is helpful in suggesting the diagnosis.

LABORATORY TESTS

The laboratory tests useful in the diagnosis of the autoimmune diseases are shown in Figure 26–8. Tests of primary immune function should include a complete blood count and differential. An elevated white blood count provides the first laboratory clue in all the multisystem diseases, with the exception of systemic lupus erythematosus in which leukopenia is seen in approximately 80 per cent of the cases. An elevated sedimentation rate is another useful finding in all the autoimmune diseases, with the exception of dermatomyositis in which it may be normal in approximately half of the cases.

Other tests that should be performed include tests of humoral (antibody) function, such as the quantification of the immunoglobulins, which usually reveals a diffuse polyclonal hypergammaglobulinemia.

Tests of tertiary immune function should be performed and should form the backbone of all laboratory testing procedures. These include the Coombs test, antinuclear factors, rheumatoid factor, ENA, LE cell preparations, and serum complement levels. Where indicated, specimens for tissue biopsy may be obtained from appropriate tissues, e.g., muscle and kidney.

From these studies and the history and physical examination, a diagnosis can often be established. For example, in a patient with multiple joint involvement, elevated sedimentation rate, leukocytosis, and positive rheumatoid factor, a diagnosis of rheumatoid arthritis would be most likely. If joint fluid is available, the additional finding in joint fluid of a lowered complement, a polymorphonuclear leukocyte response, and an increased protein would establish the diagnosis. On the other hand, in a patient presenting with transient arthritis, elevated

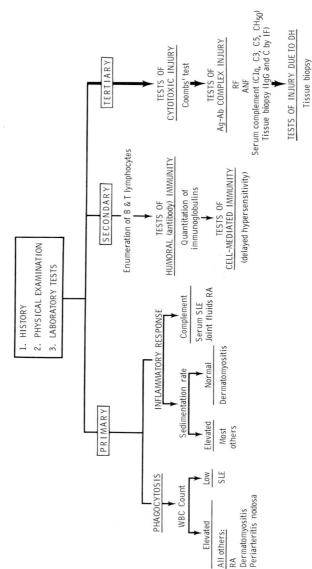

Figure 26–8. Scheme of approach in the investigation of the patient who presents with musculoskeletal (autoimmune) disorders.

sedimentation rate, leukopenia, positive antinuclear factor, and lowered complement, a diagnosis of systemic lupus erythematosus should be considered. If joint fluid is available, it would classically show a lowered complement, fewer cells, and lowered protein. In some cases, the use of tissue biopsy is required for additional substantiation of the diagnosis. For example, in periarteritis nodosa, the diagnosis would be established by a muscle, nerve, and blood vessel biopsy, particularly in a male patient. In dermatomyositis, a biopsy of skin and muscle, in addition to enzyme studies and electromyography, would help establish the diagnosis. The recent discovery of associations of HLA types with certain autoimmune diseases (Chapters 3 and 20C) suggests that histocompatibility typing may provide another diagnostic aid, e.g., ankylosing spondylitis.

Appendix 6 _____

PROBLEM: USE OF IMMUNOLOGY
IN DIAGNOSIS OF INFECTIOUS
DISEASES

Many immunologic tests are available to the physician that aid in the diagnosis of infectious diseases. Listed in Table 26–9 are examples of immunologic techniques that are commonly used. These consist of (1) determination of antibodies, which can be used either to identify an organism in the laboratory or to demonstrate an infection in the patient through a rise in serum antibody titer and (2) demonstration of delayed-hypersensitivity skin tests, which are particularly useful in the diagnosis of chronic bacterial, fungal, and some viral diseases (Table 26–9).

In addition to these tests, there are a number of other laboratory procedures that rely on serologic cross-reactivity or heterogenetic responses (Chapter 4). These are listed in Table 26–10 with examples of each.

The prominent macroglobulin response characteristic of the fetal and newborn immune responses has been used in the diagnosis of intra-uterine and perinatal infections. Both direct measurement of IgM immunoglobulins and the measurement of IgM-associated antibodies have been useful in this regard. These are shown in Table 26–11.

REFERENCES

Alford, C. A., Jr.: Immunoglobulin determinations in the diagnosis of fetal infection. Pediat. Clin. North Amer., *18*:99, 1971.

Overall, J. C., Jr., and Glasgow, L. A.: Virus infections of the fetus and newborn infant. J. Pediatr., 77:315, 1970.

Sever, J. L.: Immunologic responses to perinatal infections. J. Pediatr. Vol. 75, Part 2, December 1969.

TABLE 26–9. Types of Immunologic Procedures That Are Used in Diagnosis of Infectious Diseases

| TYPE OF INFECTION | ANTIBODY | | SKIN TEST | | |
	Assay Procedure	Example	Immediate	Delayed	Other
Bacterial	Agglutination Precipitation (flocculation) Complement fixation Fluorescent antibody	Salmonella O & H agglutinins Kahn Wassermann Streptococcal		Tuberculosis Infections with atypical mycobacteria	Toxin neutralization (Schick test)
Viral	Neutralization Complement fixation Hemagglutination inhibition Fluorescent antibody ELISA	Poliovirus Mumps Rubella Variola		Mumps	
Fungal	Precipitation (flocculation) Agglutination Complement fixation Fluorescent antibody	Histoplasmosis Coccidioidomycosis Blastomycosis	Skin test in cases of atopic disease caused by fungi	Coccidioidomycosis Blastomycosis Histoplasmosis	
Parasitic	Precipitation Complement fixation Hemagglutination Fluorescent antibody	Schistosoma	Trichinella		

TABLE 26–10. Serologic Procedures in Diagnosis of Infectious Diseases Based Upon Serologic Cross-Reactivity

DISEASE	NONSPECIFIC TESTS	SPECIFIC TESTS
Primary atypical pneumonia	Cold agglutinins (anti-I)	*M. pneumoniae* antibody (CF, growth inhibition)
Rocky Mountain Spotted Fever (RMSF)	Weil-Felix (OXK, OX19) agglutinins	RMSF CF test
Infectious mononucleosis	Heterophil antibody	EB fluorescent antibody
Syphilis	Wassermann, VDRL	FTA-Ab

TABLE 26–11. Serologic Procedures for Diagnosis of Intrauterine and Perinatal Infections Based on Prominent IgM Responses

DISEASE	TESTS
Toxoplasmosis	Fluorescent antibody Quantification of immunoglobulins
Syphilis	Fluorescent treponema antibody test (FTA) Quantification of immunoglobulins
Rubella	Fluorescent antibody Quantification of immunoglobulins
Cytomegalic inclusion disease	Fluorescent antibody Quantification of immunoglobulins
Herpes simplex	Fluorescent antibody Quantification of immunoglobulins
Acute bacterial infections	Quantification of immunoglobulins Tests of specific IgM antibody
Hepatitis B	Test for HB_sAg, e.g., radioimmunoassay or HB_sAgAb

INDEX

Note: Page references in *italics* indicate illustrations; page references to tables include the designation (t).

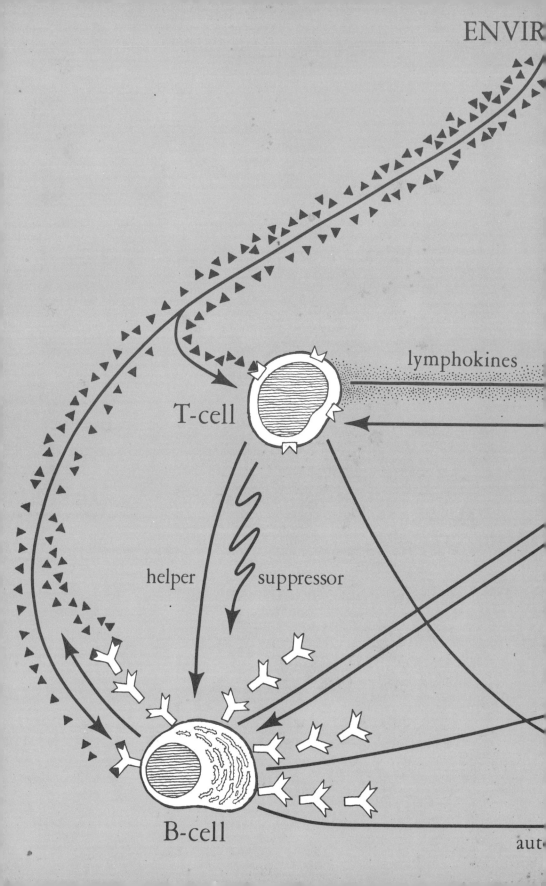